Oral Medicine and Pathology

A Guide to Diagnosis and Management

Editors

Saman Warnakulasuriya OBE BDS FDSRCS Dip Oral Med PhD DSc
Professor, Department of Oral Medicine and Experimental Pathology
King's College London, UK
Honorary Consultant Oral Medicine
King's and Guy's Hospitals
London, UK

WM Tilakaratne BDS MS FDSRCS PhD FRCPath
Professor, Department of Oral Pathology
Faculty of Dental Sciences
University of Peradeniya
Sri Lanka

Foreword

Poul Erik Petersen

JAYPEE

JAYPEE BROTHERS MEDICAL PUBLISHERS (P) LTD

New Delhi • London • Philadelphia • Panama

Jaypee Brothers Medical Publishers (P) Ltd.

Headquarters
Jaypee Brothers Medical Publishers (P) Ltd.
4838/24, Ansari Road, Daryaganj
New Delhi 110 002, India
Phone: +91-11-43574357
Fax: +91-11-43574314
Email: jaypee@jaypeebrothers.com

Overseas Offices

J.P. Medical Ltd.
83, Victoria Street, London
SW1H 0HW (UK)
Phone: +44-2031708910
Fax: +02-03-0086180
Email: info@jpmedpub.com

Jaypee-Highlights Medical Publishers Inc.
City of Knowledge, Bld. 237, Clayton
Panama City, Panama
Phone: + 507-301-0496
Fax: + 507-301-0499
Email: cservice@jphmedical.com

Jaypee Medical Inc.
The Bourse
111, South Independence Mall East
Suite 835, Philadelphia, PA 19106, USA
Phone: + 267-519-9789
Email: joe.rusko@jaypeebrothers.com

Jaypee Brothers Medical Publishers (P) Ltd.
17/1-B, Babar Road, Block-B, Shaymali
Mohammadpur, Dhaka-1207
Bangladesh
Mobile: +08801912003485
Email: jaypeedhaka@gmail.com

Jaypee Brothers Medical Publishers (P) Ltd.
Shorakhute, Kathmandu
Nepal
Phone: +00977-9841528578
Email: jaypee.nepal@gmail.com

Website: www.jaypeebrothers.com
Website: www.jaypeedigital.com

Inquiries for bulk sales may be solicited at: jaypee@jaypeebrothers.com

Oral Medicine and Pathology: A Guide to Diagnosis and Management

First Edition: **2014**

ISBN: 978-93-5025-221-5

Printed at : S. Narayan & Sons

Dedicated to

Our teachers and parents

My wife Ranjini
and
Daughter Roshini

Saman Warnakulasuriya

My wife Aruni
and
Son Praveen

WM Tilakaratne

Contributors

Andrew J Sidebottom BDS MBChB FRCS FRCS(OMF)
Consultant, Oral and Maxillofacial Surgeon
Nottingham University Hospitals NHS Trust, UK
E-mail: andrew.sidebottom@nuh.nhs.uk

Andrew Sadler BDS MBBS FDSRCS FRCS
Formerly
Clinical Lecturer and Consultant Oral Surgeon
School of Medicine and Dentistry
Queen Mary, University of London
Consultant Oral and Maxillofacial Surgeon
United Lincolnshire Hospitals, UK
E-mail: andrewsadler@ntlworld.com
sadler@sorejaw.co.uk

Anwar R Tappuni BDS LDSRCS PhD MRACDS (OM) FHEA
Clinical Senior Lecturer/Honorary Consultant
Department of Oral Medicine
School of Medicine and Dentistry
Queen Mary, University of London, UK
E-mail: a.r.tappuni@qmul.ac.uk

Christoph A Ramseier MAS (Periodontology)
Dr Med Dent
Periodontist SSP EFP
Assistant Professor
Department of Periodontology
School of Dental Medicine
University of Bern, Switzerland
E-mail: christoph.ramseier@zmk.unibe.ch

GJ Thomas BDS FDSRCS MScD PhD FRCPath
Professor, Experimental Pathology
Consultant, Head and Neck Pathology
Southampton Medical School, UK
E-mail: G.Thomas@soton.ac.uk

Helen McParland BDS FDSRCS
Department of Oral Medicine
Guy's and St Thomas' NHS Foundation Trust
London, UK
E-mail: Helen.McParland@gstt.nhs.uk

Induwara Goonerathne BDS MSc MPhil LLM Dip Forensic Med
Senior Lecturer in Forensic Medicine
Faculty of Medicine
University of Peradeniya, Sri Lanka
E-mail: induwarag@yahoo.com

Jimmy Makdissi DDS MMedSc FDSRCS DDRRCR
Senior Lecturer and Honorary Consultant
Department of Dental Radiology
School of Medicine and Dentistry
Queen Mary, University of London, UK
E-mail: j.makdissi@qmul.ac.uk

John Eveson BDS FDSRCS PhD FRCPath
Professor, Department of Oral Pathology
University of Bristol, UK
E-mail: J.W.Eveson@bristol.ac.uk

Josiah Eyeson BDS FDSRCS
Consultant Oral Surgeon
Eastman Dental Hospital
London, UK
E-mail: Josiah.Eyeson@uclh.nhs.uk

KA Moutasim BDS MSc MFD RCSI PhD
Faculty of Medicine
University of Southampton, UK
E-mail: K.A.Moutasim@soton.ac.uk

Kobkan Thongprasom BSc DDS MSc
Professor, Department of Oral Medicine
Chulalongkorn University, Bangkok, Thailand
E-mail: Kobkan.T@chula.ac.th

Lakshman Samaranayake DSc Hon FDSRCS (Edin) BDS DDS FRCPath (UK) FHKCPath MIBiol FCDSHK FHKAM (Path) FHKAM (DSurg)
Dean, Faculty of Dentistry
Chair of Oral Microbiology
Tam Wah-Ching Professor in Dental Science
The University of Hong Kong
King James IV Professor, Royal College of Surgeons
Edinburgh, Scotland, UK
Director, Prince Philip Dental Hospital, Hong Kong
E-mail: lakshman@hku.hk

MAO Lewis BDS PhD FDSRCPS FRCPath FFGDP(UK)
Professor and Honorary Consultant
Department of Oral Surgery
Medicine and Pathology
Dean, School of Dentistry
Cardiff University/Cardiff and Vale NHS Trust, UK
E-mail: lewisMAO@cardiff.ac.uk

Nalin Thakker BDS MSc PhD FRCPath
Professor of Molecular Pathology and Genetics
School of Dentistry, University of Manchester, UK
E-mail: n.thakker@manchester.ac.uk

Nipuna Parahitiyawa MBBS D Med (Micro) PhD
Senior Lecturer in Microbiology
Faculty of Dental Sciences
University of Peradeniya, Sri Lanka
E-mail: nipunabp@graduate.hku.hk

Paula Farthing BSc BDS FDSRCS PhD FRCPath FHEA
Professor of Oral and Maxillofacial Pathology
School of Clinical Dentistry
University of Sheffield, UK
E-mail: p.farthing@sheffield.ac.uk

Philip M Preshaw BDS FDS RCSEd PhD FDS (Rest Dent) RCSEd
Professor, Department of Periodontology
School of Dental Sciences and
Institute of Cellular Medicine
Newcastle University, Newcastle upon Tyne, UK
E-mail: p.m.preshaw@newcastle.ac.uk

Philip McLoughlin BDS MBBS FDSRCS FRCS
Consultant Oral and Maxillofacial Surgeon
Department of Maxillofacial Surgery
Ninewells Hospital, Dundee, UK
E-mail: philip.mcloughlin@nhs.net

Ranjit Mendis BDS PhD FDSRCS FFDRCSI
Former Professor
Department of Oral Pathology
Faculty of Dental Sciences
University of Peradeniya, Sri Lanka
Honorary Visiting Fellow
Division of Stomatology and Oral Surgery
School of Dental Medicine
Faculty of Medicine, University of Geneva
Switzerland
E-mail: ranjitm@bluewin.ch

Richard J Cook BDS MBBS FDSRCS PhD
Senior Lecturer in Oral Medicine
King's College London
Guy's and St Thomas' NHS Foundation Trust
London, UK
E-mail: richard_james.cook@kcl.ac.uk

Saman Warnakulasuriya OBE BDS FDSRCS Dip Oral Med PhD DSc
Professor
Department of Oral Medicine and
Experimental Pathology
King's College London, UK
E-mail: s.warne@kcl.ac.uk

Sol Silverman Jr MA DDS
Professor
Department of Oral Medicine
School of Dentistry
University of California
San Francisco, USA
E-mail: sol.silverman@ucsf.edu

Stefano Fedele MD
Senior Lecturer
Department of Oral Medicine
Eastman Dental Hospital
London, UK
E-mail: s.fedele@ucl.ac.uk

Tommaso Lombardi MD DMD PD
Professor and Head
Laboratory of Oral and Maxillofacial Pathology
Division of Stomatology and Oral Surgery
Faculty of Medicine, University of Geneva
Switzerland
E-mail: Tommaso.Lombardi@unige.ch

Vinay Hazarey BDS MDS
Dean and Professor
Department of Oral Pathology
Government Dental College
Nagpur, Maharashtra, India
E-mail: vinay.hazarey@gmail.com

WM Tilakaratne BDS MS FDSRCS PhD FRCPath
Professor, Department of Oral Pathology
Faculty of Dental Sciences
University of Peradeniya, Sri Lanka
E-mail: wmtilak@pdn.ac.lk

Foreword

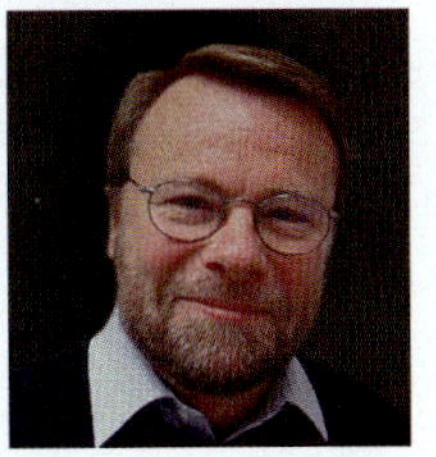

It is a pleasure to have been asked to write a foreword to this excellent book written by well-known experts in the field of oral medicine and pathology. This book has drawn them together in a unique collaboration to provide an outstanding resource on the subject. The book comprises of 24 chapters and includes extensive tables, clinical photographs, microscopic and radiological figures to aid in the understanding of the text.

Diagnosis and management of oral disorders is an exciting and thought-provoking discipline in dentistry. This text is a welcome addition to the available resources in the field and has been produced at low-cost with the needs of the postgraduate students in mind. A complete understanding of oral disorders requires sound clinical knowledge to arrive at a differential diagnosis that needs to be underpinned by information from investigative techniques. This reference book provides a comprehensive approach to both diagnosis and management, thereby making this a singular work. The management of disorders is evidence-based (when available) and will facilitate a good grounding for the trainees as well as for both generalists and specialists to become familiar with current approaches to patient care.

The text is edited by two senior colleagues practicing oral medicine and pathology with a broad understanding of the needs of low and middle-income countries, thereby facilitating the educational needs of trainees from many countries while retaining the dynamic knowledge base acquired from high-income countries. Thus, the text provides a global approach to patient care in the field of oral medicine and pathology.

I highly recommend this valuable book. Readers engaged in diagnosis and management of oral disorders will feel most enriched by the basic information and the practical guidelines provided in this field important to public health. The book is not only helpful in clinical practice but also it will be most instrumental to postgraduate training as well.

Poul Erik Petersen
Chief
Global Oral Health Programme
World Health Organization
Chronic Disease and Health Promotion
20 Avenue Appia CH-1211
Geneva, Switzerland

Preface

Oral Medicine and Pathology: A Guide to Diagnosis and Management is aimed at postgraduate students, specialist trainees, interns and all practitioners treating patients with oral diseases or those presenting with manifestations of systemic diseases in the oral cavity. Our undergraduate students have a minimum exposure to pathological disorders other than dental caries and periodontal diseases and the book provides a useful resource to their early learning. Our objective is to present a comprehensive book on patient management, to improve skills and expertise on oral diagnosis replete with a basic knowledge on both soft and hard tissue pathology.

Its concise and easy-to-read format will permit the readers to discuss the case presentations with specialists in the field, and will enable them to make accurate diagnoses in order to jointly manage patients even if they have not had extensive previous experience in oral medicine. We hope, the book will benefit practitioners responsible for the care of the oral cavity and will save them time going to one concise, authoritative source for diagnosis and treatment options, without having to wade through several texts, or in thousands of journal articles.

We have endeavored to maintain a basic format and content of clinical manifestations with numerous illustrations, to help in the diagnosis or in making a differential diagnosis. We as the editors have edited chapter contents to maintain consistency in format, depth, and style and to keep up with the advances in management of oral diseases.

The book will reflect the many years of our practical experience as well as the extensive clinical and research expertise of the various chapter contributors. We have selected authors from various prestigious institutions from all over the globe. They are well-known experts in their respective fields and this book has drawn them together in a unique collaboration to provide the reader an all-encompassing appraisal of the current state of our knowledge in oral diagnosis and management of pathological conditions that we encounter in day-to-day practice.

Saman Warnakulasuriya
WM Tilakaratne

Acknowledgments

We take this opportunity to express our gratitude to the people, who have been instrumental in the successful completion of this book. First of all our chapter contributors for accepting our invitation and for their excellent authorship in their respective fields reflecting an up-to-date knowledge and writing succinct text, which made our job as editors much easier. We thank Dr Michael Escudier of King's College London, for his contribution by revising and re-drafting Self-Assessment Questions that appear at the end of each chapter. Christine Bell helped us with initial formatting of chapters and illustrations and we thank her for attention to detail. We acknowledge several colleagues, who have helped us in proofreading Chapters 5–7; Dr BSMS Siriwardena, Dr Rasika Ekanayaka, Dr RLPR Liyanage and Dr S Wadusinghaarachchi. In addition to those named for contributing illustrations, we acknowledge Professor Edward Odell and others, who have contributed to this publication. We wish to thank Dr Shankargouda Patil for his invaluable logistic support during preparation of this volume.

Our thanks are due to Shri Jitendar P Vij (Group Chairman), Mr Ankit Vij (Managing Director), Mr Tarun Duneja (Director-Publishing), Mr KK Raman (Production Manager), Mrs Chetna Vohra (Senior Manager, Business Development) and Samina Khan (PA to Director-Publishing) of M/s Jaypee Brothers Medical Publishers (P) Ltd, New Delhi, India, and their production team for achieving an excellent standard in producing the first edition of this book.

Contents

Chapter 1

Anomalies of Teeth

Nalin Thakker

Chapter Outline

INTRODUCTION

This chapter describes some of the main developmental and nondevelopmental abnormalities of teeth.

Developmental abnormalities of teeth can arise through either inherited mutations in genes involved in tooth development or exposure to environmental factors during the development of teeth, that disrupt or modify the development process. The genes involved in tooth development can be classified into two main groups: genes whose function is critical in tooth development but not other tissues and genes whose function is critical in development of many tissues, including teeth. Pathological mutations of the former result in nonsyndromic conditions in which there are only abnormalities of teeth. In contrast, mutations of the latter result in syndromic conditions in which the abnormalities of teeth are associated with a range of other phenotypic changes. There are numerous syndromic, single gene- or Mendelian disorders that present with abnormalities of teeth. For brevity, only some of the more common conditions are described below. Their systemic manifestations are not described in detail here but are readily available from Online Mendelian Inheritance in Man (OMIM).

The nondevelopmental abnormalities of teeth are those that arise through the action of the environment (e.g. mechanical wear, chemical erosion) on fully developed teeth. The description given below excludes an account on dental caries (see Chapter 2).

DEVELOPMENTAL ABNORMALITIES OF ENAMEL

Amelogenesis Imperfecta

Amelogenesis imperfecta is the term given for a group of genetically and phenotypically heterogeneous disorders affecting the enamel. These abnormalities can occur in isolation (nonsyndromic) or as part of a syndrome and generally, affect all teeth resulting in altered structure and appearance of the teeth. The reported prevalence of amelogenesis imperfecta varies between 1 in 700 and 1 in 14,000.

The abnormalities and the resultant clinical and histological appearances in amelogenesis imperfecta vary (**Table 1.1, Figs 1.1 and 1.2**).

The consequences of poorly formed or mineralized enamel are rapid breakdown, poor esthetics, predisposition to caries and thermal sensitivity. Management is focused on exclusion of any systemic features, preservation of tooth structure and improvement of esthetics by restorative care such as prosthetic crowns or plastic restorations, prevention of dental caries and maintenance of good oral hygiene, psychological well-being of the individual and genetic counseling.

Nonsyndromic Amelogenesis Imperfecta

A number of classifications of the amelogenesis imperfecta based either on morphology, mode of inheritance and/or genetic or biochemical defect have been proposed. Classifications based just on morphology or modes of

▪ Table 1.1
Phenotypes in amelogenesis imperfecta

Defect	*Definition*	*Clinical appearances*
Hypoplastic	Reduced thickness or absence of enamel	Pitted and ridged enamel
Hypomineralized (hypocalcified)	Normal thickness of the organic matrix that is variably under-mineralized	Discolored, rough soft enamel
Hypoplastic and hypomineralized	Combination of the two	Combination of the two
Hypomature	Areas of poorly formed enamel in otherwise normal enamel	Discrete white patches

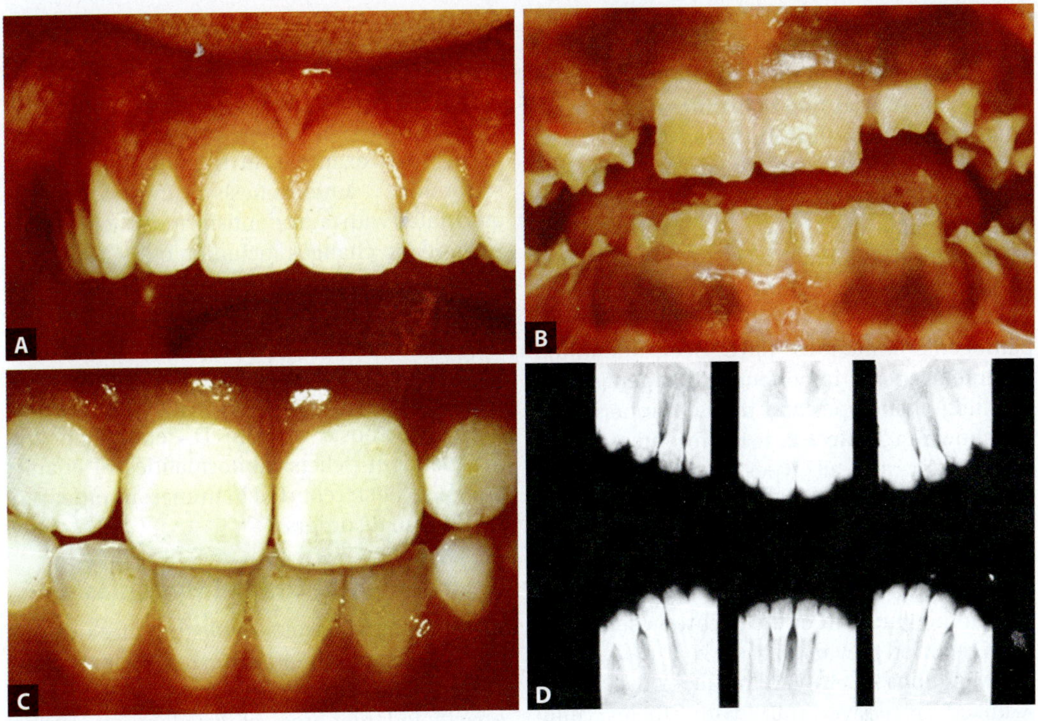

Figs 1.1A to D: Amelogenesis imperfecta. (A) Hypoplastic-hypomineralized amelogenesis imperfecta with discolored, rough soft enamel with pits and ridges; (B) Hypomineralized amelogenesis imperfecta with discolored, rough soft enamel; (C) Hypomaturation type amelogenesis imperfecta with whitish patches; (D) Radiographic appearances of hypomineralized amelogenesis imperfecta showing poorly mineralized enamel (*Courtesy:* Professor I Mackie)

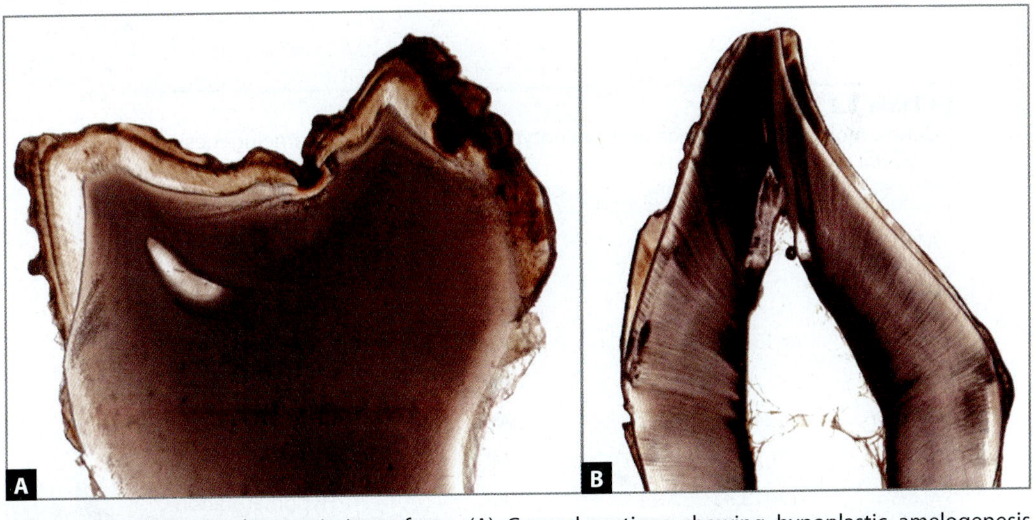

Figs 1.2A and B: Amelogenesis imperfecta. (A) Ground sections showing hypoplastic amelogenesis imperfecta with thin irregular enamel; (B) Hypomineralized amelogenesis imperfecta with enamel of relatively normal thickness but with poor mineralization (*Courtesy:* Dr K Hunter)

inheritance as primary discriminants are inadequate because of phenotypic and genetic heterogeneity and gene dose dependency of some of the traits resulting in different modes of inheritance. A classification based on molecular pathology provides a sound but possibly somewhat incomplete basis to consider this group of conditions.

Amelogenesis imperfecta can be inherited as X-linked or an autosomal recessive or dominant trait. A number of genes with pathogenic mutations have been identified in amelogenesis imperfecta. The genes, the resulting phenotypes and mode of inheritance are shown in **Table 1.2**. It is presently unclear whether or not all types of nonsyndromic amelogenesis imperfecta reported to date can be attributed to mutations in one of the genes listed in **Table 1.2**. At least one other type of amelogenesis imperfecta mapping to the distal part of the long arm of the X chromosome has been reported previously.

Mutations in *AMELX* result in a classical X-linked recessive trait with males fully expressing the phenotype whilst females show alternate banding of normal and affected enamel due to Lyonization. Mutations in *ENAM* can result in either dominant or recessive traits with either localized or generalized hypoplasia respectively suggesting dose-dependency of the trait.

Syndromic Amelogenesis Imperfecta

Amelogenesis imperfecta also occurs as part of several Mendelian conditions often with abnormalities of other ectodermal derived tissues. For example, in tricho-dento-osseous syndrome amelogenesis imperfecta is associated with taurodontism and other variable phenotypic changes including curly hair, bony sclerosis and brittle nails. In Jalili syndrome, amelogenesis imperfecta is associated with con-rod dystrophy. Amelogenesis imperfecta is also seen in some syndromes with abnormalities of calcium metabolism or regulation such as nephrocalcinosis, vitamin D dependent- and independent-rickets. Abnormalities of enamel have also been reported in numerous other rare Mendelian disorders.

Environmental Enamel Hypoplasia

Environmental insults or disturbances during tooth development are associated with enamel defects. These can range from small area of opacity to larger areas of discoloration, pitting, grooves and involvement of the whole crown (**Figs 1.3A to C**). Change may be distinctive or nonspecific. The timing of disturbance in development is indicated by the position of the defects on the crown and the teeth affected. Thus, disturbances *in utero* present on deciduous teeth, disturbances in the first two

▪ Table 1.2
Genes, modes of inheritance and phenotypes in nonsyndromic amelogenesis imperfecta

Gene	*Chromosomal location*	*Inheritance*	*Phenotype*
AMELX	Xp22.2	XR	Hypoplasia Hypomineralization Hypomaturation
ENAM	4q13.3	AD	Localized hypoplasia
		AR	Generalized hypoplasia
FAM83H	8q24.3	AD	Hypomineralization
MMP20	11q22.2	AR	Hypomaturation
KLK4	19q13.33	AR	Hypomaturation

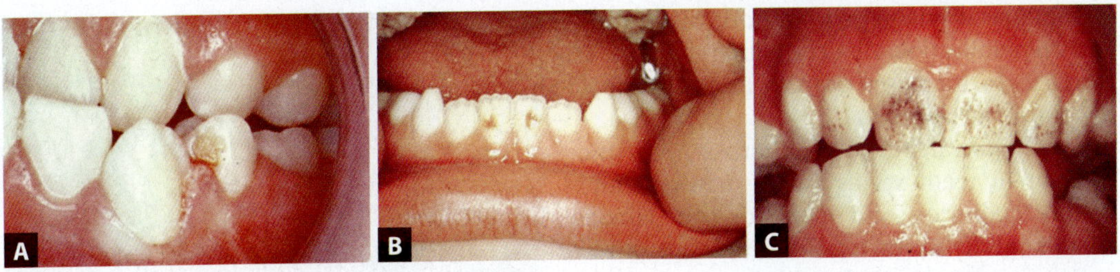

Figs 1.3A to C: Environmental hypoplasia. (A) Enamel hypoplasia localized to one tooth; (B) Enamel hypoplasia of the permanent lower central incisors as result of trauma to deciduous lower central incisors at 18 months (Turner hypoplasia); (C) Enamel hypoplasia characterized by pits affecting upper central and lateral incisors

years present on permanent anterior and first molar teeth, and disturbances in years 4 and 5 on canines, premolars and second molars.

A variable prevalence of enamel hypoplasia has been reported but most accounts suggest between 10 and 15 percent in the adult population. In a majority of cases this affects a single tooth, usually buccal surface of anterior teeth.

Nonspecific Abnormalities

A variety of environmental factors have been reported to be associated with enamel hypoplasia. These include low birth weight, viral infections, fever, prenatal or neonatal respiratory insufficiency/distress, malabsorption syndromes such as celiac disease, malnutrition, cytotoxic therapy, other drugs, metabolic disorders, parathyroid disorders.

Some specific types of environment-induced hypoplasia are also recognized and are described below.

Turner Hypoplasia

This is enamel hypoplasia of variable severity thought to be associated with periapical infection or trauma associated with preceding deciduous teeth (**Figs 1.3A to C**). Hypoplasia associated with periapical infection is most commonly seen in permanent premolars whilst that due to trauma is more commonly seen in maxillary permanent incisors.

Molar Incisor Hypomineralization

This is defined as hypomineralization of variable severity associated with systemic factors and affecting one or more permanent first molars with or without incisors involvement. The reported prevalence of molar incisor hypomineralization (MIH) varies between 2.5 and 25 percent. The etiology is unknown but is thought to be associated with many of the factors described above including infections of upper aerodigestive tract, exanthamatous fevers and antibiotics. MIH presents as well delineated white, yellow or brown opacities usually on the buccal or occlusal surfaces. The lesions are asymmetrical in contrast to amelogenesis imperfecta and fluorosis. The teeth are prone to thermal sensitivity and caries. Management includes early diagnosis, remineralization, caries prevention, restorations, extractions if necessary and orthodontic care.

Dental Fluorosis

This is defined as developmental abnormality of enamel due to excessive fluoride exposure during tooth development. Excessive intake of fluoride anytime after birth up to the age of approximately 8 years can result in fluorosis with the severity, number and type of teeth involved determined by the dose, the period and the timing of exposure. The key sources of fluoride in this respect are fluoride in the water, supplements and dentrifices.

Fluorosed enamel shows both maturation and mineralization defects with retention of amelogenin, increased porosity and subsurface hypomineralization.

The prevalence of fluorosis in the permanent teeth varies widely between and within countries and depends on factors such naturally occurring fluoride levels of the water supply, water fluoridation and other supplementation schemes. Some studies indicate that between approximately 10 and 20 percent of the population in areas with water fluoridation may have fluorosis that is of esthetic concern.

Clinically the appearances of fluorosis can vary depending on the severity of the fluorosis (**Fig. 1.4**). Mild changes consist of a few small white specks or streaks to larger opaque areas. More severe changes range from small stained pits to large confluent areas of pitting with prominent brown staining. The defects are symmetrical and diffuse, unlike changes associated with other environmental enamel defects.

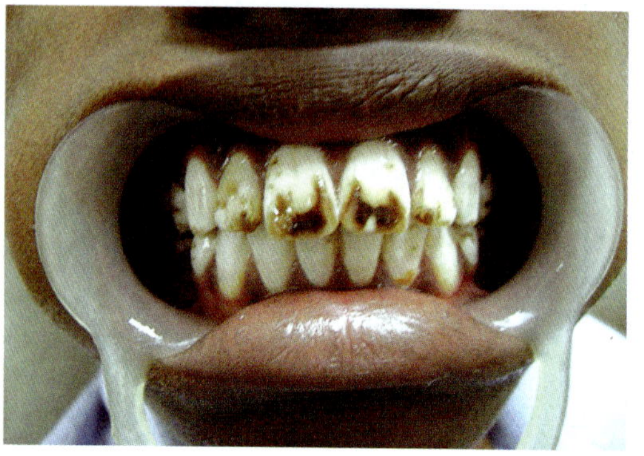

Fig. 1.4: Fluorosis. Teeth are chalky white in appearance with some teeth showing brown discoloration (*Courtesy:* Dr Manil Fonseka). Management of fluorosis is focused on improving the esthetics. In mild and moderate fluorosis, combinations of microabrasion, bleaching and restorations will usually suffice. For severe fluorosis, prosthetic crowns may be necessary

DEVELOPMENTAL ABNORMALITIES OF DENTINE

Classically, inherited defects of dentine have been classified into two main broad groups: dentinogenesis imperfecta and dentine dysplasia (**Table 1.3**).

Dentinogenesis Imperfecta

The prevalence of dentinogenesis imperfecta is thought to be between 1 in 6000 and 1 in 8000 whilst dentine dysplasia is much rarer with reported incidences of about 1 in 100,000.

Dentinogenesis imperfecta is further subdivided into three types: dentinogenesis imperfecta occurring with osteogenesis imperfecta (type I) or in isolation (type II

Table 1.3
Genes, modes of inheritance and phenotypes in dentinogenesis imperfecta and dentine dysplasia

Gene	*Inheritance*	*Phenotype*
COL1A1 *COL1A2*	AD	Dentinogenesis imperfecta type I Bone fractures Joint hyperextensibility Scleral hue Short stature Deafness
DSPP1	AD	Dentinogenesis imperfecta type II Dentinogenesis imperfecta type III Dentine dysplasia type II
Unknown	AD	Dentine dysplasia type II

and III). Dentine dysplasia is subdivided into two types based on phenotypic differences: type I or radicular and type II or coronal. However, it is now apparent that dentinogenesis imperfecta types II and III, and dentine dysplasia type II represent a spectrum of phenotypes resulting from mutations in the same gene (*DSPP*) encoding dentin sialophosphoprotein. Dentinogenesis imperfecta type I arises as part of osteogenesis imperfecta with mutations almost always (but not exclusively) in the two genes (*COL1A1* and *COL1A2*) encoding collagen type 1. The genetic defect in dentine dysplasia type I has not been identified as yet.

The specific features of each these conditions are described below. The principle consequences of poorly formed dentine are discoloration of the teeth, shearing of enamel from the dentine, rapid breakdown of teeth, pulpal exposure, and pulpal and periapical infection, and early loss of teeth in association with poorly developed roots. Surprisingly, despite widespread exposure of dentine, thermal sensitivity is not a prominent feature because of dentinal sclerosis. The key principles in management are exclusion of systemic features such as osteogenesis imperfecta, preservation of teeth through protective restorations such as prosthetic crowns, prevention of dental caries and periodontal disease, and genetic counseling.

Nonsyndromic Dentinogenesis Imperfecta (Types II and III)

Dentinogenesis imperfecta is a term used to define defects of dentine affecting both primary and secondary dentition resulting in characteristic clinical, radiographic and histological appearances. These include blue-gray or brown opalescent teeth that show rapid and marked attrition after eruption (**Figs 1.5A and B**). Radiographically, the teeth have bulbous crowns, narrow roots and pulp canals obliterated by pulp stones (**Fig. 1.5C**). Histologically, the dentine is abnormal with areas of interglobular dentine, irregular and variably reduced number of tubules, and pulpal calcifications (**Fig. 1.5D**). These characteristic changes are seen in dentinogenesis imperfecta type II.

In dentinogenesis imperfecta type III, instead of the pulpal obliteration, prominent pulpal enlargement due to hypotrophy of dentine is seen with consequent multiple pulpal exposures and apical infection. Radiographically, the teeth appear as 'shell teeth' and mandibular incisors often have apical radiolucent areas due to pulpal exposure and infection. Initially, this phenotype was thought to be limited to a dentinogenesis imperfecta occurring in a tri-racial population of Brandywine, Maryland, USA. However it is has been observed in unrelated families elsewhere and only seen in 2 percent of the Brandywine dentinogenesis imperfecta cohort suggesting this phenotype does not represent a distinct entity but is part of the variable expressivity of dentinogenesis imperfecta.

Syndromic Dentinogenesis Imperfecta

Dentinogenesis imperfecta associated with osteogenesis imperfecta (Type I)

Dentinogenesis imperfecta is most commonly observed as part of osteogenesis imperfecta and is classified as dentinogenesis imperfecta type I with features that are identical to nonsyndromic dentinogenesis imperfecta type II. It can occur in all types of osteogenesis imperfecta but is most commonly seen in types III and IV and only with missense mutations in either *COL1A1* or *COL1A2*. Occasionally, dentinogenesis imperfecta may be the most penetrant feature of this condition and thus, it is important to seek relevant history and features of osteogenesis imperfecta in all cases of dentinogenesis imperfecta.

Dentinogenesis imperfecta associated with other conditions

Dentinogenesis imperfecta may be observed as part of other rare conditions with mutations in *COL1A1* (Goldblatt syndrome) or *COL1A2* (Ehlers Danlos syndrome type VII). It is also observed in other rare syndromes associated with mutations in other genes or for which the genes have yet to be identified.

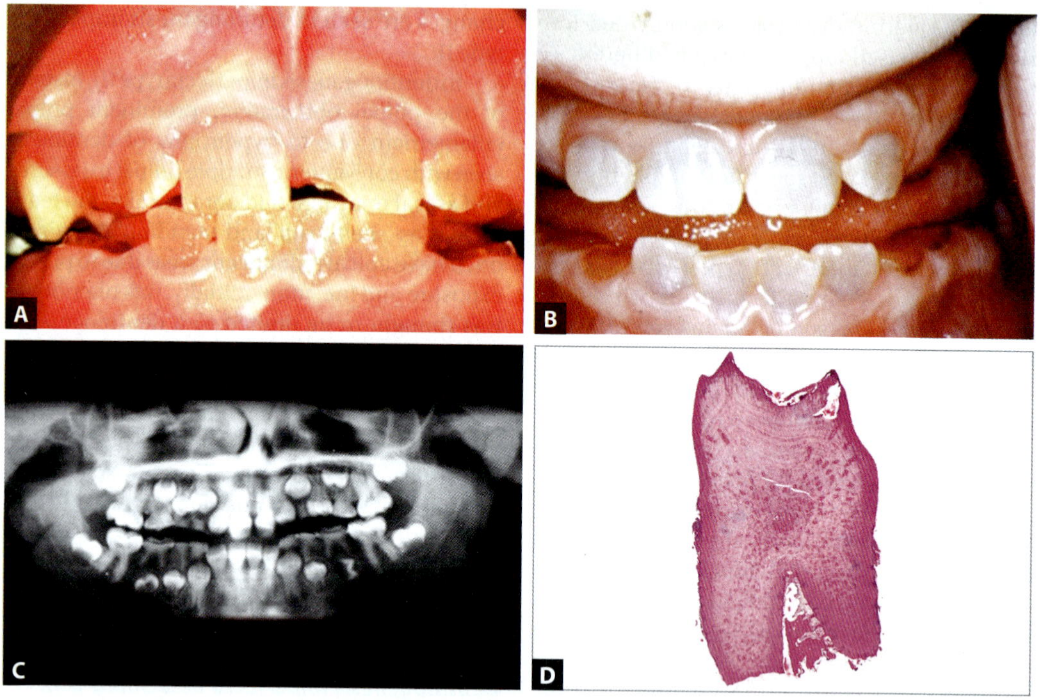

Figs 1.5A to D: Dentinogenesis imperfecta. (A and B) Clinical appearances of opalescent teeth with rapid breakdown of the crowns; (C) Radiographic appearances showing bulbous crowns with short narrow roots with obliterated pulp chambers and root canals (*Courtesy* for Figure 1.5C: Professor K Horner); (D) Histological section of decalcified tooth showing poorly formed dentine with irregular tubules and obliterated pulp chamber (*Courtesy* for Figure 1.5D: Dr K Hunter)

Dentine Dysplasia

Dentine Dysplasia Type I

This is the rarest of inherited dentine disorders and is characterized by teeth with virtually normal crowns but abnormal root development hence the alternative name for this condition of radicular dentine dysplasia. Both deciduous and permanent dentitions are affected and clinically presents as mobility of teeth and early tooth loss. The condition is usually diagnosed by radiographic examination either as an incidental finding or following history of early tooth loss. The teeth have short, conical roots with either completely obliterated pulp chambers (deciduous teeth) or almost completely obliterated pulp chambers (permanent teeth). Histologically, teeth have normal enamel with an adjacent narrow zone of normal appearing dentine beyond which there are whorled masses of dysplastic tubular and atubular dentine (**Figs 1.6A and B**). Apically, the whorled dentine masses are replaced by a less uniform arrangement of dysplastic dentine. Apical radiolucencies are also seen.

Dentine Dysplasia Type II

This condition is virtually identical to dentinogenesis imperfecta type II but largely only affects deciduous dentition (**Fig. 1.7**) with the permanent teeth either unaffected or having thistle shaped pulp chambers with multiple pulp stones. Thus, differential diagnosis of opalescent primary teeth should include dentine dysplasia (DD) type II in addition to DG.

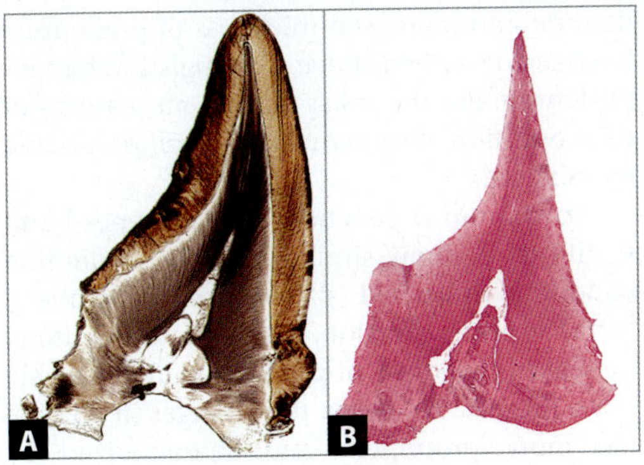

Figs 1.6A and B: Dentine dysplasia type I. (A) Ground section; (B) Decalcified section; of an affected permanent incisor showing lack of root development, normal enamel with an adjacent zone of normal appearing dentine beyond which there are whorled masses of dysplastic tubular and atubular dentine partially obliterating the pulp chamber (*Courtesy*: Dr K Hunter)

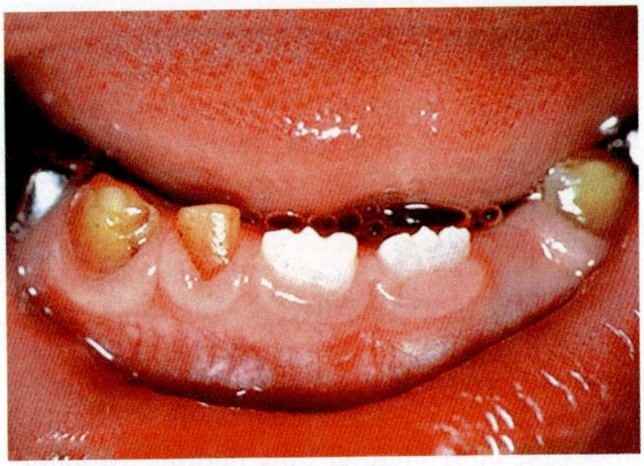

Fig. 1.7: Dentine dysplasia type II. Deciduous teeth show discoloration and rapid breakdown of the crowns whilst the permanent dentition is unaffected (*Courtesy*: Professor M Dixon)

Dentine Dysplasia Associated with Other Conditions

Dentine dysplasia is seen in association with other conditions including disorders of phosphate and/or calcium metabolism.

In familial hypophosphatemic vitamin D-resistant rickets, an X linked dominant condition, enlarged pulp chambers with prominent pulp horns, marked interglobular dentine and increased thickness of predentine (**Figs 1.8A and B**) are seen in association with bone deformities, osteomalacia and growth retardation. The condition often presents with multiple periapical dental abscesses due to early exposure of the pulp horns in anterior teeth.

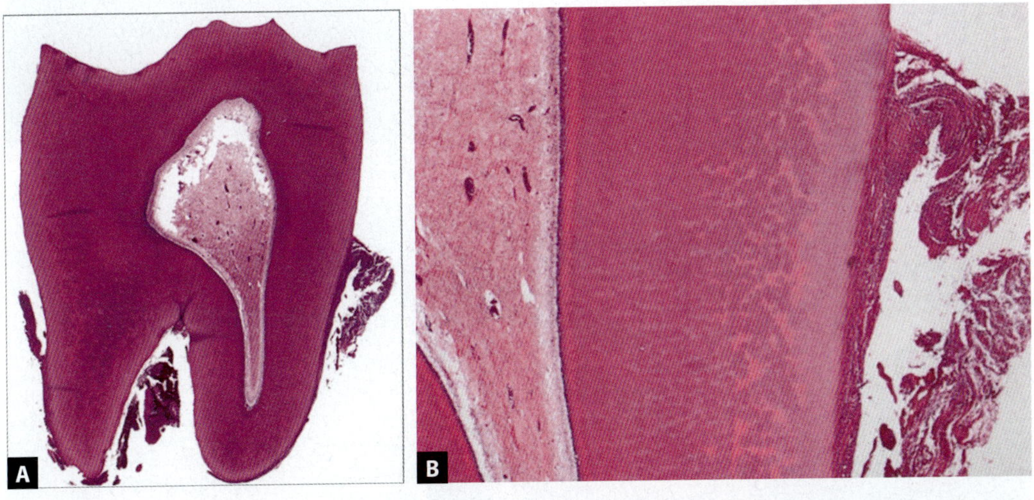

Figs 1.8A and B: Familial hypophosphatemic vitamin D resistant rickets. (A) Decalcified section of a permanent molar showing abnormal dentine involving the whole tooth; (B) Higher magnification view; showing in detail the marked interglobular dentine and increased thickness of predentine

Dentine dysplasia with short bulbous roots, pulp stones and partial obliteration of the pulp cavity occurs in hyperphosphatemic tumoral calcinosis, an autosomal recessive disorder, characterized by progressive deposition of calcified masses in soft tissues.

DEVELOPMENTAL ABNORMALITIES OF ENAMEL AND DENTINE

Composite developmental abnormalities involving both enamel and dentine probably occur in many Mendelian syndromes but have not been defined adequately. They have been described in Mendelian disorders of calcium and phosphate metabolism, and collagen some of which are describe below. Non-syndromic composite abnormalities also occur in regional odontodysplasia, a nonhereditary segmental condition of unknown etiology.

Syndromic Composite Abnormalities of Enamel and Dentine

The X linked dominant condition familial hypophosphatemic vitamin D-resistant rickets characterized by enlarged pulp chambers with prominent pulp horns, marked interglobular dentine and increased thickness of predentine has been described above. Although the changes in dentine are the most prominent features of this condition, the enamel also displays variable hypoplasia.

In vitamin D dependent rickets types I and II, the teeth show similar changes in dentine including increased size of pulp chambers, variable mineralization, interglobular dentine, increased thickness of predentine and variably sized tubules. However, the changes in enamel are more prominent and characterized by hypoplastic/hypomineralized yellow-brown enamel. In addition, the teeth do not appear to have the predisposition to early pulpal exposure and development of multiple periapical abscesses seen in familial hypophosphatemic vitamin D-resistant rickets.

Ehlers-Danlos syndrome (EDS) is a genetically heterogeneous connective tissue disorder resulting from mutation of genes encoding some types of collagen or proteins necessary for collagen assembly. There are six types of EDS showing either autosomal dominant or recessive modes of inheritance. There is broad spectrum of clinical features ranging from mild to severe that include joint hyperextensibility, skin laxity (**Fig. 1.9A**), and

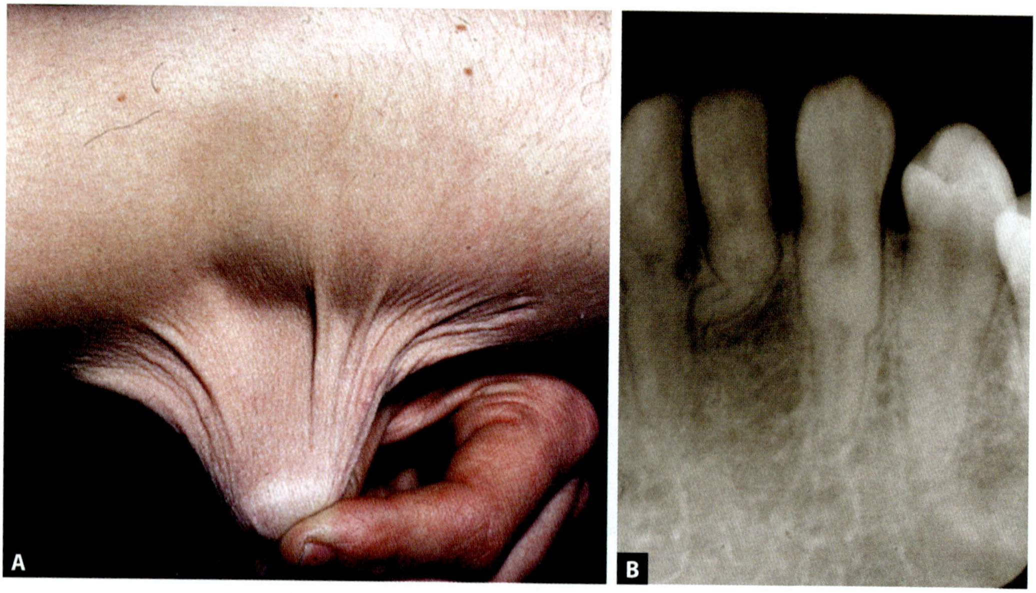

Figs 1.9A and B: Ehlers-Danlos syndrome. (A) Skin laxity; (B) Periapical radiograph of teeth showing roots with pulp stones and dilacerations

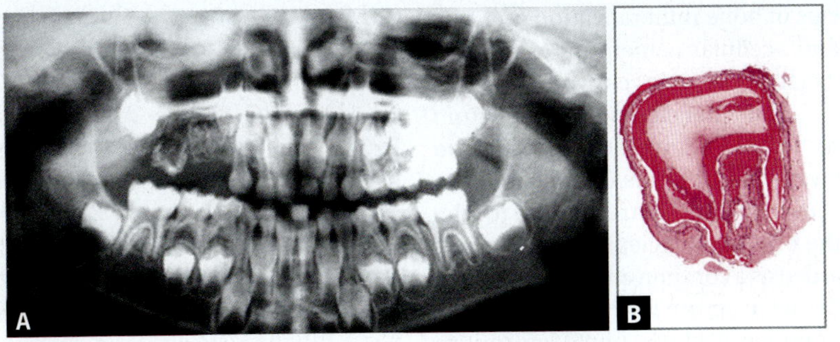

Figs 1.10A and B: Regional odontodysplasia. (A) Panoramic radiograph of the jaws showing 'ghost teeth' in the upper right quadrant; (B) Histological section of decalcified tooth showing malformed tooth with poorly mineralized enamel lacking normal prism structure and atypical dentine with interglobular dentine and increased width of predentine (*Courtesy* for Figure 1.10A: Professor K Horner)

tissue and organ fragility leading to aneurysms, bowel rupture or retinal detachment. A wide range of dental anomalies have been reported in EDS. Most commonly these include enamel hypoplasia, large pulpal calcifications or pulp stones, and shortened dilacerated roots (**Fig. 1.9B**). The dentine is reported to have abnormal tubular structure. The posterior teeth often have accentuated cusps and fissures. Hypodontia and microdontia and failure of eruption of teeth have also been reported.

Regional Odontodysplasia

This is a nonhereditary localized condition of the jaws with characteristic clinical and radiographic features. The condition involves several adjacent teeth most commonly in a single arch; however, involvement of more than one arch and all teeth has been reported. Deciduous or permanent dentition can be affected and in about half the cases both are involved. There appears to be a slightly higher incidence in females than in males and the maxilla is more commonly involved than the mandible. Association with vascular nevi, hemangioma, epidermal nevus syndrome and hemifacial hypoplasia has been reported in several cases previously.

The most characteristic anomaly is marked hypoplasia of enamel and dentine. Clinically, the teeth are discolored, soft and prone to rapid breakdown. Radiographically, the enamel and dentine are much reduced and the distinction between the two is lost due to poor mineralization, giving appearance of "ghost teeth" (**Figs 1.10A and B**). The pulp chambers are enlarged with open apices. Teeth may be missing or fail to erupt. The surrounding soft tissues are often inflamed and there may be periapical inflammation and abscess formation.

Histologically the enamel is thinned and has abnormal prism structure. The dentine is also thinned, with increased width of predentine and presence of interglobular dentine (**Figs 1.10A and B**).

The etiology of regional odontodysplasia is unknown. The association with vascular nevi, hemangioma, epidermal nevus syndrome and hemifacial hypoplasia raises the possibility of somatic mutation. Other theories include exposure to teratogenic drugs, vascular or metabolic disturbance, and viral infections.

There is a lack of consensus about the management of regional odontodysplasia. A number of factors need to be considered including the state of the affected teeth, presence of apical infection, whether deciduous or permanent dentition is affected, the need to preserve space for permanent dentition and the compromise in esthetics and function.

DEVELOPMENTAL ABNORMALITIES OF CEMENTUM

Abnormalities of cementum are usually only seen in hypophosphatasia. This is characterized by deficiencies of bone mineralization and lack of cellular and acellular cementum associated with a deficiency of the enzyme alkaline phosphatase. The deficiency arises from mutations in the *ALPL* gene and gives rise to several different clinical forms of the condition of varying severity that corresponds to the severity of the enzyme deficiency. The features are best regarded as a continuum and range from early-onset lethal or severe forms characterized by stillbirth, craniosynostosis, bony deformities hypercalcemia and renal damage to milder, late-onset types characterized by stress fractures and pseudofractures. Premature exfoliation of primary dentition can be seen in isolation (known as odontohypophosphatasia) in the mildest form of the condition or in combination with other features.

DEVELOPMENTAL ABNORMALITIES OF NUMBER OF TEETH

Hyperdontia

Hyperdontia is characterized by increase in one or more teeth in the normal dentition (supernumerary teeth). It can arise in isolation (nonsyndromic) or together with other abnormalities (syndromic). Both primary and secondary dentition may be involved. The prevalence in the Caucasian populations is between 1 and 3 percent but is reported to be higher in Mongoloid races. Presence of multiple supernumerary teeth especially nonsyndromic, is rare. Cases with one or two supernumerary teeth commonly involve the anterior maxilla whilst multiple supernumerary teeth most commonly involve premolar regions in both jaws.

The teeth can be supplemental or rudimentary. Supplemental teeth are of normal size and shape. The most common supplemental teeth are maxillary lateral incisors followed by premolars and molars. Rudimentary teeth are of small size and have an abnormal shape, e.g. conical. The most common supernumerary tooth is mesiodens, a rudimentary conical tooth arising between the permanent maxillary incisors.

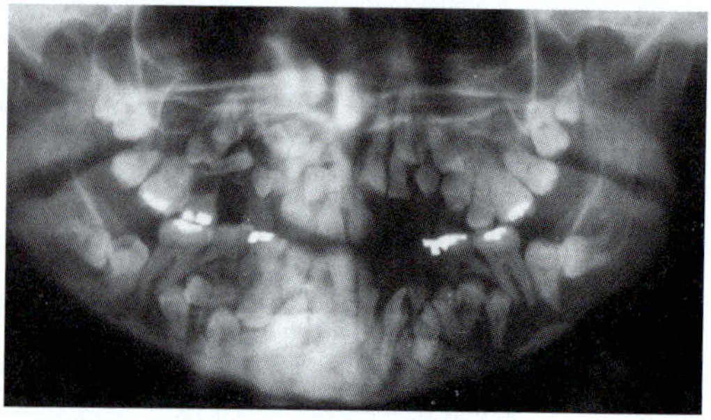

Fig. 1.11: Cleidocranial dysplasia. Panoramic radiograph of the jaws showing multiple unerupted supernumerary teeth (*Courtesy:* Professor K Horner)

Many Mendelian syndromes are associated with supernumerary teeth. The most common of these include cleidocranial dysplasia (**Fig. 1.11**), familial adenomatous polyposis, orofacial digital syndrome type I, Nance-Horan syndrome, tricho-rhino-phalangeal syndrome, Rothmund-Thomson syndrome and Hallerman-Streiff syndrome.

Supernumerary teeth are often detected as incidental findings on clinical or radiographic examination. However, they can be associated with a number of clinical problems including interference with eruption, displacement, resorption or dilacerations of adjacent teeth, crowding or spacing (diastema), dentigerous cysts and eruption into nasal or antral cavities.

Hypodontia

Hypodontia is characterized by decrease in one or more teeth in the normal dentition. Some authors differentiate this further into complete absence of dentition (anodontia), absence of more than 6 teeth (oligodontia) and absence of less than 6 teeth (hypodontia). The absence of teeth can be in isolation (nonsyndromic) or as part of constellation of features (syndromic).

Hypodontia can affect both primary and permanent dentition. The prevalence in primary dentition is low (about 0.5%) and most commonly involves maxillary incisors lateral incisors followed by mandibular lateral incisors. There is a strong correlation between hypodontia in primary dentition and hypodontia in the permanent dentition.

The prevalence of hypodontia in the permanent dentition is between 2 and 10 percent. This most commonly (~80% of cases) involves only one or two teeth. Loss of six or more teeth is extremely rare (<0.3% of population). There are racial differences in the pattern of missing teeth; third molars are the most common missing teeth in Caucasians followed by maxillary second premolars and lateral incisors. In contrast, in Mongoloid races, the mandibular incisors are the most common missing teeth. Most studies show a slightly greater incidence of hypodontia in females compared to males.

Hypodontia can occur as result of environmental factors such as local infections, radiotherapy or chemotherapy or other drugs. However, in most cases it is likely to have a genetic etiology. It is often transmitted as an autosomal dominant trait with incomplete penetrance and mutations have been identified in two genes (*MSX1* and *PAX9*) in nonsyndromic hypodontia (**Fig. 1.12A**). It is also seen in many Mendelian syndromes including the ectodermal dysplasias (including incontinentia pigmenti) where it is associated with abnormalities of shape of teeth (e.g. conical teeth) (**Fig. 1.12B**), in association with predisposition to colorectal cancer, Down syndrome and hemifacial microsomia.

Hypodontia is often associated with other abnormalities such as microdontia (e.g. peg shaped lateral incisors), transposition of permanent teeth, taurodontism and ectopic impacted canines. The principle clinical problems with lack of teeth are lack of function and esthetics coupled with malocclusion.

DEVELOPMENTAL ABNORMALITIES OF ERUPTION OF TEETH

Early Eruption Including Natal Teeth

Early eruption of teeth can occur in isolation or rarely secondary to hyperthyroidism, precocious puberty or as part of a Mendelian syndrome such as Sotos syndrome and pachonychia congenita.

Natal teeth occur in between 1:2000 and 1:3500 live births and more common in females than males. A small percentage (<10%) of these are supernumerary teeth but most are early erupted teeth from the primary dentition. Mandibular central incisors are overwhelmingly the most commonly affected tooth followed by maxillary central incisors. Although natal teeth tend to have a normal shape, they are often smaller, and have dysplastic enamel and dentine with short poorly developed roots with consequent tooth mobility.

The main problems associated with isolated natal teeth are of discomfort to mother when suckling and traumatic sublingual ulceration.

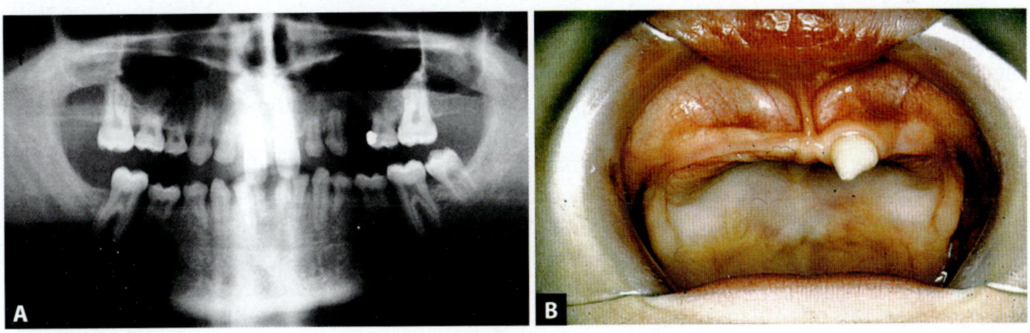

Figs 1.12A and B: Hypodontia. (A) Panoramic radiograph of the jaws showing a case of nonsyndromic hypodontia with lack of most permanent teeth; (B) Hypohidrotic ectodermal dysplasia with oligodontia and conical tooth

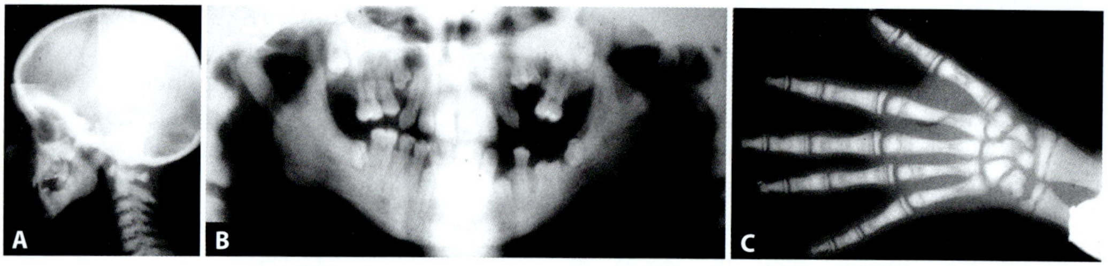

Figs 1.13A to C: Osteopetrosis. (A) Lateral skull radiograph showing generalized osteosclerosis of the calvarium and skull base, and loss of the frontal sinus; (B) Panoramic radiograph of the jaws showing generalized osteosclerosis with multiple unerupted teeth; (C) Dorsal view radiograph of left hand showing generalized osteosclerosis, and transverse striations and 'bone-in-bone' appearance in the phalanges and metacarpus

Delayed or Failure of Eruption of Teeth

This can be syndromic or occur in isolation, can involve single or multiple teeth and affect primary and/or secondary dentition.

Delayed or failure of tooth eruption is seen in many Mendelian syndromes. Some of them can be very loosely grouped into those associated with bony or calcification abnormalities such as osteopetrosis (**Figs 1.13A to C**) and cleidocranial dysplasia (*see* **Fig. 1.11**), and those associated with growth retardation or atrophy such as hemifacial atrophy, focal dermal hypoplasia and GAPO (growth retardation, alopecia, pseudoanodontia, and optic atrophy). However in other syndromes, e.g. familial adenomatous polyposis (**Fig. 1.14**), there appears to be no common mechanism of failure of eruption.

Failure of eruption of single teeth is most commonly associated with simple local mechanical obstruction because of dental crowding. Isolated abnormality of eruption without any local or systemic causes and without a family history is known as primary failure eruption. This more commonly affects posterior teeth of both primary and secondary dentition, the involved teeth may fail to erupt completely or may erupt partially and then cease to erupt. This often leads to bony ankylosis of the unerupted or partially erupted tooth.

The main problems associated with failure or delayed eruption, are malocclusion, loss of function, and bony ankylosis of teeth.

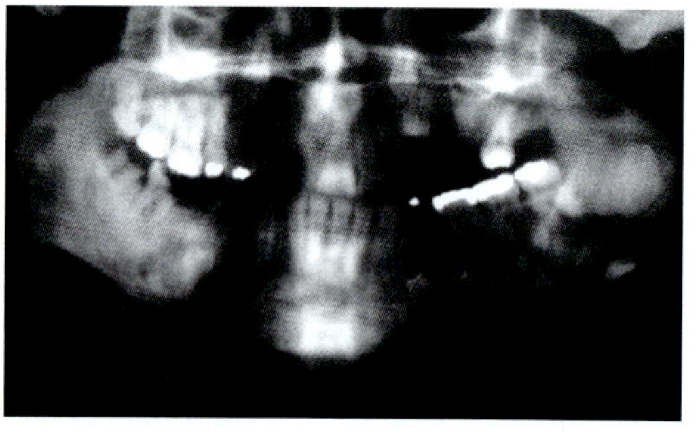

Fig. 1.14: Familial adenomatous polyposis. Panoramic radiograph of the jaws showing multiple unerupted teeth together with osteomata

DEVELOPMENTAL ABNORMALITIES RESULTING IN EARLY LOSS OF TEETH

These can be broadly divided into three main groups:

1. Inherited defects in structure of cementum or periodontium
2. Inherited or acquired immune deficiencies of phagocytes
3. Stunted or abnormal root development.

There are also forms of early-onset periodontitis where the defect is as yet uncharacterized.

Deficiency of cementum in hypophosphotasia has been described above. Structural abnormality of periodontium resulting in susceptibility to periodontitis and early loss of teeth is seen in some types of Ehlers-Danlos syndromes.

Immune deficiencies of phagocytes, particularly of neutrophil number and function, are also characterized by gingivitis and destructive early-onset periodontitis. Inherited deficiencies of neutrophil number include congenital neutropenias, cyclic neutropenia and several other syndromes. Acquired neutropenias are associated with hematological malignancies, infections and cytotoxic therapies.

Deficiencies of neutrophil function include defects in chemotaxis (leukocyte adhesion molecule deficiencies), oxidative metabolism (e.g. lack of superoxide dismutase in chronic granulomatous disease, myeloperoxidase deficiency) and protease mediated bactericidal activity (e.g. lysosomal trafficking defects in Chediak-Higashi syndrome, cathepsin C deficiency in Papillon Lefevre syndrome). These conditions usually present in childhood with recurrent infections of skin, lung, liver and bone with pathogenic and normally nonpathogenic bacteria and fungi. Clinical features include fever, recurrent abscesses, lymphadenopathy, hepatosplenomegaly and apthous ulceration.

Stunted or abnormal root development is seen in dentine dysplasia type I, occasionally in dentinogenesis imperfecta and is associated with early loss of teeth.

DEVELOPMENTAL ABNORMALITIES OF TOOTH FORM AND SIZE

Microdontia and Macrodontia

Generalized macrodontia (increase in size of teeth) or microdontia (decrease in size of teeth) is very rare. However, changes in size affecting one or more teeth occur as part of various Mendelian syndromes. For example, conical teeth are observed together with hypodontia in some types of ectodermal dysplasia, a genetically heterogeneous group of disorders characterized by abnormalities of at least two ectodermal derived tissues (commonly skin, hair, nail, eccrine glands and teeth). Similarly, macrodontia involving canine and molar teeth is seen in otodental syndrome together with sensorineural deafness and coloboma. Isolated microdontia is observed in about 1 percent of population and commonly affects 3rd molars and maxillary lateral incisors.

Dens Invaginatus

Dens invaginatus or dens-in-dente is developmental malformation thought to arise by infolding of the dental papilla and characterized by enamel-lined cavity extending to a variable depth into the body of the tooth (**Figs 1.15A and B**). In its least severe form, it forms a

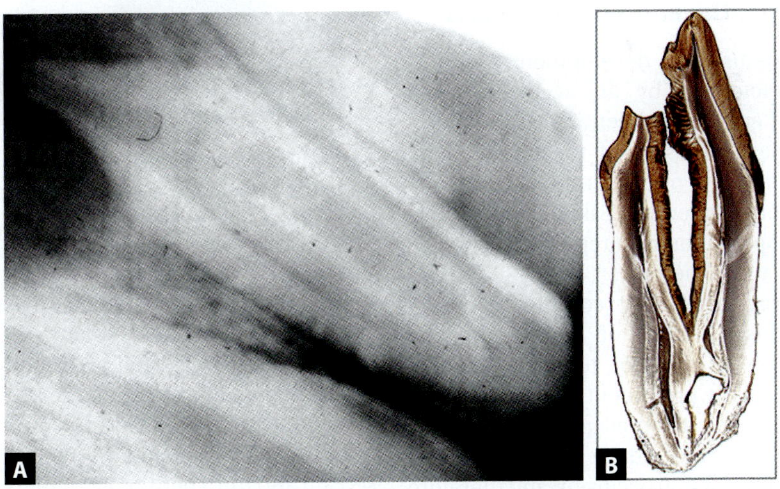

Figs 1.15A and B: Dens-in-dente. (A) Periapical radiograph showing tooth inside a tooth appearance; (B) Longitudinal histological ground section showing tooth dilated by an enamel lined cavity extending into the pulp space (*Courtesy* for Figure 1.15B: Dr K Hunter)

small pit in the enamel or an enamel-lined sac that extends into the dentine and is confined with the crown. In the more severe form, the inversion extends into the pulp and may, or may not communicate with pulp. In the most severe type, the inversion extends through the root laterally or apically and forms a second foramen in the periodontium or at the apex respectively.

The reported prevalence of the dens invaginatus in full mouth surveys is between 0.5 and 10 percent. The anomaly is usually seen in permanent teeth although occasionally it has been reported in deciduous and even supernumerary teeth. The most commonly affected teeth are maxillary lateral incisors followed by maxillary central incisors and canines.

Clinically the first presentation is often because of pulpitis or periapical infection due to communication between the pulp and invagination or secondary to caries in the invagination. Depending on the severity of the invagination, the tooth may appear to have normal morphology or may be markedly expanded to accommodate the invagination. Similarly, changes on radiographic examination may be quite subtle or marked. Endodontic treatment is normally required but may be difficult because of quite complex root morphology.

Dens Evaginatus and Enamel Pearls

Dens evaginatus is a developmental abnormality characterized by an accessory cusp consisting of enamel and dentine and in about half the cases, extension of the dental pulp. This abnormality is more common in people of Asian, North American Eskimo and Native American populations with reported incidence between 0.5 and 15 percent.

Dens evaginatus most commonly occurs on the occlusal surface of molars and the lingual surface of anterior teeth. Where the cusp is particularly prominent in anterior teeth it is referred to as a talon cusp (**Fig. 1.16**). The clinical significance of dens evaginatus is that because of its site, it is in occlusion and therefore suffers wear or fracture due to occlusal pressure resulting in pulp exposure.

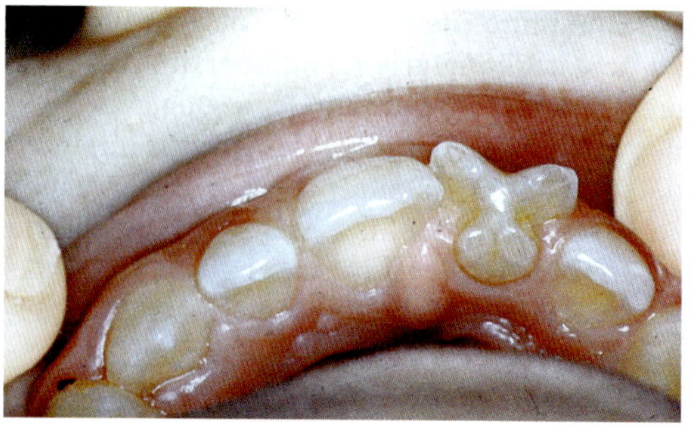

Fig. 1.16: Talon cusp. Accessory cusp on the lingual aspect of upper left central incisor

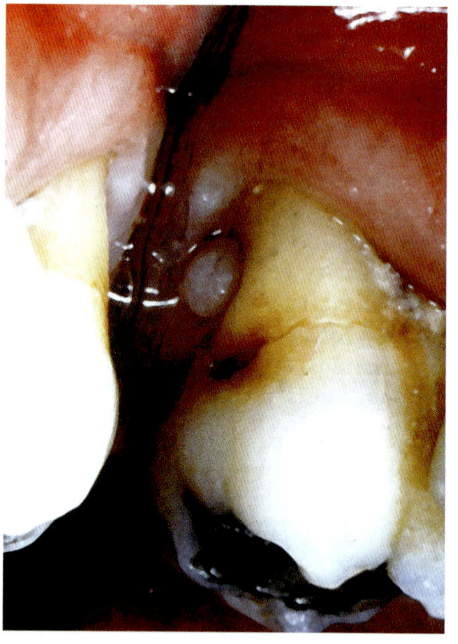

Fig. 1.17: Enamel pearl. Solitary small hard tissue nodule consisting of enamel at bifurcation of a maxillary second molar

Enamel pearls are small hard tissue nodules consisting of enamel usually with a core of dentine rarely pulp, and are found on roots of deciduous and permanent teeth (**Fig. 1.17**). They are usually solitary and commonly found at bifurcation of molars particularly maxillary, second and third permanent molars. Prevalence of between 1 and 10 percent has been reported. Clinically they are of little significance although a few studies suggest that they may act as plaque retention factors and predispose to local gingivitis or periodontitis.

Taurodontism

Taurodontism is characterized by increase in size of pulp chamber with apical displacement of the pulp chamber floor and loss of cervical constriction (**Fig. 1.18**). The anomaly most commonly occurs in isolation but is also seen in many chromosomal and Mendelian syndromes including Down syndrome, Klinefelter's syndrome and tricho-osseous-dental syndrome.

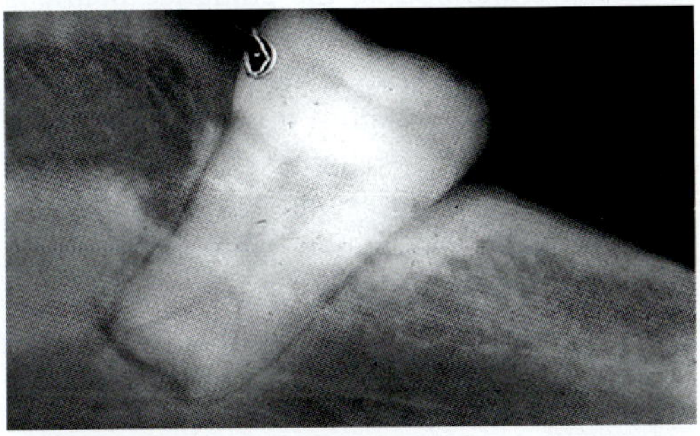

Fig. 1.18: Taurodontism. Periapical radiograph showing molar tooth with increase in size of pulp chamber, apical displacement of the pulp chamber floor and loss of cervical constriction

The reported prevalence of the condition varies markedly (5.4–65%) probably due to differences in the diagnostic criteria, and the teeth and the populations assessed.

As the crown morphology is normal, taurodontism is most commonly detected as an incidental finding on radiographs taken for routine dental care. Taurodontism is of little clinical significance other than exclusion of any syndromes and possible difficulties in endodontic treatment of affected teeth.

Gemination

Gemination is defined as an attempt by a single tooth bud to form two teeth resulting in a bifid crown with a single root (**Figs 1.19A and B**). There is no variation in the number of teeth if the bifid tooth is counted as a single tooth. Prevalence is reported to be less than 1 percent and few bilateral cases have been reported. As with fusion, gemination is largely in the anterior dentition and gemination in the primary dentition is followed in about half the cases with gemination of the succedaneous permanent teeth.

Fusion

Dental fusion is defined as a union of two adjacent teeth involving dentine and/or

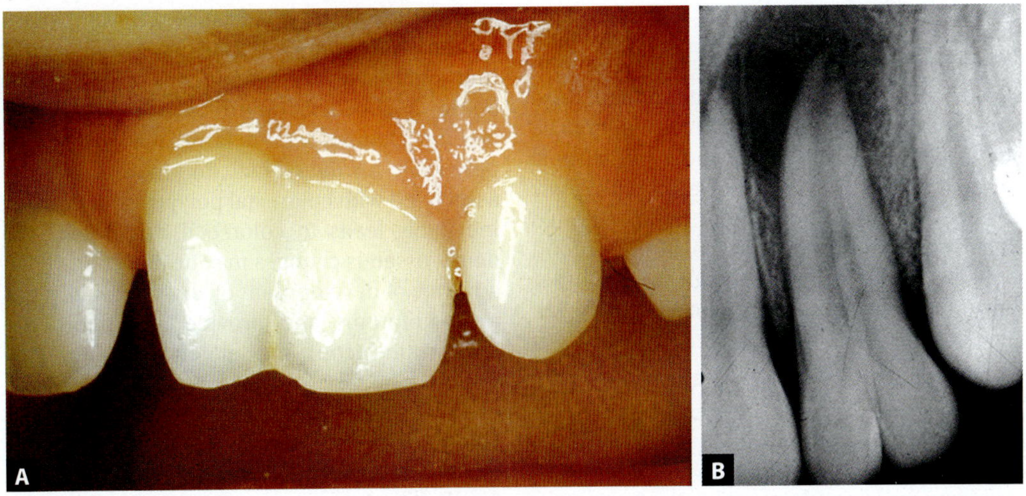

Figs 1.19A and B: Gemination. (A) Bifid crown upper lateral incisor; (B) Periapical radiograph showing bifid crown with partial single root in upper lateral incisor

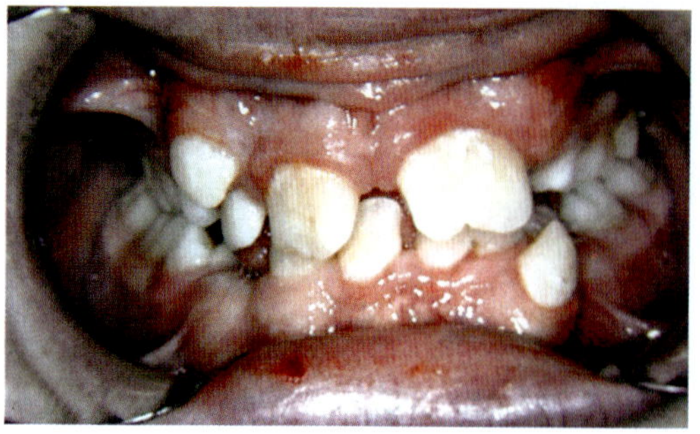

Fig. 1.20: Dental fusion. Fusion of upper anterior teeth in oculocardiofacial dental syndrome

enamel. The fusion is usually between teeth in the normal dentition although occasionally involves a supernumerary tooth. Depending on the timing of the fusion can be total or partial, the latter just involving the roots. The primary dentition is more commonly affected and the prevalence is reported to be 0.5 to 2.5 percent. It is seen almost exclusively in the anterior dentition and fusion in the primary dentition is followed in about half the cases with fusion of the succedaneous permanent teeth.

Dental fusion usually occurs in isolation but is also observed in one Mendelian syndrome, oculocardiofacial dental syndrome, an X-linked male-lethal, recessive condition with widespread abnormalities (**Fig. 1.20**).

Concresence

Concresence is fusion of the roots of teeth by hypercementosis. This is a rare condition usually affecting maxillary second and third molars. Cause is unknown but it is thought to be due to hypercementosis, secondary to chronic apical inflammation or associated with roots of impacted third molars that are positioned in close proximity to the roots of the second molars. There is no clinical significance other than difficulty in extraction of the teeth involved.

BASIC PRINCIPLES AND MANAGEMENT OF PATIENT WITH DEVELOPMENTAL ANOMALIES OF TEETH

Management of a patient presenting for the first time with a developmental abnormality of the teeth will naturally depend on the abnormality. However, we can define some basic principles that are important in management of such patients. Detailed exposition of the treatment of all developmental anomalies of teeth is beyond the scope or remit of this chapter and only a very general guidance is provided.

It is important at the outset to appreciate that the management of patients with these conditions requires multidisciplinary expertise and input. A good clinician will recognize his, or her own limitations and seek help from other relevant specialists.

Commonly, the first presentation of any significant developmental abnormality of teeth is during childhood so the guidance below is provided in this context. Additionally, often the phenotype is distinctive, and will indicate the diagnosis and define the relevant course of management. The clinical pathway through which the patients present will depend on the nature and severity of the condition. Patients with more severe phenotypes (i.e. those with more marked systemic features) are likely to present with a possible or definitive diagnosis by referral from specialist medical practitioners. In contrast, those with predominantly dental changes or with latent or subtle (but not necessarily insignificant) system manifestations may present first to the dental practitioner. Thus it is important that the dental practitioner is able to not only recognize the dental phenotype but also appreciate the significance of these changes in the wider context and the implications they may have on the patient's general well-being. A good example of this is the dento-osseous changes seen in familial adenomatous polyposis, an autosomal dominant condition associated with colorectal polyposis that almost inevitably leads to colorectal carcinoma. The dento-osseous changes may be detected well in advance of development of any colorectal signs and symptoms and provide an opportunity for prophylactic and potentially lifesaving intervention.

Comprehensive history is vital to ascertain whether the condition is acquired or genetic, isolated or part of a syndrome and sporadic or familial. In determining whether the condition is acquired or genetic, unless the phenotype is so distinctive as to suggest the diagnosis, it is important to establish history of relevant exposure to environmental agents (infections or drugs for example) during the developmental phase of the teeth affected. For primary dentition, this will of course include history of exposure of the mother during pregnancy.

A full medical history is essential in determining whether the condition is part of a syndrome. It should include eliciting history of specific features associated with the suspected condition even if medical treatment has not been sought for this, as the parent may not recognize this as significant or associate them with oral or dental changes.

A detailed family history should be elicited tracing back if possible at least two generations and a pedigree constructed indicating age and status if known of all members. This will help identify the mode of inheritance and also members of the family who may be at risk of having the condition or being carriers of the condition.

Nature of examination of patient will depend on the setting and expertise of the dental practitioner. At the very least, any obvious dysmorphic features or other general abnormalities should be noted. Examination of teeth should include accurate description of abnormality and teeth affected. Special tests will depend on the nature of the abnormality, age of the patient and nature of the condition. In young children, intrusive tests should only be pursued if there is possibility of therapeutic benefit or need for surveillance. Otherwise consideration should be given to postponing the tests until child is old enough to understand and able to consent.

For patients with a genetic condition, referral to a clinical geneticist is essential so that patients and their families can receive genetic counseling and information about recurrence risks. This is particularly important for conditions associated with potentially significant systemic features. Definitive diagnostic information for such conditions should be given to the patients together with, or by a clinical geneticist.

Treatment will clearly depend on the nature of the abnormality and may involve one or more dental specialists. Prevention of caries and/or periodontal disease is likely to be essential in many of the conditions.

ACQUIRED ABNORMALITIES OF TEETH

Attrition

Physiological attrition is an irreversible loss of dental hard tissue by wearing away of the tooth surface by tooth-to-tooth contact. Pathological attrition resulting in excessive loss of tooth surface is seen in association with parafunctional habits such as bruxism. The prevalence of severe attrition (involving dentine) in adults increases from about 3 percent at age of 20 years to 17 percent at age of 70 years. In children, a wide variation in prevalence has been reported for severe wear of the deciduous dentition ranging from 0 to 82 percent.

Clinically attrition is seen as matching wear facets on opposing teeth (**Fig. 1.21**). Commonly these are on the occlusal surface but can affect buccal and lingual surfaces with certain types of malocclusions. Excessive loss may result in a loss of occlusal face height (or vertical dimension of occlusion), thermal sensitivity due to exposure of dentine and poor esthetics.

Treatment for attrition will depend on the extent of tooth surface loss, etiology, symptoms, whether loss is progressive or stable, and the level of compromise of esthetics. Management of etiological factors such as correction of malocclusion and treatment of parafunctional habits should precede any restorative

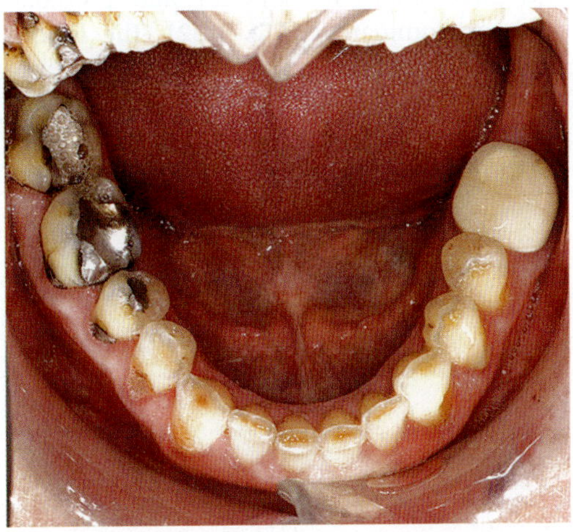

Fig. 1.21: Dental attrition. Excessive loss of tooth surface seen as wear facets on the occlusal and incisal surface of teeth (*Courtesy:* Dr S Al-Salehi)

procedures. Sensitive dentine may be treated by topical application of varnishes and use of desensitizing toothpastes.

Abrasion

Abrasion is an irreversible loss of dental hard tissue by mechanical wear of tooth substance by factors other than tooth-to-tooth contact such as food, toothpastes or toothbrushing. The prevalence of tooth loss solely due to abrasion is difficult to determine from the reported literature. It is now widely recognized that abrasion and erosion probably act in concert to cause tooth loss. Clinical and laboratory evidence suggests that abrasion alone is unlikely to cause significant tooth wear. The prevalence of noncarious cervical wear classically attributed to toothbrush abrasion is reported to be between 5 and 85 percent. This wide discrepancy is due to different parameters used to assess the loss. Loss of tooth surface limited to enamel is relatively common with prevalence ranging from 13 to 100 percent. However, prevalence of loss involving dentine is likely to be much lower at ≤5 percent.

Clinical presentation of lesions resulting from abrasion (together with erosion) depends on the etiological factors. As mentioned above, noncarious cervical lesions are associated with toothbrush abrasion. They are almost always on the outer or vestibular surface of teeth, and affect maxillary anterior and premolar teeth predominantly (**Fig. 1.22**). The lesions can have variable depth and either smooth or sharp profiles. They are usually associated with dentinal sensitivity.

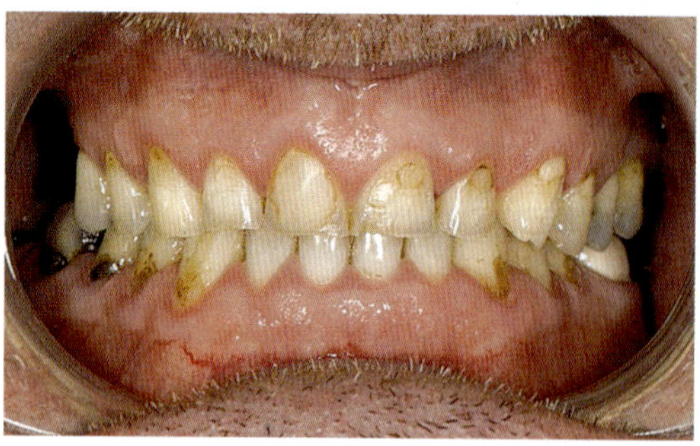

Fig. 1.22: Dental abrasion. Partly restored abrasion cavities on the cervical margins of the buccal surfaces of teeth (*Courtesy:* Dr S Al-Salehi)

Treatment involves correction of etiological factors, application of dentine bonding agents to reduce sensitivity and restorative treatment depending on the depth of the lesions.

Erosion

Erosion is irreversible loss of dental hard tissue by action of chemicals but not involving dental plaque acids or caries. As mentioned above, erosion co-exists with abrasion and attrition, and contribution of any individual component may be difficult to determine. Erosion is seen in both children and adults. Primary dentition is thought to be more susceptible to erosion than permanent dentition because of the thinner layer of enamel in the former. The reported prevalence figures vary greatly; the incidence in younger children is thought to be approximately ≤10 percent rising with age to approximately 50 percent.

There are a number of proposed intrinsic and extrinsic sources of acids. The former include gastroesophageal reflux and persistent vomiting. Gastroesophageal reflux disease or GORD is a fairly common condition reported in up to 20 percent of the population in the developed countries. It is widely accepted amongst the dental community that GORD is associated with dental erosion and an increased prevalence of dental erosion has been reported previously in patients with GORD. However a recent systemic review suggested that there is no evidence of a strong link between GORD and dental erosion.

Self-induced or spontaneous persistent vomiting can also result in erosion of tooth surface. Recurrent spontaneous vomiting is relatively uncommon. In children and more rarely in adults, cyclic vomiting (known as cyclic vomiting syndrome) is associated with migraine, abnormal gastrointestinal motility or several other disorders. Self-induced vomiting is more common and is usually observed in female teenagers or young adults as part of anorexia and bulimia nervosa.

There are several extrinsic factors in the etiology of dental erosion. Consumption of acidic drinks and to a lesser extent, acidic foods is emerging to be a significant factor. Acidic medications or illicit drugs such as ecstasy have also been reported to be associated with dental erosion. There is likely to be a greater susceptibility to dental erosion with long term drug therapy, with xerostomia-inducing drugs and consequent loss in the buffering effect of the saliva although there is no strong evidence to support this. A systemic review of occupational exposure to acids concluded that evidence of association with dental erosion is limited to battery and galvanizing workers (with limited data to support association with exposure in other areas such as chemical and pharmaceutical industries).

Clinically, dental erosion shows variable appearances. These include a smooth shiny rounded surface, surface depressions often with irregular ridges, cusp or incisal tip thinning and fracture, exposure of dentine with change of tooth color from white to yellow and at later stages thermal sensitivity. Commonly maxillary anterior teeth are involved; the most common sites on the teeth are palatal, incisal and occlusal surfaces (**Figs 1.23A to C**).

Cornerstone of management is identification and removal of the etiological factor(s). Where a systemic cause is suspected, liaison with an appropriate specialist is important. Dietary monitoring (using diet diaries) and counseling, oral hygiene instruction, remineralization of the tooth surface with fluoride toothpastes, mouthwashes and varnishes, and application of dentine bonding agents to reduce sensitivity all have a role in treatment. In the more severe cases, restorative treatment may be necessary (O'Sullivan and Milosevic, 2008).

Abfraction

Abfraction is defined as the pathological loss of tooth substance caused by biomechanical loading forces that result in flexure and failure of enamel and dentin at a location away from loading. This is thought by some to be the primary etiological factor for wedge shaped cervical lesions traditionally attributed to abrasion and erosion. It is postulated that tensile stress on teeth during mastication, in malocclusion and parafunctional habits such as bruxism can concentrate at the cemento-enamel junction and lead to tooth breakdown at this site. In addition, the tensile stresses can pull apart the enamel prisms making the surface more vulnerable to acid erosion. The evidence for this is largely based on engineering models. There is no convincing evidence that abfraction acts as a primary factor in inducing cervical lesions and it is widely accepted that these lesions arise through a multifactorial etiology with erosion and abrasion playing a significant role.

INTERNAL AND EXTERNAL ROOT RESORPTION

Pathological root resorption is defined as loss of tooth surface on the inside or outside of the root (internal or external root resorption respectively) by clastic activity.

Root resorption is thought to consist of two phases, injury and stimulation. The first phase is injury to the nonmineralized tissues such as predentine and precementum on the tooth surface with exposure of mineralized tissue to

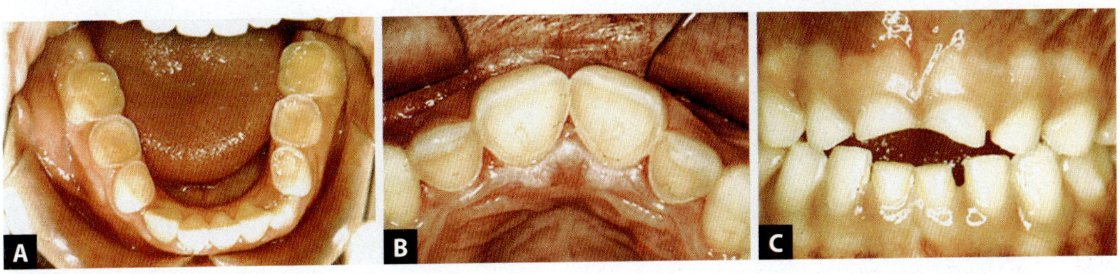

Figs 1.23A to C: Dental erosion affecting occlusal, palatal and incisal surfaces (*Courtesy:* Dr S Al-Salehi)

clastic cells of monocyte-macrophage series. This leads to colonization of the tooth surface by clastic cells and limited resorption of the hard tissues. However, this will only continue in presence of stimulation of clastic activity by, e.g. inflammation or pressure.

Several different types of processes are involved in root resorption:

- Inflammatory resorption associated with marked inflammation
- Replacement resorption associated with mild inflammation and characterized by attempted repair with metaplastic hard tissues
- Surface resorption associated with sustained pressure
- Ankylosing resorption associated with severe trauma resulting in exposure of a large area of mineralized dentine to osteoclasts with consequent root resorption and replacement by bone.

Internal Root Resorption

Internal root resorption can be apical or intraradicular. The former is the more common and seen together with apical external root resorption in up to 75 percent of teeth with periapical infection and inflammation. Intraradicular root resorption is relatively rare in permanent dentition and may be associated with pulpitis, trauma or autotransplantation. This type of resorption is characterized by replacement with metaplastic osteocementum.

Early internal resorption often has no specific features and may be detected as an incidental finding on radiographs. The presenting signs and symptoms may be those associated with the etiological factors, i.e. pulpitis, periapical inflammation or trauma. In more advanced internal root resorption, there may be pink discoloration of the crown associated with coronal intraradicular root resorption, sinus tracts associated with root perforation, or mobility of the crown associated with root fracture.

External Root Resorption

Several specific types of external root resorption are seen.

Cervical external root resorption is thought to be associated with inflammation in the periodontium. This may be a consequence of bacterial irritation or mechanical trauma. It has also been reported to occur more frequently in endodontically treated teeth where a bleaching agent was used in preparation of the root canal. It is thought that the bleaching agents leach through the dentinal tubules into the periodontium causing local injury. In most cases with early cervical lesions, there are no symptoms. In teeth with more advanced lesions with larger resorption cavities, there may be thermal sensitivity or pink discoloration of the crown at the cervical margin as the enamel is undermined by granulation tissue. Affected teeth have vital pulp and exposure of the pulp and symptoms of pulpitis may only occur at a late stage. Radiographically, cervical external root resorption is detected as an irregular cervical radiolucency through which the mineralized intact outline of the pulp chamber and root canals is visible (**Figs 1.24A and B**). Management of cervical external resorption involves exposure of the erosion

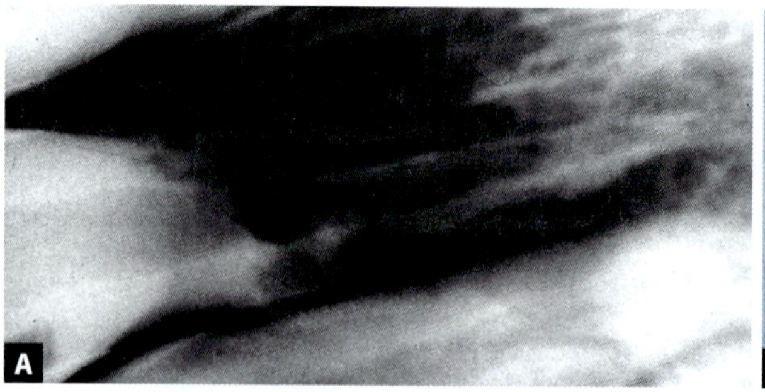

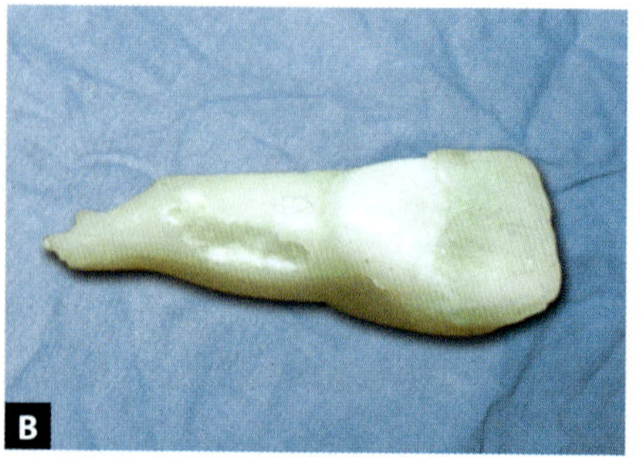

Figs 1.24A and B: External root resorption. (A) Extracted upper central incisor with external root resorption; (B) Periapical radiograph showing an upper central incisor with external root resorption

cavity, debridement, treatment with calcium hydroxide and placement of restoration. Endodontic treatment is only necessary where there is pulpal involvement.

Inflammatory external resorption along the length of the root and at the apex of the tooth can also occur in association with pulpitis and apical periodontitis. Radiographically, this is seen as irregular erosions of root surface. Management is by endodontic treatment.

Pressure-related symmetrical external root resorption in the apical third of teeth is sometimes seen as a consequence of orthodontic treatment. There may be significant shortening of the roots but the teeth are vital and symptomless. Similarly, resorption due to pressure from tumors, cysts or impacted teeth results in localized resorption in an area of pressure but the affected teeth are vital and symptomless.

Ankylosing-type of external root resorption occurs as a consequence of severe trauma such as intrusive luxation or reimplantation after lengthy delay following avulsion. The affected tooth is symptomless and may show reduced physiological mobility. Radiographically, the resorption cavities on the root surface are filled in by bone and there is a loss of periodontal ligament space.

TOOTH DISCOLORATION AND STAINING

Changes in the appearance of the color of the teeth may be due to intrinsic tooth discoloration, external staining or internalized discoloration.

Intrinsic Discoloration

This can arise from:

- Developmental structural abnormalities of teeth
- Incorporation of color imparting substances in the hard tissues during development.

Inherited and acquired developmental structural abnormalities of enamel and dentine that alter the appearance of teeth have been discussed above. These include amelogenesis imperfecta, environmental enamel hypoplasia including fluorosis, dentinogenesis imperfecta and dentine dysplasia.

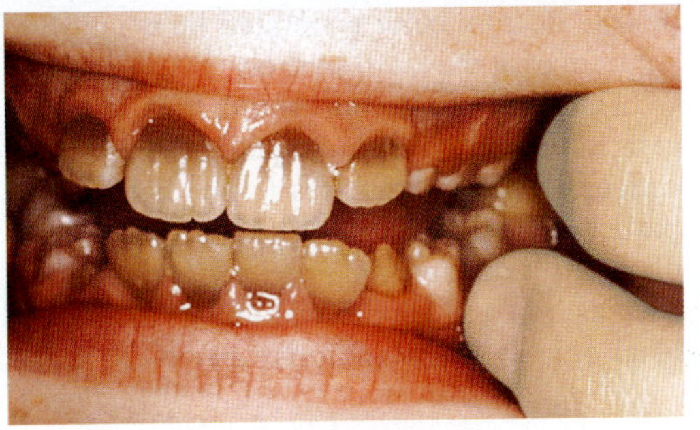

Fig. 1.25: Intrinsic discoloration of teeth. Tetracycline staining of teeth imparting yellow discoloration to newly erupted teeth that changes to gray-brown discoloration on exposure to sunlight

Color imparting substances derived from intrinsic and extrinsic sources may be incorporated into the developing dentition. Extrinsic substances include tetracycline that complexes with calcium ions on the surface of hydroxyl apatite crystals. The discoloration will depend on the type of tetracycline, dose and the period of use. Most commonly the staining will appear as a discrete bright yellow to gray or brown band at eruption but will change over time on exposure to sun (**Fig. 1.25**).

Intrinsic sources of discoloration include metabolic products. In alkaptonuria, an autosomal recessive condition characterized by a deficiency of enzyme involved in tyrosine breakdown results in accumulation of homogentisic acid which imparts a brown discoloration to teeth. In congenital erythropoietic porphyria, an autosomal recessive condition in which there is deficiency of enzyme necessary for heme production, there is build of porphyrin precursors that impart red-brown discoloration to teeth and red fluorescence under UV light. Similarly conditions in which there is extensive hemolysis or hyperbilirubinemia during the period of dental development can lead to deposition of biliverdin in teeth and yellow discoloration.

Extrinsic Staining

This can arise from either from the intrinsic color of substances incorporated into the dental pellicle or from color generated by reaction of substances at the tooth surface.

There are numerous sources of chromogens in the mouth including foods, drinks (tea, coffee, wine), mouthrinses (chlorehexidine in particular) and medications such as iron supplements. Occupational exposure to metal salts such as iron and copper can impart distinctive black or green discoloration respectively.

Internalized Staining

Unlike intrinsic discoloration, this arises through internalization of chromogens into the tooth substance after development of the tooth is complete. Factors that increase the porosity of the surface enamel or expose dentine such as acquired or inherited developmental defects, or dental caries can predispose to internalized staining. In addition to chromogens in foodstuffs, drinks, etc. tin from dental amalgam can also be internalized and discolor teeth with longstanding restorations.

SELF-ASSESSMENT QUESTIONS

1. Define amelogenesis imperfecta and explain how the clinical presentation reflects the underlying genetic basis.
2. Define environmental enamel hypoplasia and describe three common examples.
3. Define dentinogenesis imperfect and describe the three most common types.
4. Describe two conditions which result in abnormalities of both enamel and dentine.
5. Classify, and describe with examples, abnormalities of tooth number.
6. Discuss the causes of delayed or failure of eruption of teeth.
7. Describe the causes of early loss of teeth.
8. Describe five developmental abnormalities of tooth size and form.
9. Describe the four forms of noncarious tooth surface loss.
10. Discuss the causes of intrinsic staining.

SUGGESTED READING

1. Brook AH. Multilevel complex interactions between genetic, epigenetic and environmental factors in the aetiology of anomalies of dental development. Archives of Oral Biology. 2009;54(Suppl 1): S3-S17.
2. I Bailleul-Forestier, Molla M, et al. The genetic basis of inherited anomalies of the teeth: Part 1: Clinical and molecular aspects of non-syndromic dental disorders. European Journal of Medical Genetics. 2008;51(4):273-91.
3. I Bailleul-Forestier, Berdal A, et al. The genetic basis of inherited anomalies of the teeth: Part 2: Syndromes with significant dental involvement. European Journal of Medical Genetics. 2008;51(5):383-408.
4. Thesleff I. The genetic basis of tooth development and dental defects. American Journal of Medical Genetics. 2006;Part A 140A(23): 2530-5.

Chapter

2

Pathology of Dental Caries

Ranjit Mendis, Tommaso Lombardi

Chapter Outline

INTRODUCTION

Dental caries is one of the most common human diseases, is wide spread among all communities and is described as a chronic disease or process that progresses very slowly. It is considered as infectious disease, initiated by microbial activity on the tooth surface. The WHO has estimated that more than 5 billion people have experienced tooth decay.

The disease is expressed as a localized destruction of the tooth hard tissues by acids in the microbial deposits (biofilms) adhering to the teeth, producing cavities in the tooth crown (**Fig. 2.1**). The cavities start at the enamel surface and penetrate the enamel and dentine, or cementum and dentine and eventually extend to the pulp cavity. The deciduous and permanent dentitions are both affected by caries. In the absence of treatment, dental caries progress until the tooth crown is destroyed. Until recently both the prevalence, and the incidence of dental caries has steadily increased in many populations, but some countries have noted a decline in recent decades.

Various different techniques have been used to demonstrate the caries process but diagnosis of dental caries is by visuotactile examination using standard probes and routine radiography **(Fig. 2.2)**. This chapter will focus on the histopathological and ultrastructural changes seen in the enamel, dentine and cementum, and the hard tissue response to caries. To be comprehensive, the etiology and microbiology of dental caries, methods of detection and the approaches for preventing dental caries will also be discussed.

Dental caries may be classified according to the location affected on the individual tooth as pit and fissure caries (occlusal caries) and interproximal caries (smooth surface caries). If it is a new attack, it is referred to as primary caries and if it occurs around the margins of an existing restoration it is referred to as secondary (recurrent) caries.

Pit and fissure caries develops in the occlusal surfaces of molars and premolars, in the buccal surfaces of molars and premolars, and in the palatal surfaces of maxillary incisors. Pits and fissures affected by early caries may appear stained brown or black and will feel slightly soft and 'catch' a fine dental probe point. Caries usually develops in the walls of the fissure.

Smooth surface caries affects the proximal surfaces of the teeth, also referred to as interproximal caries gingival third of the buccal and lingual surfaces, also referred to as cervical caries.

Recurrent caries occurs in the immediate vicinity of a restoration. It is due to inadequate extension of the prepared cavity to self cleansing areas or poor adaptation of the restoration to the prepared cavity, which produces a 'leaky margin'.

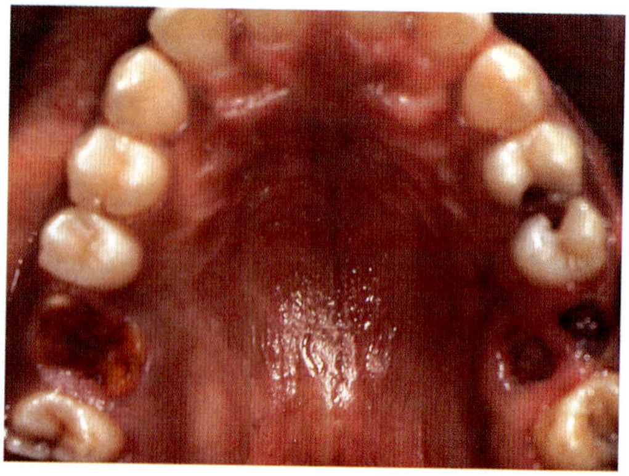

Fig. 2.1: Extensive caries in relation to the upper left premolars. The upper right first molar and the upper left first molar are destroyed due to dental caries

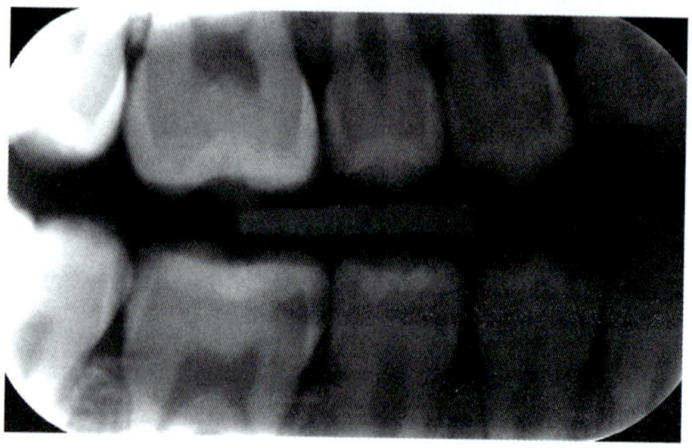

Fig. 2.2: Bite-wing radiograph to show a mandibular first molar tooth with mesial caries involving the enamel and dentine and the second premolar tooth with early distal enamel caries

ETIOLOGY AND MICROBIOLOGY OF DENTAL CARIES

Dental caries is a multifactorial disease in which there is an interplay of the four principal etiological factors. All four factors must act together for the development of dental caries. These factors are—susceptible tooth surface, saliva (host factors), dental plaque or dental biofilm, and fermentable bacterial substrate such as sugar or fermentable carbohydrate which comes from the diet. In addition, a fourth factor - time, must be considered as the etiology. Diagrammatically these four factors can be portrayed in a Venn diagram as four overlapping circles (**Fig. 2.3**).

The Venn diagram also allows us to understand ways of caries prevention, based upon attempts to:

1. Increase the resistance of the host (fluoride therapy, fissure sealants, immunization).
2. Reduce the numbers of microorganisms in contact with the tooth plaque (biofilm) control.
3. As the substrate is important, attempts should be made to select noncariogenic or less cariogenic foodstuffs.
4. Reduce the time that the substrate is in the mouth by reducing the frequency of intake of food and performing adequate oral hygiene measures soon after food intake.

Tooth morphology is an important determinant. Pit and fissure areas of molars and premolars are highly susceptible to caries as food debris and bacteria collect within these pits and fissures. In addition, irregularities in arch form, crowding and overlapping of teeth favor the accumulation of plaque. Saliva plays an important role in attenuating caries by mechanical washing of some of the food debris, bacteria and their soluble products. The saliva also has a buffering action which tends to neutralize acids produced by the biofilm bacteria on tooth surfaces. Saliva also has several different antibacterial factors. Further, saliva is supersaturated with calcium and phosphorus ions, which are important in the remineralization of white-spot lesions.

Dental caries is a chronic endogenous infection caused by the normal oral commensal flora. Hence, dental caries is a bacterial disease.

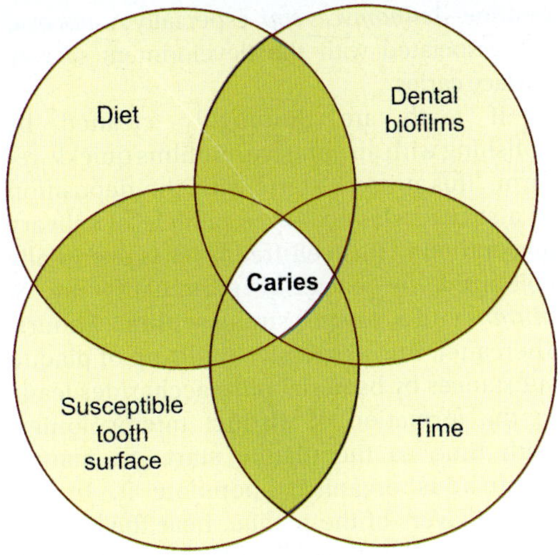

Fig. 2.3: The interplay of major etiologic factors in dental caries (all four factors must act together for dental caries to occur)

Cariogenic bacteria are acidogenic and produce a pH low enough (usually pH less than 5) to decalcify tooth substance. They must possess attachment mechanisms for firm adhesion to smooth tooth surfaces and be able to produce adhesive, insoluble plaque polysaccharides (glucans). Glucans are mostly used as a major bacterial food source.

Present evidence indicates that the viridans streptococci are essential for the development of caries. This group includes different species of streptococci such as *Streptococcus mutans, S. sanguis, S. sobrinus, S. salivarius* and *S. mitior*.

In persons with high caries activity, due to high dietary sucrose intake *S. mutans* strains predominate in the dental plaque. *Streptococcus mutans* produce lactic acid from sucrose and lives at a pH as low as 4.2. It forms large amounts of extracellular, sticky and insoluble glucan plaque matrix. Further *S. mutans* adheres to the pellicle and contributes to the biofilm formation. Other bacteria including lactobacilli and other strains of streptococci are only weakly cariogenic or noncariogenic despite being able to produce acid. It is believed that lactobacilli are more involved in the progression of the deep enamel carious lesion rather than in its initiation. They are also pioneer organisms in the advancing caries front, especially in the dentine. *Actinomyces spp.* especially *A. viscosus* are associated with the development of root surface caries.

If teeth are thoroughly cleaned by polishing with an abrasive, biofilms quickly reform. This process starts with the deposition of a structureless cell-free pellicle of salivary glycoprotein. This cell-free layer is eventually colonized by bacteria, particularly by *S. mutans* and *S. sanguis* strains within 24 hours. Thereafter, the progressive build-up of plaque substances by bacterial polysaccharides leads to the formation of distinct microcolonies. With time as the plaque starts to mature filamentous organisms populate it. In the deeper layers of the plaque, near the enamel surface, a low plaque pH is continually maintained. This low pH is responsible for the demineralization of the tooth enamel surface.

CARIES OF ENAMEL

Basic Enamel Structure

Mature enamel is highly mineralized consisting of approximately 96 percent mineral and 4 percent organic material and water. The inorganic component of enamel is a crystalline calcium phosphate (hydroxyapatite). Ions such as strontium, Mg, Pb and fluoride if present during enamel formation may be incorporated into the crystals. Enamel varies in color from light yellow to gray white and varies in thickness from 2.5 mm over the working surface to a knife edge at the cervical line. When demineralized sections are examined, an empty space can be seen in the area previously occupied by enamel. The main organizational units are the enamel rods (prisms) and interrod enamel (interprismatic substance). The rods are 60 to 70 nm wide and 25 to 30 nm in thickness. It is believed that the length of the crystals actually spans the entire thickness of the enamel layer. The relationship of the enamel rod and the interred enamel has been shown by scanning electron microscopy and transmission electron microscopy. In longitudinal ground sections, a series of dark lines extending from the dentinoenamel junction towards the tooth surface are seen and these are called the striae of retzius.

Macroscopic Features

Pit and Fissure Caries

Pit and fissure caries develops in the occlusal surfaces of molars and premolars, on the buccal surface of molars and on the palatal surfaces of maxillary incisors. Occlusal fissures are deep invaginations of enamel. These fissures are diverse in shape and have been described as broad or narrow funnels, constricted hourglasses, multiple invaginations with inverted Y shaped divisions and also with irregular shapes. Pits and fissures affected by early caries may appear stained brown or black and will feel slightly soft and 'catch' a fine dental probe point. Caries usually develops in the wall of the fissure on both sides, rather than at the base of the fissure. The lesion is described as cone-shaped with the base directed towards the dentine and the apex towards the enamel surface.

Smooth Surface Caries (Interproximal Caries)

Smooth surface caries develops on the proximal surfaces of the teeth or on the gingival one-third of the buccal surface of molars. This is also called cervical caries.

Interproximal caries begins just below the tooth contact area and appears in the early stage as a faint white, kidney shaped opacity of the enamel without apparent loss of continuity of the enamel surface. This is referred to as a white spot lesion.

Microscopic Features

Evidence supports the concept that in its early stages caries causes minimal damage to the outer smooth surface of the enamel but considerable demineralization occurs below the surface. The histopathological features of the typical smooth surface lesion, in enamel as seen in ground sections mounted in Canada Balsam (**Fig. 2.4**), consists of four clearly distinguishable zones. Commencing from the inner advancing front of the lesion, these are:

1. Translucent zone
2. The dark zone which separates

3. The body of the lesion from the translucent zone
4. The surface zone (layer), which remains relatively unaffected except for some demineralization (**Figs 2.4 to 2.7**). There is no sudden changes from zone to zone but rather a gradual series of changes within the lesion. Under polarizing light microscopy (**Fig. 2.5**) it has been shown that the appearance of these four zones together with the normal enamel depend on minute spaces within the tissue.

The translucent zone lies deep to the dark zone, separating it from the normal enamel

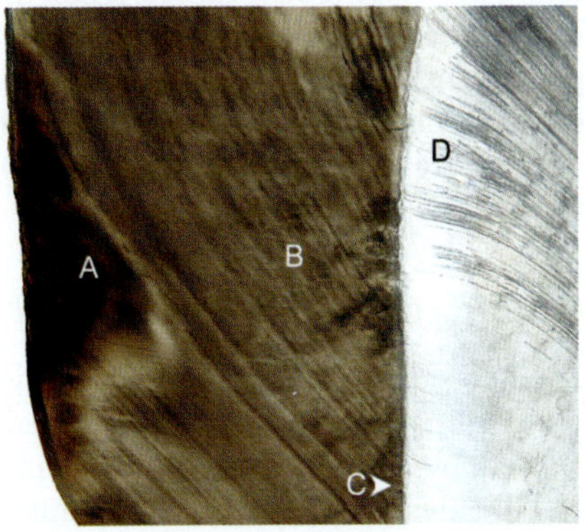

Fig. 2.4: Carious lesion of interproximal enamel before break down of the enamel surface. A. the carious lesion, B. normal enamel, C. amelodentinal junction and D. normal dentine. Ground longitudinal section, 100 μm thick, photographed in transmitted light microscopy, mounted in balsam. (Magnification X 75)

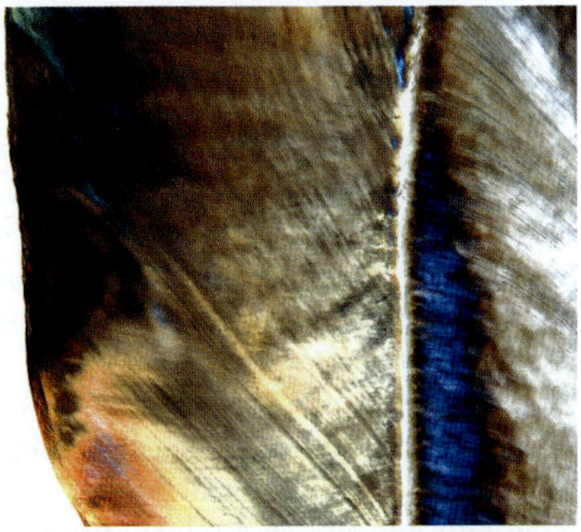

Fig. 2.5: The same ground section shown in Figure 2.4 viewed by polarized light mounted in balsam. The body of the lesion and the intact surface layer are seen. The translucent zone and the dark zone are not clearly seen

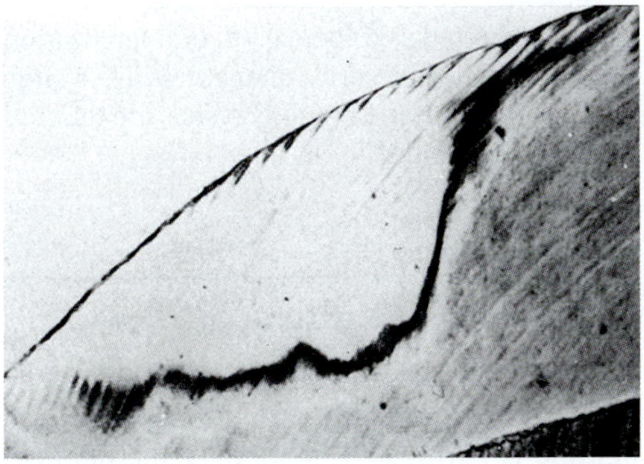

Fig. 2.6: Early interproximal carious lesion of enamel. Ground longitudinal section, 75 μm thick, photographed in quinoline RI-1.62 and viewed by polarized light. (Magnification X 75) (*Courtesy:* Late Professor AI Darling, University of Bristol, England)

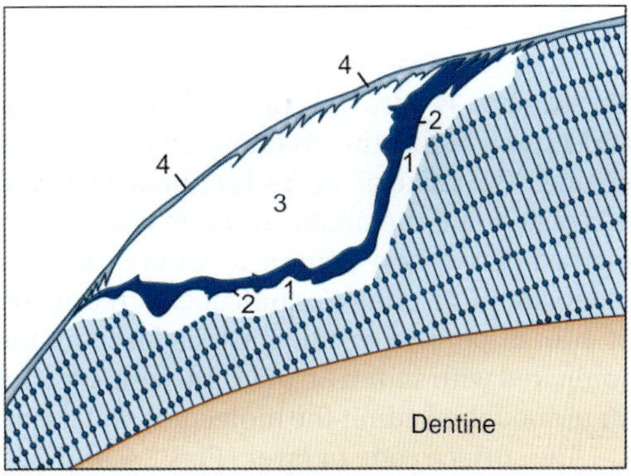

Fig. 2.7: Diagrammatic representation of the early interproximal carious lesion (smooth surface carious lesion) of enamel, shown in Figure 2.6, demonstrating the four major zones. From deeper down, the normal enamel is shaded blue. (1) the translucent zone; (2) the dark zone; (3) the body of the lesion and (4) the surface zone (layer) with slight demineralization

(**Figs 2.6 and 2.7**). The translucent zone and dark zone are best seen in quinoline viewed by polarized light microscopy. In the translucent zone, the normal structural appearances of the enamel are lost. The interprismatic markings, the striae of retzius and the cross striations of the prisms are absent or less conspicuous. The formation of the translucent zone appears to be the earliest change in enamel at the advancing front of the lesion. The translucent zone is characterized by approximately 1 to 2 percent loss of mineral. In normal enamel, adjacent to the translucent zone, the spaces are a few in number, comprising probably less than 0.5 percent of its total volume. The translucent zone is broader in progressive active caries and is narrow or absent in arrested or remineralized lesions.

The dark zone (**Figs 2.6 and 2.7**) is found as a band on the deep aspect of the body of the lesion and superficial to the translucent zone and appears as a dense, brown, opaque zone in which a little structure can be seen. It shows positive birefringence in polarized light whereas normal enamel has a negative intrinsic birefringence relative to the prism direction. The dark zone stretches over the whole aspect of the body of the lesion and appears to spread back into the surface zone along the striae of retzius. An average reduction of 2 to 4 percent of mineral per unit volume has been reported for enamel sampled from the dark zone.

The body of the lesion (**Figs 2.6 and 2.7**), the largest zone, is positively birefringent (**Fig. 2.5**) and extends from the enamel surface into the enamel. The striae of retzius is enhanced within this region and the prism structure is also well-marked, showing a pattern of cross striations. Microchemical analysis indicates a reduction of 4 to 25 percent in mineral per unit volume compared with sound enamel. These spaces are large enough to admit the molecules of Balsam.

The surface zone or layer (**Figs 2.6 and 2.7**) ranges between 20 and 100 μm in thickness and appears relatively unaffected in the initial lesion as compared with the subsurface zones. The surface zone has 1 percent mineral loss. Like normal enamel the surface zone retains a negative birefringence in polarized light. In microradiographs, the surface zone is radiopaque and is sharply demarcated from the underlying radiolucent areas. By scanning electron microscopic observations, minute pathways have been shown in the surface layer.

The organic structures found at the amelodentinal junction, the enamel lamellae and the enamel tufts may play some part in the spread of the carious process but their significance is less than has been thought earlier. When the carious lesion reaches the amelodentinal junction, prominent lateral spread of caries occurs, thereby undermining the enamel (**Figs 2.10 and 2.11**).

The features of these four zones are summarized in **Table 2.1**.

Ultrastructural Changes in Enamel

The first change found in enamel, based upon nondemineralized sections of caries of enamel viewed by transmission electron microscopy, is the destruction of the apatite crystals, both within the enamel prisms as well as the interprismatic substance. The progressive dissolution of the apatite crystals results in a broadening of the intercrystalline spaces so that small gaps appear. These gaps become filled with an amorphous material. Some of this amorphous material gives a positive histochemical reaction to carbohydrates.

Peripheral arcade like defects can be seen in a transverse section (**Fig. 2.8**) between rows of crystals. The crystals at the prism junction appear larger and more electron dense (**Fig. 2.9**). This has been interpreted as evidence for remineralization taking place during caries of enamel. These large and rhombohedral, irregular crystals are referred to as 'caries crystals.'

CARIES OF DENTINE

Basic Dentine Structure

When dentine is viewed microscopically several structural features can be identified. The dentine is permeated by tubules, the dentinal tubules, that traverse from the pulpal surface to the amelodentinal and cementodentinal junctions. In transverse sections, the tubules are approximately circular although their appearance is dependent on the plane in which

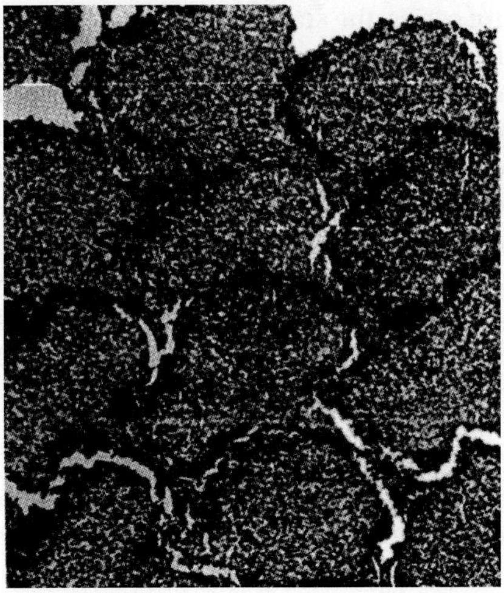

Fig. 2.8: Early caries in enamel. Slight gaps have developed between rows of crystals. Transmission electron microscopy, original magnification X 6500 (*Courtesy:* DB Scott and Quintessence Publishing Co. Inc,1989)

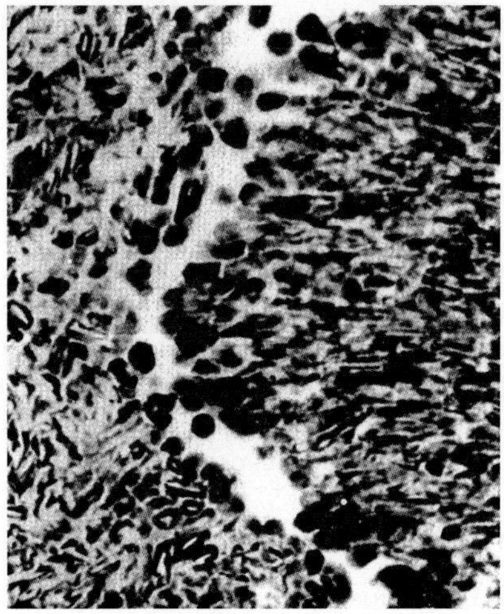

Fig. 2.9: Early caries in enamel. Higher magnification of the junction between prisms showing a cleft bordered by lager crystals. Transmission electron microscopy, original magnification X 30,000 (*Courtesy:* DB Scott and Quintessence Publishing Co. Inc, 1989)

▪ Table 2.1
Pathology of dental caries of enamel—a summary

Zone	*Features*
Translucent zone	The earliest change seen in enamel caries Seen at the advancing front of the carious attack Normal structural appearance of enamel is lost in this zone 1–2% mineral loss Best viewed in quinoline under polarized light
Dark zone	Narrow in advancing lesion Broader in arrested or remineralized lesions 2–4% mineral loss seen Best viewed in quinoline under polarized light
Body of the lesion	Broader in progressing caries Broad body of the lesion in arrested or remineralized lesions 4–25% mineral loss seen The striae of retzius is enhanced in the body of the lesion
Surface zone (layer)	A zone of remineralization 20–100 μm thick 1 percent mineral loss seen Radiopaque in microradiography

the tissue is sectioned. The dentine between the tubules is termed intertubular dentine.

The dentinal tubules are tapered structures measuring approximately 2.5 μm in diameter near the pulp, 1.2 μm in the midportion of the dentine and 900 nm in diameter near the amelodentinal junction. Their number range from 59000 tubules per square millimeter at the coronal surface of the tooth to about 76000 tubules per square millimeter at the pulpal surface. The dentinal tubules branch and these branches anastomose giving the dentine a high degree of permeability.

Macroscopic Features

The caries in dentine could be classified into acute, i.e. rapidly progressive and arrested (chronic or slow) caries. The acute caries, commonly seen in young individuals is soft to the probe and yellowish in color. The chronic caries, usually seen in adults is harder to the probe and brownish-black in color.

Microscopic Features

When the occlusal carious process in the enamel reaches the amelodentinal junction, the caries spreads laterally (**Fig. 2.10**) due to the increased amounts of organic material at the enamel tufts and enamel lamellae present in this region. As a result of this spread, the enamel becomes undermined (**Fig. 2.11**). This is the reason why the enamel crumbles during cavity preparation due to the lack of underlying dentine support. Both in smooth surface caries and pit, and fissure caries, the superficial dentine is involved before the breakdown of the enamel surface.

In ground sections, these affected dentine areas would appear slightly more translucent if the occlusal carious process has progressed slowly. In early enamel caries, the translucent zone is formed almost at the amelodentinal junction in the region of the mantle dentine. With progressive spread of caries the translucent zone spreads to the outer and inner circumpulpal dentine and surrounds the area of carious demineralization in the dentine along the sides and the floor of the cavity (**Fig. 2.10**). This translucent zone is an area seen in the dentine all round the lesion as if it were trying to localize the carious attack. When ground sections are prepared from this area for optical microscopy, the organic constituents of tubules are destroyed and only the mineral components remain. This reactive translucent zone, when examined in air, by transmitted light microscopy, appears bright or translucent, while in reflected light, it appears dark. The extent and the degree of translucency vary with the size and position of the carious lesion (**Fig. 2.10**).

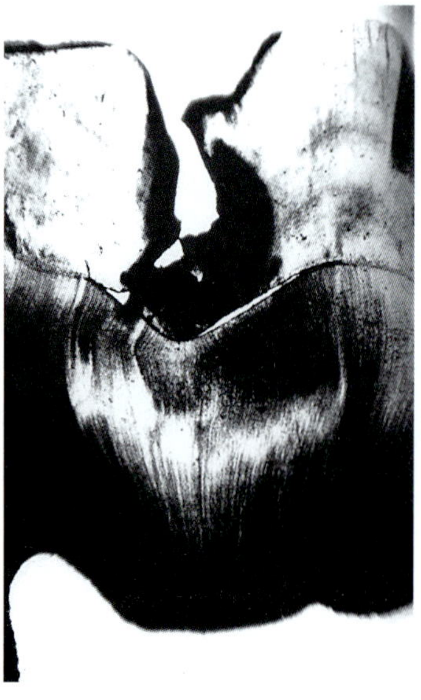

Fig. 2.10: Ground longitudinal section, 75 µm thick, of an early occlusal enamel pit and fissure carious lesion showing the translucent zone reaction in dentine. Photographed by transmitted light microscopy in air. The adjacent tubules appear opaque Magnification X 30

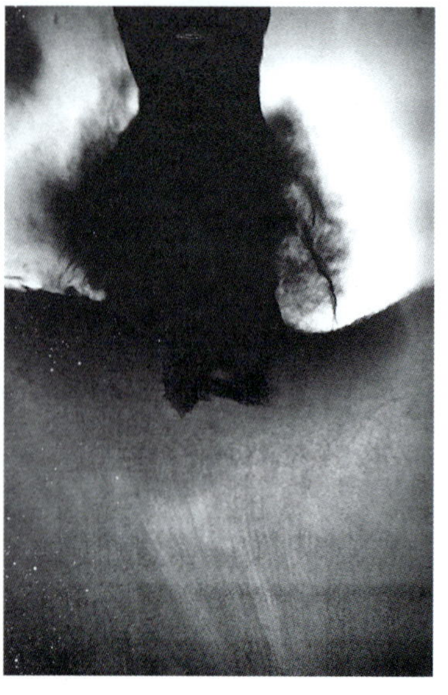

Fig. 2.11: Microradiographic appearance of the tubules in the translucent zone in longitudinal section in Figure 2.10. The area representing the translucent zone shows increased radiopacity and this radiopacity seems to spread towards the pulp. Magnification X 30; exposure 20 kV, 30 mA using 649-0 plates

Demineralized sections of dentine fail to show the translucent zone because the calcium salts have been removed from the tissue during specimen preparation. Thus, the translucent zone and the normal dentine will appear similar and no conclusions can be made about this zone.

The evidence for the increased mineral content in the translucent zone is supported by the use of polarized light microscopy, where it appears as a zone of intense negative birefringence due to the mainly inorganic framework. With advancing demineralization, this zone is removed and the positive fiber birefringence of the underlying collagen matrix occurs.

By far, microradiography remains the best method available to determine the presence of mineral salts. In longitudinal sections, the translucent zone is hypercalcified and radiopaque as shown in **Figure 2.11**. It is also known that the area of radiopacity so obtained, corresponds to the distribution of the translucent zone as seen in ground sections examined using transmitted light microscopy. After examining transversely cut tubules in the region of the translucent zone by microradiography, it has been shown that this hypercalcification is confined to the lumen of the tubules.

Observations made of the undemineralized translucent zone under transmission electron microscopy have shown that the tubules are completely closed in this region by mineralized material. The mineral salts were more densely packed within the tubules than in the intertubular dentine.

From all this laboratory evidence and indeed from clinical experience of arrested caries, it can be appreciated that the translucent zone is calcified and the increase in calcification is confined to the dentinal tubules in this region.

In the interproximal carious lesion, as opposed to the occlusal carious lesion, the most common reaction is the production of dead tracts. This dead tract follows the tubules that are affected and terminate in the pulp chamber in a knob of reparative dentine. A lateral translucent zone reaction is evident on either side parallel to the dead tract. The optical properties of the translucent zone are similar to those described for the translucent zone of occlusal dental caries.

As the carious lesion progresses, the dentine becomes increasingly stained with a yellow to brown discoloration together with the partial demineralization of the dentine which precedes invasion of microorganisms into the dentinal tubules. It has been shown that the extent of this demineralization is always greater than the area of altered dentine seen in histological preparations. The appearance of carious destruction of dentine is shown in **Figure 2.12**, by hematoxylin and eosin staining and in **Figure 2.13** by periodic acid-Schiff (PAS) staining. Under higher magnification, the bacterial plaque, attached tightly on the dentine surface, can be seen together with microorganisms

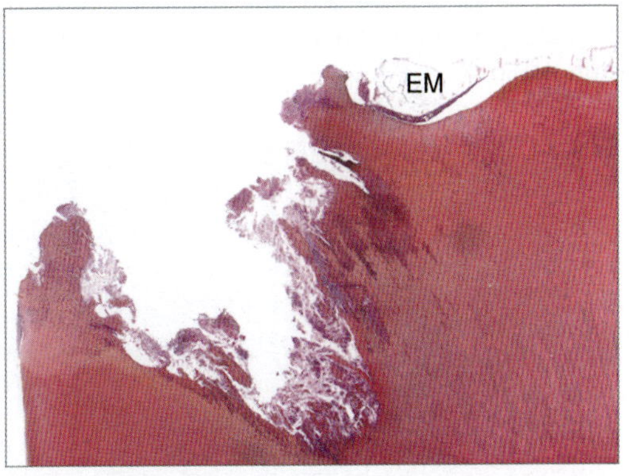

Fig. 2.12: Carious destruction of dentine. Hematoxylin and eosin stained section to show the enamel matrix (EM) and cavitation in the dentine, magnification X 20

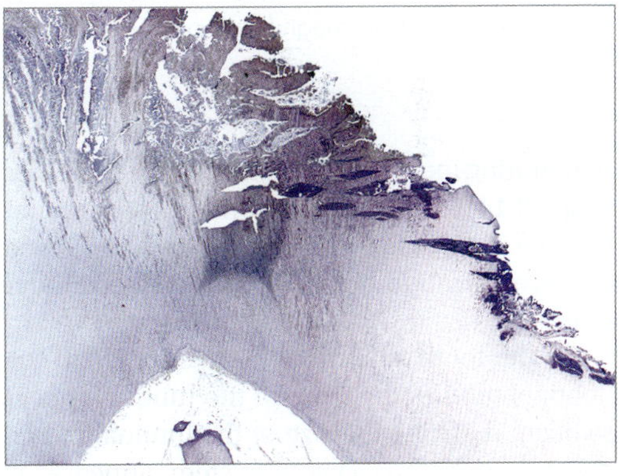

Fig. 2.13: Caries in dentine with transverse cleft formation. These clefts are filled with bacteria and occur at right angles to the tubules. Periodic acid-Schiff staining magnification X 20

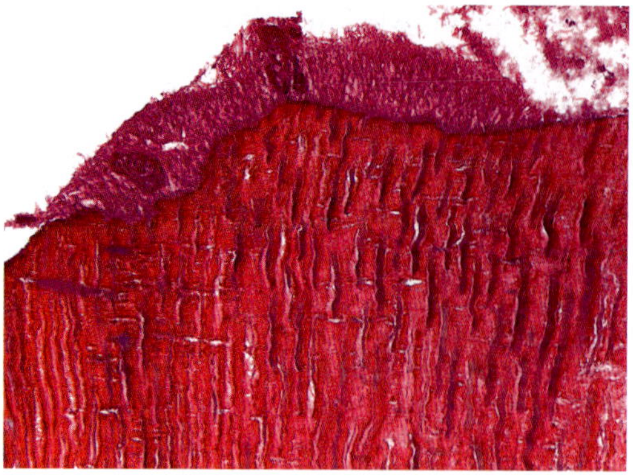

Fig. 2.14: Caries of dentine with bacterial plaque (biofilm), attached tightly on the dentine surface and organisms invading the dentinal tubules. Hematoxylin and eosin stained section magnification X 180

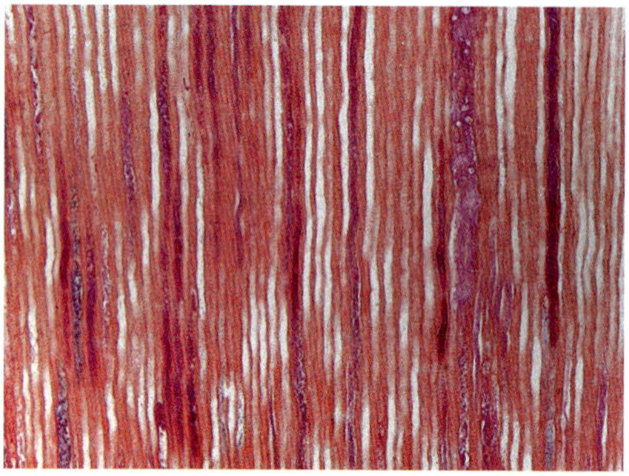

Fig. 2.15: Microorganisms penetrating deeper down inside the dentinal tubules. Hematoxylin and eosin stained section magnification X 180

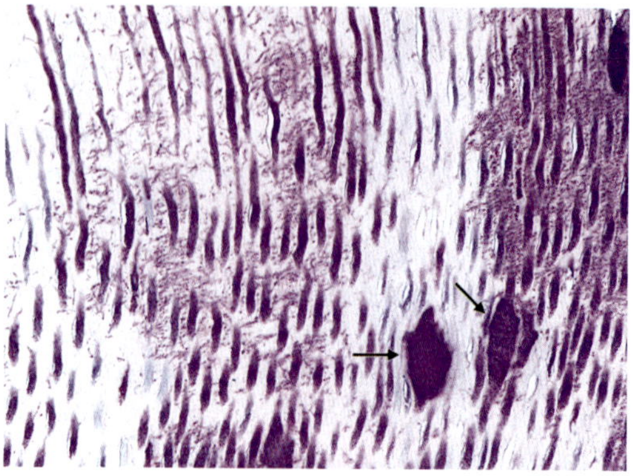

Fig. 2.16: Microorganisms penetrating dentine. Periodic acid-Schiff stain showing two varicosities (arrows) magnification X 180

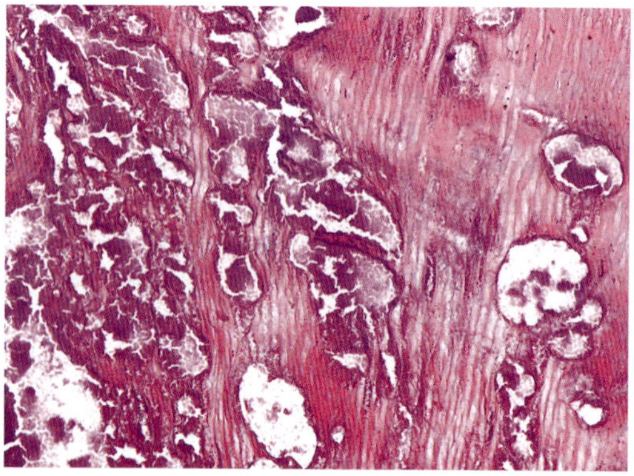

Fig. 2.17: Further advanced caries in dentine under higher magnification showing tubules packed with bacteria causing displacement of adjacent tubules with bending of the tubules. Hematoxylin and eosin stained section magnification X 140

penetrating into and within the dentinal tubules (**Fig. 2.14**). The dissolution of peritubular dentine seems to occur first and this is followed by decalcification and lysis of the intertubular matrix.

If the tooth is sectioned transversely to the dentinal tubules the walls of the tubules appear swollen, reducing the size of the lumina and an effect described as 'clay pipe stem' appears. As microorganisms penetrate further, the dentine becomes decalcified and also stained with a brownish color. The bacterial proliferation through the tubules can be seen in longitudinal sections. The bacteria grow within the tubules forming colonies that cause distension of the tubules (**Figs 2.14 to 2.16 and 2.36**). The distensions give the tubules a ballooned or dilated appearance variously described as beading, varicosities, moth-eaten pattern or rosary pattern (**Figs 2.16 and 2.17**). In a transverse section of the tubules, some tubules contain no bacteria. In older literature these areas have been called 'liquefaction-foci'. This terminology is incorrect

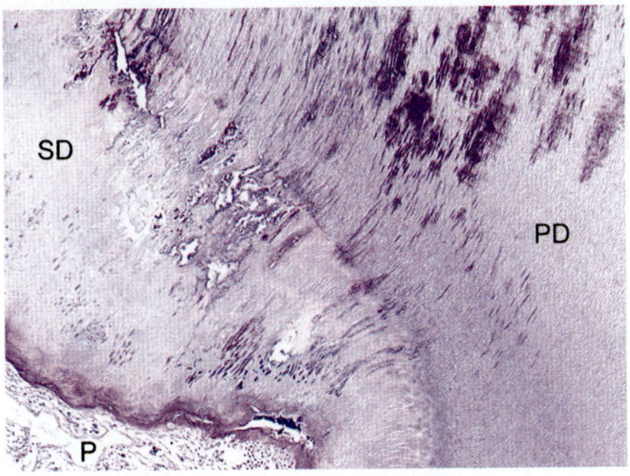

Fig. 2.18: Carious destruction of the secondary dentine. PD: Primary dentine; SD: Secondary dentine; P: Pulp tissue periodic acid-Schiff staining, magnification X 20

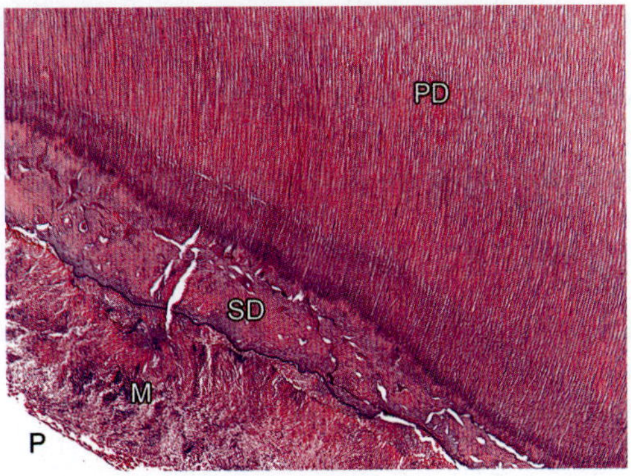

Fig. 2.19: Carious destruction of secondary dentine. PD: Primary dentine with no caries of dentine; SD: Secondary dentine; P: Pulp chamber. M: Plaque (biofilm) build up within the pulp chamber and producing caries of secondary dentine from the pulpal aspect. Hematoxylin and eosin stained section, magnification X 20

as there is no liquid inside these areas but only bacteria and tissue debris.

These distensions cause displacement of adjacent tubules (**Fig. 2.17 and Fig. 2.37**). As the walls of the tubules near these distensions are broken down by bacterial action, the tubules burst into the surrounding intertubular dentine and the microorganisms proceed to proteolyze this area. In these areas clefts are found running at right angles to the tubules (**Figs 2.13, 2.17 and 2.37**) and they are referred to as transverse clefts. Some researches feel that the cleavages follow the contour of Lines of Owen. It is not known whether these clefts occur naturally or are artifacts but they run parallel to the general direction of the collagen fibers of the organic matrix. With further breakdown of the enamel and cavitation, together with further access to microorganisms and food debris, the dentine becomes completely destroyed. The cleavages which contain bacteria, necrotic masses and debris coalesce, thereby creating a clinical defect in the dentine.

When the carious process reaches the secondary dentine or reparative dentine, there is bacterial penetration of this tissue and carious destruction of the secondary dentine can be seen (**Fig. 2.18**). If microorganisms enter the pulp the carious process can reach the secondary dentine through the pulpal aspect too, as shown in **Figure 2.19**.

CARIES OF CEMENTUM OR ROOT SURFACE CARIES

Basic Cementum Structure

The cementum immediately adjacent to the root dentine is called primary cementum or acellular cementum and extends from the cervical margin of the tooth to the apical area. Its primary function is to anchor the tooth to the bone via the periodontal ligament. From the middle towards the apical third of the root and in the root bifurcation area there is also the secondary cementum or cellular cementum. This cementum has the main function of adaptation and repair, with cellular cementum increasing in teeth with age and in various other pathological situations. The cells in cellular cementum are called cementocytes.

Macroscopic Features

Caries of cementum usually occurs in older persons who suffer from gingival recession. This gingival recession may be due partially to age but mainly to the presence of chronic inflammatory periodontal disease. As a result, the cemento-enamel junction is exposed.

The carious process begins at the primary cementum with the formation of several small discolored areas to extensive yellowish brown zones on the surface of the cementum along the cementoenamel junction. These lesions may coalesce and spread over the surface. Microbial plaques may be adherent to the defective zone. The surface then becomes soft on probing with a leatherly texture. These lesions may or may not be cavitated. In arrested (inactive) root surface lesions, the surface is shiny in appearance and is smooth and hard on probing with a yellowish to brown or black discoloration.

Microscopic Features

In active root surface carious lesions, sectioned in longitudinal section as shown in the illustrations, there would be an active bacterial plaque on the surface of the cementum layer (**Figs 2.20 to 2.22**). Cementum would show gradual destruction with the loss of the surface layer. Pieces of cementum would fracture either horizontally (**Fig. 2.20**) or parallel to the incremental lines (**Fig. 2.21**). Clefts would appear in the cementum (**Fig. 2.22**). Microorganisms appear to invade the cementum either along calcified Sharpey's fibers or between the bundles of fibers, pausing at the

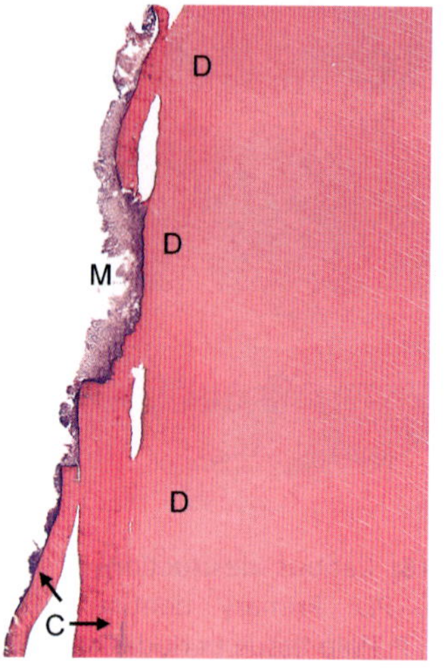

Fig. 2.21: Caries of cementum showing stepwise destruction of cementum (C) along incremental lines. The section also shows lifting away of bacterial plaque (M) covered cementum from the dentine surface (D). Hematoxylin and eosin stained, magnification X 180

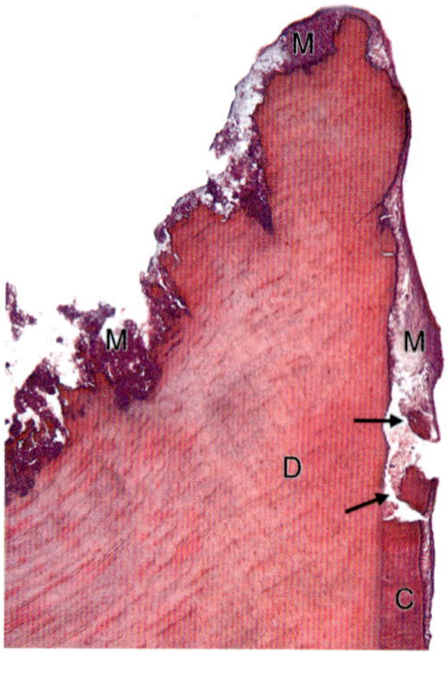

Fig. 2.20: Caries of cementum. Photomicrograph of a decalcified section showing caries of dentine (D) and cementum (C) with bacterial plaque (M) on the cementum surface and dentine surface. Pieces of cementum have separated off due to the carious attack (arrows). Hematoxylin and eosin stained, magnification X 180

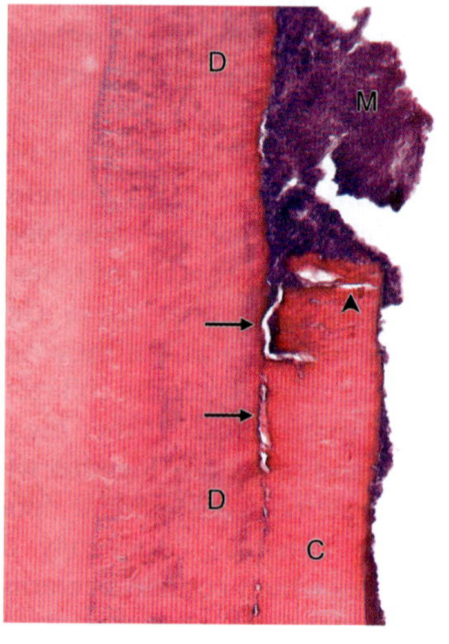

Fig. 2.22: Caries of cementum. Photomicrograph of a decalcified section showing exposed dentine (D) covered by a layer of microorganisms (M) and the fracture of cementum (C) arrowhead. Microorganisms seem to spread between the cementum and the dentine (arrows).

Note: There is no evidence of bacterial penetration into the peripheral dentine. Hematoxylin and eosin stained, magnification X 180

incremental lines and at times spreading along them. Since cementum is formed in concentric layers and presents a lamellated appearance, the microorganisms tend to spread laterally between the various layers. When secondary cementum is involved the pattern becomes less regular.

After decalcification of the cementum, proteolysis of the remaining matrix occurs similar to the process in dentine with the ultimate destruction of the tissue.

RESPONSE OF THE PULPODENTINAL COMPLEX TO CARIES PROGRESSION

In this chapter, caries of enamel and caries of dentine are described separately. This is explainable, as the two tissues differ markedly from each other, both in their development and structure. The enamel is developed from the ectodermal component of the tooth germ while the pulpodentinal complex is derived from the mesodermal component. The enamel has no cells and blood vessels and cannot respond to injuries while the dentine and the odontoblasts are integral components of the pulpodentinal complex with specific defense reactions to external stimulation. Any stimulus which affects the dentine would give rise to a defense reaction in the pulpodentinal complex.

The most common defense reaction by the pulpodentinal complex to caries progression is tubular sclerosis which is a deposition of mineral within the dentinal tubules resulting in gradual tubule closure.

In normal life, the tooth in the oral cavity is subjected to bacterial plaque (biofilm) activity and natural routine physiologic processes such as age changes, attrition, reactions to hot and cold, occlusal stress and various other stimulations including dental caries.

Age changes in the dentine occur throughout life, with no obvious microscopic changes seen in the intertubular dentine, but with gradual mineralization of the peritubular dentine with centripetal deposition of peritubular dentine and with gradual tubule obliteration. The biology of the human dentinal tubule in transverse section is shown and explained in **Figure 2.23**. With physiologic attrition and pathologic attrition as a result of bruxism and traumatic occlusion, this process is speeded up resulting in further obliteration of the dentinal tubules. Caries on the other hand, speeds up this process and such affected dentine is seen as sclerotic dentine in the area under the influence of caries and reparative dentine (reactive dentine) under the influence of the dental pulp (**Fig. 2.24**). Further, the speed of the carious process varies greatly in different environments and in different teeth. If the carious process is slow, there is time for effective tubule obliteration and formation of the translucent zone around the lesion by the pulodentinal complex defence mechanisms. The carious attack is being contained within the dentine by the defense mechanisms of the tooth. However, the carious attack is rapid the pulp would be involved early, resulting in a pulpitis.

In order to demonstrate the response of the pulpodentinal complex to caries, dentinal tubules can be studied in ground section preparations of teeth by light microscopy, microradiography and also electron microscopy. Both transverse sections of teeth and longitudinal sections can be used. As explained under caries of dentine, the tubules traverse from the pulp to the amelodentinal junction. These tubules are shown in **Figures 2.25 to 2.27** with ground sections mounted in balsam. Tubule directions in a longitudinal ground section are shown in **Figure 2.25** adjacent to a dead tract. Higher magnification of the area in transmitted light is shown in **Figure 2.26** and the same area under reflected light is shown in **Figure 2.27**. The thickness of the ground section and the mounting technique effect the penetration of balsam into the tubules. Thin balsam penetrates the tissue better.

There are many different types of dentinal tubule morphology as shown by microradiography in **Figure 2.28**. Generally, tubules will have a certain amount of peritubular dentine formed depending from which site in the tooth the section is prepared and also the age of the tooth. At the same level tubules could be seen with no peritubular dentine, while some tubules are open, others are partly open and still others are closed. All these tubules lie adjacent to one another **Figure 2.28**. There could be some tubules with abnormal morphology too. With dental caries and with a slowly progressing carious lesion, peritubular dentinogenesis is accelerated

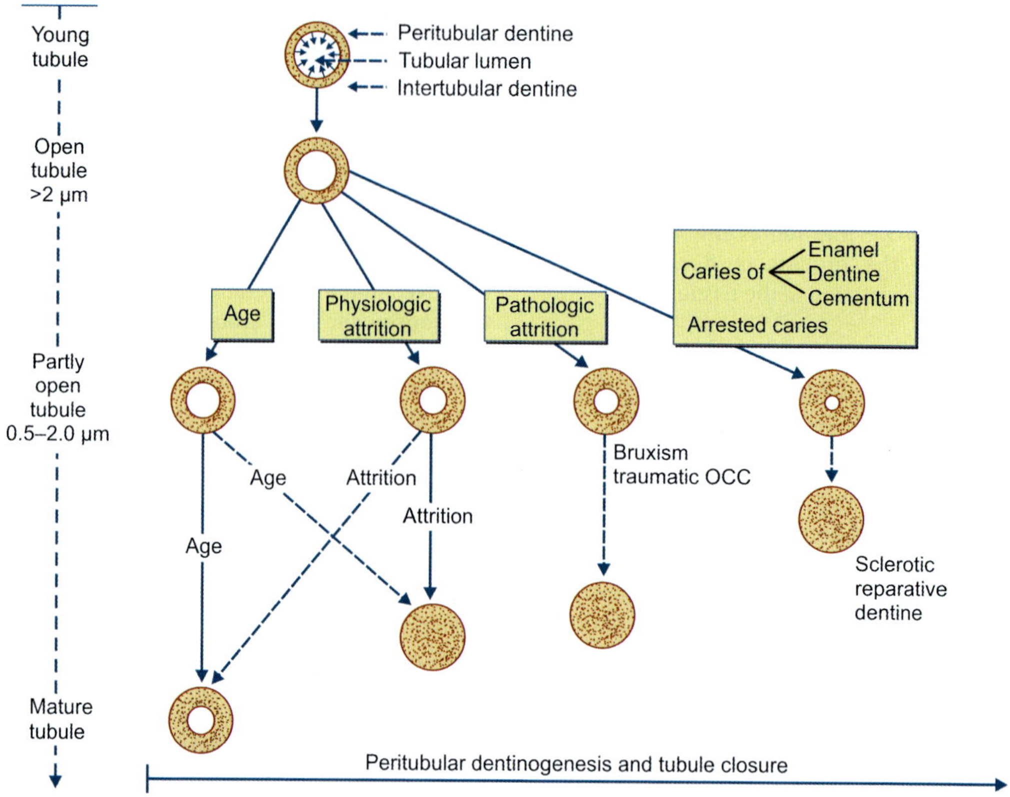

Fig. 2.23: The biology of the human dentinal tubule showing the tubular lumen and peritubular dentinogenesis with age, attrition and caries

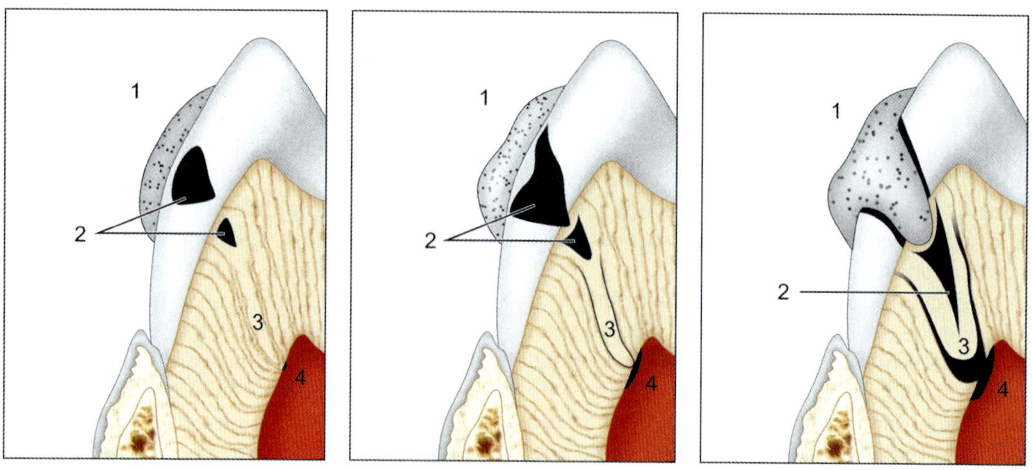

Fig. 2.24: Diagrammatic representation of dentine reaction to progressive caries. (1) bacterial plaque (biofilm), microorganisms penetration, and destruction of enamel and dentine, (2) zone of demineralization, (3) sclerotic reaction or translucent zone trying to localize the lesion and in the pulp (4) reparative dentine (reactive dentine) formation

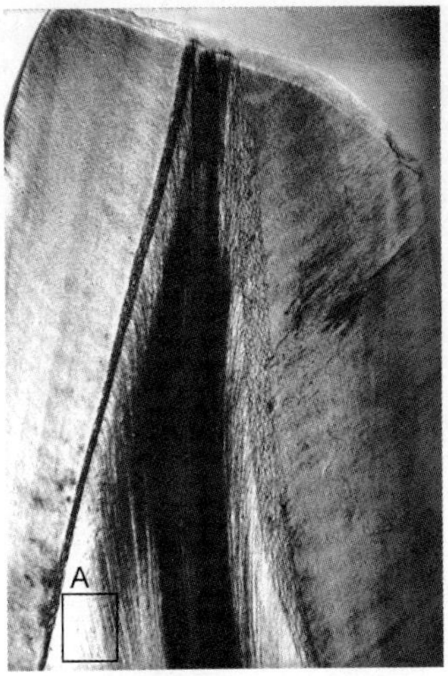

Fig. 2.25: Photomicrograph of dentinal tubules in longitudinal ground section adjacent to a dead tract to show the direction of individual dentinal tubules (Transmitted light in air magnification X 35)

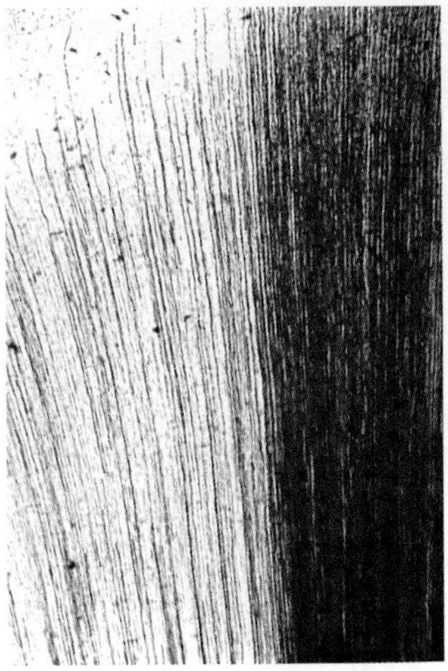

Fig. 2.26: High power view of the area marked (A) in Figure 2.25, in transmitted light to show the dentinal tubules. (Magnification X 80)

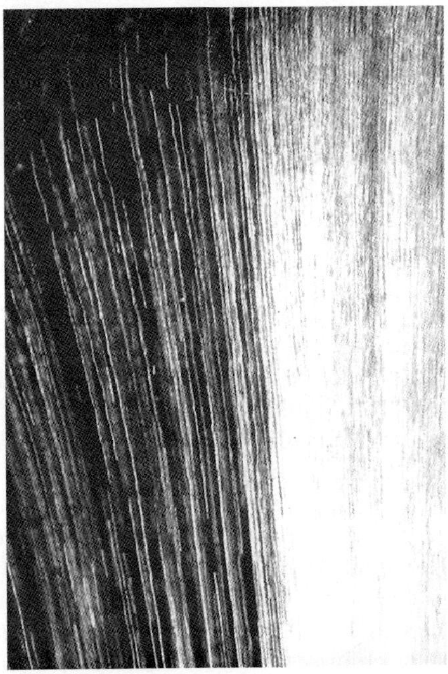

Fig. 2.27: High power view of the area marked (A) in Figure 2.25, in reflected light to show the appearance of the same tubules (Magnification X 80)

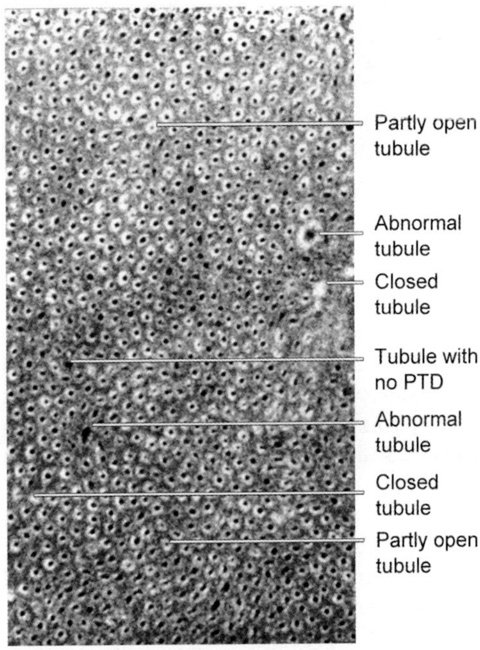

Fig. 2.28: Photomicrograph illustrating the dentinal tubules in transverse section to show variation in tubular morphology (Microradiography specimen. Magnification X 1200)

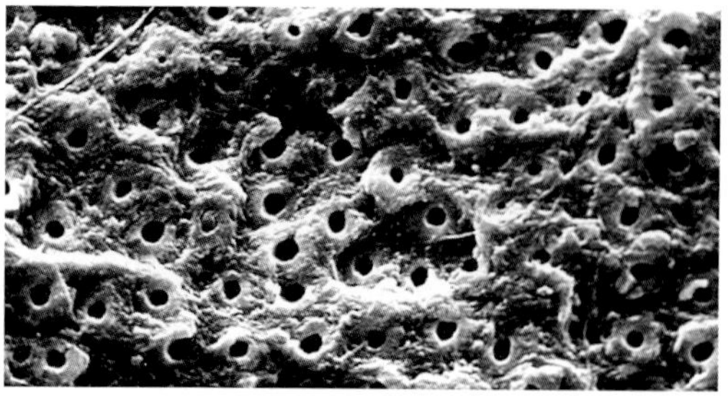

Fig. 2.29: Transverse section of fractured coronal dentine to show the appearance of the dentinal tubules unaffected by caries. Scanning electron microscope photograph. Magnification X 2000

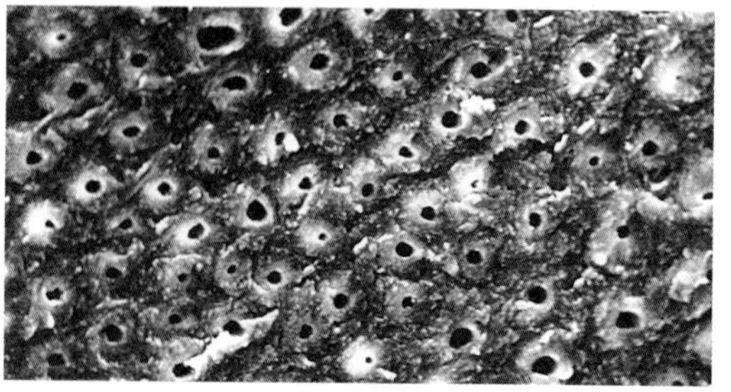

Fig. 2.30: Transverse section of fractured coronal dentine nearer to the carious lesion on the lateral translucent zone to show gradual peritubular dentinogenesis. Scanning electron microscope photograph. Magnification X 2000

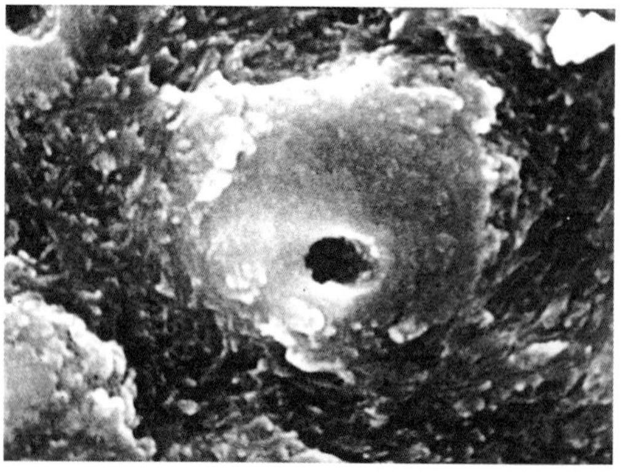

Fig. 2.31: To show one dentinal tubule under higher magnification. Scanning electron microscope photograph. Magnification X 10,000

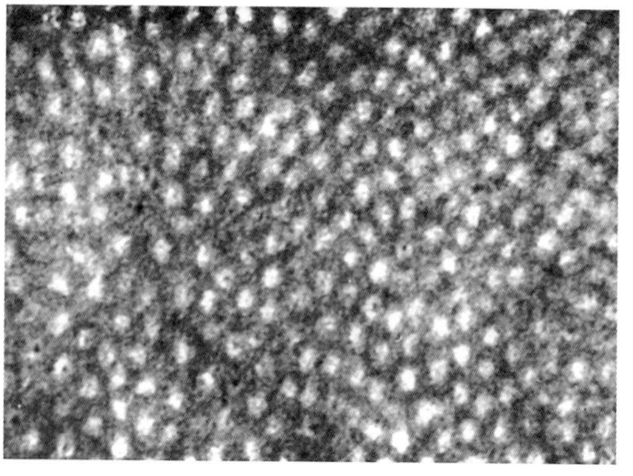

Fig. 2.32: Photomicrograph illustrating the closed dentinal tubules in transverse section. Microradiography specimen. Magnification X 800

as shown by scanning electron microscopy in **Figures 2.29 to 2.31**. In the established translucent zone the tubules are obliterated, shown by microradiography in **Figure 2.32** and in **Figures 2.33 and 2.34** shown by scanning electron microscopy.

Besides peritubular dentinogenesis, in relation to caries of dentine, dentinal tubules could be obliterated with other mineral material and other mineralizing mechanisms.

PATHOPHYSIOLOGIC DYNAMICS OF THE CARIOUS PROCESS

Minerals are exchanged between the superficial enamel surface and the oral environment. The minerals can move from the tooth surface into the saliva and from the saliva into the enamel surface depending on the mineral concentration and the pH at the interface. There are two processes taking place almost simultaneously—demineralization and remineralization.

In demineralization, minerals move out from the enamel surface into the adjacent environment over a long period of time, thus producing the incipient carious lesion or the 'white spot' lesion. This lesion could be reversed under appropriate conditions both in the mouth and in laboratory sections. When large amounts of crystallites are removed the integrity of the structural protein matrix breaks down and the resulting collapse of the matrix results in the production of an irreversible lesion with cavitation. At this stage, restorative dental

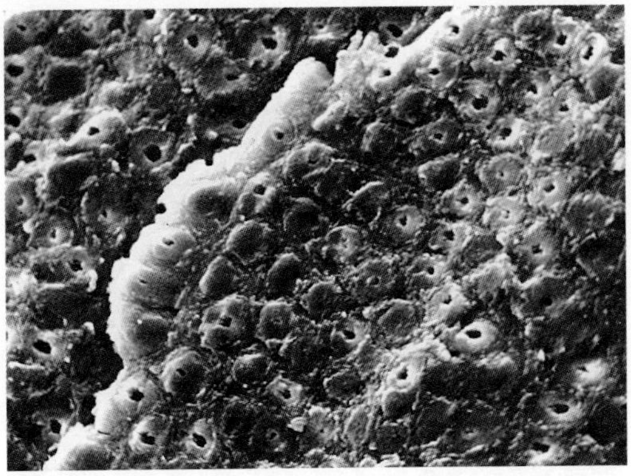

Fig. 2.33: Transverse section of fractured coronal dentine over the lateral translucent zone to show closed dentinal tubules. Scanning electron microscope photograph. Magnification X 2,000

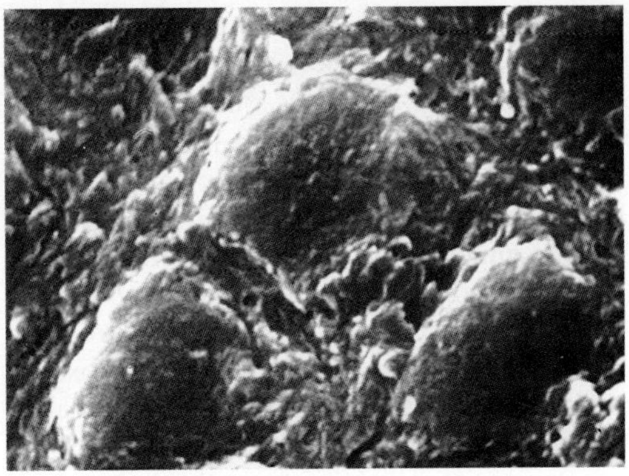

Fig. 2.34: To show a closed dentinal tubule under higher magnification. Scanning electron microscope photograph. Magnification X 10,000

treatment becomes mandatory. Until cavitation occurs minerals are able to ebb and flow, both from the enamel surface into the oral fluids and from the oral fluids into the enamel surface without the production of a clinical cavity. This is what happens in the arrested carious lesion.

In the remineralization phase crystallites are reformed within the microcavities that were created during the demineralization process. The crystallites deposit haphazardly in the deeper cavities and this could be demonstrated as a layer, a few microns in thickness by microscopy. This hypermineralized layer retards the effect of transient caries on the enamel surface. This process can go on simultaneously around different places of the same lesion. Saliva is the source of minerals for the remineralization process. This requires intact, disease free and functional salivary glands. In salivary gland pathology such as xerostomia, rapid and widespread dental caries follows, unless appropriate therapy is given, such as saliva substitutes.

ARREST OF THE CARIOUS LESION

The interstitial carious lesion (white spot) may become arrested when the adjacent tooth is lost and the stagnation area is removed. Dentine caries may be arrested if the carious cavity becomes saucerized and a wide area of dentine becomes exposed. This is usually seen in children's teeth when, by reason of breakdown of the walls of an occlusal cavity, the lesion becomes self-cleansing. Regular tooth brushing would prevent plaque buildup and also somewhat arrest the progress of the lesion. The softened carious dentine is removed by attrition and abrasion, leaving behind a very hard, smooth, usually dark stained and highly polished dentine surface. In such cases the pulp is still vital even though it may have receded. Since this exposed dentine is harder and more mineralized than normal, it could be presumed that these changes occurred by sclerosis or mineralization of the tubules with peritubular dentine. To achieve this, the odontoblasts must remain active. Thus, there must have been a combination of slow advance, small stimuli and efficient pulpodentinal reaction. This has been referred to as eburnation of the dentine.

RAMPANT CARIES

Rampant caries is a widespread, rapidly spreading, destructive type of caries which results in early involvement of the pulp. When the patient presents to an oral health care provider there would be active carious lesions present in almost all teeth including the usually caries resistant canine teeth, both in the maxillary arch and in the mandibular arch. The condition is of rapid onset and usually affects girls in the younger age groups more than boys. Both the deciduous teeth and the permanent teeth are affected.

The initial lesion usually appears on the labial surface of maxillary incisors close to the gingival margin, as a white area of decalcification on the enamel surface soon after eruption. These lesions become pigmented to a light yellow and also extend to the interproximal surfaces. The palatal surfaces, usually caries resistant, may also be involved.

Rampant caries involves the permanent dentition of teenagers because of their frequent intake of cariogenic snacks and sweet drinks between meals. Typical rampant caries in adolescents is characterized by buccal and lingual caries of premolars and molars and interproximal and labial caries in mandibular incisors.

Nursing bottle caries is a form of rampant dental caries in the deciduous dentition of infants and children. This is due to infants falling asleep with a baby bottle filled with sugar containing substances.

A special form of rampant caries may occur in those who have a reduced salivary flow as a result of radiotherapy for the treatment of cancer of the head and neck region. This is called radiation caries. Aplasia of salivary glands also could lead to rampant decay in early ages.

PATHOLOGY OF THE PULP AND PULP REACTION

As a result of deep caries of enamel, caries of dentine and caries of cementum involving the dentine, the pulp becomes inflamed due to bacterial penetration through the dentinal tubules, into the pulp tissue, resulting in a pulpitis (**Figs 2.14 to 2.18**). This pulpitis may be either acute or chronic. In acute pulpitis the painful response may be initiated by hot, cold, sweet and sour stimulae and the patient may sometimes not be in a position to easily localize the tooth. The patient may complain of a severe throbbing pain, at times lancinating in type and the patient may have pain while lying down. In chronic pulpitis there could be spontaneous attacks of dull pain. Chronic pulpitis could also be symptomless till an acute exacerbation

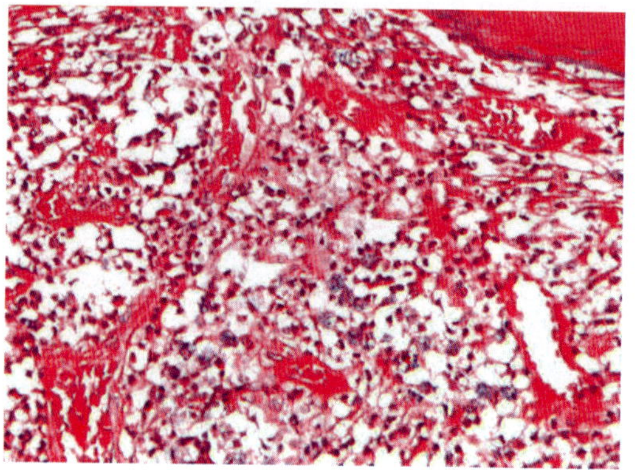

Fig. 2.35: To show pulpal hyperemia. The pulp of the tooth shows diffuse dilated blood vessels, vascular congestion and red blood cells

Note: The focal absence of the odontoblast cell layer on the dentine surface in the upper right part of the illustration. Decalcified section, hematoxylin and eosin stained. Magnification X 170

sets in, triggering off the pain. In order to treat an effected tooth, clinicians tend to divide clinical pulpitis into 'reversible pulpitis' and 'irreversible pulpitis'.

The diagnosis of reversible pulpitis is made when the pain evoked by hot, cold or sweet and sour stimuli are of short duration, about 1 to 2 seconds and which disappears when the stimulus is removed. The underlying pulpal pathology is one of very mild inflammation and pulpal hyperemia (**Fig. 2.35**), which would resolve once the tooth is treated by restorative procedures. If pain occurs suddenly and persists for sometime (several minutes to hours), after removal of the stimulus, a clinical diagnosis of irreversible pulpitis is made. Irreversible pulpitis progresses from reversible pulpitis. The pathology is one of severe inflammation of the dental pulp accompanied by exudation. There is minimal chance of spontaneous recovery. The pain is severe and at times poorly localized. The pain may radiate to the ear, face or neck. Treatment is by either endodontic therapy or extraction of the tooth. It must be appreciated however, that these are only clinical guidelines.

Acute Pulpitis and Pulp Abscess

Acute inflammation of the dental pulp follows either focal reversible pulpitis with pulp

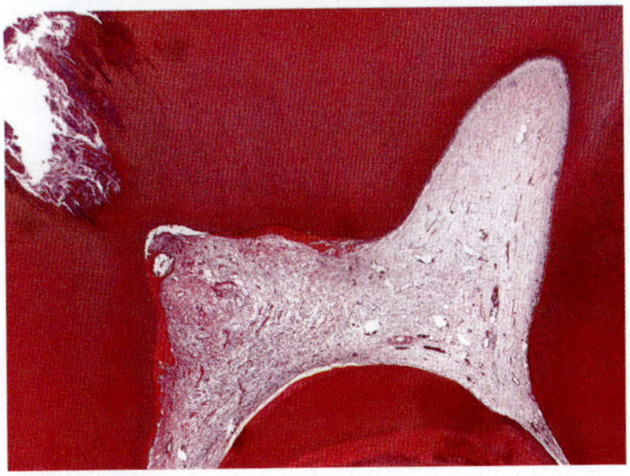

Fig. 2.36: Acute pulpitis in relation to a deep carious lesion in the dentine. Beneath the caries, a dense inflammatory infiltrate is seen. The adjacent pulp cornua is normal (Decalcified section, hematoxylin and eosin stained, magnification X 16)

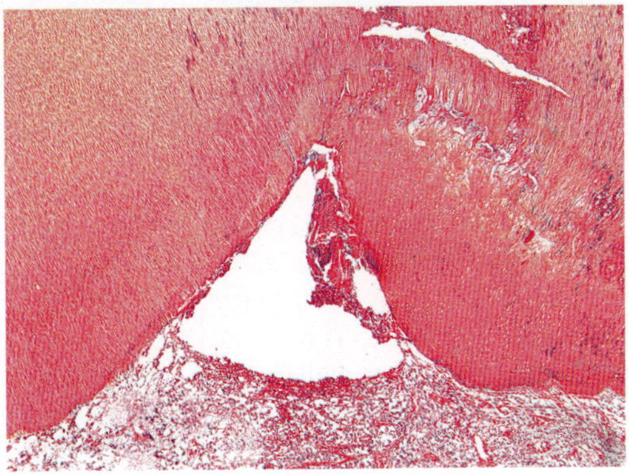

Fig. 2.37: Higher magnification to show details of early pulp abscess formation. A cornual abscess is present, bordered by a pyogenic membrane, containing some tissue debris. Decalcified section, hematoxylin and eosin stained, magnification X 40

hyperemia, or as an acute exacerbation of an already established chronic inflammatory process within the pulp. The pulpitis may be total if it involves the entire pulp and partial if only the pulp adjacent to the pulp cornua (pulp horn) is inflamed (**Figs 2.36 and 2.37**). The pulp tissue becomes inflamed with the dilatation of blood vessel walls, accumulation of edema fluid in the tissues and the accumulation of polymorphonuclear leukocytes (**Fig. 2.37**).

When this happens the odontoblasts in the area are usually destroyed. If the carious process has been slow in progression some reparative dentine would also form below the primary dentine. With the progress of acute pulpitis, there is more localized destruction of pulp tissue, with the formation of a pulp abscess containing pus, bacteria and remnants of tissue digestion (**Fig. 2.37**).

With time, and further progression of the carious process, the entire pulp becomes involved in the inflammatory process. The entire odontoblast layer then gets destroyed and the pulp rapidly disintegrates and becomes necrotic and gangrenous. This is referred to as acute suppurative pulpal necrosis.

Chronic Pulpitis

Chronic pulpitis is characterized by the infiltration of the pulp tissue by chronic inflammatory

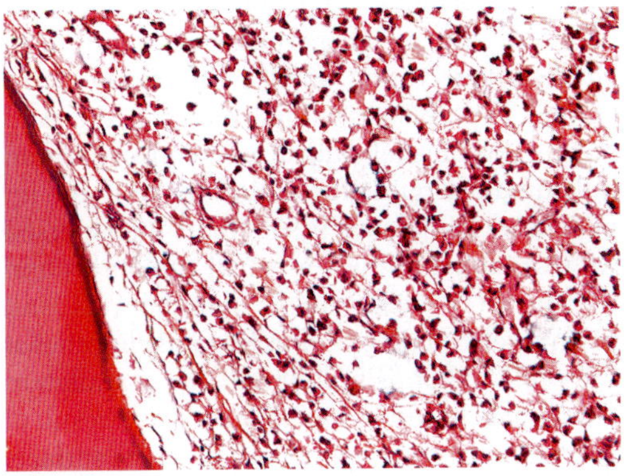

Fig. 2.38: To show generalized chronic pulpitis. The pulp of the tooth shows diffuse involvement by chronic inflammatory cells mainly lymphocytes and plasma cells together with fibrosis
Note: The absence of the odontoblast cell layer. Decalcified section, hematoxylin and eosin stained. Magnification X 170

cells, mainly lymphocytes and plasma cells (**Fig. 2.38**) together with a marked fibrous tissue proliferation.

Chronic Hyperplastic Pulpitis, Pulp Polyp

If there is a connection between the dental pulp and the oral environment through a large carious lesion with pulp exposure, the pulp tissue grows

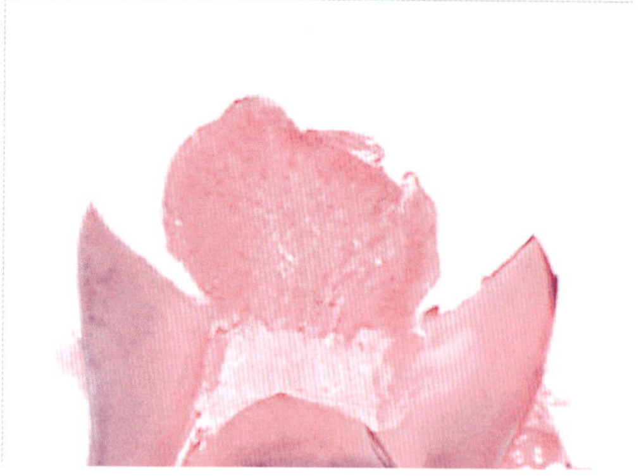

Fig. 2.39: Chronic hyperplastic pulpitis (pulp polyp). A nodule of granulation tissue is covered by epithelium. Decalcified section, hematoxylin and eosin stained. Magnification X 10

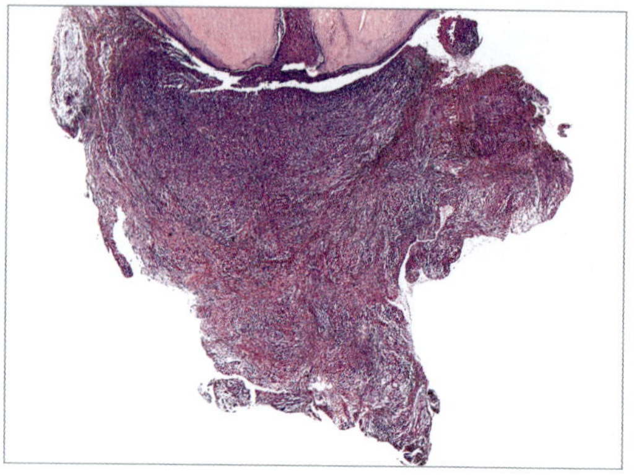

Fig. 2.40: Chronic periapical granuloma. The tissue mass attached to the root of the tooth is composed of granulation tissue. Decalcified section, hematoxylin and eosin stained. Magnification X 10

out into the oral cavity through the exposure. This occurs in the molar teeth, both in the deciduous dentition and in the permanent dentition, in children and young adults. This results in a chronic hyperplastic pulpitis also called a pulp polyp. The normal pulp tissue converts to an inflammatory pulp granulation tissue made up of delicate connective tissue fibers interspersed with variable numbers of small capillaries and inflammatory cells, chiefly lymphocytes and plasma cells. At times, fibroblast and endothelial cell proliferation is prominent. The granulation tissue mass becomes epithelialized as a result of implantation of the epithelial cells on its surface. The epithelium is stratified squamous in type and are desquamated oral mucosal epithelial cells carried to the surface of the growing pulp polyp by saliva. The tissue reaction is an inflammatory hyperplasia (**Fig. 2.39**).

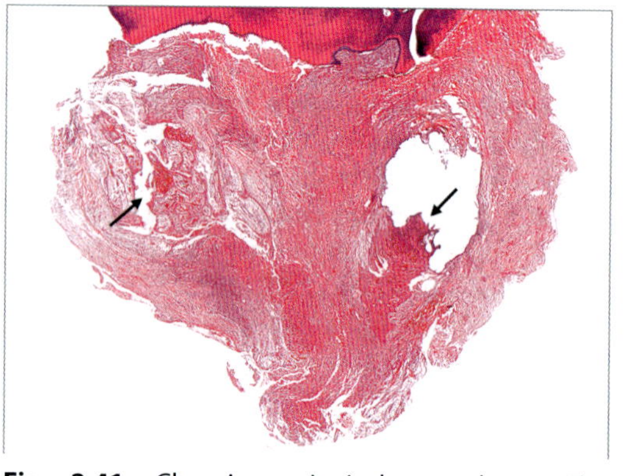

Fig. 2.41: Chronic periapical granuloma. The tissue mass attached to the root of the tooth shows epithelial proliferation within induced by inflammation. This shows an early periapical cyst formation (arrows). Decalcified section, hematoxylin and eosin stained. Magnification X 2

PERIAPICAL INFLAMMATION OF TEETH

Once the pulp becomes necrosed the inflammation spreads to the periapical region of the tooth. An apical periodontitis would develop with the gradual formation of a chronic periapical granuloma (**Figs 2.40 and 2.41**).

It begins as a chronic process from the onset and is associated with a localized sac attached to the root of the tooth containing granulation tissue, lymphocytes and plasma cells. The inflammation induces resorption of the supporting bone adjacent to the granuloma. The granuloma contains proliferating fibroblasts and endothelial cells with the formation of tiny vascular channels in a delicate connective tissue fibrillar matrix. There is abundant infiltration by mononuclear phagocytes. There are also, foam cells and cholesterol clefts. With time, within the granuloma epithelial proliferation takes place (**Fig. 2.41**). This epithelium originates from the epithelial cell rests of Malassez and is seen as sheets of stratified squamous epithelium and as anastomosing cords of epithelium. **Figure 2.41** illustrates the formation of an early radicular (periapical) cyst.

The periapical pathology as a sequel to pulp infection is a common finding. The infection remains localized but occasionally it spreads to the adjacent bone terminating as an acute dentoalveolar abscess which becomes chronic after drainage. Further complications would be the formation of a cyst, its gradual expansion (see Chapter 5), infection and osteomyelitis of the jaw bone (see Chapter 4).

DETECTION AND ASSESSMENT OF DENTAL CARIES

The human tooth is a unique tissue of soft and mineralized tissue coexisting side by side. Enamel is the hardest nonvital calcified tissue in the body. Dentine is the hardest vital tissue and the dental pulp is a connective tissue lined by an odontoblast layer that functions throughout the life of the tooth. As such defense mechanisms are built into the tooth, mainly to the pulp and dentine, in order protect the tooth against dental caries. If the oral environment is reversed by disrupting dental plaque biofilms and by reducing dietary sugars and cariogenic bacteria, the enamel lesions could be reversed and the dentine and pulp protected from carious destruction. In the beginning of this chapter, the serious ravages of carious destruction of tooth enamel, dentine and the cementum was explained. If left unmanaged, the pulp would be infected and the patient would lose the tooth, besides suffering from unnecessary severe pain.

Detection of Dental Caries

Accordingly, the detection of the carious lesion is important. At the chair side, visual methods and visuotactile methods are used. These methods are augmented by radiographic techniques for caries detection.

Dentists often fail to adopt the proper means for detecting early caries formation. Early detection of developing lesions may permit curative rather than restorative procedures to be employed. The group of early lesions clinically undetectable may be in a reversible state. It can be arrested and potentially reversed.

Typically, to evaluate the caries status of a patient, we make a dichotomous decision (absence or presence) based on subjective signals such as color, translucency and hardness using relatively crude instruments such as explorers and radiographs. These methods lack sensitivity. The most recent development, the International Caries Detection and Assessment System (ICDAS), is meant to be a unifying set of predominantly visual criteria that can be used to describe the characteristics of clean, dry teeth at both the enamel and dentinal caries level and to assess caries activity. Studies indicate that ICDAS is repeatable, and has good sensitivity and specificity when compared with polarized light microscopy.

More technologically advanced measures to detect incipient dental caries include quantitative laser or light fluorescence (QLF), electrical conductance measurements (ECM), infrared (IR) laser induced fluorescence, Fiberoptic transillumination (FO-TI) Digital imaging fiberoptic transillumination (DI-FO-TI). Both QLF and the TI methods enable imaging detection of enamel caries that can be digitally stored and viewed later. The QLF method also includes image analysis software which measures the difference in fluorescence between sound and demineralized enamel. Changes in fluorescent radiance and lesion area can be followed over time to measure lesion development.

Transillumination of enamel with near-infra light (NIR) light is a promising technique for the detection and imaging of occlusal and approximal lesions. Application of repeatable, nonionizing radiation of the tooth allows the Transillumination method to be used without restriction to monitor the caries process. The LF method generates a simple numerical index of de- and remineralization in enamel and dentin that can be recorded in the patient's file and monitored over time.

National Institutes of Health (NIH) Consensus Development Conference on Diagnosis and Management of Dental Caries in 2001 and in 2004 concluded that there is an adequate body of evidence supporting the use of fiberoptic transillumination (FOTI) for the detection of interproximal lesions. DIFOTI is a more recent development combining FOTI with a charge-coupled device digital intraoral camera. One *in vitro* study indicated that the method has higher sensitivity than does a radiographic examination for detecting lesions on interproximal, occlusal and smooth surfaces.

Each of these caries detection tools has certain advantages and disadvantages. NIH Consensus Conference (2004) concluded that "the current diagnostic practices are inadequate to achieve the next level of caries management in which noncavitated lesions are identified early so that they can be managed by nonsurgical methods". Therefore, one must evaluate the findings from early caries detection methods carefully before making clinical diagnostic decisions solely on the basis of the test values provided. Not all methods can detect early lesions accurately, and false positive and false negative results may occur. There is also a strong operator influence on the performance of the methods with different operators obtaining different results.

One popular technique currently being researched is the DIAGNOdent device that measures laser fluorescence within the tooth structure. As the incident laser light is propagated into the site, two-way handpiece optics allows the unit to simultaneously quantify the reflected laser light energy. At the specific wavelength that the device operates (655 nm), clean healthy tooth structure exhibits little or no fluorescence, resulting in very low scale readings on the display. Carious tooth structure exhibits fluorescence.

At the current state of development, early caries detection tools such as QLF, ECM, DIAGNOdent, DIFOTI or FOTI should be used as adjuncts to clinical decision making and they serve primarily as supporting tools for making preventive treatment plan decisions in conjunction with caries risk assessment. However, the key question as to whether they improve patients' dental health outcomes has yet to be answered.

Assessment of Dental Caries

In order to assess current caries activity and caries risk status, the following should be noted on clinical examination:

a. How many carious lesions are present?
b. The location of these lesions
c. Presence of active carious lesions in self-cleansing areas like the buccal surfaces of mandibular molars which would indicate high caries activity
d. Visible plaque and gingivitis indicating poor oral hygiene.

The current understanding of the dynamic nature of the caries process, in which lesion progression can be arrested at any stage of the process, supports the importance of clinically assessing caries activity. The diagnosis process should include assessing if early lesions are active (progressing), arrested or regressing. Diagnosing caries activity permits dentists to make informed decisions regarding the use of sealants and topical fluoride varnish treatment on a tooth surface-specific basis. Evidence of clinically evident active disease is a strong indicator that caries is occurring elsewhere in the dentition at a subclinical level. Thus, the early diagnosis of dental caries disease activity also can increase the reliability of caries risk assessment so that appropriate whole-mouth preventive intervention can be initiated.

The assessment of the caries activity status of early lesions is challenging. It is an important element in practice protocols. The challenge for clinicians is that careful visual and tactile inspection is required to assess lesion activity. Clinical diagnostic criteria have been developed and validated in a high prevalence caries population to assess lesion activity. Caries activity criteria are being evaluated as part of ICDAS. The criteria are based on the physical properties of surface reflection and texture of early lesions, with chalky rough surfaces being active, and smooth, shiny surfaces being inactive. The color of the lesion also can be used to make the distinction between arrested and active lesions, with arrested lesions having an internal brown pigmentation and surface stain and active lesions retaining their white appearance. A recent study pointed out the difficulty in trying to differentiate active lesions from inactive lesions in one appointment without specific training or calibration. Given the highly site specific nature of caries, it is possible to have areas that are arrested and active on the same tooth surface. There is also the possibility of lesions being in a transitional stage, either going from active to inactive or from inactive to active. When there is uncertainty about the diagnosis, the clinician has the option to defer giving a definitive diagnosis until the next recall visit. The future holds promise for the development of clinically useful tools to help dentists make decisions about the activity status of carious lesions.

Caries Indices

The indices for dental caries assess the severity of dental caries and are used in population studies. The universally accepted index for dental caries status is the DMF Index (Decayed-Missing-Filled- Index).

It can be used as DMFT for calculation of the index for permanent teeth of an individual or a group.

Individual DMFT: Total each component, i.e. D, M and F separately, then sum it all (D + M + F).

Group average can be obtained:

$$\frac{\text{Sum of D + M + F}}{\text{Number of individuals in the group}}$$

Percent needing care can also be estimated by:

$$\frac{\text{Total number of decayed teeth}}{\text{Total number examined}}$$

For children, an index of past caries experience based upon the number of decayed, missing and filled surfaces of deciduous (indicated by lower case letters dmfs) or permanent (indicated by capital letters DMFS) teeth gives a more accurate estimate.

Other caries indices are also available such as Stone's Index (1949), caries severity index (1960), Caries susceptibility index (1961) and functional measure index (FMI) 1987.

Microbiological Tests to Predict Caries Activity

These tests have been used to predict sites or individuals at risk of developing caries. The numbers of *Streptococcus mutans* and *Lactobacillus spp* are estimated by plate counts in the laboratory from saliva samples. Semi-quantitative, commercially-available, chair side detection kits for estimation of both *S. Mutans* and *Lactobacillus spp* could also be used.

A paraffin wax stimulated sample of saliva is obtained from the patient and sent to the microbiology laboratory. The saliva is diluted and cultured on selective commercially available media. After incubation the number of colonies are counted and then quantified to obtain the count per milliliter of saliva. For high caries activity : $>10^6$/mL *S. mutans* and/or > 100000/mL *Lactobacillus spp* for low caries activity: < 100000/mL *S. mutans* and < 10000/mL *Lactobacillus spp.*

APPROACHES FOR PREVENTING DENTAL CARIES INCLUDING DENTAL CARIES VACCINES

Caries is a disease process that needs to be managed over a person's lifetime. The theory is predisposition to dental caries may change during the life time of an individual patient and that while practicing the least invasive dentistry with the objective of good preservation of the dentition should be the practitioner's approach. This approach relies on accurate diagnosis of the disease and lesions, caries prevention, just-in-time restorations, minimally invasive operative procedures, and the prevention of recurrence.

There are many approaches to the prevention of dental caries. These could be summarized as follows:

1. The mechanical removal of the dental plaque or biofilms by efficient and effective oral hygiene measures could almost prevent dental caries. This can be achieved by conventional oral hygiene practices such as tooth brushing and flossing.
2. Use of various plaque control measures, such as the use of mouth washes and tooth pastes containing antimicrobial agents such as chlorhexidine and surfactants, which can reduce formation of biofilms and thereby reduce dental caries. Chlorhexidine can be delivered either by gel, e.g. as a 1 percent gel in custom-fitted vinyl applicators, as a mouth rinse or as a varnish.

3. Application of fluoride supplements. These include fluoridated water supplies, salt and milk fluoridation, use of fluoride containing tooth paste, fluoride tablets, fluoride varnishes applied by the dentist especially for children who at high-risk and fluoride mouth rinse program in school. For self-administered care, fluoride toothpaste is the most powerful intervention for caries prevention because it has high clinical effectiveness and social acceptability. A cochrane review of randomized or quasi-randomized controlled trials with blind outcome assessment, comparing fluoride toothpaste with placebo in children aged 16 years or more for at least 1 year, concluded that fluoride toothpastes are clearly effective in prevention of caries. This conclusion is supported by more than 50 years of research. Fluoride functions posteruptively by favorably influencing the kinetics of de- and re-mineralization. Fluoride interacts with the enamel of erupted teeth to form fluorapatite. Fluorapatite is more resistant to acid dissolution than hydroxyapatite.
4. Regular dental care with professional prophylaxis at the dentist's office by the dentist or dental hygienist, with good oral hygiene instructions.
5. For occlusal pits and fissures that are most vulnerable to dental decay, fissure sealants could be used at the dentist's office.
6. Reduction in the amount and frequency specially reducing between meal consumption of carbohydrates and sugar intake and the use of sugar substitutes such as artificial sweeteners. These sweeteners include cyclamate, aspartame, saccharin, sorbitol and xylitol. Advice to restrict the consumption of sugary snacks and drinks should also be given to all patients as part of general dietary counseling.
7. For the future:
   a. Replacement therapy and probiotics. Probiotics are live microorganisms which, when administered in adequate numbers, confer a health benefit on the host. There are two main approaches: (a) pre-emptive colonization where key functions within the biofilm are filled by beneficial microorganisms before the undesirable strain has had a chance to colonize or become established. The initial colonizer becomes integrated into the ecosystem and then excludes the pathogen from gaining a foothold. (b) To derive a more competitive strain that would displace a pre-existing organism from the biofilm.
   b. Active and passive vaccination. Despite the abundance of experimental evidence for the effectiveness of dental caries vaccines, none exist yet for human use. The mutans streptococci are confirmed pathogens, fulfilling most of Koch's postulates and carried by around 98 percent of individuals around the world. There is evidence that *Streptococcus sobrinus* may also contribute to the carious process. A vaccine against dental caries using mutans streptococci (whole cell vaccines), or molecules derived from these bacteria (subunit vaccines), has been proposed for many years. The major factors that are thought to contribute to cariogenicity of mutans streptococci are—acidogenecity, aciduricity, sucrose-independent adhesion and sucrose-dependent adhesion. These properties are required for biofilm formation. These factors are therefore important in the development of appropriate antibodies. Interest has been focused on three groups of antigens in the bacteria- (a) cell-wall proteins, a high molecular weight protein that acts as an adhesin binding to a salivary glycoprotein (b) glucosyltransferases (GTFs) and (c) glucan-binding proteins in the production of suitable and effective anticaries vaccines.
8. Photodynamic therapy. Cariogenic bacteria such as mutans streptococci are susceptible to killing by low power laser light once cells have been treated with low concentrations of a photosensitizer dye such as toluidine blue. When activated, the dye liberates free radicals which are lethal to neighboring cells. Photodynamic therapy has been shown to work well on dental caries biofilms.

However, without proper public education on preventive measures prevention of caries is a challenge. Parents and children should be educated on dietary practices and on oral health maintenance by adequate daily plaque removal.

For patients with low salivary flow due to dry mouth arising from conditions such as Sjögren's syndrome, rheumatoid arthritis, diabetes and use of drugs producing xerostomia as a side effect, suitable salivary substitutes could be provided to reduce the development of caries.

SELF-ASSESSMENT QUESTIONS

1. Describe the etiology and microbiology of dental caries.
2. What laboratory methods are available to study the pathology of dental caries?
3. Describe the detection, clinical appearance and histopathology of caries in enamel.
4. Describe the pathology of caries in dentine and explain the sequelae.
5. Describe the response of the pulpodental complex to caries progression.
6. Describe the underlying pulpal changes occurring in the progression from acute pulpitis through chronic pulpitis to chronic open hyperplastic pulpitis and its sequelae.
7. Describe the changes observed in enamel, dentine and cementum with advancing age.
8. Explain why some superficial enamel cavities cause pain while some deep cavities can be pain-free.
9. Describe the methods available for the detection of caries in a clinical setting.
10. Describe five approaches to the prevention of dental caries.

SUGGESTED READING

1. Berkovitz BKB, Holland GR, Moxham BJ. Oral Anatomy, Embryology and Histology, 3rd edn. Mosby International Ltd; 2002.
2. Blanaid D, Watt RG, Batchelor P, Treasure ET. Essential Dental Public Health. OUP, Oxford; 2002.
3. Darling AI. Dental Caries, Chapter 5. In: Gorlin RJ, Goldman HM (Ed). Thoma's Oral Pathology, Volume 01, 6th. edn. The CV Mosby Company, St. Louis; 1970.
4. Fejerskov O, Nyvad B, Kidd E AM. Pathology of Dental Caries, Chapter 3. In: Fejerskov O, Kidd EAM (Eds). Dental Caries - The disease and its clinical management. 2nd edn. Oxford: Blackwell Munksgaard; 2008.
5. Le Charpentier Y, Auriol M. Histopathologie bucco-dentaire et maxillo-faciale, Chapter 3. Masson, Paris, 1997.
6. Mendis BRRN, Darling AI. A Scanning electron microscopic and microradiographic study of closure of human coronal dentinal tubules related to occlusal attrition and caries. Archs. Oral Biol. 1979;24:725-33.
7. Samaranayake L. Essential Microbiology for Dentistry, 3rd edn. Churchill Livingstone, Edinburgh; 2006.

Chapter 3

Periodontal Diseases

Philip M Preshaw

Chapter Outline

INTRODUCTION

Periodontal disease is a common, chronic inflammatory disease of the tooth supporting structures. It is one of the most common diseases known to mankind, and its sequelae, mobile teeth and loss of teeth, can have a major impact on quality of life and nutrition. Good oral health is an essential prerequisite for maintaining good general health. The dental team therefore have a major role in contributing to the health and wellbeing of their patients. Given that periodontal diseases are, for the most part, largely preventable and the tissue destruction that ensues is largely irreversible, it remains the responsibility of the dentist to examine patients carefully, to reach an accurate diagnosis, to communicate their findings to the patient, and to provide appropriate therapy. The first step in improving our management of periodontal diseases is to ascertain the prevalence of these conditions in the population.

EPIDEMIOLOGY OF PERIODONTAL DISEASE

Epidemiology describes the study of the distribution of disease in human populations. It is important to distinguish between the incidence of a disease and the prevalence of a disease. Incidence refers to the number of new cases of a disease that develop over a given time period in a population. However, we are unable to identify the exact point in time at which a patient develops periodontitis, and therefore in periodontal epidemiology we do not attempt to measure disease incidence. Instead, we rely on disease prevalence, which refers to the proportion (percentage) of people in a population affected by the disease at a given point in time.

To ascertain the prevalence of periodontal disease, we need to be able to accurately and reproducibly define whether or not a patient has the disease. But, how is periodontitis diagnosed or defined? Many studies in the 1960s and 1970s used a very low threshold for defining the presence of periodontitis, or even failed to distinguish between gingivitis and periodontitis, which resulted in very high reported prevalence rates in the periodontal literature. Data from research conducted at the time suggested that periodontitis inevitably commenced in early adulthood, and that almost the entire population was affected by the time individuals reached their 40s. Tooth loss was thought to increase gradually with age, in a relatively linear fashion. These observations led to a theory of periodontal disease that we might now refer to as the 'Old Theory of Periodontitis' (**Box 3.1**).

Box 3.1: Theories of periodontitis

The old theory of periodontitis

- Periodontal disease is inevitable following gingivitis
- Periodontal disease is uniformly distributed in the population
- Disease severity is correlated with plaque levels
- There is a linear, progressive loss of attachment over time
- The severity of periodontitis increases with age

The new theory of periodontitis

- Gingivitis and mild periodontitis are common, and gingivitis is present in a majority of most populations
- Approximately 10 to 15 percent of most populations exhibit advanced periodontitis
- Gingivitis precedes periodontitis but not all sites with gingivitis develop periodontitis
- Periodontitis is not a natural consequence of ageing (but older people may present with more loss of attachment as a result of a lifetime of tissue breakdown events)
- In some patients, periodontitis may progress with episodes of disease activity interspersed with periods of quiescence, in a nonlinear manner.

Today, we can recognize the methodological shortcomings of these early studies. Guidelines for assigning a diagnosis for the presence of periodontal disease in epidemiological studies have been developed (see reading list). We now realize that although gingivitis and mild periodontitis (characterized by isolated shallow pockets of 4–5 mm) are common, advanced periodontitis (characterized by multiple deep pockets of 6 mm or greater) is much less prevalent than previously thought. Although estimations of the prevalence of advanced periodontitis vary according to the population studied, a consistent finding is that advanced periodontal disease affects approximately 10 to 15 percent of adults in most populations. Though this is less than estimates of disease prevalence that were reported previously, this still represents a very large proportion of most populations, with large numbers of people affected. Furthermore, plaque and calculus are almost ubiquitous, and are found in the vast majority of adults.

In addition to studying the epidemiology of periodontal disease, researchers have investigated the nature of periodontitis progression. Early studies considered that loss of attachment and alveolar bone destruction continued in a linear fashion over time, and that once periodontitis was initiated, its progression was inevitable. More recent longitudinal monitoring studies have revealed that, for the majority of periodontitis patients, most sites are stable at any given time, and only a relatively small proportion demonstrate disease progression. It must be remembered, however, that these findings are based on repeated examination of patients using a periodontal probe. The periodontal probe is a somewhat crude diagnostic tool. The probe is attempting to identify tissue breakdown events at the base of the pocket that are resulting in microscopic alterations in the epithelial and connective tissue attachment to the tooth, and therefore it is unsurprising that we are unable to identify with any degree of reliability which periodontal sites are actively undergoing breakdown when we examine a patient. Nonetheless, we can summarize the findings of more recent epidemiological surveys into what we can call the 'New Theory of Periodontitis,' as shown in **Box 3.1**. This theory reveals that severe forms of periodontitis are found in approximately 10 to 15 percent of most populations, representing a very large number of individuals across the world.

HISTORY, EXAMINATION AND ASSESSMENT OF RISK FACTORS

A thorough history and a careful examination are fundamental to making the correct diagnosis. During the history, patients should be allowed to explain the problem from their perspective, and the dentist should ask open questions to encourage the patient to talk freely. The dentist should be nonjudgemental and should be sympathetic to the patient. Many patients consider that periodontal disease is 'all their own fault,' but given what we know about the importance of the host inflammatory responses in determining the progression of disease (see below), we know this is simply not true. The dentist should be supportive, while also communicating effectively and clearly with the patient so that the patient will understand their role in managing the condition.

History

It helps, when taking a history, to follow a structure so that important questions are not missed. A suggested scheme is presented in **Table 3.1**. Given that most cases of periodontitis do not cause pain, many patients may not be aware that they have a problem until the condition is very advanced. Therefore, the onus for detection of disease rests firmly with the clinician. Gingival bleeding is one of the most common complaints of patients with periodontal disease, usually when toothbrushing or eating. If the condition is more advanced, and has been present for a number of years, patients may present with mobile teeth, or teeth that have drifted, opening up spaces between teeth. Teeth drift when their periodontal support is compromised to such an extent that the teeth are no longer in equilibrium with forces from occlusion and the adjacent soft tissues.

Many patients are very concerned about bad taste in the mouth and halitosis. Halitosis is a common finding in patients with periodontitis and can result from many causes including:

- Accumulation of plaque and calculus

Table 3.1
Structured history taking

Presenting complaint	• In the patient's own words. • Patients will typically mention bleeding gums, bad breath, mobile teeth, drifting of teeth, gingival recession. However, pain is not usually reported in gingivitis or periodontitis.
History of presenting complaint	• How long has there been a problem? • Has the patient been aware of this for weeks, months, years?
Previous dental history	• Is the patient a regular dental attender? • Has any periodontal treatment been provided in the past? If so, by whom (e.g. dentist, hygienist, periodontist)? • How long did the treatment appointments last? • Was the treatment a simple 'scale and polish' or was it more thorough root surface debridement? • If teeth have been lost, why was this?
Use of oral hygiene products	• What is the patient using? • Frequency of tooth brushing? • Are interdental cleaning brushes being used?
Family history	• Do any other family members have periodontal problems (this could potentially indicate aggressive periodontitis, which has a familial aggregation)
Social history	• Is the patient employed? What do they do? • Sources of stress in life?
Smoking history	• If a current smoker, how many cigarettes per day, and for how many years have they smoked? • If an ex-smoker, when did they quit? For how many years did they smoke, and how many cigarettes did they used to smoke per day?
Medical history	• Record and update the medical history at each visit. • Are there risk factors for periodontal disease, e.g. diabetes? • Are there medical conditions that impact on dental management or provision of periodontal treatment? • Are there nutritional deficiencies or dietary problems? • Which medications does the patient take, and can these impact on periodontal status or treatment?

- Food debris
- Purulent exudate from a periodontal pocket
- Excessive bacterial growth on the dorsum of the tongue
- Necrotizing ulcerative gingivitis.

If pain is present, it may indicate necrotising ulcerative gingivitis, or an acute periodontal abscess. Gingival recession that has resulted in exposure of the roots may also result in dentine sensitivity. Pain is not otherwise a typical feature of chronic periodontitis.

Examination

The intraoral examination should include several components. An initial assessment of the level of oral hygiene and plaque control is important. The degree of gingival inflammation should be also assessed. All patients should be screened for periodontal disease by probing, and the quickest method is to record the basic periodontal examination (BPE), also known as the Community Periodontal Index of Treatment Needs (CPITN).

A WHO (World Health Organization) periodontal probe should be used: this has a 0.5 mm diameter ball end and a colored band extending 3.5 to 5.5 mm from the tip. The dentition is divided into sextants, the periodontium around each tooth is probed and the highest score in each sextant is recorded. The score codes assigned are used as a guide to determine the need for periodontal treatment **(Table 3.2)**. If the results of the screening examination indicate the presence of periodontitis (i.e. BPE code 3 or code 4), then a detailed periodontal examination should be undertaken (i.e. full charting). If there is only one tooth in a sextant, no score is recorded for that sextant, and instead, the tooth is assessed together with the teeth in the neighboring sextant.

For those patients requiring a full periodontal examination, this should be performed at 6 sites per tooth, together with measurement of gingival recession (and calculation of loss of attachment by addition to the probing depth measurements) and bleeding on probing. Bleeding on probing results from the trauma caused to the epithelial pocket lining and connective tissue by the probe, but given that many factors can affect whether the tissue bleeds in addition to the degree of inflammation (such as the force of probing, sharpness of the probe tip), presence of bleeding on probing has a low sensitivity for periodontal disease progression. However, absence of bleeding on probing is a good indicator of periodontal stability.

Furcation involvement should be assessed with a curved furcation probe (Nabers probe). Classification is as follows:

- *Class I:* The tissue destruction does not exceed more than 3 mm (or not more than one-third the tooth width) into the furcation
- *Class II:* The tissue destruction is >3 mm (or more than one-third the tooth width) into the furcation but does not completely pass through the furcation
- *Class III:* It has through-and-through involvement, and the lesion extends across the entire width of the furcation.

A tooth with a furcation involvement is a compromised tooth. It has been estimated that the surface area of the root trunk of the first maxillary molar is approximately 30 percent of the total root surface area. In other words, by the time the furcation can be detected, a significant

▪ Table 3.2
The basic periodontal examination (BPE)

*Code**	*Probing*	*Treatment needs*
0	Colored band on the probe is completely visible No calculus detected No bleeding on probing	No need for periodontal treatment
1	Colored band on the probe is completely visible No calculus detected Bleeding on probing	Oral hygiene instruction (OHI)
2	Colored band on the probe is completely visible Calculus detected (supra- or subgingival), or overhanging restoration(s)	*OHI:* Elimination of plaque-retentive areas, scaling, root surface debridement (RSD)
3	Colored band on probe is partly visible, indicating probing depth of >3.5 mm but <5.5 mm	OHI, RSD
4	Colored band on probe completely disappears into pocket, indicating probing depth of >5.5 mm	OHI, RSD. Complex additional treatment may be required. Referral to a periodontal specialist may be necessary.

* The symbol (*) should be added to the score when furcation involvement is present. The score should then be recorded, for example, as 4*, or 3*, etc.

degree of periodontal breakdown has already occurred.

Tooth mobility should also be assessed by applying a labiolingual, horizontal force to each tooth, using the handles of dental mirrors. A mobility index can be recorded as:

- 0 Normal, physiological mobility (<0.3 mm)
- 1 Horizontal mobility > 0.3 mm to 1.0 mm
- 2 Horizontal mobility 1.0 to 2.0 mm
- 3 Horizontal mobility > 2.0 mm and/or vertical mobility.

Occlusal examination should be undertaken when indicated. Many patients with periodontitis present with mobile teeth, and occlusal interferences may contribute to this. It is important to note that trauma from occlusion does not cause periodontitis; however, in the presence of pre-existing periodontitis, trauma from occlusion may exacerbate mobility and lead to an increased rate of alveolar bone loss. Fremitus should be assessed, and the presence of traumatic incisal relationships should be determined. Traumatic incisal relationships are classified by the Akerly classification:

1. Lower incisors in compete overbite, contacting palatal mucosa but distal to the palatal gingival margins of the upper anterior teeth.
2. Lower incisors in complete overbite, contacting palatal gingival margins of the upper anterior teeth (can result in localized trauma and recession at the palatal gingival margins of the maxillary anterior teeth).
3. As for class 2, but there is also shearing trauma of the gingival margins at the labial aspects of the lower anterior teeth as the upper incisors slide past the lower incisors (predisposed by lack of posterior support, and class II division 2 overbite).
4. Palatal attrition, i.e. dental trauma as the lower incisors contact the palatal surfaces of the upper incisors.

Occlusal trauma can be defined as injury to the attachment apparatus of the teeth as a result of occlusal forces, and is classified as primary occlusal trauma or secondary occlusal trauma. Primary occlusal trauma is occlusal trauma that affects periodontally healthy teeth (i.e. those with normal attachment and bone support), and is usually caused by excessive occlusal forces (e.g. as a result of an occlusal interference). Secondary occlusal trauma is that which affects periodontally compromised teeth (which have pre-existing attachment loss and bone loss), and may result from either normal or excessive occlusal forces.

A classic appearance of a periodontally compromised tooth that also is subject to trauma from occlusion (i.e. secondary occlusal trauma) is that of a crater-like defect with extensive bone loss and a very mobile tooth (**Fig. 3.1**). This is distinct from the radiographic appearance of a periodontally healthy tooth subject to a traumatic occlusion (i.e. primary occlusal trauma). In the healthy situation, trauma from occlusion (primary occlusal trauma) may result in widening of the periodontal membrane space and increased mobility, but will not cause periodontitis. If the traumatic interference is removed, then the periodontal membrane space returns to normal and mobility decreases.

Radiographic investigation is an essential part of the assessment of patients with periodontitis. Modern panoramic machines provide high quality images at reduced radiation exposure compared to full mouth periapicals. Radiographic features that can be identified include:

- Pattern of bone loss: horizontal or vertical, localized or generalized, irregular or regular extent of bone loss, usually described as a proportion or percentage of the root affected
- Furcation bone loss

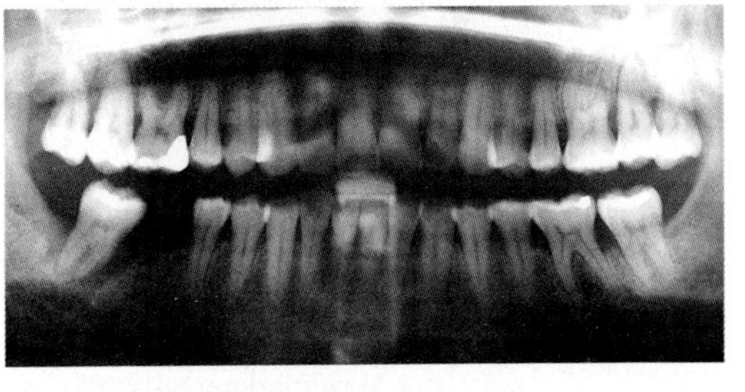

Fig. 3.1: Trauma from occlusion resulting in exacerbation of pre-existing periodontal disease. Radiograph showing generalized horizontal alveolar bone loss affecting between one-third and one-half the root length, being most advanced at molar sites and the maxillary incisors. Extensive vertical defects/crater defect at tooth 47, in traumatic occlusal relationship

- Variations in root anatomy
- Interproximal calculus
- Widening of the periodontal membrane space
- Overhanging restorations.

A decreased alveolar bone height on a radiograph is a historical record of previous periodontal involvement and provides no information on current disease activity.

Risk Factor Assessment

Assessment of risk factors (or predisposing factors) is one of the most important parts of the assessment of a patient with periodontitis, yet is often overlooked. Risk factors can be broadly classified as systemic risk factors or local risk factors.

Systemic risk factors include smoking and diabetes. Smoking is the most important systemic risk factor for periodontitis and a detailed smoking history must always be recorded. Patients must always be informed of the importance of this risk factor and encouraged to quit. Smoking has wide ranging impacts on inflammation and immune responses, and is a significant negative modifier of multiple types of periodontitis. It is important to record in the patient notes that the importance of smoking as a risk factor has been explained to the patient. Similarly, poorly controlled diabetes is a major risk factor for periodontitis. However, patients with well controlled diabetes do not appear to be at increased risk for periodontitis. Local risk factors include multiple anatomic and iatrogenic factors that typically are plaque retentive (e.g. overhanging margins of restorations, orthodontic appliances, etc).

DIAGNOSIS, TREATMENT PLANNING AND EMPOWERING THE PATIENT

A correct diagnosis is essential for correct treatment planning. It is important not to adopt a 'one size fits all' approach to periodontal treatment. The treatment must be individualized to the patient, and that starts with a thorough history to understand the needs of the patient, and requires a correct diagnosis. A diagnosis can be assigned based on the disease criteria established by the American Academy of Periodontology in 1999 (**Table 3.3**). Reaching a correct diagnosis is dependent on

Table 3.3
Classification of periodontal diseases

Gingival diseases	**A. Plaque-induced gingivitis:** This is the most common type of gingival condition, and may be associated with plaque only, or further modified by, for example, systemic drugs (e.g. those that cause drug induced gingival overgrowth), or hormonal variations (e.g. those seen in pregnancy) **B. Nonplaque induced gingivitis:** This includes specific infections (e.g. primary herpetic gingivostomatitis), gingival manifestations of conditions such as lichen planus, and traumatic gingival lesions
Chronic periodontitis	This is the most common form of periodontitis. It is characterized by some/all of the following: • Most prevalent in adults but can occur in children/adolescents • Subgingival calculus commonly found • Associated with a variable microbial pattern • Slow/moderate rate of progression, but may have periods of rapid progression • Can be classified on basis of extent (e.g. localized or generalized) or severity (e.g. amount of attachment loss) • Can be associated with local predisposing factors (e.g. plaque retentive features such as overhangs) • Can be modified by/associated with systemic exposures such as smoking, or conditions such as diabetes

Contd...

Contd...

Aggressive periodontitis	'Aggressive periodontitis' (AP) replaces previously used terms such as 'rapidly progressive periodontitis' or 'juvenile periodontitis'. The primary characteristics of AP are: • Except for the presence of periodontitis, patients are otherwise clinically healthy • Rapid attachment loss and bone destruction (often characterized by very irregular pattern of alveolar bone loss, multiple vertical defects, extensive bone loss) • Familial aggregation (which is why it is important to ask about family members when examining patients with suspected aggressive periodontitis) Secondary characteristics of AP are: • Plaque levels are sometimes less than might be expected given the severity of the periodontal disease (this situation might be typically seen in a very concerned and motivated patient who clearly has a genetic susceptibility and is maintaining good oral hygiene, yet still has advanced disease) • Elevated levels of *Aggregatibacter actinomycetemcomitans* (especially in localized AP) and *Porphyromonas gingivalis* • Phagocyte abnormalities and a hyper-responsive macrophage phenotype, including elevated levels of PGE_2 and IL-1β (though there is no diagnostic test for a hyper-responsive phenotype and this is essentially a research finding only) AP can be further classified as localized (localized to the first molars and incisors, and typically has a circumpubertal onset) or generalized (affecting at least 3 permanent teeth other than first molars and incisors, usually affecting people <30 years, but patients may be older, and with a pronounced episodic nature of attachment loss and alveolar bone loss).
Periodontitis as a manifestation of systemic disease	This includes periodontitis associated with **hematological disorders** (such as acquired neutropenia and leukemias) and periodontitis associated with **genetic disorders** (such as cyclic neutropenia, leukocyte adhesion deficiency syndromes, Papillon-Lefèvre syndrome, Chediak-Higashi syndrome, Ehlers-Danlos syndrome, hypophosphatasia.
Necrotizing periodontal diseases	**A. Necrotizing ulcerative gingivitis (NUG)** Characterized by gingival necrosis, with 'punched-out' papillae, pain, gingival bleeding, halitosis, pseudomembranous sloughing. Predisposing factors include stress, smoking, poor diet, HIV infection. **B. Necrotizing ulcerative periodontitis (NUP)** Characterized by necrosis of the gingiva, PDL and alveolar bone. Most typically seen in patients with significant systemic illness, e.g. HIV, severe malnutrition, immunosuppression.
Abscesses of the periodontium	**A. Gingival abscess,** localized to the marginal gingiva or interdental papilla **B. Periodontal abscess,** localized abscess in the pocket, may result in bone loss **C. Pericoronal abscess,** also known as pericoronitis
Periodontitis associated with endodontic lesions	These are combined periodontal-endodontic lesions, typically referred to as 'perio-endo lesions'. Either the periodontal or endodontic lesion may be the cause or the result of the other, or both lesions may develop independently on the same tooth, until they coalesce into a single lesion.
Developmental or acquired conditions	**A. Localized tooth related factors** (e.g. anatomic factors, iatrogenic factors such as overhangs, root resorption, root fractures) **B. Mucogingival deformities around teeth** (e.g. localized recession defects, lack of keratinized gingiva, high frenal attachment) **C. Mucogingival deformities on edentulous ridges** (e.g. reduced ridge height or width) **D. Occlusal trauma** (primary occlusal trauma or secondary occlusal trauma)

having taken a thorough history, a detailed and accurate clinical examination with appropriate radiographic assessment and interpretation, and assessment of risk factors.

Having made a diagnosis, it is then necessary to formulate a treatment plan. The treatment plan should be comprehensive in scope, and should include management of risk factors in addition to conventional periodontal therapies. Aspects that can be considered in the treatment plan are indicated in **Table 3.4**.

It is clear that successful periodontal therapy requires a motivated and compliant patient as well as a motivated clinician. Periodontal management should be considered a team effort, and it should be made clear to the patient that they have a role to play in managing their condition, and they will be supported in this by the dental team. Most periodontal conditions are chronic, representing long-term problems that require long-term solutions. Most importantly, behavior change is required of patients (e.g. to improve their plaque

Table 3.4
Aspects to consider when formulating a treatment plan

Plaque control	Plaque control is the essential component of any periodontal therapy. Without plaque control, any form of periodontal treatment will fail. Oral hygiene instruction (OHI) should be provided that is relevant to the patient and is achievable. Don't overload the patient with too much information at once. Demonstrate toothbrush use in the patient's mouth. Explain the rationale for cleaning subgingivally. Reassure the patient that bleeding on brushing is not a reason to stop brushing. Suggested oral hygiene aids include: • Manual brush—use with crevicular technique to ensure bristles penetrate subgingivally • Powered brush—very different technique from manual brush, ensure patient is using correctly • Single tufted brush—excellent in recession defects, around single standing teeth, at areas of crowding • Floss—for interproximal cleaning, usually at sites with no attachment loss • Bottle brushes—essential for interproximal cleaning at sites with recession in periodontitis patients • Mouthrinses—may be used to supplement brushing but must not be used instead of brushing
Root surface debridement (RSD)	The cornerstone of periodontal therapy. The focus of RSD is the disruption of the subgingival biofilm and removal of plaque and calculus. Calculus is plaque retentive but otherwise does not directly contribute to periodontitis. Disruption of the biofilm is essential to reduce the bacterial challenge. This should then result in resolution of inflammation in the periodontal tissues, leading to shrinkage of the tissues, formation of a long junctional epithelium, and a reduction in probing depths. Shallower pockets are easier to maintain and clean than deep pockets, and inflammation is easier to control at shallow sites compared to deep sites. RSD can be undertaken with hand or ultrasonic instruments. Root planing is no longer an appropriate therapy, as it is clear that planing away the root surface does not benefit the patient, and can result in tooth sensitivity. For this reason RSD is the treatment of choice and involves multiple light strokes to disrupt the biofilm.
Risk factor management	Risk factor management complements OHI and RSD, and can take many forms: • Elimination of local risk factors (e.g. replacing overhanging restorations) • Smoking cessation (essential, but difficult to achieve) • Liaison with the medical practitioner to assist in medical management (e.g. of diabetes)
Periodontal surgery	Periodontal surgery may be the primary therapy in specific situations, e.g. connective tissue grafts to cover recession defects or gingivectomy surgery for drug induced gingival overgrowth. Periodontal surgery may also be indicated at specific nonresponding sites after effective nonsurgical management, and the aim of such surgery is to improve access for cleaning (for the clinician and the patient).
Adjunctive treatments	Adjuncts may be local (e.g. placement of local drug delivery systems) or systemic (e.g. systemic antibiotics or host modulating agents)

control, to quit smoking, to attend long-term for periodontal maintenance care). In order for behavior to change, the patient must know the reason for the change, and therefore needs to be educated about periodontal disease and its management. This involves spending time talking to the patient to ensure they understand what is expected of them. The patient must be empowered to manage their problem, and must be supported by the dentist and hygienist.

The best way to empower and motivate a patient is to give them personalized biofeedback about their condition. This involves explaining the periodontal problem as is relevant to the patient, demonstrating problem areas in the mouth, and demonstrating solutions to those problems. Important areas to cover as part of this process include:

- Identifying the patient's long-term goals for their periodontal health, i.e. what do they want to achieve? For many patients, they will have goals such as preventing tooth loss, reducing bleeding or mobility, eliminating halitosis. The treatment plan must aim to achieve these goals, as this is the best way to achieve compliance.
- Set targets, based on the patient's goals as well as the clinician's goals. For example, set targets for plaque reduction, for probing depth reductions (such as: aim to reduce the number of pockets 5 mm or greater by 90%).
- Assess baseline oral hygiene habits (methods, frequency, duration) and then introduce better techniques (revise methods, frequency, duration), making new oral hygiene technique relevant to the clinical situation for that patient.
- Explain about periodontal disease by providing structured information about what has happened so far, the consequences if untreated, what can be expected following treatment, and the importance of plaque control.
- Explain about the importance of modifying behavior, such as quitting smoking and the benefits that can be expected.
- Reassure the patient, provide a supportive environment for them.
- Continually motivate and support the patient, help them to achieve the goals they want to achieve.

All of this takes time, but ultimately is much more likely to result in a successful outcome.

GINGIVITIS

Gingivae have a distinctive appearance that is clearly different from the inflamed gingival tissues seen in gingivitis. In this healthy patient, the gingival tissues are pink and noninflamed. The interdental papillae fill the interdental spaces below the contact point.

Gingivitis is defined as the inflammation of the gingival tissues. The most common form of gingivitis is plaque-induced gingivitis. The gingiva become erythematous, edematous, shiny, and soft or spongy in texture. Sulcus depths increase (false pockets) as a result of tissue swelling from inflammatory edema. The interdental papillae and marginal gingiva are initially involved before inflammation spreads to the attached gingiva. The gingival tissues may bleed on gentle probing. The clinical appearance of gingivitis (**Fig. 3.2**) is quite distinct from that of healthy gingival tissues (**Fig. 3.3**).

The inflammatory response that characterizes gingivitis is confined to the gingival tissues, and does not involve the other periodontal tissues. The condition may persist indefinitely.

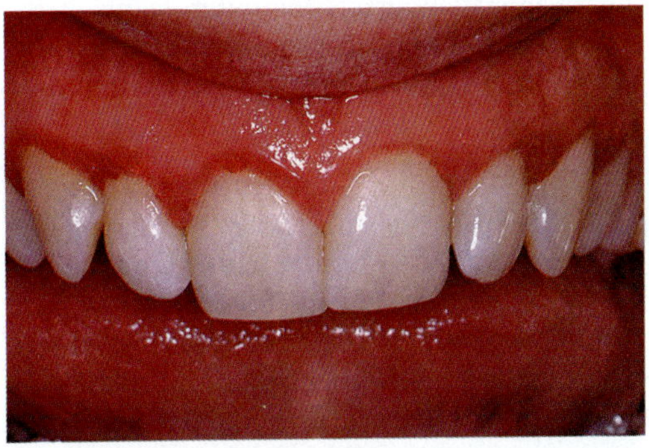

Fig. 3.2: Clinical appearance of gingivitis. There is generalized erythema of the marginal gingival tissues as a result of plaque accumulation. The interdental papillae are swollen, and the interdental papilla between 13 and 12 is particularly inflamed

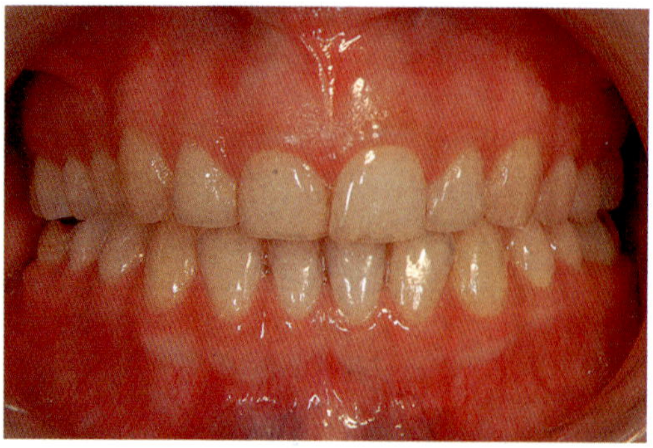

Fig. 3.3: Clinical appearance of healthy gingiva. There is no gingival edema and no bleeding

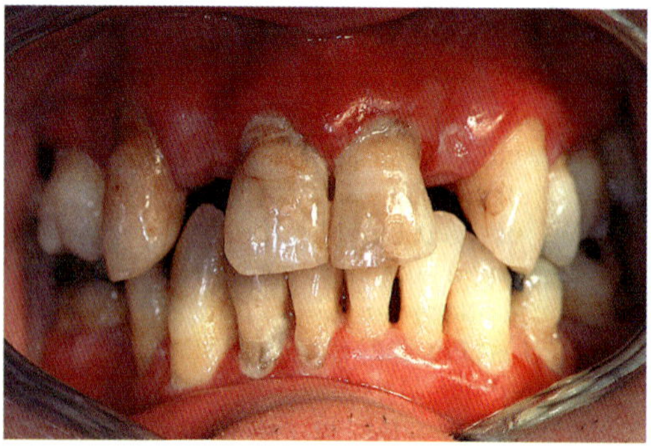

Fig. 3.4: Clinical appearance of desquamative gingivitis associated with lichen planus. The inflamed tissues are fiery red in appearance and the inflammation affects the entire width of the keratinized gingiva. Lacy white striations typical of lichen planus can be seen at other anatomical sites

Gingivitis is reversible with effective plaque control and is so common within populations as to be almost considered a physiological condition rather than a disease state. This is a controversial statement, but is supported by the finding that even in clinically healthy tissues, if these are examined histologically, infiltrating inflammatory cells can always be identified (albeit in reduced numbers compared to gingivitis or periodontitis).

Treatment for gingivitis focuses around patient education to improve plaque control, together with necessary instrumentation:

- Instruction in toothbrushing and use of interdental cleaning aids
- Supra- and subgingival instrumentation (including any combination of ultrasonics, hand instruments, prophylaxis, etc.) to remove plaque and calculus and to disrupt the biofilm
- Elimination of plaque retentive factors.

Some other forms of gingivitis are reviewed in **Box 3.2**. These are much less common than plaque-induced gingivitis, but nonetheless are not rare. Among them desquamative gingivitis is a particular presentation of both oral lichen planus (**Fig. 3.4**) and mucous membrane pemphigoid.

PERIODONTAL DISEASES

The most frequently occurring form of periodontal disease is chronic periodontitis. The other important form of periodontitis that dentists must be aware of is aggressive periodontitis.

Chronic Periodontitis

According to the classification proposed by the American Academy of Periodontology in 1999, chronic periodontitis can be defined as 'an infectious disease resulting in inflammation within the supporting tissues of the teeth, progressive attachment and bone loss.' The authors went on to say that chronic periodontitis is initiated and sustained by bacterial plaque, but host defence mechanisms play an integral role in its pathogenesis. Previous descriptions of periodontitis in the 1960s and 1970s focused solely on the etiological role of bacteria in their definitions. The fact that definitions of this common disease have changed over time reflects our improving understanding of the pathogenesis of the condition. Perhaps a reasonable definition of chronic periodontitis based on current understanding would be:

Chronic periodontitis is bacterially-induced inflammation of the periodontium.

This definition confirms the role of bacteria in initiating and perpetuating the condition, but firmly underscores the importance of inflammation in the pathogenesis of the disease. Indeed, the inflammatory response is responsible for the majority of tissue destruction seen in patients with periodontitis. Some of the characteristics of chronic periodontitis are indicated in **Table 3.3** and the clinical appearance

Box 3.2: Different types of gingivitis

Pregnancy gingivitis

Etiology	Increased levels of circulating estrogen and progesterone during pregnancy exacerbate existing gingivitis. The hormones increase capillary permeability leading to increased erythema and edema.
Clinical features	Severity tends to increase throughout pregnancy. Often a degree of resolution during 3rd trimester and after parturition. A local gingival overgrowth (i.e. pregnancy epulis) may result from chronic irritation or mild trauma to the tissues.
Treatment	Prevention, education, plaque control, instrumentation.

Plasma cell gingivitis

Etiology	Precise details unclear, but is a contact hypersensitivity reaction often caused by dietary components (e.g. cinnamon). Microscopically, the epithelium is atrophic with massive infiltrate of plasma cells in the connective tissues.
Clinical features	Gingival tissues are fiery red, and the lesion involves the entire width of the attached gingiva. The lesion is also very sore.
Treatment	Identify the causative allergen. May require involvement of dermatologist for patch testing. Plaque control, gentle cleaning techniques.

Desquamative gingivitis

Etiology	Not a discreet clinical entity, but is a term used to describe a gingival manifestation common to plasma cell gingivitis and mucocutaneous disorders such as lichen planus and benign mucous membrane pemphigoid.
Clinical features	Fiery red, desquamative lesions affecting the entire width of keratinized gingiva and may be localized or generalized throughout the mouth **(Fig. 3.4)**
Treatment	Liaise with oral medicine specialist. Plaque control essential. Topical steroids may be required, potentially systemic steroids in advanced cases.

Necrotizing ulcerative gingivitis (NUG)

Etiology	A fusiform-spirochetal complex is traditionally associated with NUG. Ulceration of the gingival epithelium occurs with necrosis of the connective tissues. Superficially, deposits of fibrin are intermeshed with dead and dying epithelial cells, neutrophils and bacteria (creating the characterizing pseudomembranous sloughing). Deeper tissues demonstrate a dense infiltrate of neutrophils, characteristic of nonspecific inflammation.
Clinical features	'Punched out' ulcers covered with a yellow-gray pseudomembranous slough. The tips of the interdental papillae are affected first, rapidly followed by the marginal gingiva. NUG is very painful and there is also marked halitosis. A pre-existing gingivitis is usually also present. Fever and regional lymphadenopathy are associated with severe disease.
Risk factors	Pre-existing gingivitis (confirming a poor standard of plaque control). Smoking (major risk factor, favors gram-negative flora, impacts on immune responses). Mental stress (NUG often seen in college students and army personnel). Malnutrition (predisposes to infection and severe NUG, and may extend onto the external face, resulting in the very serious condition noma or cancrum oris). HIV infection (may also predispose to NUG that may progress to necrotizing ulcerative periodontitis)
Treatment	Reduce/stop smoking. Oral hygiene instruction, soft brush, mouthrinses useful if brushing very painful. Metronidazole 200 mg three times per day for 3 to 5 days. *Instrumentation:* Ultrasonics useful when pain starts to subside, careful prophylaxis. *Note:* Incomplete treatment can result in recurrence and eventually, loss of gingival contour, which may create esthetic problems.

of a patient with chronic periodontitis is shown in **Figure 3.5**.

Clinical characteristics of chronic periodontitis include pocket formation, loss of attachment, bleeding on probing and alveolar bone loss. Pocketing results from apical migration of the junctional epithelium, and a pocket is generally said to exist (as opposed to a healthy sulcus or gingival crevice) if the probing depth is 4 mm or greater. Bleeding on probing results from penetration of the inflamed, ulcerated tissues lining the pocket by the probe as it is inserted into the pocket. Migration of teeth may occur following attachment loss, and a typical presentation is of maxillary incisors that drift labially, resulting in increased overjet and formation of diastemata. Affected teeth also have a tendency to overerupt (**Fig 3.5**).

Alveolar bone resorption occurs concurrently with pocket formation and attachment loss. Two distinct patterns of bone destruction are recognized radiographically. Horizontal bone loss occurs when the entire width of interdental bone is resorbed. Vertical bone defects are produced when the interdental bone adjacent to the root surface is more rapidly resorbed, leaving an angular, uneven morphology. Frequently, both patterns of bone resorption are seen at different sites in

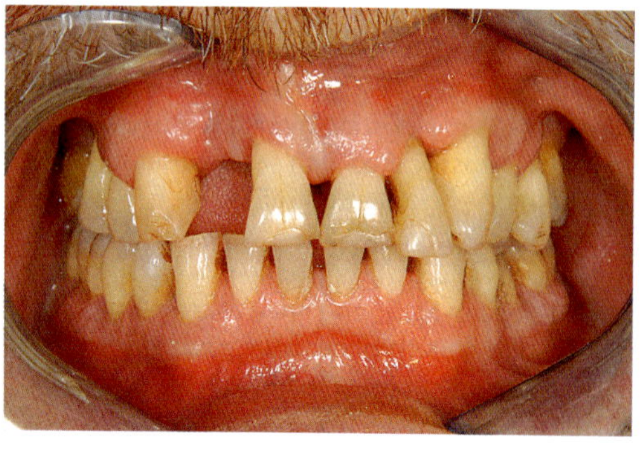

Fig. 3.5: Clinical appearance of chronic periodontitis. The gingival tissues appear to be relatively noninflamed. However, the gingival anatomy is very abnormal as a result of periodontal breakdown, particularly in the maxilla. There is marked gingival recession

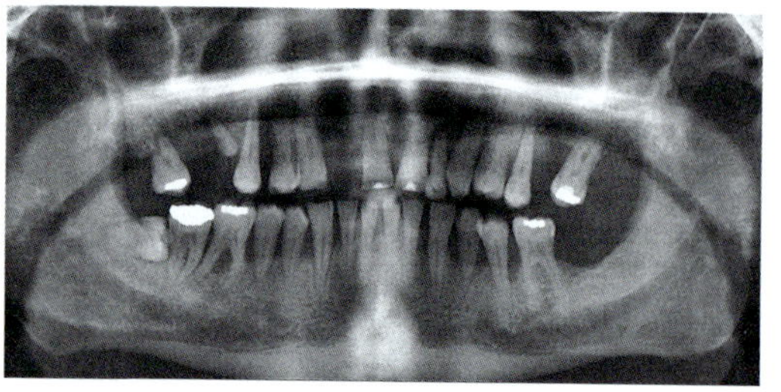

Fig. 3.6: Radiographic appearance of chronic periodontitis showing alveolar bone loss. Generalized horizontal bone loss: 50 to 75 percent of root length, irregular pattern of bone loss. Vertical bone defects: 15 m, 22 m, 23 m, 35 d, 34 md. Furcation bone loss: 46. Possible combined periodontal—endodontic lesion: 22

the same patient **(Fig. 3.6)**. For those areas at which the radiographic appearance is not clear (e.g. apical periodontitis at some teeth), long cone periapical images would be necessary to provide further information. Infrabony defects can also be classified according to the number of remaining bony walls; one-, two- or three-walled defects **(Fig. 3.7)**. Of course, the number of bony walls can only be confirmed by direct vision during flap surgery.

As a result of progression of periodontitis, there may be generalized gingival recession. Treatment of periodontitis also can result in gingival recession as a result of shrinkage of the tissues following resolution of gingival inflammation.

Aggressive Periodontitis

Aggressive periodontitis (AP) is characterized by rapid attachment loss, rapid bone destruction and a familial aggregation. Apart from the presence of periodontitis, patients are otherwise healthy. The term 'aggressive periodontitis' is now used in preference to the term 'early onset periodontal disease' (which comprised prepubertal periodontitis, juvenile periodontitis and rapidly progressive periodontitis). AP can be localized or generalized **(Table 3.3)**. Aggressive forms of periodontitis can also be seen in children, or in association with certain

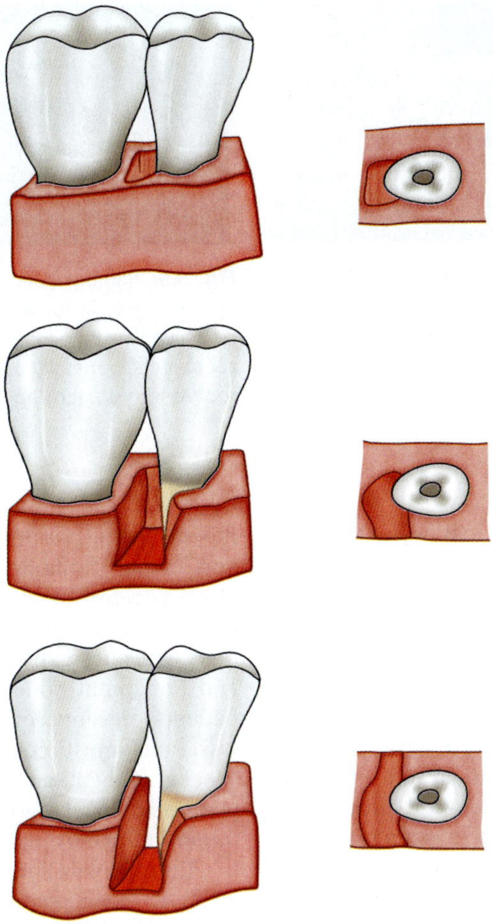

Fig. 3.7: Diagrammatic representation of infrabony defects. The so-called number of walls of a defect refers to the number of bony walls remaining. The 3-walled defect (top) is an enclosed bony space adjacent to the root, and provides the best opportunities for bony regeneration by GTR/GBR as any bone graft material would be retained in the defect. The 2-walled defect (middle) is less favorable as a candidate for GTR/GBR surgery as retention of bone graft material in the defect is less predictable. Similarly, the 1-walled defect (bottom) develops when the bony lesion expands through the cortical plate, and has a very poor prognosis for regenerative procedures. The crater defect (not shown) is a circumferential bone defect that wraps around the tooth. It should be remembered that the anatomy of any particular bone defect is very difficult to assess from radiographs or clinical assessment alone, and usually, the defect shape only becomes apparent once a surgical procedure has begun

syndromes and medical conditions. Given the familial link for AP, the family history is especially important when evaluating patients, and if appropriate, the brothers and sisters of affected individuals should also be examined.

Localized AP typically affects the permanent dentition and has an onset around puberty. The prevalence varies and has been reported to be anywhere from around 0.1 percent (e.g. UK) to 0.5 to 0.8 percent (certain populations, e.g. Afro-Caribbeans). There is no predilection for either sex. Localized AP is characterized by pocketing, bleeding on probing and attachment loss localised to the incisor and first molar regions. There is rapid bone loss and destruction of soft tissues. There is a distinctive

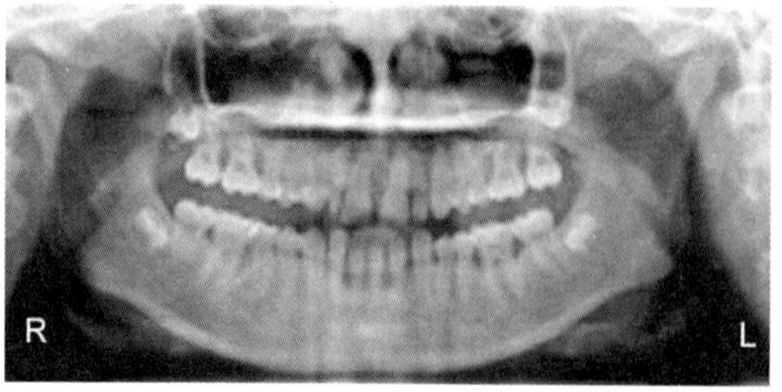

Fig. 3.8: Radiograph appearance of localized aggressive periodontitis. There is extensive alveolar bone loss affecting the first molars and the incisors, particularly the mandibular incisors. Note the vertical bone defects/angular defects at the mesial and distal surfaces of the first molars. Patient age is 16

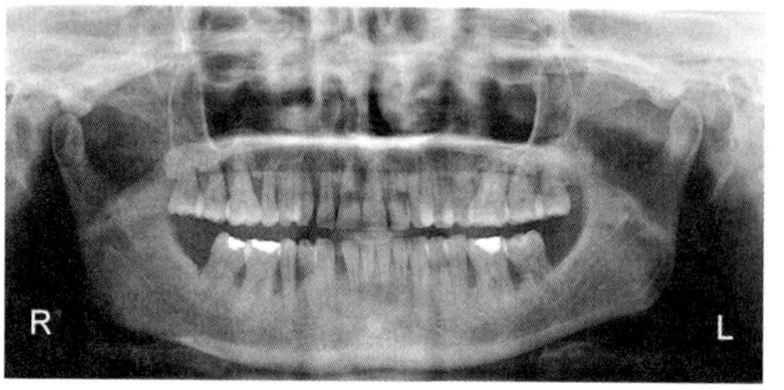

Fig. 3.9: Radiographic appearance of generalized aggressive periodontitis. There is extensive generalized alveolar bone loss, irregular with multiple vertical defects, generally up to 50 to 75 percent of the root length. Patient age is 28

pattern of alveolar bone loss with, typically, bilateral angular defects around first molars and horizontal bone loss around incisors **(Fig. 3.8)**. Up to two other permanent teeth may also be affected within the definition of localized aggressive periodontitis. Increased levels of Aggregatibacter actinomycetemcomitans are typically found in localized AP cases, and this organism has the ability to invade epithelial cells and connective tissues and produces a number of potent virulence factors such as leukotoxin (kills polymorphonuclear leukocytes and macrophages), epitheliotoxin (toxic to epithelial cells) and collagenase (degrades collagen).

The ability of *A. actinomycetemcomitans* to invade the gingival tissues represents a reservoir of infection that is difficult to eradicate by conventional treatment strategies alone. In the past, root surface debridement (RSD) was combined with systemic tetracycline (250 mg four times per day for 2 weeks). However, strains of *A. actinomycetemcomitans* have become resistant to tetracycline, and therefore a combination of amoxicillin (250 mg three times per day) and metronidazole (400 mg three times per day) for 7 days, to coincide with the RSD, is preferred.

Generalized AP is usually identified in individuals somewhere between 25 and 35 years of age. It is characterized by marked gingival inflammation, deep probing depths, bleeding on probing, extensive attachment loss, multiple mobile teeth, purulent exudate from pockets, and often, multiple periodontal abscesses. There is rapid bone resorption, resulting in a generalized, irregular pattern of alveolar bone loss, typically with a combination of vertical and horizontal bone defects (**Fig. 3.9**). Many patients present with a history of prior tooth loss, and most complain of drifting teeth, spacing of teeth, and sometimes displacement or exfoliation of a tooth following a relatively minor traumatic episode.

The microbial flora is typically gram-negative, with *A. actinomycetemcomitans* a common finding, and also *Porphyromonas gingivalis*. There is typically a poor serum antibody response to the bacteria, and it is possible that defects in neutrophil function are present, though this is not routinely tested for. Affected individuals typically have a more aggressive inflammatory host response, characterized by production of elevated levels of inflammatory mediators such as prostaglandin E_2 (PGE_2), interleukin-1β (IL-1β), and tumor necrosis factor-α (TNF-α) in response to the bacteria.

Treatment for generalized AP focuses on extracting any hopeless teeth. RSD is then performed, typically with systemic antibiotic therapy (amoxicillin and metronidazole for 7 days as described earlier) prescribed to coincide with the RSD. Surgical treatment may be indicated to improve access for RSD, assuming that plaque control is of a sufficient standard. In some cases, the disease may eventually become quiescent, or it may progress to a presentation more similar to a slower progressing chronic periodontitis.

MICROBIOLOGY, HISTOLOGY AND PATHOGENESIS

Microbiology

Confirmation of the etiological role for bacteria in causing gingival inflammation was demonstrated in experimental gingivitis studies in the 1960s. Prior to this, the etiology of periodontitis was not known, although calculus was considered to be an irritant to the gingival tissues. The nonspecific plaque hypothesis was postulated, which considered that periodontal disease results from the physical mass of bacteria present, and periodontitis develops once a certain threshold has been reached. In other words, it is the quantity of plaque that is important, rather than the quality. Subsequent research led to the specific plaque hypothesis, which suggested that specific bacteria are causative for periodontal disease, particularly species such as *P. gingivalis*, *A. actinomycetemcomitans* and *Tannerella forsythia* (then known as *Bacteroides forsythus*).

More recently, cluster analysis of subgingival species has demonstrated that certain species commonly occur together in 'complexes'. These have been color coded (red, orange, green, yellow, etc.) representing a progression from health (characterized by a predominantly gram-positive, aerobic, nonmotile microflora) to disease (characterized by a gram-negative, anaerobic, motile microflora). The red complex species (*P. gingivalis, T. forsythia, Treponema denticola*) are strongly associated with advanced periodontitis. The orange complex species (including *Prevotella intermedia, Fusobacterium nucleatum, Peptostreptococcus micros, Campylobacter rectus*) is also associated with periodontitis, but less strongly than the red complex species. Plaque in patients with periodontitis tends to contain a higher proportion of red and orange complex species compared to those who are periodontally healthy.

A major development in the understanding of periodontal microbiology was the concept that plaque bacteria exist in biofilms, which can be defined as matrix enclosed populations adherent to each other and/or surfaces or interfaces. Biofilms are complex bacterial communities that form in aqueous environments where there is a regular nutrient source. Biofilms serve to protect individual bacterial species, and within the biofilm are fluid channels which function almost as a primitive circulatory system (supplying nutrients and removing waste). Quorum sensing allows communication between bacterial species and within the biofilm there is a degree of metabolic cooperation. Biofilms have evolved to protect bacteria, and the matrix within which the bacteria are embedded protects against killing, for example, by phagocytes or antimicrobials. For this reason, the biofilm must always be disrupted by root surface debridement, and if antibiotics are used, they must be used as an adjunct to RSD.

Awareness of the importance of biofilms, together with knowledge gained from the cluster analyses of the microflora has given rise to the most current concept of the role of bacteria in periodontitis, the environmental plaque hypothesis. This suggests that the entire subgingival microbial environment is the important determinant of the role of bacteria in the development of disease, and that disease results from interactions between the subgingival microbial environment and the inflammatory host response. Approximately 300 to 500 bacterial species have been identified in the periodontal pocket, and many more may exist that are, as yet, unknown.

Following professional tooth cleaning, plaque formation occurs within a predictable sequence of events.

Acquired pellicle formation occurs immediately after cleaning as salivary glycoproteins selectively adsorb onto the tooth surface. Acquired pellicle functions as a protective, lubricating layer, but it also allows for bacterial adherence.

Early colonizers (0–7 days after cleaning) begin to colonize the surface. gram-positive cocci (e.g. *Streptococcus* species) and rods (e.g. *Actinomyces* species) predominate at first, and as time progresses, the biofilm becomes increasingly complex with gram-negative cocci (e.g. *Veillonella* species) and rods (e.g. *Capnocytophaga* species) beginning to appear. As the thickness of the biofilm increases, the deeper layers become increasingly anaerobic, and conditions favor the growth of anaerobic species such as *Fusobacterium* species and *Prevotella intermedia*.

Late colonizers adhere and maturation occurs from 7 days onwards. Late colonisers do not adhere directly to the tooth surface and are often virulent species that have been implicated as specific periodontal pathogens, including *P. gingivalis*, motile gram-negative rods, and spirochetes.

Prolonged accumulation of plaque leads to calculus formation (i.e. plaque that has become mineralized by calcium and phosphate ions). Brushite forms first ($CaHPO_4.2H_2O$) and is followed by octacalcium phosphate [$Ca_8(HPO_4)_4$]. Mature calculus contains predominantly crystals of hydroxyapatite [$Ca_{10}(PO_4)_6.OH_2$] and tricalcium phosphate [$Ca_3(PO_4)_2$]. Calculus crystals grow in close proximity to the tooth, gaining mechanical retention in surface irregularities. Supragingival calculus forms as yellow-white deposits at, or just coronal to, the gingival margin, that are frequently stained by tobacco and foods or drinks, and commonly found close to the openings of the ducts of major salivary glands. Subgingival calculus forms apical to the gingival margin, particularly at interproximal surfaces, and appears as dark brown-black deposits on the root surface. It is important to note that calculus is not the cause of periodontal disease. However, it does form a plaque retentive surface that keeps plaque in close contact with the periodontal tissues and compromises oral hygiene.

Bacterial species associated with specific periodontal conditions are indicated in **Box 3.3**. Bacteria must possess a variety of properties in order to colonize periodontal sites. These include adherence, invasion, and tissue damage/evasion strategies. Bacteria must first adhere via surface fimbriae which adhere to components of the acquired pellicle or to other bacteria. Adherence allows bacteria to accumulate and to withstand the mechanical cleaning effects of the oral soft tissues, and saliva and gingival crevicular fluid flow. Certain species have the ability to invade the gingival soft tissues, particularly *A. actinomycetemcomitans* and *P. gingivalis*, which allows for the direct

Box 3.3: Plaque bacteria associated with specific periodontal conditions

Periodontal health

Total recovery of organisms is low, and mainly comprises gram-positive species such as *Streptococcus sanguis, Streptococcus mitis, Actinomyces naeslundii, Actinomyces viscosus*. The predominance of these species may be protective by preventing colonization by more pathogenic species (e.g. *S. sanguis* produces H_2O_2 which is toxic to *A. actinomycetemcomitans*).

Gingivitis

A more complex flora develops, including a mixture of gram-positive and gram-negative species, and aerobic and anaerobic organisms. gram-positive species include the *Streptococcus* and *Actinomyces* species found in health. Gram-negative organisms include *Prevotella intermedia, Fusobacterium nucleatum, Eikenella corrodens* and *Capnocytophaga* species.

Chronic periodontitis

Chronic periodontitis is associated with a complex microflora, and species that are commonly recovered include *Porphyromonas gingivalis, Aggregatibacter actinomycetemcomitans, Tannerella forsythia, P. intermedia, A. naeslundii, Campylobacter rectus, E. corrodens, F. nucleatum, Treponema* and *Eubacterium* species.

Aggressive periodontitis (AP)

A. actinomycetemcomitans is strongly associated with localized AP, and may comprise the majority of cultivable bacteria at affected sites. Other species associated with localized AP include *P. gingivalis, P. intermedia* and *Capnocytophaga* species. Generalized AP is associated with increased prevalence of *P. gingivalis, A. actinomycetemcomitans, T. forsythia, P. intermedia* and *E. corrodens*.

delivery of toxic bacterial products into the tissues. Additionally, bacteria that have invaded the tissues can represent a reservoir of organisms that are not removed by root surface debridement. Many bacteria produce toxic substances as metabolic waste products, such as NH_3, H_2S and short chain carboxylic acids such as butyric acid. Certain species also produce enzymes such as collagenases and other proteases. *P. gingivalis* produces immunoglobulin-degrading proteases, and many strains are encapsulated which protects against phagocytosis. These organisms therefore have the ability to destroy connective tissues, inhibit host defence mechanisms and induce a marked inflammatory response.

Histology and Pathogenesis

Pathogenesis means the sequence of events leading to the occurrence of a disease. A good understanding of the pathogenesis of periodontitis is facilitated by a clear knowledge of the histological changes that occur in inflamed periodontal tissues. **Figure 3.10** shows the histological appearance of healthy gingival tissues, and this contrasts clearly with the histological appearance of inflamed gingival tissues (**Fig. 3.11**).

As plaque bacteria accumulate at the gingival margin, bacterial products (e.g. lipopolysaccharide, LPS) cross the junctional epithelium and invoke an inflammatory response in the gingival tissues. This results in vasodilatation and increased vascular permeability, with leakage of fluid and migration of defence cells into the connective tissues. For descriptive purposes, the inflammatory changes can be described as the initial, early and established gingival lesions, but it should be remembered that these are histological descriptors only, and are not diagnostic criteria to be used when examining a patient.

The *initial gingival lesion* develops after 0 to 4 days of plaque accumulation on a completely clean tooth surface and is characterized by:

- Vascular dilatation and increased vascular permeability, leading to leakage of fluid from the vessels and increased gingival crevicular

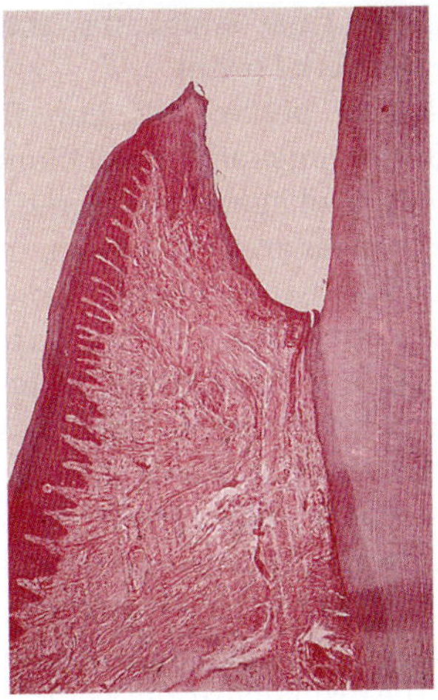

Fig. 3.10: Histological appearance of healthy gingival tissues. There is continuity of the oral epithelium, the sulcular epithelium and the junctional epithelium. The connective tissue is comprised of well ordered, densely packed, collagen fiber bundles. The free gingival margin is a well-defined knife-edge facing the enamel surface. There is no evidence of a significant inflammatory cell infiltrate. Note, the enamel has been lost from this decalcified section

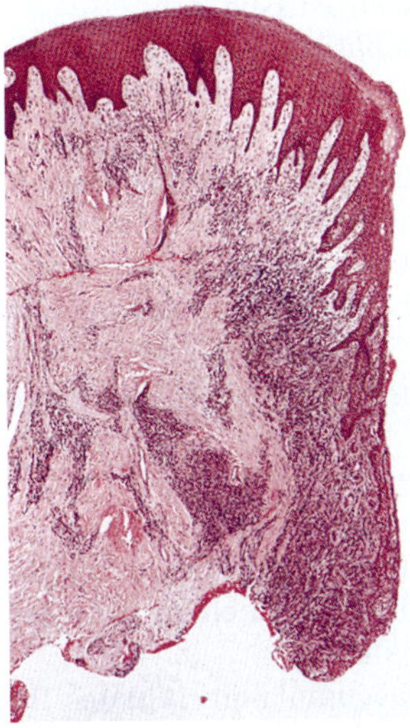

Fig. 3.11: Histological appearance of inflamed gingival tissues. Following plaque accumulation at the gingival margin, there has been infiltration of the connective tissues by numerous defence cells, particularly neutrophils together with plasma cells, monocytes/macrophages and lymphocytes

fluid (GCF) flow, which has the effect of diluting bacterial toxins

- Migration of neutrophils into the tissues through the junctional epithelium and into the sulcus, to phagocytose bacteria.

These changes are evident even in clinically healthy gingival tissues. In other words, even in healthy gingival tissues, there is always evidence of a low grade inflammatory response, with transmigrating neutrophils progressing from the vasculature, up a chemotactic gradient, to enter the sulcus to phagocytose bacteria.

The early gingival lesion develops approximately 4 to 7 days after plaque accumulation and corresponds to the early clinical signs of gingivitis. The histological characteristics are:

- Continued vasodilatation and increased permeability, with increased fluid exudation and continued transmigration of neutrophils
- Breakdown of collagen adjacent to the junctional epithelium
- Accumulation of lymphocytes (particularly T lymphocytes) and macrophages
- Cytotoxic changes in fibroblasts, resulting in reduced capacity for repair
- Proliferation of the junctional and sulcular epithelium into collagen depleted zones of the connective tissue.

The *established gingival lesion* develops after 14 to 21 days of plaque accumulation and corresponds to the clinical signs of chronic gingivitis. Histopathological changes include:

- Further engorgement of blood vessels, resulting in venous stasis and the superimposition of a dark blue tinge over the erythematous gingiva
- Migration of plasma cells into the connective tissues
- Continued transmigration of large numbers of neutrophils
- Significant collagen depletion and proliferation of the epithelium into the collagen depleted areas.

Plaque accumulation initiates the inflammatory responses seen in the gingival tissues. As the plaque matures, the subgingival environment alters to favor the growth of gram-negative species. Edema results in gingival swelling, and a slight deepening of the sulcus, which creates an environment even more favourable for gram-negative species. The inflammatory lesion in the gingiva results in increased GCF flow and products from the tissues are utilised as nutrients by pathogenic organisms. The inflammatory changes also result in increased permeability of the junctional epithelium, allowing bacterial products to penetrate the tissues more easily, resulting in further inflammation. Therefore, there is a dynamic relationship between the subgingival biofilm and the host inflammatory response, and a chronic cycle of inflammation develops.

Chronic gingivitis may persist indefinitely, and the precise mechanisms that convert the lesion to periodontitis are not known. It is likely that alterations in the balance between the biofilm and the host response are important, though at present these are not well defined. The transition from gingivitis to periodontitis is recognized histologically by the development of the advanced inflammatory lesion which is characterized by:

- Vascular proliferation and vasodilatation, vessels are engorged with blood
- Transmigration of the connective tissues by large numbers of neutrophils, plasma cells, lymphocytes and macrophages
- Pocket epithelium becomes very thin and ulcerated, and is very permeable to bacterial products, inflammatory mediators and defence cells
- Extensive collagen depletion and apical migration of the junctional epithelium, resulting in deepening of the pocket
- Osteoclastic bone resorption, driven primarily by host derived mediators such as PGE_2 and IL-1β.

Specific pathogenic mechanisms important in periodontitis are indicated below:

Direct Injury by Plaque Bacteria

Many species produces substances harmful to the tissues, including enzymes such as proteases and collagenases, and metabolic by-products such as NH_3, H_2S and butyric acid. It is clear, however, that direct injury by bacterial products contributes relatively little to the tissue destruction seen in periodontitis, and most of the tissue breakdown results from the activation of host inflammatory and immune processes in response to the presence of bacterial products in the tissues.

Lipopolysaccharide (LPS) is a potent stimulator of immune-inflammatory responses and is found in the outer membrane of gram-negative bacteria. The immune system has evolved to recognise LPS via toll-like receptors (TLRs), a family of cell surface molecules that recognise microbe associated molecular patterns (MAMPs). MAMPs are conserved molecular structures located on diverse pathogens, and TLRs are pattern recognition receptors (PRRs) that recognise MAMPs. TLR-4 recognizes LPS from gram-negative bacteria, and functions as part of a complex of cell surface molecules including CD-14 and MD-2. Interaction of LPS with this CD-14/TLR-4/MD-2 complex triggers a series of intra-cellular events, the net result of which is increased production of inflammatory mediators (most notably cytokines) and the differentiation of immune cells (e.g. dendritic cells) for the development of effective immune responses against the pathogens. It is noteworthy that *P. gingivalis* has an atypical form of LPS which is recognized by both TLR-2 and TLR-4. Lipoteichoic acid (LTA), a component of the cell wall of gram-positive bacteria also signals through TLR-2. LPS and LTA are released from bacteria present in the biofilm and stimulate inflammation in the tissues, leading to vasodilatation, increased vascular permeability, recruitment of inflammatory cells by chemotaxis, and release of proinflammatory mediators by the leukocytes that are recruited to the area.

Proteases produced by bacteria break down structural proteins such as collagen, thereby providing peptides for bacterial nutrition. *P. gingivalis* produces two classes of cysteine proteases which are particularly important in periodontal pathogenesis known as the gingipains. These include the lysine specific gingipain Kgp and the arginine specific gingipains RgpA and RgpB. The gingipains can disrupt immune-inflammatory responses, leading to increased tissue breakdown and can stimulate cytokine secretion via the activation of protease-activated receptors (PARs).

Host Derived Inflammatory Mediators

The inflammatory and immune processes that develop in the periodontal tissues in response to the subgingival biofilm are protective by intent, but result in considerable tissue damage. It is therefore important to review the key mediators that orchestrate the host response and that lead to the observed tissue destruction. These can be broadly be divided into the cytokines, the prostanoids and the matrix metalloproteinases.

Cytokines

Cytokines are soluble proteins and act as messengers to transmit messages from one cell to another. They bind to specific receptors on target cells and initiate intracellular signaling cascades that result in phenotypic changes in the cell via altered gene regulation. They are effective at very low concentrations, are able to induce their own expression either in an autocrine or paracrine fashion, and have pleiotropic effects (i.e. multiple biological activities) on a large number of cell types. They are key inflammatory mediators in periodontitis and are produced by a large number of cell types including infiltrating inflammatory cells such as neutrophils, macrophages and lymphocytes, and also by resident cells in the periodontium such as fibroblasts and epithelial cells. Cytokines are of fundamental importance in amplifying immune responses and combating infections, but they also have profound biological effects that lead to tissue damage in chronic inflammation. For example, cytokines mediate connective tissue and alveolar bone destruction through the induction of fibroblasts and osteoclasts to produce proteolytic enzymes (i.e. matrix metalloproteinases) that break down the structural components of these tissues. Cytokines do not act in isolation but in flexible and complex networks that involve both pro-inflammatory and anti-inflammatory effects and that bring together aspects of both innate and acquired immunity. Cytokines play a key role in all stages of the immune response in periodontal disease. Key cytokines relevant in periodontal pathogenesis are listed below.

Interleukin-1β

Interleukin-1β (1L-1β) plays a key role in infection and immunity, and induces the synthesis and secretion of other inflammatory mediators such as PGE_2. IL-1β is produced by macrophages, monocytes, neutrophils, fibroblasts, keratinocytes, epithelial cells, B-cells and osteocytes. It synergizes with other pro-inflammatory cytokines and PGE_2 to induce bone resorption, and GCF concentrations of IL-1β are increased at sites of gingivitis and periodontitis.

Tumor Necrosis Factor-α

Tumor Necrosis Factor-α (TNF-α) is a key inflammatory mediator in periodontal disease that shares many of the cellular actions of IL-1β. It plays a fundamental role in immune responses, increases neutrophil activity and tissue turnover by inducing MMP secretion. TNF-α is secreted by activated macrophages and other cell types, particularly in response to LPS. TNF-α has pro-inflammatory effects including stimulating endothelial cells to express selectins that facilitate leukocyte recruitment, activation of IL-1β production and induction of PGE_2. TNF-α, though having similar pro-inflammatory activity to IL-1β has much less potent effects on osteoclasts.

Interleukin-6

Interleukin-6 (IL-6) is a member of a group of cytokines that includes IL-11, leukemia inhibitory factor (LIF) and oncostatin M that share common signaling pathways via signal transducers gp130. IL-6 is the most studied, and has multiple pleiotropic properties. IL-6 secretion is stimulated by IL-1β and TNF-α and is produced by a range of cells including T-cells, B-cells, macrophages and dendritic cells. It is also secreted by osteoblasts and stimulates bone resorption and the formation of osteoclasts.

Interleukin-1α

Interleukin-6 (1L-1α) is primarily an intracellular protein that is not normally secreted, and likely mediates inflammation only when released from necrotic cells, acting as a signal to indicate tissue damage. IL-1α is a potent bone resorbing agent, but its precise role in periodontitis is not clear.

Interleukin-1 Receptor Antagonist

Interleukin-1 Receptor Antagonist (IL-1Ra) has structural homology to IL-1β and binds to the IL-1 receptor (IL-1R1). However, binding of IL-1Ra does not result in signal transduction and therefore IL-1Ra antagonizes the activity of IL-1β (i.e. it is therefore anti-inflammatory).

Prostaglandins

The prostaglandins are a group of lipid compounds derived from arachidonic acid, a fatty acid found in the plasma membrane of most cells. Arachidonic acid is metabolised by cyclooxygenase-1 and -2 (COX-1 and COX-2) to generate a series of related compounds called the prostanoids, which include the prostaglandins, thromboxanes and prostacyclins. Prostaglandin E_2 (PGE_2) is by far the most important in periodontal pathogenesis, and results in vasodilatation, and induces cytokine secretion. COX-2 is upregulated by IL-1β, TNF-α and LPS, resulting in increased production of PGE_2 in inflamed periodontal tissues. In the periodontium, PGE_2 is primarily secreted by macrophages and fibroblasts. PGE_2 results in induction of matrix metalloproteinases and osteoclastic bone resorption and has a major role in contributing to the tissue damage seen in periodontitis.

Matrix Metalloproteinases

Matrix Metalloproteinases (MMPs) are a family of zinc-dependent enzymes that are capable of degrading extracellular matrix molecules, including collagens. MMPs play a key role in periodontal tissue destruction and are secreted by the majority of cell types in the periodontium, including fibroblasts, keratinocytes, endothelial cells, neutrophils and macrophages. In healthy tissues, MMPs are mainly produced by fibroblasts, which produce MMP-1 (also known as collagenase-1) which has a primary role in normal collagen turnover in the tissues. Transcription of genes coding for MMPs is upregulated by cytokines such as IL-1β and TNF-α. MMP activity is regulated by specific endogenous tissue inhibitors of metalloproteinases (TIMPs) and serum glycoproteins such as α-macroglobulins. In inflamed tissues, excessive quantities of MMPs are secreted by resident cells and the large numbers of transmigrating inflammatory cells, particularly neutrophils, as they migrate through the tissues. As a result, the balance between MMPs and their inhibitors is disrupted, resulting in breakdown of the connective tissue matrix. The predominant MMPs in periodontitis are MMP-8 (also known as collagenase-2 and also as neutrophil collagenase) and MMP-9 (also known as gelatinase B), both of which are secreted by neutrophils, and are very effective at degrading type 1 collagen. MMP-8 and MMP-9 levels are increased at sites of active disease and these MMPs contribute significantly to the tissue damage that occurs as periodontal disease progresses.

Increased understanding of the importance of MMPs in periodontal pathogenesis has led to the development of a systemic drug therapy to modulate the inflammatory response by inhibiting MMP levels. Doxycycline has been used for this indication, at subantimicrobial doses of 20 mg twice daily for periods of 3 months at a time. Doxycycline, like all the tetracyclines, has the ability to downregulate MMPs, and the subantimicrobial dose has been shown to inhibit collagenase activity in the periodontal tissues with no evidence of antibiotic effects. This forms the basis for the concept known as host response modulation, i.e. a treatment methodology used in addition to conventional treatment (RSD) to reduce destructive aspects of the host response.

Pathogenesis and Clinical Signs of Disease

It is important to remember how pathogenesis influences the clinical presentation. Clinically healthy gingival tissues may demonstrate signs of inflammation when histological sections are examined. Transmigrating neutrophils are evident, moving up a chemotactic gradient towards the sulcus to phagocytose bacteria. If the bacterial challenge persists, the cellular and fluid infiltration continues to develop and neutrophils and other inflammatory cells soon occupy a significant volume of the inflamed gingival tissues. Neutrophils are very important for bacterial killing and are defensive cells. However, they release large quantities of destructive enzymes such as MMPs as they migrate through the tissues, resulting in collagen depletion in the connective tissues. They also release potent lysosomal enzymes and reactive oxygen species (ROS, for example, superoxide, $\bullet O_2^-$, and hydrogen peroxide H_2O_2) extracellularly, causing further tissue damage. Degeneration of fibroblasts limits opportunities for repair, and the epithelium proliferates apically, deepening the pocket further, which is rapidly colonised by subgingival bacteria. The very first steps in the development of the pocket result from a combination of factors including:

- Edema of the inflamed gingival tissues
- Detachment of cells at the coronal aspect of the junctional epithelium while those at the apical aspect migrate apically into the collagen depleted areas
- Intraepithelial cleavage within the junctional epithelium.

A cycle of chronic inflammation is established in which the subgingival biofilm drives inflammatory responses in the periodontium, characterised by infiltration by leukocytes, release of inflammatory mediators and destructive enzymes, connective tissue breakdown, and breakdown and proliferation of the epithelium in an apical direction. The pocket epithelium becomes thin and ulcerated and bleeds more easily (bleeding on probing). The inflamed junctional epithelium is less able to withstand penetration by a periodontal probe (probing depths increase). The bacteria in the pocket are never fully eliminated, as they are effectively outside the body. Attempts at effective oral hygiene are rendered more difficult by the deepening of the pocket, and the cycle continues.

As the advancing inflammatory front approaches the alveolar bone, osteoclastic bone resorption commences. This is protective, to prevent bacterial invasion of the bone, but ultimately contributes to tooth mobility and tooth loss. Resorption of alveolar bone occurs simultaneously with breakdown of periodontal ligament fibers. For bone loss to occur, the concentrations of inflammatory mediators in the gingival tissues must be sufficient to activate pathways that lead to bone resorption and the mediators must penetrate to within a critical distance of the alveolar bone. Histological studies have demonstrated that the bone resorbs such that there is always a width of noninfiltrated connective tissue of about 0.5 to 1.0 mm overlying the bone. Osteoclasts are stimulated to resorb bone by cytokines, prostaglandins and other inflammatory mediators, and the bone thereby 'retreats' from the advancing inflammatory front.

Bone turnover is also controlled by the RANK/RANK-L/OPG system. RANK is the receptor activator of nuclear factor-kappa, and is a cell surface receptor expressed by osteoclasts. RANK-L (RANK-ligand) is a ligand that binds to RANK, and is expressed by bone stromal cells, osteoblasts and fibroblasts. Binding of RANK-L to RANK results in osteoclast differentiation and activation, leading to bone resorption. OPG (osteoprotegerin) is another ligand that binds to RANK. Hence, RANK-L and OPG are both cytokines that bind to RANK. However, whereas RANK-L promotes activation and differentiation of osteoclasts, OPG has the opposite effect, inhibiting osteoclast differentiation. The balance between OPG and RANK-L activity can therefore drive bone resorption or bone formation. IL-1β and TNF-α regulate the expression of RANK-L, leading to activation of osteoclasts via RANK and therefore bone resorption. It has been reported that RANK-L levels are higher, and OPG levels are lower, in patients with periodontitis compared to those with healthy gingiva. The balance between RANK-L and OPG is an example of the importance of balance between pro-inflammatory and anti-inflammatory mediators in periodontal homeostasis, and factors that act to tip the balance in favor of inflammation and tissue destruction will contribute to progression of periodontal disease.

PERIODONTAL—SYSTEMIC INTERFACE

A number of systemic diseases have been associated with periodontal disease in epidemiological studies. These include diabetes and cardiovascular disease, and also the impact of periodontal disease on the risk for adverse pregnancy outcomes.

Diabetes

Many studies have reported that type 2 diabetes mellitus (T2DM) is a major risk factor for periodontal disease, particularly if the diabetes is poorly controlled. In T2DM, the main causal processes are insulin resistance (i.e. an inability of the body to respond normally to insulin) and a failure of pancreatic β cells to produce sufficient insulin. This results in hyperglycemia which in turn has wide ranging molecular and cellular effects resulting in oxidative stress, upregulation of proinflammatory responses and vascular changes that collectively predispose patients to the complications of diabetes. T2DM is regarded as an inflammatory disease, and inflammation underpins the mechanisms that link T2DM and periodontal disease.

Plasma levels of IL-6 and TNF-α are increased in patients with T2DM, and a major source of these cytokines is the adipose tissue. Adipose tissue used to be considered a passive storage system for lipids, but is now recognized as an active endocrine organ, secreting a variety of hormones and mediators, collectively known as adipokines, including IL-6 and TNF-α. Other important adipokines include leptin (proinflammatory) and adiponectin (anti-inflammatory). In T2DM, there are elevated levels of circulating cytokines and adipokines, and these may contribute to a heightened inflammatory state in the periodontal tissues, contributing to increased periodontal disease in individuals with diabetes.

Impaired or dysregulated PMN function may be a further mechanistic link between T2DM and periodontal disease. Altered PMN function has been reported in patients with T2DM, and studies have correlated both periodontitis and diabetes with defective PMN chemotaxis. Diabetes may also increase susceptibility to periodontitis via impaired PMN apoptosis. Apoptosis (programmed cell death) is a mechanism by which superfluous or damaged cells are selectively removed by phagocytic cells without resulting in inflammation. However, PMN apoptosis is defective in diabetes, resulting in increased retention of neutrophils in the periodontal tissues, which could result in increased tissue breakdown by prolonged release of MMPs and ROS from the neutrophils.

In the hyperglycemic state, structural proteins undergo a nonenzymatic glycosylation process to form advanced glycation endproducts (AGEs). The receptor for AGE, RAGE, on macrophages leads to upregulation of proinflammatory cytokines such as IL-1β, IL-6 and TNF-α upon binding to AGEs, and this results in increased inflammation in the tissues. AGEs also enhance the respiratory burst of PMN NADPH oxidases, which are active in the phagosome during phagocytosis.

There are therefore a variety of mechanisms which are likely to link periodontal disease and diabetes. Given that both are inflammatory conditions, there is the potential that periodontal treatment in patients with diabetes could possibly improve glycemic control, but this remains to be definitively proven. However, it is clear that all patients with diabetes should be very carefully examined to check for the signs of periodontitis, and asked about their level of glycaemic control. Patients with well controlled diabetes do not appear to be at increased risk for periodontitis compared to nondiabetic individuals. For those patients with periodontitis and poorly controlled diabetes, it is worth liaising with the medical practitioner to highlight the problem of periodontitis, and to provide support for improving diabetes control as well as providing the necessary periodontal treatment.

Coronary Heart Disease

A number of studies have been published that have demonstrated an apparent link between the presence of periodontitis and the risk for coronary heart disease (CHD). Reviews of the causality of these relationships have been inconclusive, however. The main problem is the confounding variables, and periodontal disease shares known risk factors for CHD, particularly smoking. Accounting for confounding variables such as smoking, stress and other lifestyle factors is very difficult when assessing risk, given that both diseases are chronic inflammatory conditions that affect a large number of individuals. It is reasonable to suggest that there may be an increased risk for CHD in periodontitis patients, but this is far from proven at the present time. Some of the mechanisms that potentially link periodontitis and CHD are described below, and all may play a role in linking the two conditions.

Direct bacterial effect: Patients with periodontitis have a large surface area of inflamed, ulcerated pocket epithelium that interacts with the subgingival biofilm. Within the biofilm are a number of species that could gain access to the circulation and lead to coronary events. *P. gingivalis* has been found in carotid and coronary atheromatous plaques, giving rise to speculation that it could precipitate rupture of the fibrous membrane and lead to either unstable angina or a further myocardial infarction.

Indirect inflammatory effects: Periodontitis induces an inflammatory response that elevates levels of acute phase proteins such as C-reactive protein (CRP) and fibrinogen. CRP and fibrinogen are independent risk factors for CHD and both have been related to poor periodontal health. Other inflammatory mediators such as cytokines produced during periodontal inflammation may also gain access to the circulation, resulting in proinflammatory effects elsewhere in the body.

Common genetic predisposition: Interest has also focused on the so-called hyperinflammatory phenotype, and this may provide both a cellular and molecular link between periodontal disease and CHD. A hyperinflammatory immune response could increase the susceptibility to both conditions. In the context of periodontitis, a hyperinflammatory trait would result in increased production of cytokines and other inflammatory mediators in response to LPS challenge, resulting in increased periodontal breakdown. In the context of CHD, mediators such as IL-1β, TNF-α and thromboxane A_2 (TxA_2, released following arachidonic acid metabolism) can initiate platelet aggregation and promote the formation of lipid-laden foam cells and the deposition of cholesterol in the vascular intima. Monocyte activity can also be influenced by various lipid transport molecules, with low density lipoproteins upregulating secretion of IL-1β, TNF-α and TxA_2.

Shared risk factors: Shared risk factors such as smoking and stress may also contribute to associations between periodontitis and CHD, and future studies must control for these. Oral hygiene could also be a surrogate indicator for lifestyle factors that impact on personal hygiene and healthcare.

Pregnancy Outcomes

Some studies have identified associations between adverse pregnancy outcomes, such as preterm low birth weight babies and periodontal disease. However, many studies that have investigated this issue have found no association. Therefore, at present there is insufficient evidence to determine whether periodontal disease truly has an impact on pregnancy outcomes and research is ongoing. Preterm birth refers to delivery before 37 weeks, and low birth weight means <2,500 g. There are potentially two mechanisms by which periodontal disease may affect pregnancy outcomes. The first is that periodontal bacteria gain access to the circulation (via the inflamed pocket epithelium in patients with periodontitis), and cause inflammation elsewhere in the body. The second is that inflammatory mediators released in periodontal disease (such as cytokines and prostaglandins) gain access to the circulatory system, and these affect placental viability and initiate contractions prematurely. Risks for preterm birth include the age of the mother (greater risk if <18 or >35 years old), genetic predisposition, being over- or underweight before pregnancy, short stature, low socioeconomic status, infection, stress and obesity. It is clear that several of these risks are also risk factors for periodontal disease. At the present, there is no convincing evidence of a strong link between adverse pregnancy outcomes and periodontal disease. No studies have demonstrated causality, and in general in those studies that report an association, the associations are weak. Most of the studies are underpowered and more research is necessary. It has been confirmed, however, that periodontal treatment in pregnant mothers is safe.

TREATMENT OF PERIODONTAL DISEASE

Treatment of periodontal disease is unlike any other form of dental treatment, and this is for one reason: the patient must be an active partner in the management of their condition. For just about all other forms of dental treatment (extractions, restorations, etc.), the onus of responsibility rests firmly with the clinician. All the patient is needed to do is sit in the dental chair while the work is performed. It is understandable, therefore, that many patients feel that the dentist is responsible for the management of all their dental problems. However, this just won't work for periodontal disease. Patients must be educated about the importance of their role in managing their condition, and must work together with the dental team to achieve the shared objectives of therapy. The dental team must spend the time to educate the patient, perform excellent treatment, and also support the patient during the longer term. Periodontal disease is a chronic disease, and its management should also be regarded as a chronic management strategy. It is also very important to avoid blame, and be empathetic and supportive of patients with periodontal disease.

It is very important to ask the question "why do we do periodontal treatment?". The aim is resolution of inflammation, and this can be achieved through a variety of means: plaque control, RSD, adjunctive treatments. Resolution of inflammation will result in reductions in probing depths through shrinkage of the tissues, reduced penetration of the probe tip, and formation of a long junctional epithelium. Shallower pockets favor a less pathogenic microflora, and importantly, are easier to keep clean (both by the patient and the clinician). Inflammation drives the destructive processes forwards, so resolution of inflammation should have the effect of halting disease progression. A variety of factors will determine the success of treatment, including compliance, plaque control, the quality of treatment provided, the patient's inflammatory responses, genetic factors, and exposure to risk factors such as smoking. Historically, periodontal treatment has focussed solely on plaque control and the therapy provided by the clinician (nonsurgical or surgical). However, it is clear that there are many aspects of the pathogenic process that could be targeted as part of periodontal therapy (e.g. risk factor modification, resolution of inflammation) in addition to the traditional approaches of oral hygiene instruction and RSD.

Some key aspects of modern periodontal therapy are:

- *Patient education and empowering*—essential for successful management, achieved via personalized biofeedback.
- *Setting targets*—shared targets with the patient, such as prevention of tooth loss (specific teeth), reducing the number of pockets that are 5+ mm to, for example, <10 percent of the number of 5+ mm pockets that the patient presented with, eliminating bleeding on probing, eliminating halitosis.
- *High quality therapy*—multiple, frequent episodes of RSD, ideally with ultrasonics.
- Long-term maintenance care, with frequent recall and monitoring.

Plaque Control

Without effective plaque control, all periodontal treatments are doomed to failure. Plaque control is a shared responsibility between the patient and the clinician. Instructing patients in plaque control techniques should be done in their mouth using a mirror (personalized biofeedback), and should be reviewed on a regular basis. It is useful to take digital photos of the patient performing the necessary techniques in their own mouth and printing them to give to the patient so they can copy the same techniques when they get home. Key aspects of plaque control are listed below.

Manual Toothbrush

Bass technique is appropriate for most patients: toothbrush is placed at gingival margin with bristles orientated at 45° to the long axis of the tooth, pointing apically. Short vibratory strokes are applied (this forces the bristles interproximally and approximately 1 to 2 mm subgingivally, resulting in gingival blanching). After about 20 strokes the brush is repositioned to the next section of teeth. A horizontal scrubbing action should be avoided, as this can result in abrasion cavities and gingival recession. Hard bristles should be avoided for the same reason. Soft bristles will reach subgingivally more effectively.

Single Tufted Toothbrush

One of the most useful brushes money can buy! Useful in recession defects, around single standing teeth, around appliances, at areas of crowding, and as a general purpose brush throughout the dentition (in addition to manual brush). Should be used with the same 45° orientation as the manual brush, so the bristles penetrate subgingivally (**Fig. 3.12**).

Powered Brush

Usually have compact heads, which can improve access. Studies have confirmed, in general, slight superiority compared to manual brushes in terms of plaque removal. Can be very beneficial for those with limited dexterity. Method of use is completely different from manual brush. Powered brush head is placed against the tooth surface next to the gingival margin, and then held in place while the brush action cleans the surface.

Dental Floss

Essential for interproximal cleaning, particularly in patients with no recession or attachment loss and tight contacts between teeth. Toothbrushes

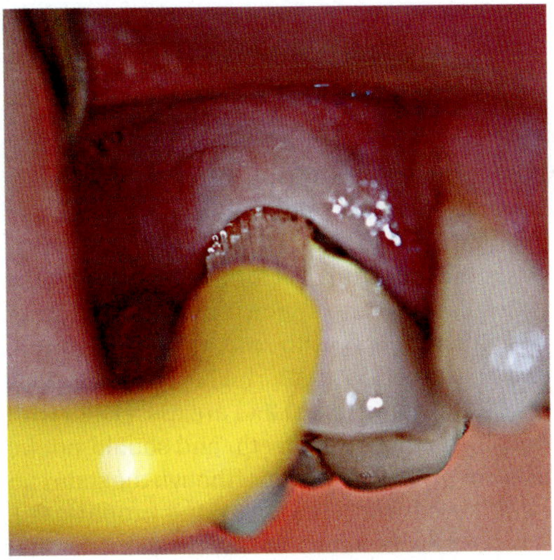

Fig. 3.12: Single tufted toothbrush

generally are unable to reach fully into the interproximal surfaces, therefore floss should be used. Remember, most patients who say they can't use floss are really saying that they won't use floss. Therefore, careful patient education is necessary.

Bottle Brushes

Used for interproximal cleaning where there is space to do so, i.e. in patients with recession and attachment loss. As a general rule, the largest bottle brush that will fit through a given interproximal space should be used, and the brush should be slightly curved with the curve pointing in an apical direction to facilitate subgingival cleaning in the interproximal space. These brushes should not be used with toothpaste, because of the tight confines of the interproximal space that would result in interproximal abrasion defects if paste were used.

Toothpastes

Toothpastes are used as aids for cleaning tooth surfaces, and contain abrasives (e.g. silica), water, preservatives, flavoring, coloring, detergents, and therapeutic agents (e.g. fluoride). Abrasives can constitute 20 to 40 percent of the paste, and enhance plaque removal, but can also contribute to abrasion if brushing is overzealous. Smokers' pastes and tooth powders are particularly abrasive and should not be used.

Mouthrinses

Mouthrinses are a means of chemical plaque control, and the most effective agents are chlorhexidine and the essential oils mouthrinses (Listerine). Binding of chlorhexidine to bacterial cell walls causes disruption of the osmotic barrier and interference with membrane transport, resulting in cell death. The higher concentrations of chlorhexidine (e.g. 0.2%) are associated with brown staining of the teeth, and should not be used for prolonged periods (though the stain can be removed with ultrasonics and prophylaxis). Lower concentrations of chlorhexidine do not suffer from the same problems.

Root Surface Debridement (RSD)

Root surface debridement (RSD) (sometimes referred to as root surface instrumentation) is the preferred term for the procedures that used to be referred to as scaling and root planing (SRP), *see* **Box 3.4**. RSD is generally undertaken with various hand instruments and/or ultrasonic instruments (**Box 3.5**). As a result of RSD, the biofilm is disrupted, there is a reduction in the bacterial challenge by removal of plaque, and calculus is removed. This leads to shrinkage of the gingival tissues (as edema resolves), increased resistance of the tissues at the base of the pocket to penetration by the probe tip (as inflammation resolves), and the formation of a long junctional epithelium. All of these mechanisms contribute to the reduction in probing depths observed after effective nonsurgical therapy, although gingival shrinkage and resolution of inflammation contribute most to the probing reductions observed after RSD.

The magnitude of the probing depth reductions and attachment gains that can be expected following RSD depend on the depth of the pocket prior to treatment:

- Pockets initially 4 to 6 mm deep will demonstrate probing depth reductions of 1.0 to 1.5 mm and attachment gains of 0 to 0.5 mm following RSD
- Pockets initially ≥ 7 mm will demonstrate probing depth reductions of 2.0 to 3.0 mm and attachment gains of 1.0 to 2.0 mm following RSD.

It is important to note that in healthy sites (probing depths ≤ 3 mm), vigorous instrumentation may result in probing depth increases and attachment loss as a result of trauma, and therefore instrumentation in healthy sites should be undertaken very carefully and gently.

It is also important to leave sufficient time following RSD before probing again to evaluate the outcome. Periodontitis is a chronic disease and requires a chronic, long-term approach to management. Resolution of inflammation is a slow process that requires commitment and compliance by the patient and the clinician. Therefore, probing too soon after undertaking RSD is likely to be a disappointing experience because the improvements that are yet to be

Box 3.4: What is in a name? RSD vs. SRP

Scaling and root planing (SRP) is no longer considered an appropriate term to describe the non-surgical instrumentation of root surfaces as part of periodontal therapy. Root planing is not a procedure that dentists should be performing. Root planing derives from a time when it was considered necessary to remove a substantial amount of cementum from the root surface to 'detoxify' the root. Accordingly, dentists spent considerable efforts laboriously planing away the root surface to achieve a 'glassy hard smooth surface'.

However subsequent research identified the following:

- Periodontal healing can occur equally well on rough surfaces as smooth surfaces
- No matter what form of instrumentation is used, some calculus always remains, so the argument of planing the root to achieve total calculus removal is not valid
- It is not necessary to plane the root surface to remove the majority of the LPS in the cementum, indeed, most can be removed by simple polishing.

Furthermore, planing the root removes substantial quantities of cementum, which over time can result in tooth sensitivity. It has been estimated that 10–12 strokes with a manual instrument to plane the root surface removes approximately 100 µm of cementum (i.e. one-tenth of a mm), whereas 10–12 strokes with an ultrasonic instrument removes approximately 10 µm of cementum. It is easy to imagine that a patient undergoing long term periodontal maintenance care would lose all of their cementum to root planing if it were performed at every maintenance visit.

Therefore, the term **root surface debridement (RSD)** is now preferred. The aims of RSD are:

- Disrupt the subgingival biofilm
- Remove plaque and calculus
- Create an environment more compatible with healing.

RSD can be performed equally well with ultrasonics, hand instruments or a combination of both. The key technique is *multiple, overlapping, light strokes* with the instrument being used. The aim is not to plane the root surface. Ultrasonics are quicker than hand instruments, and may be better tolerated by patients. Clinical outcomes are similar, but speed of treatment is an advantage with ultrasonics.

A disadvantage with ultrasonics is that they are universal instruments, i.e. designed to be used at most areas in the mouth, whereas many hand instruments (e.g. Graceys) are area specific, with different instruments being designed specifically for different areas. A combination of ultrasonics and hand instruments is therefore desirable when treating patients.

Scaling is a term used to describe removal of mainly supragingival calculus, and again this can be undertaken with ultrasonic and/or hand instruments. In many ways, scaling is almost a cosmetic procedure, and is not a therapy for periodontitis in the same way that RSD is.

realised will not be fully evident. Furthermore, inappropriate decisions about the need for further treatment may then be made. Therefore, a minimum of 3 months should be allowed before probing to evaluate the treatment outcome. The patient must not be 'abandoned' during this time, but must be supported to maximize their plaque control with frequent short recall appointments, e.g. monthly, for reinforcement of oral hygiene instruction and prophylaxis.

Full mouth disinfection (FMD) is a treatment strategy that involves performing all the instrumentation required within a short time period, typically within 24 hours. The original hypothesis that led to this approach was that quadrant-by-quadrant treatment, with quadrants being instrumented at weekly intervals, could lead to compromised outcomes as a result of recolonization of treated quadrants by bacteria from as yet untreated quadrants. Research has indicated that typically, the outcomes following FMD are similar to those achieved by quadrant RSD, and therefore the decision to perform FMD or not is based on patient and operator preference. Many patients prefer this more efficient treatment strategy, and ultrasonics should be mainly used to further improve efficiency. The original FMD protocols

Box 3.5: Periodontal instruments

Periodontal explorer: Used to detect subgingival calculus deposits, typically are very light instruments (to improve tactile sensitivity) with fine curved tips to reach subgingivally.

Sickle scaler: Strong, heavy instruments used to remove supragingival calculus. Have two cutting surfaces that converge in a sharp tip. Should not be used subgingivally because of likely trauma to the soft tissues. Inserted under ledges of calculus and used with a pull stroke to remove the calculus.

Curettes: Fine instruments, used for subgingival RSD. They are designed to adapt to the root surface and provide good access to deep pockets without causing trauma. They have a spoon-shaped blade with a rounded tip, and two cutting surfaces. They can be area specific, i.e. designed to adapt to specific anatomical areas of the dentition and are used to instrument specific surfaces. Or, they can be universal curettes that afford access to any/all root surfaces by altering the position and angulation of the instrument.

Periodontal hoes: Used for removal of calculus from broad, flat root surfaces. Inserted into the pocket, placed against the tooth surface and pulled coronally to remove calculus. Should not be used in furcations as they will traumatize the root surface and create plaque-retentive grooves.

Chisels: Used to clean interproximal surfaces of teeth such as the mandibular anterior teeth (also referred to as push scalers). They are inserted from the buccal and pushed lingually (with protection for the tongue provided by a mouth mirror)

Ultrasonic instruments: An alternating current in the handpiece creates an alternating magnetic field that results in slight expansion and contraction of the metal coil, so that the tip vibrates at up to 50,000 Hz. A variety of inserts (tips) are available for instrumentation. Water cooling is essential to dissipate the heat generated by the vibrations, and for the same reason, the tip must be kept moving (to prevent heat build-up and gouging). The vibrating tip shatters cementum attached to the root surface, and all sides of the tip are working. Within the water spray, water droplets collapse creating microscopic vacuums, releasing energy (this process is called cavitation) which enhances the removal of deposits.

also called for the use of chlorhexidine to reduce bacteria in the pockets after instrumentation (by irrigation into the pockets), and also in other anatomical niches such as the dorsum of the tongue, buccal mucosa and tonsils (by using chlorhexidine mouthrinse and spray for the tonsils). The contribution of chlorhexidine to the improvements observed following FMD is not completely clear, however, and again, it remains a personal choice whether it is used as part of FMD protocols. In all cases, excellent plaque control must be achieved.

Adjunctive Treatments

The use of adjunctive systemic antibiotics in the management of periodontal disease should be limited to the following conditions:

- Necrotizing ulcerative gingivitis
- Multiple or severe periodontal abscesses with involvement of regional lymph nodes
- Some cases of aggressive periodontitis (including localized and generalized forms).

In all cases, systemic antibiotics should be used as an adjunct, i.e. in addition to conventional forms of periodontal therapy. The bacteria in the subgingival biofilm are much more resistant to killing by antibiotics than free floating planktonic bacteria, and therefore, to derive maximal benefit from systemic antibiotics, RSD must also be performed to disrupt the biofilm. There is no indication to prescribe antibiotics for the treatment of chronic periodontitis as there are no clear benefits over and above those achieved by RSD alone, and given the prevalence of chronic periodontitis, such a treatment strategy would greatly increase the risk of antibiotic resistance at a population level.

Antimicrobials (e.g. chlorhexidine, doxycycline) have also been incorporated into slow release delivery systems administered directly into the periodontal pocket. This results in a high concentration locally with minimal systemic exposure, and potentially, a prolonged duration of action. However, GCF flow will tend to wash away these products if they are too fluid, which can limit their efficacy. Typically, these tend to be used after an initial course of RSD in which the majority of sites might have improved but there are still some remaining deeper pockets. Further RSD is provided at those sites together with placement of a local delivery system.

Host response modulation is a treatment concept in which an adjunctive systemic therapy is used to modify destructive aspects of the host response. Doxycycline has been investigated for this indication, as, like all tetracyclines, it inhibits MMP activity, even at low doses which have no antibiotic effect. Therefore, 20 mg twice daily for periods of 3 months at a time has been shown to improve outcomes following RSD by about 30 percent, whether considering mean probing depth reductions, or percent of sites demonstrating clinically significant reductions in probing depths. The use of this dose of doxycycline (referred to as subantimicrobial dose doxycycline) has not been associated with the development of antibiotic resistance.

Risk Factor Management

Risk factor management must be an integral part of all periodontal therapy. This can include management of local risk factors (e.g. removal of overhangs) or systemic risk factors such as smoking. Smoking has multiple negative impacts on immune-inflammatory responses that increase susceptibility to periodontitis including:

- Altered neutrophil chemotaxis, phagocytosis and oxidative burst
- Increased levels of proinflammatory mediators (TNF-α, PGE_2) and MMPs in GCF
- Vasoconstrictive effects on gingival vasculature and reduced GCF flow.

Patients must be educated about the importance of eliminating risk factors, and must be helped to quit smoking. It has been estimated that more than half of the cases of periodontitis (in the US population) are attributable to smoking. Smoking cessation must be an integral part of the management of dental patients who smoke, and the dental team is ideally placed to support patients as they attempt to quit.

Maintenance Care

Periodontitis is a chronic disease, and its treatment must be regarded as a chronic management process. It is not sufficient to provide one course of RSD and assume that the problems are over. Patients need many years of therapy, including, usually, an initial intensive period of periodontal treatment, and then prolonged phases of periodontal maintenance care, interspersed with more active phases of treatment when indicated clinically. In many ways, the long term maintenance care is the most important part of treatment. It is during this phase that the improvements achieved in the initial therapy (e.g. reductions in probing depths) can be capitalised upon, or alternatively, if the patient is not adequately supported, then treatment can start to fail. Communication is yet again the key: patients must be aware of their need for long term periodontal therapy, and the dental team must support patients during this difficult time. The research literature confirms that if patients are seen regularly for many years, receiving appropriate support, motivation and empowerment, together with correct clinical management (frequent prophylaxis, repeated instrumentation) then their periodontal condition can be stabilised. Key aspects of periodontal maintenance care include:

- Regular and frequent recall period, usually every 2 to 3 months after the initial treatment is completed, and can later be lengthened to every 3 to 4 months if patient demonstrates good plaque control and good resolution of inflammation
- Regular and repeated reinforcement of oral hygiene instruction, focusing on the patient's specific needs
- *Regular prophylaxis:* Full mouth polishing (ideally with rubber cup to go slightly subgingival) at every maintenance visit
- *Ultrasonic instrumentation:* Repeated, gentle (multiple light strokes) instrumentation with ultrasonics to disrupt the subgingival biofilm and remove reforming calculus deposits

- *Monitoring of probing depths:* Annual full periodontal charting required. Don't rely on the BPE as this is not a good system for monitoring patients post-treatment.

Surgical Therapy

One of the limitations of RSD is that the subgingival environment is not visible during the treatment procedure. Therefore, the main reason for performing periodontal surgery is usually to improve access for cleaning—both for the operator during the surgical procedure, and also for the patient and the clinician postsurgery, to improve access for brushing and for professional cleaning. Most patients will usually undergo a course of nonsurgical treatment (RSD) and then enter the periodontal maintenance phase. For those sites that fail to respond to the initial therapy (e.g. because of complicated local anatomy, furcation involvement, etc.), the decision may be taken to improve access via a surgical approach. It is important not to progress to surgery too swiftly, however, as many sites continue to improve for several months after the initial nonsurgical treatment. Therefore, most patients should undergo RSD, and then a period of at least 6 months during which intensive and effective periodontal maintenance care is provided, including more focussed nonsurgical treatment at nonresponding sites, before making a decision about whether to progress to surgery. All periodontal treatment will fail in the absence of plaque control, and therefore, surgery must not be undertaken unless the patient is able to maintain an excellent standard of oral hygiene.

It is not within the scope of this chapter to provide detailed instruction in periodontal surgical techniques. However, some common periodontal surgical techniques are briefly discussed below.

Periodontal Flap Surgery

Flap surgery involves raising a periodontal flap to directly visualize the root surface. Following debridement of the root, the flap is replaced and sutured. Healing primarily occurs by formation of a long junctional epithelium. This results in probing depth reductions so that pockets are easier to maintain and keep clean. A new connective tissue attachment may form following flap procedures, but this is not predictable with certainty. The long junctional epithelium that forms following periodontal surgery is more susceptible to inflammation-induced breakdown than the original connective tissue attachment, and therefore, postoperative plaque control must be of a very high standard.

A variety of flap procedures can be performed:

- *Replaced flap:* Flap is replaced at the level of the presurgical position. This provides good access to the root with (usually) fairly minimal postoperative problems of esthetics or hypersensitivity, and the width of keratinized gingiva is maintained.
- *Apically repositioned flap:* Flap is apically repositioned and sutured just coronal to the alveolar bone crest. This can create significant cosmetic concerns if performed at anterior teeth (because of the appearance of recession postsurgery). However, this technique can be very useful at posterior teeth where esthetics are not a concern, as it provides greater probing depth reductions than the replaced flap procedure.
- *Apically repositioned flap with bone removal:* As above, but with bone recontouring to eliminate infrabony defects. May be useful in isolated circumstances where there is a deep infrabony pocket that is limiting oral hygiene access, although in general, it is best to maintain bone and to not remove bone by alveolar recontouring.

Crown Lengthening

Crown lengthening procedures are essentially apically repositioned flaps with bone removal, usually undertaken to increase crown length prior to placement of restorations. It is important to preserve the biologic width, which is a requirement for a distance of about 2.0 to 2.5 mm between the margins of the intended restorations and the alveolar bone crest to allow for the soft tissue attachment (i.e. epithelial and connective tissue attachment) to the root surface. If restorations are placed that encroach upon this space, inflammation and attachment loss may occur. Indications for crown lengthening include:

- Short clinical crowns requiring increased retention for the placement of restorations such as crowns or composite build-ups in wear cases
- Subgingival caries, to allow for restoration
- Root fracture or root resorption in the coronal third of the root
- To improve esthetics of anterior teeth that have short clinical crowns in a patient with a high smile line.

Gingivectomy

Gingivectomies are primarily used to remove excess gingival tissue in cases of drug induced gingival overgrowth (DIGO). Most patients with DIGO have difficulty with oral hygiene as a result of the abnormal anatomy of the enlarged gingival tissues. Therefore, there is usually also a strong inflammatory component to the condition as a result of plaque accumulation. Patients should therefore first undergo nonsurgical treatment to improve oral hygiene and remove plaque and calculus. This usually leads to a reduction in the size of the enlarged tissues as a result of resolution of inflammation, which makes the subsequent surgery safer and easier.

Guided Tissue Regeneration/Guided Bone Regeneration (GTR/GBR)

Following periodontal surgery, the newly instrumented surface is rapidly colonized by epithelial cells that form a long junctional epithelium, which prevents the formation of new connective tissue attachment to the root surface. GTR aims to prevent the epithelial cells from colonizing the root, thereby providing space for pluripotential cells from the periodontal ligament to proliferate and migrate into the area. These have the capacity to differentiate into fibroblasts, cementoblasts, and osteoblasts, and thus can generate new connective tissue attachment. GTR is achieved by placing resorbable barrier membranes (typically made of collagen) over periodontal defects to exclude the epithelium and create a space in which a blood clot forms which is then colonized by cells from the periodontal ligament and the alveolar bone. Key aspects of GTR include exclusion of epithelium, preservation of space under the membrane and formation of a stable blood clot into which cells can migrate. GTR is most predictable in class II furcations in mandibular molars, and in three-walled bone defects, particularly if combined with a bone graft (guided bone regeneration—GBR). Bone grafts can be the patient's own bone harvested from another site, or, more conveniently, synthetic hydroxyapatite granules.

Mucogingival Surgery

Surgical procedures for the correction of mucogingival defects (e.g. localized recession defects) are varied, technique sensitive and challenging. As with all periodontal surgery, plaque control is of paramount importance. Techniques for covering localized recession defects include free gingival grafts, connective tissue grafts, coronally advanced flaps, pedicle sliding flaps, and pouch techniques. The most predictable procedures for covering localized recession defects are connective tissue grafts (with the CT graft taken from the palate) coupled with a coronal advancement procedure. These techniques are very demanding, and should only be undertaken by periodontal specialists who have received appropriate training.

SELF-ASSESSMENT QUESTIONS

1. Describe how you would obtain a structured history from a patient with periodontitis.
2. Summarize the Basic Periodontal Examination (BPE) classification system and outline briefly the treatment required according to each BPE code.
3. Compare and contrast the presentation and clinical features of chronic periodontitis and aggressive periodontitis.
4. Periodontists now describe periodontal instrumentation as 'root surface debridement' rather than 'scaling and root planing'. Explain why this change in terminology has come about, and list the main differences between these two treatment approaches.
5. Provide a scoring system for: (i) furcation involvements and (ii) tooth mobility and explain how the clinical examination should be performed to assign scores to a tooth.

6. Behavior change to improve oral hygiene and to eliminate risk factors is an essential component of periodontal therapy. Explain how you would achieve such change in your patients with periodontitis.
7. What do you understand by the term 'subgingival biofilm'?
8. Briefly elaborate on the role on matrix metalloproteinases in the pathogenesis of periodontal disease.
9. Discuss, with specific examples, the "periodontal-systemic interface".
10. Outline the treatment of periodontal disease paying particular attention to adjuvant treatments and risk factor management.

SUGGESTED READING

1. Armitage GC. Development of a classification system for periodontal diseases and conditions. Annals of Periodontology. 1999;4:1-6.
2. Cobb CM. Clinical significance of non-surgical periodontal therapy: an evidence-based perspective of scaling and root planing. Journal of Clinical Periodontology. 2002;29(Suppl. 2):6-16.
3. Jonsson B, Ohrn K, Oscarson N, Lindberg P. The effectiveness of an individually tailored oral health educational programme on oral hygiene behavior in patients with periodontal disease: a blinded randomized-controlled clinical trial (one-year follow-up). Journal of Clinical Periodontology. 2009;36:1025-34.
4. Kornman KS, Page RC, Tonetti MS. The host response to the microbial challenge in periodontitis: assembling the players. Periodontology 2000. 1997;14:33-53.
5. Kuboniwa M, Lamont RJ. Subgingival biofilm formation. Periodontology 2000. 2010;52: 38-52.
6. Page RC, Eke PI. Case definitions for use in population-based surveillance of periodontitis. Journal of Periodontology. 2007;78: 1387-99.
7. Ryder MI. The influence of smoking on host responses in periodontal infections. Periodontology 2000. 2007;43:267-77.
8. Socransky SS, Haffajee AD. Periodontal microbial ecology. Periodontology. 2000. 2005;38:135-187.
9. Tomasi C, Wennstrom JL. Full-mouth treatment vs. the conventional staged approach for periodontal infection control. Periodontology. 2000. 2009;51:45-62.
10. Tonetti MS, Claffey N. Advances in the progression of periodontitis and proposal of definitions of a periodontitis case and disease progression for use in risk factor research. Group C consensus report of the 5th European Workshop in Periodontology. Journal of Clinical Periodontology. 2005;32:210-3.

Chapter

4

Inflammatory Disorders of Jaws including Necrosis

Stefano Fedele, Josiah Eyeson

Chapter Outline

INTRODUCTION

Osteonecrosis of the jaws is a pathological process characterized by ischemic (avascular) bone necrosis. Although bone necrosis can be asymptomatic, individuals with jawbone osteonecrosis can present a constellation of clinical features including pain, fistulas, bone enlargement, trans-mucosal exposure and infection.

Bone necrosis can have many different causes such as radiotherapy, infection, medications and other chemicals, thrombosis, and can occur in the context of pre-existing bone disorders such as osteopetrosis and bone dysplasia.

This section of the chapter focuses on osteonecrosis of the jaws associated with bisphosphonate medications (osteochemonecrosis) and radiotherapy (osteoradionecrosis). A brief summary of osteonecrosis associated with other causes is also provided.

OSTEONECROSIS

Bisphosphonate-associated Ostenecrosis (BONJ-Osteochemonecrosis)

Bisphosphonates are orally—and intravenously administered agents which act as potent inhibitors of bone resorption via powerful inhibition of osteoclastic activity. Bisphosphonates are used to prevent bone complications (pain and fracture) of osteoporosis, multiple myeloma, and metastasizing breast, prostate and other solid cancers. Bisphosphonates are generally considered relatively safe and burdened by few adverse effects. These include: acute phase reaction (fever, chills, flushing, bone pain) during infusion, hypocalcemia, oral-esophageal ulceration, and more recently low-energy spontaneous (atraumatic) femoral fracture.

Definition and Diagnostic Criteria

Definition of Bisphosphonate-related osteonecrosis of the jaws (BONJ) is important as it impacts on epidemiological studies and design on novel clinical trials. BONJ is usually defined as the presence of trans-mucosal (intraoral) or transcutaneous (facial) exposure of areas of maxillary or mandibular bone, persisting over 6 to 8 weeks, in a patient who is receiving, or has been exposed to, bisphosphonates, with radiotherapy to the head and neck regions being an exclusion criterion. Infection of the exposed bone with or without the formation of abscesses, fistulas, and possibly pathologic fracture often complicate the clinical picture, giving rise to disfigurement, chronic pain and recurrent orofacial infections. Current epidemiological data are largely based on this classic definition of exposed BONJ.

There is increasing evidence that osteochemonecrosis can present, in some instances, with jawbone symptoms and signs in the absence of bone exposure. Jawbone pain, sinus tract, gingival swelling and bone enlargement and rarely pathological fracture with no frank bone exposure have been reported to occur in patients using bisphosphonate medications in the absence of dental infection or other jawbone disease. These symptoms/signs are currently included in some of the available classifications/definitions as temporary features of developing osteonecrosis and are regarded as features of “probable BONJ”. It is not known whether nonexposed osteochemonecrosis represents a separate clinical variant *per se*—i.e. without progressing into frank bone exposure—and how its inclusion in current definitions would influence epidemiological data. As diagnosis of BONJ is largely based on clinical features, presence of radiological abnormalities, as well as histopathological evidence of avascular bone necrosis, can further support BONJ diagnosis but is not considered a necessary diagnostic criterion.

Epidemiology

Current epidemiological figures indicate that since 2003 more than 1000 cases of BONJ have been documented in the literature. However, more than 3500 cases have been reported to Food and Drug Administration (FDA) in US alone, hence the actual number of patients affected by BONJ worldwide is likely to be significantly under-reported. Differences in BONJ definition and in the examination of data of patients (e.g. Oral Health Care specialist vs Oncologist) would further explain flaws and lack of homogeneity of current epidemiological data. Most studies reported the incidence of BONJ to be approximately 5 to 9 percent in cancer patients exposed to intravenous high-potency bisphosphonates. Osteonecrosis is much less likely in individuals receiving oral bisphosphonates (e.g. for osteoporosis) than those on intravenous bisphosphonates, having a reported prevalence of <1 percent.

Etiopathogenesis

Little is known about the etiopathogenesis of BONJ. BONJ has been suggested to be caused by marked over-suppression of bone metabolism, which may result in accumulation of physiologic microdamage in the jawbones, compromising biomechanical properties and ability to repair injury (e.g. dental extraction or masticatory forces). Indeed this hypothesis is supported by the recent reports of increased risk of atraumatic spontaneous femur fractures in patients exposed to long-term bisphosphonates therapy.

Other authors have suggested that BONJ may result from vascular insufficiency with damage to the microcirculation, resulting in predisposed individuals, in bone ischemia and subsequent necrosis. Finally, bisphosphonates are well known to inhibit epithelial cell migration, and the consequent delayed wound healing after dental extraction has been suggested to trigger jaw bone infection and necrosis. None of these theories has been demonstrated or supported by experimental evidence.

Recent animal studies demonstrated the presence of areas of nonexposed intrabony medullar avascular necrosis in dogs exposed to bisphosphonates, suggesting that the primary event of BONJ may occur within the bone and that exposure may develop at a later stage.

Risk Factors

Studies have reported a number of risk factors to be associated with higher risk of BONJ occurrence. These include potency of the bisphosphonates, history of surgery to the jawbones, history dental infections, use of dentures, previous corticosteroid therapy, use of antiangiogenesis medications, diabetes, and smoking.

Length of therapy (and relative cumulative dose) is another important factor determining the risk of BONJ. The mean time to BONJ development after treatment with high-potency bisphosphonates is approximately 1 to 2 years, whilst it takes an average of 3 to 5 years for oral bisphosphonate to cause jaw osteochemonecrosis.

Clinical Features

Previous studies reported that patient's with BONJ typically present with a nonhealing socket after dental extraction. Intraoral exposure of greyish-brownish necrotic bone via transmucosal fenestration is the most common clinical feature (**Figs 4.1 and 4.2**). The mandible is significantly more affected than the maxilla. Associated features include sinus tract, pus discharge, bone enlargement, pathological fractures, extraoral or antral fistulas, abscesses and cervical lymphadenopahty. Immunocompromised patients can experience secondary severe infection of the head and neck region, including cellulitis, deep neck infections, and necrotizing fasciitis.

The area of bone necrosis can be significantly larger than the extent of transmucosal bone exposure and indeed cases of pathological fracture associated with minimal bone exposure have been reported.

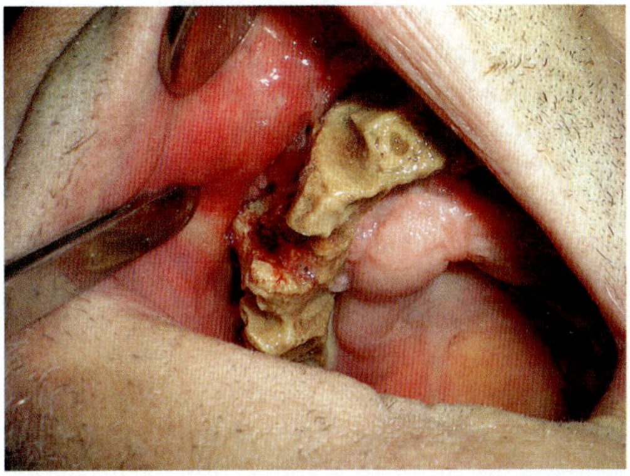

Fig. 4.1: Bisphosphonate-associated ostenecrosis of jaw.
Note: The large area of maxillary bone exposure associated with infection, swelling, and erythema of surrounding soft tissues. (*Courtesy:* Professor Giuseppe Colella, Second University of Naples, Italy)

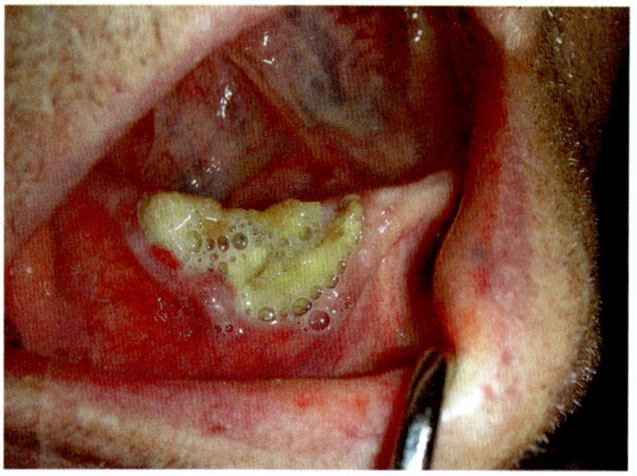

Fig. 4.2: Bisphosphonate-associated ostenecrosis of the jaws. Note a 4 to 5 cm area of mandibular bone exposure associated with pus discharge and mucosal erythema. These lesions are often associated with paraesthesia/anesthesia of the homolateral lip (*Courtesy:* Professor Giuseppe Colella, Second University of Naples, Italy)

Pain, which is typically associated with secondary infection, can range from mild to severe. There remain however, patients who have minimal bone necrosis/exposure, no obvious sign of infection, and report no significant discomfort. Sharp-edged exposed mandibular bone can also cause painful trauma and ulceration to surrounding soft tissues (e.g. tongue).

More recent studies have clarified that a significant portion of patients (up to 50%) will experience spontaneous development of BONJ (without a history of dental extraction or other dento-alveolar surgery).

There is also increasing evidence that early-phase osteochemonecrosis may present with sinus tract, toothache-like or jawbone pain, and/or bone/gingival swelling in absence of bone exposure. Although a significant percentage of these patients would subsequently progress to frank bone exposure, there remain individuals who will not do so, thus suggesting the existence of a separate variant of nonexposed BONJ. The American Association of Oral and Maxillofacial Surgeons suggested a clinical classification of BONJ into 4 stages (**Table 4.1**).

▪ Table 4.1
Clinical classification of BONJ

Stage	*Clinical features contributing to four stages*
At risk	No apparent necrotic bone in patients who have been treated with either oral or IV bisphosphonates
Stage 0	No clinical evidence of necrotic bone, but non-specific clinical findings and symptoms
Stage 1	Exposed and necrotic bone in asymptomatic patients without evidence of infection
Stage 2	Exposed and necrotic bone associated with infection as evidenced by pain and erythema in region of exposed bone with or without purulent drainage
Stage 3	Exposed and necrotic bone in patients with pain, infection, and one or more of the following: pathologic fracture, extraoral fistula, oral antral/oral nasal communication, or osteolysis extending to the inferior border of the mandible or the sinus floor

(Modified from Ruggiero et al. J Oral Maxillofac Surg. 2009;67(5 Suppl):2-12)

Histopathology

Osteochemonecrosis is histopathologically characterized by:

- Central areas of bony structure showing wide acellular necrotic regions with large and scalloped Haversian canals surrounded by
- Peripheral areas of bone tissue loss filled with an inflammatory infiltrate, mostly composed by polymorphonuclear phagocytes, plasma cells, monocytes and lymphocytes, acellular necrotic debris, thin-walled and dilated blood vessels.

A variety of oral cavity pathogens can be detected on histological or microbial examination (specially *Actinomyces*, but also *Entercoccus, Candida albicans, Haemophilus influenza, α-haemolytic streptococci, Lactobacillus, Enterobacter* and *Klebsiella pneumonite*). It is generally accepted that infection has little, or no role in BONJ pathogenesis although it may contribute significantly to its morbidity (pain and bone resorption).

Imaging

Radiography (panoramic or periapical), computed tomography (CT), magnetic resonance imaging (MRI), and nuclear bone scans can identify areas of osteochemonecrosis, although relevant features are typically nonspecific and mimic those of other bone disorders such as osteomyelitis, osteoradionecrosis, and cancer metastasis.

Frank advanced BONJ shows a number of X-ray and CT findings including osteosclerosis, osteolysis (**Figs 4.3 and 4.4**), sequestra, periostal thickening, and cortical erosion, with CT being superior to panoramic in terms of detectability and definition of necrosis extent. Widening of periodontal ligament space, thickening of lamina dura and periapical mixed radiolucent-radiopaque lesion have been reported as potential X-ray signs of early nonexposed osteochemonecrosis of alveolar bone surrounding vital healthy teeth.

MRI and nuclear bone scans are highly sensitive and have the potential to identify bone marrow inflammation and bone necrosis, especially in early phases when no obvious bone exposure is clinically apparent.

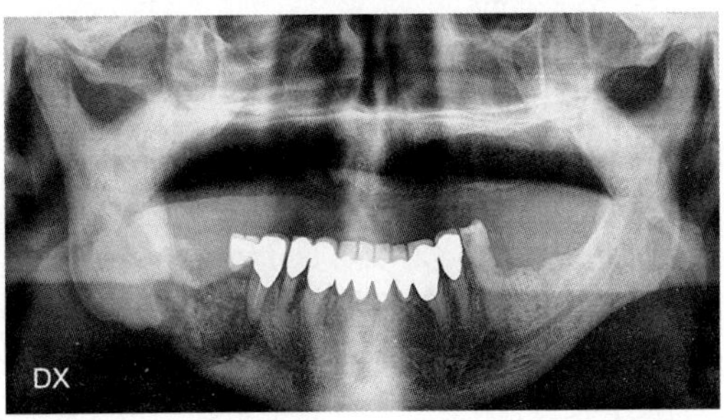

Fig. 4.3: Radiological features of bisphosphonate associated osteonecrosis of the jaws: panoramic. *Note:* Full-thickness osteolysis, pathological fracture, and diffuse osteosclerosis of the right mandible. (*Courtesy:* Professor Giuseppe Colella, Second University of Naples, Italy)

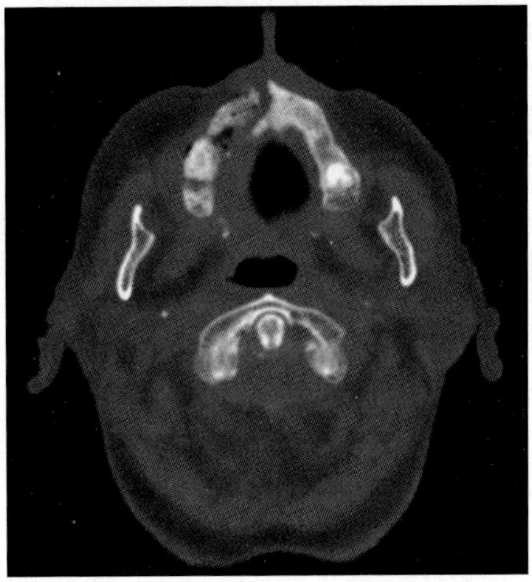

Fig. 4.4: Radiological features of bisphosphonate-associated osteonecrosis of the jaws: CT scan. *Note:* Osteolysis, osteosclerosis, fistula tracts and soft tissue swelling to the right maxilla. (*Courtesy:* Professor Giuseppe Colella, Second University of Naples, Italy)

Treatment

Management strategies need to consider both prevention and treatment. Efforts should be made to prevent BONJ via risk factor-reducing strategies. These include: performing dental surgery before bisphosphonate therapy, providing preventive dentistry during bisphosphonate therapy (e.g. noninvasive restorative dental treatment to avoid jawbone infection and extraction), and reducing the cumulative dosage and duration of bisphosphonate therapy.

Avoidance of extraction has no impact on the 30 to 50 percent of individuals with spontaneous BONJ.

Once osteochemonecrosis has developed, it is often intractable. However, most affected patients can benefit from palliative treatment pharmacological control of secondary infection and pain is the mainstay of therapy, although there remains no evidence regarding the most effective antibiotic and analgesic regimen (**Table 4.2**).

Aggressive surgical resection of the necrotic bone has been traditionally reported to be unsuccessful and counterproductive, and has been recommended only for symptomatic patients who do not respond to pharmacological

▪ Table 4.2
Treatment indicated for each stage of disease

Stage	*Treatment indicative for each stage*
At risk	No treatment indicated
Stage 0	Systemic management, including use of pain medication and antibiotics.
Stage 1	Antibacterial mouth rinse Clinical follow-up on quarterly basis
Stage 2	Symptomatic treatment with oral antibiotics. Pain control. Oral antibacterial mouth rinse. Superficial debridement to relieve soft tissue irritation.
Stage 3	Antibacterial mouth rinse Antibiotic therapy and pain control. Surgical debridement or resection for longer term palliation of infection and pain.

management, such as those with pathologic fractures of the mandible or persistent infection. More recently, however, an increasing number of reports have shown positive results of surgical intervention (either traditional bone resection or with neodimium: yttrium-aluminium-garnet (Nd:YAG) laser), especially in patients exposed to low-potency oral bisphosphonates, as long as appropriate identification of healthy bone margins and primary soft tissue closure is performed. Hyperbaric oxygen has demonstrated no beneficial effects. Discontinuation of bisphosphonates seems to offer no beneficial effects due to the extremely long half-life of these agents.

Prognosis

Osteochemonecrosis is a potentially severe complication of bisphosphonate therapy. Prognosis can be very variable. If left untreated, BONJ can impact severely onto the quality of life of affected individuals because of disfigurement, chronic pain, and recurrent orofacial infections. Some patients seem to have milder form of osteochemonecrosis with little discomfort and no functional impairment. Progression to severe life-threatening infection can rarely occur in immuno-compromised individuals.

Management is often challenging and consists mainly of pharmacological control of infection and pain. Resection of the necrotic bone has shown to be of little benefit although an accurate presurgical planning with detailed surgical margin identification seems to increase significantly the success rate.

OSTEOCHEMONECROSIS ASSOCIATED WITH MEDICATIONS OTHER THAN BISPHOSPHONATES

Jaw osteonecrosis has been reported in individuals exposed to novel antiresorptive agents including the receptor tyrosine kinase (RTK) inhibitor sunitinib and receptor activator of nuclear factor-kappa B (RANK) ligand inhibitor denosumab. Denosumab-associated jaw osteonecrosis seem to have similar incidence figures as necrosis associated with zoledronic acid, one of the most used bisphosphonates. In addition, the antiangiogenic monoclonal antibody bevacizumab, which inhibits vascular endothelial growth factor-A (VEGF-A), has been reported to cause jaw necrosis.

Box 4.1: Bisphophonate-associated osteonecrosis (BONJ)

Key features helpful in diagnosis

- BONJ most commonly is associated with high potency intravenous bisphosphonates.
- A history of dental extraction/surgery to the jawbone is observed in at least 50 percent of affected patients.
- Most common presentation of frank BONJ is trans-mucosal/cutaneous exposure of necrotic bone.
- Early stage BONJ can present with toothache-like pain, sinus tract and bone enlargement in absence of frank bone exposure.
- Biopsy and histopathological confirmation of suspected BONJ is usually not needed. Exclusion of metastases be the jawbones (via bone biopsy) can be however be necessary in occasional patients.
- Imaging techniques, although nonspecific, can support diagnosis of osteonecrosis. CT, MRI and bone scintigraphy/PET scans are typically more detailed than plain radiology and may identify areas of non-exposed and asymptomatic early BONJ. Other antiresorptive and antiangiogenic agents have been reported to cause jawbone necrosis.

Radiotherapy-associated Osteonecrosis (ORN-Osteoradionecrosis)

The management of advanced cancers of the head and neck region including oral cavity, naso and oropharynx and larynx, has traditionally relied on radiotherapy alone or in combination with surgery and/or chemotherapy. All these treatments are associated with substantial adverse effects. Radiotherapy is conventionally given in daily fractions of 1.8 to 2.0 Grays (Gy), up to total doses of 66 to 70 Gy over 6 or 7 weeks. Radiotherapy to the head and neck region typically causes both acute and long-term complications because of the adverse effects upon normal tissue. Frequently seen acute side-effects are mucositis, dysphagia, erythema and desquamation of the skin. Late complications are primarily the results of chronic injury to salivary glands, connective tissue and bone, leading to xerostomia, soft tissue fibrosis, and bone hypovascularity which can further progress to osteoradionecrosis. Osteoradionecrosis of the jaws can cause intolerable pain, fracture, secondary infection and fistulas, which have the potential to cause permanent disfigurement and impairment of orofacial functions.

Definition and Diagnostic Criteria

Osteoradionecrosis (ORN) of the jaws is defined as an area of necrotic bone exposed through the overlying mucosa or skin for longer than 2 to 3 month (6 months for some authors) in a previously irradiated field and in the absence of tumor recurrence.

Epidemiology

It is commonly agreed that osteoradionecrosis is infrequently observed. Its real incidence is however unclear, as a wide variable range of 1 to 37.5 percent has been described. These data however come from short-term studies performed on small cohorts of patients. Longer and larger studies have in fact reported an incidence of approximately 5 to 15 percent, which is probably most representative.

Etiopathogenesis

Irradiation of the bone causes release of free radicals from water molecules that react with DNA, RNA and enzymes of intrabony endothelial cell and lead to impaired function and finally cell death. Over time, this leads to thrombosis, hypovascularity, tissue hypoxia, destruction of bone-forming cells and marrow fibrosis which exceed normal homeostasis of bone tissue repair, creating either spontaneous tissue breakdown (spontaneous ORN) and/or reduced healing potential after trauma (ORN triggered by extraction or other surgical procedures). An infectious component is often present but is believed to be a contaminant rather than an etiological factor. The mandible is more susceptible than is the maxilla because of the nature of its vasculature (i.e. it obtains its main blood supply from one single artery).

Risk Factors

The risk of ORN depends on a number of factors that include: type of radiotherapy, cumulative radiation dose, the tumor stage and close proximity to bone, poor oral health, smoking and alcohol abuse, gender and age. Hyperfractionation and intensity-modulated radiotherapy (IMRT) seem to be associated with a much lower risk of ORN development, but there remains a need of long-term studies to confirm this preliminary observation.

Clinical Features and Histopathology

Osteoradionecrosis can occur anytime from 1 month to 14 years after radiotherapy. Although it can occur spontaneously, most cases are triggered by surgical procedure to the jawbones (e.g. dental extraction). Osteoradionecrosis usually starts as an asymptomatic exposure of necrotic bone that may progress to pain, abscess, fistula formation, trismus, paraesthesia and pathologic fracture. Although a number of classification systems based on clinical features and/or response to hyperbaric oxygen have been introduced, none of them has been validated in well-designed studies. Histological features of ORN include hypovascularity, destruction of osteocytes, absence of osteoblasts and lack of new osteoid. Inflammation and infection are commonly observed. With respect to prognosis, ORN can cause persistent pain, impair nutrition in a patient group who are often already nutritionally deprived, and can lead to disfiguring surgery.

Imaging

Computerized tomography is typically superior to panoramic radiography in visualizing the features of ORN such as dimension, margins, central necrosis and sequestration, cortical interruption and soft tissue thickening. There remains however, a consistent overlap with the radiological features of other bone disorders (e.g. osteomyelitis and metastases). MRI can support further identification of abnormalities of bone marrow and soft tissues adjacent to necrotic jawbone, whereas scintigraphy is typically characterized by high sensitivity but low specificity for the diagnosis of ORN.

Management

Osteoradionecrosis is recognized as one of the most severe complications of radiation therapy. It is difficult to treat and often leads to poor outcome and deformity.

Prevention

Prevention is the mainstay of ORN management and indeed improved dental care of cancer patients receiving radiotherapy to the head and neck has largely contributed to a reduction in the incidence of ORN during the last few years. Most patients nowadays complete dental extractions (all teeth with a questionable prognosis and either gross mobility or periodontal disease) before commencing radiotherapy and receive comprehensive restorative dental procedures/ oral prophylaxis during radiotherapy within the context of multidisciplinary care.

For those individuals who need dental extractions after or during radiotherapy, the risk of ORN development is significant, the estimated incidence ranging from 2 to 18 percent.

The previously established dogma upon the need of hyperbaric oxygen (HBO) before and after dental extractions is now largely abandoned due to lack of evidence. Theoretically, it was suggested that high oxygen level with HBO can induce angiogenesis in the hypoxic, hypocellular and hypovascular irradiated bone tissue, thus preventing the occurrence of ORN after tooth extraction (the so-called hypoxic–hypocellular–hypovascular tissue theory). However, a very recent systematic review has shown that there is very limited evidence that the use of hyperbaric oxygen reduces significantly the incidence of osteoradionecrosis in irradiated patients requiring tooth extraction. The only available randomized trial performed so far reports a reduction of ORN after prophylactic HBO from 7 to 4 percent, apparently supporting the use of HBO. Nevertheless, a number of practical issues remain:

a. HBO protocol requires 20 sessions of 90 min each before extraction—which translates in approximately one month of preparation before extraction.
b. Availability is often limited, and relative cost can also be significant; associated complications, although uncommon, can be severe such as pneumothorax, arterial air embolism, oxygen toxicity seizure, or acute pulmonary edema. These considerations have to be balanced with the small reduction in the incidence of ORN that could be obtained with HBO.

Indeed there is a consensus that minimal surgical trauma, alveolectomy with careful bone trimming, conservative flaps, primary closure without tension and removal of few teeth per session minimize postoperative complications and can reduce rates of ORN in the absence of hyperbaric oxygen therapy. The use of prophylactic antibiotics with the aim of reducing the risk of ORN remains highly controversial.

Therapy

Therapy of ORN largely depends on disease extent and stage.

Management of early and limited ORN is usually conservative and include local wound irrigation, oral hygiene improvement, local application of antiseptics, curettage, debridement, and superficial sequestrectomy. Antibiotic and analgesic can control relevant infection and pain and HBO could be an effective adjunct.

Advanced and widespread ORN can be effectively managed with aggressive resection and surgical reconstruction with vascularized graft. Hyperbaric oxygen does not seem to offer an additional benefit in the treatment of advanced ORN when a vascularized reconstruction is used. New therapeutic strategies based on antioxidant products such as pentoxifylline, tocopherol (vitamin E) and bisphosphonate are promising although there remains no well designed case-control studies.

Prognosis

Prognosis of osteoradionecrosis varies from small bone exposure that may cause little or no pain and remain stable for years or heal with conservative management, to severe cases necessitating surgical intervention and reconstruction.

Box 4.2: Osteoradionecrosis (ORN) of the jaws

Key features helpful in diagnosis

- Most commonly ORN is triggered by dental extraction/surgery to irradiated bone.
- Spontanoeus ORN is rare.
- Most common presentation of frank ORN is trans-mucosal/cutaneous exposure of necrotic bone.
- Biopsy and histopathological confirmation of suspected osteonecrosis is usually or metastasis to bone not needed.
- Exclusion of intra-bony cancer, recurrence (via bone biopsy) can be however necessary in occasional patients.
- Imaging techniques, although nonspecific, can support diagnosis of osteonecrosis and help to plan surgical resection (where needed).
- CT, MRI and Bone scintigraphy/PET scans are typically more detailed than plain radiography.

Neuralgia-inducing Cavitational Osteonecrosis

Neuralgia-inducing cavitational osteonecrosis (NICO) remains a very controversial entity. Some authors have suggested that NICO represents a specific type of painful osteonecrosis which results from edema of bone marrow with nonsuppurative osteomyelitis secondary to marrow ischemia within the background of inherited hypercoagulopathies (thrombophilia; hypo-fibrinolysis). It has been suggested by Bouquot *et al.* that a significant portion of patients with atypical facial neuralgia/pain could be in fact be affected by a form of jaw bone osteonecrosis caused by genetically determined intrabony thrombosis (e.g. low protein C, low stimulated tissue plasminogen activator activity and/or high lipoprotein) leading to bone marrow ischemia and edema. They also reported that such abnormalities could be diagnosed via bone scintigraphy, genetic testing and an non-validated ultrasonograph bone densitometer. Others have stressed that significant methodological issues seriously limit the quality of available evidence and questioned even the existence of such an entity. Indeed papers published about NICO mainly come from one single group of investigators and have not been reproduced or confirmed elsewhere. Further, more definition, clinical features and radiological aspects of NICO have been modified several times during the years, adding even more confusion to an already cloudy not evidence-based scenario. There remains confusion also with respect to therapy, as NICO has been suggested to respond to surgical curettage of affected bone, as well as medical therapy with warfarin, stanozolol and potentially to L-arginine.

Other Causes of Osteonecrosis

Avascular bone necrosis of the jaws has been reported in association with a number of causes and diseases including herpes zoster infection, deep fungal infection, arsenic, cocaine, thrombophilia/hypofibrinolysis, osteopetrosis, bone dysplasia, chemotherapy, antiphospholipid syndrome and diffuse sclerosing osteomyelitis. Osteonecrosis due to herpes zoster or deep fungal infections (e.g. mucormycosis) is very uncommon and likely related to infection-induced arterial compression or thrombosis. It is characterised by spontaneous otherwise unexplained tooth loss followed by exposure of and bone sequestra. Osteopetrosis, sclerosing osteomyelitis and fibro-osseous dysplasia can lead to ischemic bone necrosis due to the presence of genetically-determined hypovascular sclerotic bone and often as a consequence of tooth extraction or other invasive surgical procedures. Reduced blood supply is also the likely mechanisms behind the reported cases of jaw avascular necrosis in patients with systemic lupus eryhtematosus, antiphospholipid syndrome, or those using antineoplastic medications.

INFLAMMATORY DISEASES OF THE JAW BONES

Osteomyelitis

Definition

Osteomyelitis is an inflammatory disease of bones following infection by a pyogenic organism. It may be either an acute or chronic process. It may also be associated with pus accumulation (suppurative) or not (nonsuppurative).

Predisposing factors for the onset of osteomyelitis include virulence of the microorganism, host resistance and vascularity of the jaw. Host resistance is adversely affected by conditions such as diabetes, autoimmune disease, leukemia, sickle cell disease, acquired immunodeficiencies, syphyllis and cancer chemotherapy. The vascularity of the jaws is adversely affected by radiation, osteoporosis, osteopetrosis, Paget's disease of bone, fibrous dysplasia, bone malignancy, bone necrosis secondary to mercury, bismuth and arsenic toxicity.

Adult males are usually affected with the mandible being more commonly affected. Affected mandibular regions in decreasing frequency are body > symphysis > angle > ramus > condyle. It is thought that the maxilla is less commonly affected due to more extensive blood supply, thin cortical plates, relative paucity of medullary tissues which preclude confinement of infections resulting in their spread to surrounding soft tissues or paranasal sinuses. Osteomyelitis is rarely seen in neonates or infants and when present is in the maxilla. This is as a result of uncontrolled middle ear infection or secondary to birth injuries at the time of delivery.

Etiology

Osteomyelitis is a mixed aerobic and anaerobic bacterial infection. Bacteria that have been associated include the fusobacteria, *Porphyromonas*, *Prevotella*, streptococci and staphylococci families. Historically osteomyelitis was thought to be due to infection by *Staphylococcus aureus* species only. Osteomyelitis has also been associated with infections by herpes zoster virus, cytomegalovirus, actinomycosis, tuberculosis and syphilis.

Clinical Features

Osteomyelitis is characterized by severe throbbing, deep-seated pain and swelling. With disease progression pus accumulates initially within the medullary bone then extends to involve the cortex with eventual perforation of the cortex. The pus then accumulates under the periosteum causing distension of the periosteum. Over time there may be bone expansion due to subperiosteal bone formation with the resulting swelling becoming firm.

The overlying gingiva is red, swollen and tender. As the disease progresses, the associated teeth become loose and tender with pus exudation from the gingival crevice and mucosa. Any attached muscle in the region of the jaw affected by the osteomyelitis becomes edematous and this might give rise to trismus and difficulty in swallowing. There may be associated fever, leucocytosis, regional lymphadenopathy and cellulitis. In the case of osteomyelitis of the mandible, the inferior dental nerve may be involved resulting in altered sensation of the lower lip.

Acute osteomyelitis of less than a month's duration is associated with fever, increazed white cell count, lymphadenopathy and localized swelling. Chronic osteomyelitis is often associated with a localized swelling, pain, sinus formation, pus discharge, bony sequestrum, loosening of teeth and pathologic fractures.

Radiographic changes as a result of osteomyelitis become evident after ten days. These radiographic changes include loss of trabeculae, radiolucency, ill-defined margins with a fluffy or moth-eaten appearance. Where bony sequestra are present radiopaque areas will be seen within the radiolucent areas. Subperiosteal new bone formation may also be evident. Early bone changes are detectable with Computer Tomographic (CT) scan examination before being visible on plain radiographs. CT scans are better than plain radiographs in revealing lesion extent, extent of cortical erosion and identification of sequestra. Magnetic resonance imaging is the examination of choice in identifying medullary changes.

Pathogenesis

The process of osteomyelitis is initiated by acute inflammation and its features of hyperemia, increased capillary permeability and infiltration of granulocytes. Proteolytic enzymes are released by the granulocytes resulting in tissue necrosis, destruction of bacteria and vascular thrombosis. Intramedullary pressure increases where there is intramedullary accumulation of pus which is composed of necrotic tissue, dead bacteria with granulocytes. The increased pressure causes vascular collapse, venous stasis and consequently ischemia. As the disease progresses, pus accumulates beneath the periosteum resulting in periosteal elevation from the cortex and further compromise of blood supply. Further pus accumulation causes the cortex to be breached, giving rise to mucosal and/or cutaneous abscesses or fistulae. In the vicinity of the inferior dental canal, pus accumulation may result in the compression of the inferior dental bundle resulting in sensory impairment.

As effectiveness of host defences and therapy increases, the process of osteomyelitis may resolve. Chronic osteomyelitis may develop where effect of host defences and therapy are inadequate. In some situations as the inflammatory process regresses, granulation tissue forms around involved bone. New vascularization may result in the lyses of bone leading to separation of dead fragments of bone which become bony sequestra. The bony sequestra may be encased in a sheath of new bone thus becoming an involucrum. The sequestra may revascularize, be resorbed, be quiescent or become chronically infected requiring surgical removal.

Diagnosis

A swab of pus sent for microbiological culture would confirm the infective agent. Radiographic features of bone loss are commonly referred to as "moth eaten appearance".

Bony sequestrum, if available, is sent for histological and microbiological examination.

Management

Management includes the administration of antibiotics. The route of antibiotic administration is dependent on the presence, or not, of systemic manifestations of infection. In the presence of systemic manifestations of infection the intravenous route is preferred and the selected antibiotic (based on the culture and sensitivity reports) are administered for up to 2 weeks. In the absence of systemic signs the oral route will be adequate for up to 6 weeks. Polymethylmethacrylate beads impregnated with antibiotics such as gentamicin or tobramycin can be placed in the area of osteomyelitis as a source of local antibiotic administration for up to 3 months. Any host factors adversely contributing to the development of osteomyelitis will need to be addressed. Incision and drainage of sites of pus accumulation, removal of involved teeth, decortication, debridement of bony sequestra and necrotic material are likely. The defect arising from resection of infected bone may need reconstruction and the clinical decision will need to be made whether immediate or late bone-graft reconstruction is used.

Complications

- Altered sensation especially where the inferior dental nerve is involved.
- Pathological fracture of the involved jaw bone.
- Chronic osteomyelitis after inadequate treatment.
- Cellulitis.
- Septicemia in the immunocompromized individual.

Box 4.3: Osteomyelitis of jaw bones

Key features helpful in diagnosis

- Osteomyelitis is an inflammatory disease of bone
- Adult males usually affected
- Mandible more commonly affected
- Characteristics: deep seated pain and swelling
- Teeth may become loose
- Pus may be present
- Systemic signs such as fever, regional lymphadenopathy may be present
- Radiolucency with ill-defined margins with a moth-eaten appearance on radiographs.

Chronic Osteomyelitis

Chronic osteomyelitis is more common than the acute variant. It results from inadequately treated acute osteomyelitis. The presence of local bone sclerosis is a factor for the development of chronic osteomyelitis. However, it usually develops *de-novo* as a result of infection by virulent bacteria or in avascular bone. It is characterized by persistent pain, exposed bone and radiographic changes after florid infection. Focal sclerosing osteomyelitis which may arise in the presence of longstanding infection is commoner in the young. Chronic osteomyelitis in the presence of acute necrotising ulcerative gingivitis may result in the development of noma whose treatment comprises of antibiotics and debridement. Antibiotics of the penicillin group with established potency in bone infections in combination with metronidazole is found to be consistently useful in arresting the fulminating acute phase of noma. Overall, the "gold standard" remains that antibiotics administered at the acute phase must be sufficiently broad to cover the spectrum of aerobic and anaerobic organisms inhabiting the periodontium and oropharynx. Improved oral hygiene instructions and strategy also must accompany early phase treatment.

Actinomycosis

Actinomycosis is a slowly progressing chronic infection with granulomatous and suppurative features. Actinomycosis is caused by filamentous, gram-positive, non-acid-fast, non-spore-forming bacteria. They belong to the, genus *Actinomyces*. *Actinomyces* organisms grow slowly in anaerobic-to-microaerophilic conditions. The most common isolated species are *Actinomyces israeli*, *Actinomyces gerencseriae*, *Actinomyces turicensis*, *Actinomyces radingae*, and *Actinomyces europaeus*. In addition to these microorganisms, almost all actinomycotic lesions contain so-called companion bacteria. The most important of these bacteria is *Actinobacillus actinomycetemcomitans*. These companion bacteria appear to magnify the low pathogenic potential of actinomycetes.

Actinomycosis usually affects soft tissue and occasionally bone. It can affect the mandible and overlying soft tissues as well as the parotid gland and tongue. Cervicofacial actinomycosis is characterized in the initial stages by soft-tissue swelling of the perimandibular area. Direct spread into the adjacent tissues occurs over time forming multiple abscesses along with development of fistulas (sinus tracts) that discharge purulent material containing granules with a yellow sulfur-like appearance (termed sulfur granules).

It could be difficult to diagnose actinomycosis based on the clinical features alone, direct identification and/or isolation of the infecting organism from a clinical specimen or from sulfur granules is necessary for definitive diagnosis in most cases. A pus sample can be obtained from a draining sinus or by needle aspirate. A gram-stained smear of the specimen may demonstrate the presence of beaded, branched, gram-positive filamentous rods, suggesting the diagnosis of actinomycosis and culture under anaerobic conditions may require 2 to 3 weeks. The preliminary diagnosis of actinomycosis could also be made by examining sulfur granules crushed between 2 slides, stained with 1 percent methylene-blue solution, and examined microscopically for features characteristic of actinomycetes.

In most cases of actinomycosis, antimicrobial therapy is the only treatment required, although surgery can be adjunctive in selected cases including incision and drainage of abscesses, excision of sinus tracts. Penicillin G or V is the drug of choice for treating infections caused by actinomycetes though recalictant cases may need doxycycline or augmentin.

Infantile Osteomyelitis

Infantile osteomyelitis is a rare condition associated with *Staphylococcus aureus* infection. It occurs a few weeks after birth, in the usually involving the maxilla. It had a mortality of 30 percent in the preantibiotic era. It is thought to spread via the hematogeneous route or from perinatal trauma of oral mucosa possibly from contaminated human or artificial nipples. It is also possibly a result of spreading infection from the maxillary sinus.

Potential complications include the risk of eye involvement, extension to dural sinuses, potential facial deformities, loss of teeth due to delayed or inappropriate treatment.

Clinical features include facial cellulitis around the orbit, irritability, malaise, hyperpyrexia, anorexia, dehydration, convulsions and vomiting. Pus may be present within the nostril on the affected side. Intraorally the maxilla on the involved side will be swollen, fluctuant with the presence or not of fistulae.

CT scan examination is needed to establish the extent of the osteomyelitis. Aggressive intravenous antibiotics are required, together with incision and drainage. Oral antibiotics are advised for a further 2–4 weeks after resolution.

Box 4.4: Infantile osteomyelitis

Key features helpful in diagnosis

- Is rare
- Is associated with *Staphylococcus aureus*
- Occurs few weeks after birth
- Usually affects the maxilla.

Chronic Recurrent Multifocal Osteomyelitis of Children

Chronic recurrent multifocal osteomyelitis (CRMO) of children is an inflammatory disease of the bone which resembles infectious osteomyelitis. Its hallmark is recurring episodes of sterile osteomyelitis that affect children around fourteen years of age. Affected sites include the mandible, tibia, clavicle, fibula, spine and femur. The mandibular lesions are usually bilateral, irregular, mottled, multilocular and located in the rami. They undergo spontaneous remission with antibiotics and surgical debridement having little effect. CROM shows several similarities with synovitis, acne, pustolosis, hyperostosis, osteitis (SAPHO) syndrome and is now believed to belong to autoinflammatory syndromes, a group of genetically-determined disorders characterized by unprovoked (or triggered by minor events) recurrent episodes of systemic inflammation involving various body systems.

Proliferative Periostitis (Periostitis Ossificans)

Proliferative periostitis (Periostitis ossificans) also referred to as Garrés sclerosing osteomyelitis. Chronic nonsuppurative sclerosing osteomyelitis is an irritation induced focal thickening of the periosteum and cortical bone of the tibia as well as the mandible. Children and young adults with a mean age of 13 years are usually affected. It is thought to be as a result of an active periosteal response to low grade infection or irritation in young people. It usually manifests in the premolar and molar areas. It is characterised by the presence of a nontender unilateral bony swelling of the lateral and inferior aspects of the mandible. It is associated with a periapically involved carious tooth and history of dental pain. It can also be due to periodontal infections and trauma. The overlying skin is normal and there is no lymphadenopathy or fever present. Radiographically it presents as well-calcified layers of reactive bone proliferation with a laminated ('onion skin') appearance. The apices of involved teeth may have associated radiolucency.

Histology

There are parallel rows of highly cellular and reactive woven bone in which individual trabeculae are frequently orientated perpendicular to the surface.

Management

Initially treat it is necessary to the dental cause. If there is no improvement, or in the absence of inflammation then carry out a biopsy because conditions such as Ewing's sarcoma, osteosarcoma and cortical hyperostosis (Caffey's disease) may have a similar radiographic appearance.

Box 4.5: Proliferative periostitis

Key features helpful in diagnosis

- Chronic, nonsuppurative sclerosing
- Affects children and young adults with a mean age of 13-years
- Develops in response to low-grade infection or irritation
- Involves and molar regions.

Chronic Sclerosing Osteomyelitis

There are two types of chronic sclerosing osteomyelitis namely the diffuse type and florid osseous dysplasia type.

Diffuse Chronic Sclerosing Osteomyelitis

The diffuse type is an inflammatory, non-suppurative, painful disease with a protracted course. There may be episodes of recurrent swelling and pain. It affects the whole height of the mandible, usually on one side. It affects mainly the body of the mandible though the angle, ramus and condyle may also be affected. Young adults in the third decade are usually affected with two-thirds being female.

Radiographic features include diffuse intramedullary sclerosis, poorly defined margins, occasional areas of radiolucency and radiopacity. It is associated with *E. Corrodens, Actinomyces* and *Bacteroides infection*. Management includes the administration of high doses of antibiotics and removal of the source of infection. In some cases it may be necessary to carry out decortication or resection of involved bone and the appropriate reconstruction.

Florid Osseous Dysplasia

Radiographic features of opaque masses limited to the alveolar process. Usually present in African and Caribbean women (see Chapter 7).

Diffuse Sclerosing Osteomyelitis

Diffuse sclerosing osteomyelitis is an ill-defined group characterized by pain, inflammation, periosteal hyperplasia, sclerosis. There is an obvious infectious process causing sclerosis of bone. It occurs in adulthood with no sex predilection and usually affects the mandible.

The sclerosis tends to center on the crestal portion of the tooth-bearing part of the alveolar ridge. Radiographic examination shows radiopaque areas at sites of chronic infection such as apical inflammatory disease.

Histology

Bone sclerosis and remodelling is present. The Harversian canals are widely scattered with little marrow spaces. There is little inflammatory soft tissue component associated. In cases where inflammation involves the sclerotic bone this results in bone necrosis and subsequent sequestrum formation colonized by bacteria.

Management

The aim of treatment is to remove the foci of chronic infection. Areas of sclerosis may remodel or persist. It is important to avoid periodontitis or apical inflammatory disease.

Primary Chronic Osteomyelitis

Primary chronic osteomyelitis is characterized by recurrent episodes of pain, swelling and local induration. The active stage may be associated with lymphadenopathy and inferior dental nerve paraesthesia. No fever, pus, sequestra or sinus is present and there is no obvious odontogenic cause. It tends to have two onset peaks namely adolescence and after the fifth decade of life.

A mixed pattern of osteolytic and sclerotic areas is seen on radiographs. The osteolytic areas are not continuous as noted in suppurative osteomyelitis. The affected bone becomes thickened and overtime a more sclerotic picture is noted on radiographs.

Synovitis-acne-pustulosis-hyperostosis-osteomyelitis (SAPHO) and chronic recurrent multifocal osteomyelitis (CRMO) are reported subsets of primary chronic osteomyelitis.

SAPHO also affects multiple sites such as the anterior chest wall, sternum, clavicle, spine and ribs. It usually occurs in people < 60 years with a negative result upon microbiological examination. The osteolytic areas tend to be within sclerotic bone.

CRMO also affects multiple sites such as the clavicle, humerus, radius and tibia. There may also be skin involvement, e.g. palmoplantar pustulosis psoriasis.

Histology

There is evidence of bone remodelling in the areas of sclerosis. There is inter-trabecular fibrosis present as well as scattered lymphocytes and plasma cells. There may be foci of micro-abscesses, hyalinization around small blood vessels and subperiosteal formation. No bone necrosis, bacterial colonization or pus is associated.

Management

Treatment results are mixed. It is difficult to eliminate the infection as despite treatment there are still flare-ups and partial remissions. Various treatment modalities have been proposed with limited success. Long-term antibiotics with or without hyperbaric oxygen, corticosteroids, nonsteroidal anti-inflammatories and calcitonin have all been used. Intravenous bisphosphonates, e.g. alendronate, pamidronate and disodium clodronate are reported to show significant benefit. For example, a single intravenous dose of alendronate is reported to result in pain reduction within twenty four hours, suppression of bone turnover and lead to long-term remission.

Chronic Tendoperiostitis

Chronic tendoperiostitis is thought to be a reaction of bone to the chronic overuse of the attached masticatory muscles such as that due to parafunctional behavior.

Patients have a mean age of 40 years. It is characterized by recurrent pain, cheek swelling, trismus and no suppuration. Radiographic examination shows sclerotic areas to be related to sites of muscle attachment.

Histology

There is evidence of sclerosing and remodelling of cortical and subcortical bone resulting in increased bone volume. Chronic inflammatory cells may also be present.

Management

The results after the use of antibiotics, antibiotics-impregnated beads, surgical exploration, decortication, hyperbaric oxygen and steroids have been unsatisfactory. Another suggested treatment modality aims to reduce muscle overuse through employing relaxation techniques, soft diet, occlusal splints and muscle relaxant drugs.

Box 4.6: Chronic tendoperiostitis

Key features helpful in diagnosis

- Recurrent pain
- Cheek swelling
- Trismus
- No suppuration
- Sclerotic areas related to sites of muscle attachment.

Condensing Osteitis (Focal Sclerosing Osteomyelitis)

Condensing osteitis (Focal sclerosing osteomyelitis) is characterized by localized areas of bone sclerosis associated with the apices of teeth undergoing pulpitis or pulpal necrosis, e.g. carious teeth, teeth with deep restorations. It usually affects children or young adults. Radiographs show the presence of a radiopaque area at the apex of the tooth with probable widened periodontal ligament space or apical area. It usually involves the premolar or molar areas of the mandible. The radiopacity is not separated from the tooth apex and there is no radiolucent outline.

Management

The aim of treatment is to treat the odontogenic cause.

Box 4.7: Focal sclerosing osteomyelitis

Key features helpful in diagnosis

- Associated with teeth undergoing pulpitis or pulpal necrosis
- Usually affects children or young adults
- Radiopaque area attached to tooth apex
- Usually affects mandibular premolar and molar teeth.

Alveolar Osteitis (Dry Socket, Fibrinolytic Alveolitis)

A blood clot normally forms within the tooth socket after a dental extraction. The clot then undergoes organization and subsequently progresses with the formation of woven bone. The woven bone then develops into mature bone. Where the clot is lost healing is impaired with the development of alveolar osteitis. The clot is thought to be lost secondary to the transformation of plasminogen to plasmins. This results in lysis of fibrin and formation of kinins which are potent pain mediators. The fibrinolysis can be due to trauma, estrogens, bacterial pyrogens, poor oral hygiene, traumatic extractions, presurgical infections, spitting and smoking. The prevalence of alveolar osteitis is reported as 20 percent in those smoking > 1 pack/day and 40 percent in those who smoke on the day of operation or within 24 hours. The frequency is higher in the posterior mandible. There is no sex predilection. It is reported that alveolar osteitis occurs in 1 to 3 percent of all extractions and in 25 to 30 percent after the extraction of impacted third molars. The frequency of alveolar osteitis decreases with prophylactic removal rather than therapeutic removal of third molars. The frequency is reported to be highest in the 40 to 45 years age group with the prevalence highest in the 20 to 40 years age group.

After the loss of the blood clot there is exposure of the bare bony socket which tends to be very sensitive. There is severe pain, foul odor, lymphadenopathy and sometimes swelling. The pain may radiate to the ipsilateral ear, temporal regions and eye. Alveolar osteitis may have a duration between 10 to 40 days.

Box 4.8: Alveolar ostetitis

Key features helpful in diagnosis

- Loss of blood clot from extraction socket
- Severe pain
- Foul odor
- Lymphadenopathy
- Duration of 10 to 40 days.

Management

Radiographic examination may be needed to rule out the presence of a tooth remnant or a foreign body as the cause of poor healing. Irrigation of the socket with warm saline or chlorhexidine is advised. Prior to placement of a dressing, e.g. alvogyl, the socket should be inspected. Good oral hygiene to reduce the bacterial load may assist healing. To reduce the risk of alveolar osteitis it is suggested that the socket be irrigated postextraction with saline. Another suggested protective measure is to rinse with chlorhexidine on the day of the procedure and several days postup.

SELF ASSESSMENT QUESTIONS

1. Define bisphosphonate related osteonecrosis of the jaws, describe its epidemiology and outline the risk factors associated with its development.
2. Outline the key features which are helpful in the diagnosis of bisphosphonate related osteonecrosis of the jaws.
3. Describe a clinical classification and associated management guideline for bisphosphonate related osteonecrosis of the jaws.
4. Define radiotherapy associated osteonecrosis, describe its epidemiology and outline the risk factors associated with its development.
5. Outline the key features which are helpful in the diagnosis of radiotherapy associated osteonecrosis.
6. Describe the usual clinical presentation and histopathology of radiotherapy associated osteonecrosis.
7. Describe your approach to the prevention of radiotherapy associated osteonecrosis as well as the management of an established case.
8. Define acute osteomyelitis and outline its etiopathogenesis.
9. Describe the management of acute osteomyelitis and outline possible sequelae of the condition.
10. Describe the etiology, clinical presentation and management of alveolar osteitis.

SUGGESTED READING

1. Almazrooa SA, Woo SB. Bisphosphonate and nonbisphosphonate-associated osteonecrosis of the jaw: a review. J Am Dent Assoc. 2009;140(7): 864-75.
2. Bamias A, Kastritis E, Bamia C, Moulopoulos LA, Melakopoulos I, Bozas G, et al. Osteonecrosis of the jaw in cancer after treatment with bisphosphonates: incidence and risk factors. J Clin Oncol. 2005;23:8580-7.
3. Lyons A, Ghazali N. Osteoradionecrosis of the jaws: current understanding of its pathophysiology and treatment. Br J Oral Maxillofac Surg. 2008;46(8):653-60.
4. Marx RE, Sawatari Y, Fortin M, Broumand V. Bisphosphonate-induced exposed bone

(osteonecrosis/osteopetrosis) of the jaws: risk factors, recognition, prevention, and treatment. J Oral Maxillofac Surg. 2005;63:1567-75.
5. Pitak-Arnnop P, Sader R, Dhanuthai K, Masaratana P, Bertolus C, Chaine A, Bertrand JC, Hemprich A. Management of osteoradionecrosis of the jaws: an analysis of evidence. Eur J Surg Oncol. 2008;34(10):1123-34.
6. Silverman SL, Landesberg R. Osteonecrosis of the jaw and the role of bisphosphonates: a critical review. Am J Med. 2009;122:S33-45.
7. Sciubba JJ, Goldenberg D. Oral complications of radiotherapy. Lancet Oncol. 2006;7(2):175-83.
8. Teng MS, Futran ND. Osteoradionecrosis of the mandible. Curr Opin Otolaryngol Head Neck Surg. 2005;13(4):217-21.

Chapter

5

Cysts of the Oral and Maxillofacial Region

WM Tilakaratne

Chapter Outline

INTRODUCTION

Occurrence of cysts in oral and maxillofacial region is far more common compared to rest of the body. This is especially true when it comes to intraosseous lesions. The majority of intra bony cystic lesions occur as a result of activation of epithelial remnants from enamel organ. This type of a phenomenon of having epithelium within the bone is uncommon in bones other than the mandible and maxilla. Therefore, the prevalence of cystic lesions is common in jaws. Inflammatory odontogenic cysts are responsible for a large majority of cases due to the presence of untreated dental decay in the community (Chapter 2). With the available current scientific findings, odontogenic keratocyst (OKC) has been moved to odontogenic tumor category in 2005 WHO classification. There is still a considerable debate as to whether OKC should be regarded as a true neoplastic lesion or an unusual cystic lesion. The term fissural cyst has been used over the years to denote cystic lesions arising from entrapped epithelium during the closure of embryological lines. However, according to the recent literature such a process does not exist and the term fissural cyst has become a misnomer. Due to the above reason the existence of globulomaxillary cyst, median palatine cyst and median mandibular cyst has been abandoned. The only remaining lesions from the above category appeared to be nasopalatine cyst and nasolabial cyst. Although a true cystic lesion should have a cyst wall, lining and the lumen, there are a few lesions which do not fulfil the above criteria. Aneurysmal bone cyst and solitary bone cyst are the examples from intraosseous cysts and mucous extravasation cyst is a common soft tissue example for the above category.

The diagnosis of most cystic lesions needs clinicopathological correlation. Treatment of a cyst is either by enucleation or by marsupialisation. Recurrence of odontogenic cyst other than OKC and glandular odontogenic cyst is exceptionally uncommon and malignant transformation takes place very rarely.

ODONTOGENIC CYSTS

Radicular Cyst

Radicular cyst is the most common cyst in jaw bones accounting for 60 percent of the odontogenic cysts. It arises in relation to apical region, or less commonly to the lateral side of a nonvital tooth, as a result of stimulation of epithelial cell rests of Malassez in a chronic periapical granuloma. It is clear that necrotic pulpal tissue and bacterial products initiate inflammation in the periapical region giving rise to a periapical granuloma. With time a central cavity is formed due to necrosis of cells and subsequently the cavity is lined by proliferating cell rests of Malassez. Although the exact agent stimulating the proliferation of epithelial cell rests is not properly understood, available information suggests that it may well be due to bacterial endotoxins. Invariably inflammation takes place as a result of these toxins, and inflammatory mediators which mediate the reaction such as IL-1 and IL-6 together with other molecules stimulate cell rests of Malassez to proliferate within the periapical granuloma. It was postulated in the past that increased carbon dioxide tension and decreased oxygen tension leading to acidic pH make the surroundings favorable for cell rests to proliferate. There are various theories regarding the expansion of the cyst including increased osmotic pressure in the cavity, increased hydrostatic pressure, epithelial proliferation, various cytokines and matrixmetalloproteinases (MMPs). However, increased hydrostatic pressure within the cyst lumen is considered to be the main factor responsible for expansion of most cystic lesions. Prostaglandin E2 (PGE2), PGI2, IL-1 and IL-6 may also play a role as they are potent cytokines with bone resorbing properties.

Box 5.1: Radicular cyst

Key features helpful in diagnosis

- The most common odontogenic cyst.
- Associated with a nonvital tooth.
- Presents as a well-defined periapical radiolucency.
- Lining epithelium is nonkeratinized stratified squamous and shows arcading pattern.
- Cyst wall is inflamed and contains cholesterol clefts.

Clinical Features

Most radicular cysts are asymptomatic and are found on routine dental radiographs of nonvital teeth. The maxillary anterior region is the most common site (**Fig. 5.1**) and maxilla to mandibular ratio is 3:2. The reason for the higher frequency of maxillary involvement is the presence of more non vital teeth in the upper jaw. Although highest number of cases occur in the third decade, the majority are from third to fifth decade. There is a male preponderance which may be due to better care for the anterior teeth by females. A radicular cyst arising in deciduous teeth is a very rare event. Early lesions are bony hard in consistency as there is enough bone surrounding the cystic cavity. However with the enlargement of the cyst, thickness of the overlying bone becomes less and palpation would allow the bone to go in giving rise to "Ping pong ball sign". Further thinning would cause it to crack on hard palpation like an "Egg shell". Towards the later stage the cyst is without any overlying bone leading to fluctuant swelling. Pain is usually not a feature of a radicular cyst unless it is infected.

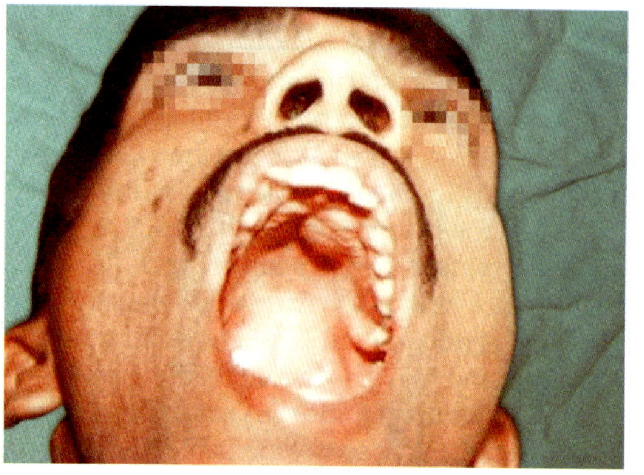

Fig. 5.1: Radicular cyst. A well-demarcated swelling of palate—a radicular cyst arising from upper left lateral incisor

Radiological Features

Historically the size of the radiolucency is considered to be of diagnostic importance to differentiate a cyst from a periapical granuloma. The diagnosis of a cyst can be made confidently when the radiolucency is more than 2 cm (**Fig. 5.2**). However, when the radiolucency is smaller it is difficult to separate a cyst from a granuloma. When the lesion is less than 1 cm in diameter the probability of that being a granuloma is much higher. Other associated features such as cortication, resorption of roots and loss of lamina dura in the apical area are common to both periapical granuloma and a cyst in most cases. Therefore, they may not be definite features to separate the two entities.

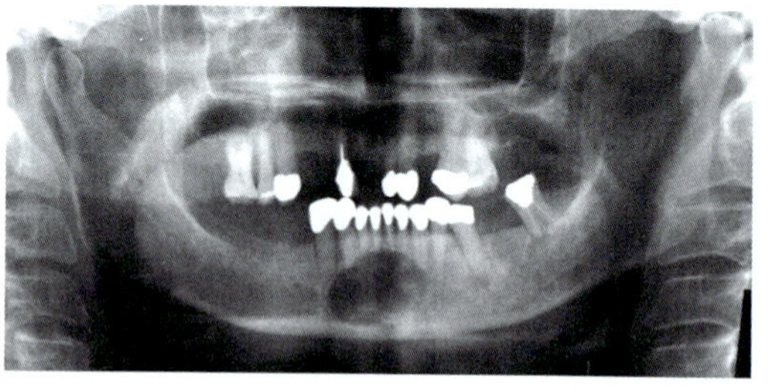

Fig. 5.2: Radicular cyst. Well-defined and well corticated radiolucency in relation to multiple nonvital lower anterior teeth (*Courtesy:* Dr Jimmy Makdissi)

Histopathology

Histologically, lining epithelium of the radicular cyst is stratified nonkeratinizing with prominent arcading pattern (**Fig. 5.3**). The thickness of the epithelium varies, with most cysts showing 5 to 20 cells. Keratinization is a very rare feature observed in long standing cysts. Metaplastic changes in the epithelium in terms of mucous cells and respiratory type of epithelium are common findings especially in maxillary cysts.

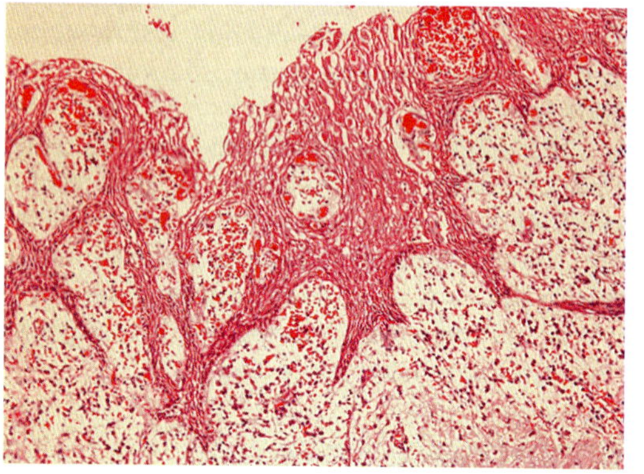

Fig. 5.3: Radicular cyst. Stratified squamous non-kerartinized epithelium showing arcading pattern and the cyst wall contains a mixed inflammatory infiltrate

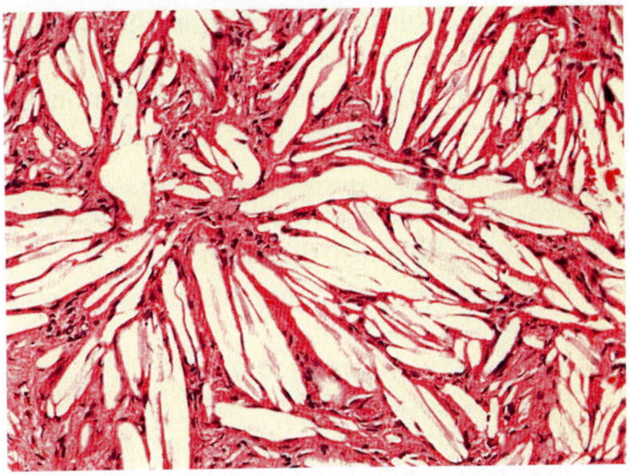

Fig. 5.4: Radicular cyst. Presence of cholesterol clefts in the cyst wall is a common finding

Hyaline bodies often referred to as hyaline bodies of Rushton are found in the epithelium in some cysts. They can rarely be found in the capsule. Although the origin of hyaline bodies was believed to be of hematogenous in the past, recent evidence shows that it is a secretory product of odontogenic epithelium. The capsule is inflamed with a dense mixed inflammatory infiltrate towards the epithelium. Cholesterol clefts with associated multinucleate giant cells are often present (**Fig. 5.4**). The lumen contains straw colored fluid containing epithelial debris, soluble proteins and cholesterol crystals. Shimmering effect can be demonstrated when the fluid is held to direct light.

Treatment

Radicular cysts have traditionally been treated by enucleation of the cyst and root canal treatment for the affected tooth if it is restorable but rarely for a larger lesion. Marsupialization is advisable in order to preserve the normal structures. However, most clinicians nowadays prefer to treat them with nonsurgical endodontics. The healing of the periapical region takes place due to acute inflammation as a result of instrumentation. There is always a controversy regarding healing of a properly formed cyst after root canal treatment. In order to answer this two types of radicular cysts have been described recently. One is called a "true cyst" where the cystic cavity has no connection with the root canal and the other type is known as a "pocket cyst" where the root canal opens into the cyst cavity. The latter type appears to be rare and it responds better to nonsurgical endodontics.

Lateral Periodontal Cyst

The lateral periodontal cyst is also of inflammatory origin. Therefore it is similar to a radicular cyst except that it arises in relation to a lateral root canal. Histological features are more or less identical.

Residual Cyst

A residual cyst is truly a radicular cyst without the causative tooth *in situ*. If the tooth is extracted without identifying the cystic lesion in the apical region the cyst can remain without symptoms. The diagnosis is usually by routine radiography performed for other treatment procedures or investigations. Histopathology is very similar to that of a radicular cyst. Long standing lesions may not show many inflammatory features as the causative tooth has been removed.

Paradental Cyst

Paradental cyst is defined as a cyst arising on the lateral aspect of a vital tooth as a result of inflammation in the periodontal pocket. The most common site of occurrence is the disto-buccal side of a partially erupted mandibular third molar. Infected mandibular buccal cyst which occurs in relation to first or second mandibular molars in children is also included in the category of paradental cyst. Recently the former has been named as a juvenile paradental cyst. The exact pathogenesis of the lesion is debatable as there are different views. However, it seems that the epithelium derives either from reduced enamel epithelium or cell rests of Malassez and the cyst forms as a result of expansion of lateral part of the follicle secondary to inflammation in the periodontal pocket.

Paradental cysts account for 1 to 4.7 percent of odontogenic cysts. There is a wide variation in the frequency in the published literature due to under diagnosis of the cyst as a result of inadequate clinical information reaching the pathologist and also due to the fact that histopathological features are similar to that of a radicular cyst.

Clinical and Radiological Features

The majority of cysts, in relation to mandibular third molars, usually occur in the third decade with significant male predilection (1:0.5). More than 60 to 70 percent of them have been diagnosed at the buccal or disto-buccal aspect of a partially erupted lower third molar. Juvenile forms of the cyst, which is common in the buccal side of the lower first molar occurs in and around 10 years of age. Most patients reveal a history of repeated attacks of pericoronitis. Pain and swelling are features in some patients and the affected tooth is vital. The above feature would exclude the possibility of an inflammatory periodontal cyst. The juvenile form is characterized by periosteal buccal bone formation in relation to the vital first mandibular molar tooth in a young child.

In radiographs, a paradental cyst shows a well defined and well corticated radiolucency on the buccal or more commonly on the disto-buccal side (**Fig. 5.5**). Lamina dura is usually intact.

Histopathology

The histopathological features of paradental cyst are identical to that of radicular cysts (**Fig. 5.3**). The lining epithelium is composed of hyperplastic non keratinized stratified squamous epithelium with the cyst wall containing a dense inflammatory infiltrate. Presence of cholesterol crystals in the capsule are a feature in some cases.

Removal of the affected tooth with enucleation of the cyst is the treatment of choice.

Box 5.2: Paradental cyst

Key features helpful in diagnosis
- Radiolucency in disto-buccal side of an impacted lower 3rd molar.
- Associated with a vital tooth.
- History of pericoronitis.
- Lining epithelium is nonkeratinized stratified squamous similar to radicular cyst.
- Cyst wall contains inflammatory infiltrate.

Dentigerous Cyst

Dentigerous cyst arises in relation to an unerupted tooth. The cyst wall encloses the crown due to expansion of the dental follicle and remains attached to the cemento-enamel junction (**Fig. 5.6**). Although there are different theories regarding the pathogenesis of dentigerous cyst, the most likely explanation is that the cyst forms as a result of accumulation of fluid between the reduced enamel epithelium and enamel. Hence, the cyst has been classified as of developmental in origin. There has been a view that periapical inflammation of the deciduous tooth may give rise to dentigerous cysts in the developing permanent tooth. However, the above cannot be applied to the most common

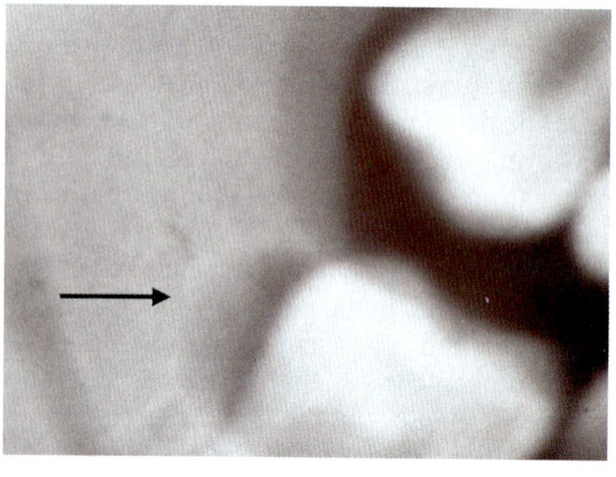

Fig. 5.5: Paradental cyst. Radiolucency on the distal aspect of a partially erupted lower-third molar is the most common presentation (*Courtesy:* Professor Jos Hille)

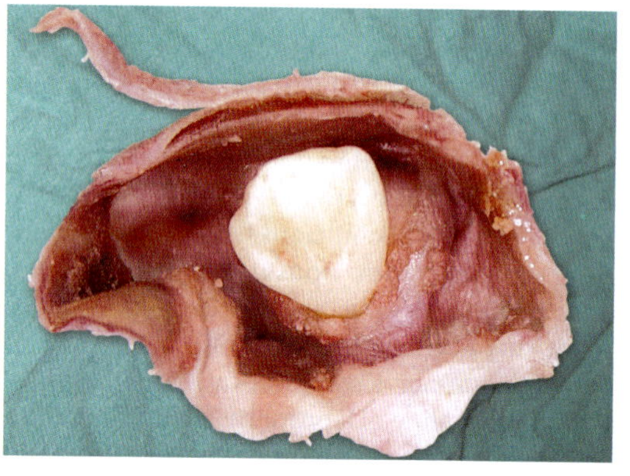

Fig. 5.6: Dentigerous cyst. Macroscopic appearance of the cyst shows attachment of the cyst lining to cemento-enamel junction

site of occurrence of a dentigerous cyst as there is no overlying deciduous in the lower 3rd molar area. Involvement of the *PTCH* gene has been implicated in the pathogenesis of the cyst but the evidence supporting the hypothesis is not confirmatory unlike in the case of odontogenic keratocyst. The expansion of the cyst is mostly similar to that of the radicular cyst with increased hydrostatic pressure and osmotic pressure within the cyst lumen. The evidence for the role of cytokine and other inflammatory mediators are lacking as dentigerous cysts expand irrespective of secondary inflammation.

Box 5.3: Dentigerous cyst

Key features helpful in diagnosis

- The most common developmental odontogenic cyst.
- Associated with an impacted tooth, frequently lower 3rd molar or upper canine.
- Presents as a well-defined radiolucency covering crown.
- Lining is thin nonkeratinized stratified squamous epithelium.
- Cyst lining is attached to cemento-enamel junction.
- Cyst wall is not inflamed unless it is infected.

Clinical and Radiological Features

Dentigerous cysts account for 16 to 24 percent of odontogenic cysts. The highest frequency is seen in the 2nd and 3rd decades. The most common site of occurrence is the mandibular 3rd molar region followed by maxillary canine, mandibular premolar and maxillary 3rd molar. Males are affected more than females (3:2). The diagnosis is mostly by radiographs when investigated for an unerupted or missing tooth. These are slow growing swellings usually without pain unless infected. Depending on the amount of overlying bone present , consistency on palpation is similar to that of a radicular cyst.

The majority present as unilocular radiolucent lesions with well defined and well corticated margins (**Fig. 5.7**). The appearance alters when the cyst is infected. Multilocularity is a rare presentation. Three different radiological patterns have been described depending on the relationship of the crown to radiolucency.

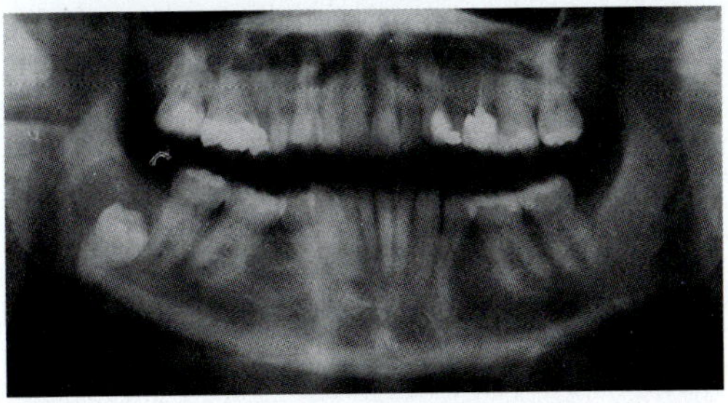

Fig. 5.7: Dentigerous cyst. Well-defined and well corticated cystic lesion associated with impacted right lower-third molar covering the crown of the tooth (*Courtesy:* Dr Jimmy Makdissi)

a. Central (whole crown is enveloped symmetrically)
b. Lateral (one aspect of the crown is enveloped)
c. Circumferential (almost the entire tooth is enveloped)

Rarely, when a radicular cyst arises from a deciduous tooth it mimics a dentigerous cyst in relation to the corresponding permanent tooth. Differentiation between dilated follicle and dentigerous cyst may not be easy radiologically. However, unless the pericoronal space is at least more than 4 to 5 mm, diagnosis of a cyst may not be reasonable.

Histopathology

Histopathological features reveal that the lining epithelium is of nonkeratinized stratified squamous and usually consists of 2 to 4 cells (**Fig. 5.8**). Presence of mucous secreting cells in the epithelium is a frequent feature in both maxillary (53%) and mandibular (36%) cysts. Together with mucous cells ciliated epithelium is also present in some lesions. Hyaline bodies of Rushton are found in the cyst epithelium occasionally. The cyst wall is composed of fibrous tissue and especially in noninflamed cysts the appearance is similar to that of follicular tissue. Odontogenic epithelial rests may be present in the cyst wall. When the cyst is inflamed the histopathological features are identical to that of a radicular cyst. Therefore, the clinical and radiological information is mandatory to arrive at the correct diagnosis. In addition, macroscopic

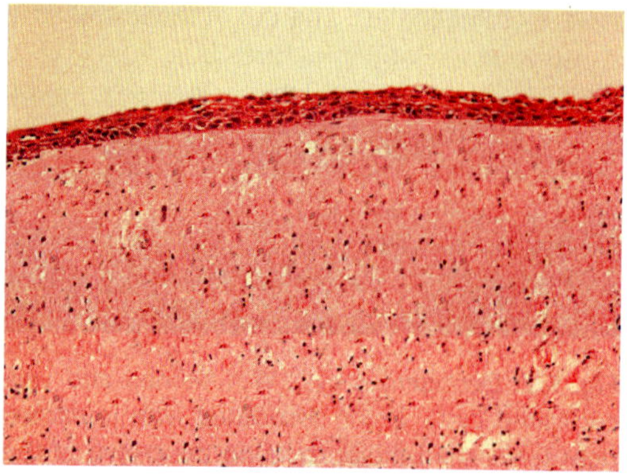

Fig. 5.8: Dentigerous cyst. The linning is composed of thin nonkeratinized stratified squamous epithelium. Fibrous cyst wall is without inflammatory cells

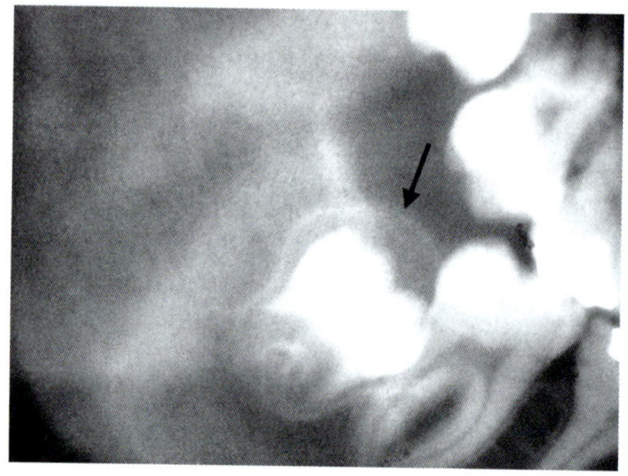

Fig. 5.9: Eruption cyst. Cyst in relation to erupting lower molar tooth shows a soft tissue shadow of the cyst (*Courtesy:* Professor Jos Hille)

examination shows the attachment of the cyst to cemento-enamel junction (**Fig. 5.6**).

Treatment and Prognosis

The majority of dentigerous cysts are enucleated together with the unerupted tooth. However, for dentigerous cysts in children if the tooth is in a favorable position to erupt partial removal of the cyst exposing the tooth followed by orthodontic traction may help to align the tooth to the correct position. Larger cysts can be treated with marsupialization allowing the cyst to decompress and complete removal of the cyst can be carried out later on with a simple surgical procedure. Ameloblastoma arising in dentigerous cyst has been reported although there are arguments for and against. Mucoepidermoid carcinoma arising from mucous secreting cells of the lining has also been reported.

Eruption Cyst

The eruption cyst is considered as the soft tissue counterpart of dentigerous cyst. Actual frequency of the cyst is difficult to determine as this is rarely biopsied and spontaneous rupture and eruption of the tooth does not indicate further treatment. Therefore, the number of cases in pathology files is much lower than the real occurrence. Pathogenesis is similar to that of dentigerous cyst and the lining epithelium is derived from reduced enamel epithelium.

Clinical Features

Although it arises in relation to any erupting tooth, maxillary first permanent molar and incisors are frequently affected. The cyst occurs in relation to both deciduous and permanent teeth. The majority are reported before the age of 10 years with a slight male predilection. Characteristic presentation is a bluish translucent swelling over the crown of an erupting tooth. Most lesions rupture due to trauma. Although there are no radiological changes in most lesions, some may show a soft tissue shadow (**Fig. 5.9**).

Histopathological Features

When a cyst is submitted for histopathological evaluation, surface epithelium is usually included overlying the cyst. Demarcation between connective tissue of the lamina propria and cyst wall is difficult to identify. The connective tissue towards the cyst epithelium is inflamed. Lining epithelium is stratified squamous with 2 to 3 cells in thickness (**Fig. 5.10**).

Treatment

Treatment is not indicated. However, eruption of the affected tooth is facilitated by simple excision of the overlying epithelium and connective tissue.

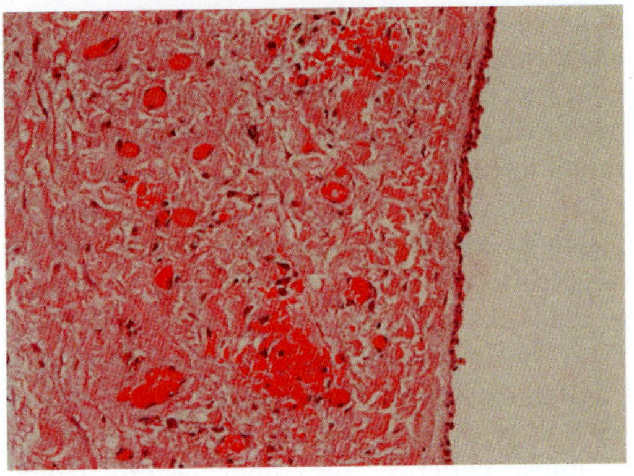

Fig. 5.10: Eruption cyst. Fibrous cyst wall is lined by thin nonkeratinized epithelium similar to reduced enamel epithelium

Odontogenic Keratocyst (Keratocystic Odontogenic Tumor)

Odontogenic keratocyst (OKC) is the second most common developmental odontogenic cyst and the most investigated cyst in terms of its pathogenesis and behavior compared to other cystic lesions. The cyst is known to recur more than all other cysts. In addition, it grows faster and to a larger size than the rest. These differences may have led the researchers to work on this and raise controversy of the nature of the lesion as to whether it is a cyst or a true neoplastic lesion. Accordingly, WHO in its 2005 classification renamed OKC as "keratocystic odnotogenic tumor". However, the debate on accepting the term is going on and it will take some more years for clinicians and pathologists to understand the issue comprehensively. OKC is also associated with nevoid basal cell carcinoma syndrome (NBCCS) or Gorlin Goltz syndrome.

OKC arises either from dental lamina or from its remnants. However, some cysts are thought to arise from basal cell proliferation of surface epithelium. Arising from the enamel organ before dental hard tissue formation is a theory that has very little evidence for justification. Identification of mutations in *PTCH* gene which is considered to be the mutated oncosuppressor gene in NBCCS has shed new dimensions to the pathogenesis of OKC. It reveals that syndromic patients as well as a minority of sporadic lesions show mutations in *PTCH* gene leading the trend towards the neoplastic nature of the lesion. The cyst has two inherent features in terms of high growth potential and ability for recurrence than other odontogenic cysts. Expansion of the cyst may have different mechanisms to those of radicular and dentigerous cysts. There may be ways other than fluid related expansion in OKC. Growth of the epithelium is shown to play a key role as the growth potential of cystic epithelium is higher than other cystic lesions and in some cases similar to ameloblastoma. Matrixmetalloproteinases (MMPs) and IL-1 have also been implicated in expansion. OKC recurs more frequently than other odontogenic cysts. There are several reasons suggested including presence of satellite or daughter cysts, thin and fragile cystic epithelium with increased possibility of leaving fragments during surgery, extension of the cyst between roots, flat epithelial connective tissue interface, intrinsic growth potential of the epithelium and cyst arising from proliferation of basal cells of the surface epithelium. In addition syndromic patients develop multiple new cysts as well as recurrences. Diagnosis of the cyst is usually by radiography and histopathology. Fine needle aspiration biopsy is not a pathognomonic investigation. Soluble protein content in the cyst fluid is usually less than 5 g/dL whilst it is more than 5 g/dL in radicular and dentigerous cyst.

Clinical and Radiological Features

It has been reported that OKC accounts for up to 4 to 10 percent of odontogenic cysts, with 40 to 60 percent of the patients in 2nd and 3rd decades. It is rare in the 1st decade. Diagnosis of OKC in syndromic patients is earlier (10–30 years) than that of nonsyndromic patients (15–45 years). Although there is a male predilection (1.5:1) for nonsyndromic patients, a slight female dominance has been reported for syndromic patients. Seventy percent of the lesions occur in the mandible with half of these located close to angle of the mandible (**Fig. 5.11**). Usually presents as a slow growing painless swelling although some may complain of pain. Large mandibular lesions tend to be associated with paresthesia of the lower lip. When a cyst shows visible swelling it has already developed to a larger lesion because of the extension within

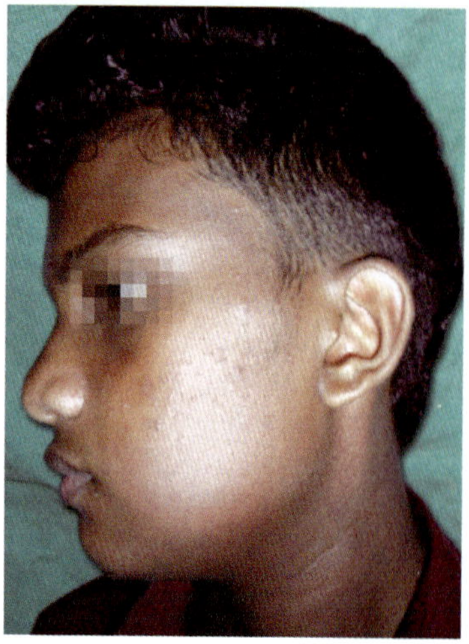

Fig. 5.11: Odentogenic keratocyst. A large bony hard swelling in the left body and angle of the mandible in a young boy

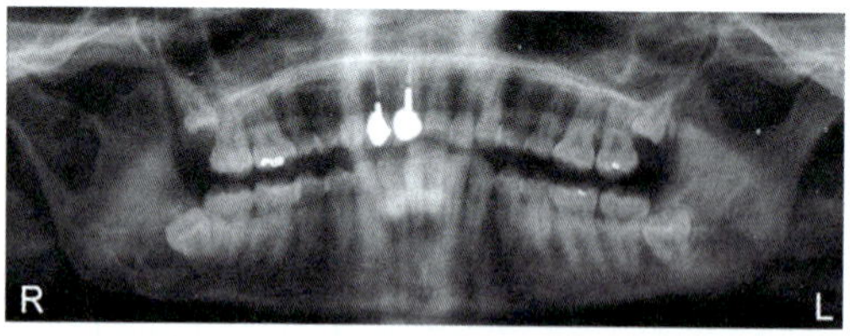

Fig. 5.12: Odentogenic keratocyst. Large multilocular radiolucency with well-defined and corticated margins in the right angle and ramus of the mandible (*Courtesy:* Dr Jimmy Makdissi)

the medullary cavity without giving rise to a swelling. For the same reason some patients are unaware of the cyst until it causes a pathological fracture. OKC in the maxilla, especially in close relation to the antrum, may give rise to proptosis and diplopia due destruction or lifting up of the orbital floor.

Radiologically, OKC presents either as a unilocular or multilocular radiolucency with well defined and well corticated margins in most patients (**Fig. 5.12**). However, some unilocular lesions with scalloped borders may be misinterpreted as multilocular. When this occurs at the angle of the mandible anteroposterior extension appears to be more pronounced than buccolingual. The inferior dental canal is usually displaced downward in larger lesions. Displacement of adjacent teeth is a feature but significant resorption of roots is not common. When the lesion is larger, perforation of the cortical plate may be seen. Multilocular radiolucency in the angle of the mandible is an important clinical scenario as several lesions should be considered in the differential diagnosis. The most important one in the list is ameloblastoma because an ameloblastoma is a true tumor, there is prominent buccolingual expansion, paresthesia of the lower lip and resorption of roots compared to OKC in most patients. The other lesions which should be excluded with clinicopathological correlation are ameloblastic fibroma, central giant cell granuloma, odontogenic myxoma and aneurysmal bone cyst. Smaller cysts in between roots of two teeth mimic the appearance of lateral periodontal cyst.

Histopathology

Histopathologically the cyst lining shows a characteristic stratified squamous parakeratinized epithelium of uniform thickness containing 5 to 10 cells. The surface of the epithelium is corrugated (**Fig. 5.13A**). Cysts with orthokeratin on the surface do not show characteristic features of OKC. Therefore it has been described as a separate entity in recent literature as orthokeratinizing odontogenic cyst. Basal budding is present in some cases. The basal cells show palisading and the nuclei are hyperchromatic (**Fig. 5.13B**). Epithelial connective tissue interface is flat. The cyst wall is composed of dense fibrous tissue and contains satellite cysts up to 7 to 25 percent of the cases. The lumen contains keratin. When the cyst is infected epithelium tends to be hyperplastic and the surface keratin is lost making confirmation of the diagnosis difficult.

Treatment

Most OKCs are treated with enucleation and surface curettage of the cystic cavity. Carnoy's solution is used for chemical cauterization of the cavity by some surgeons. However, it is not unusual to observe aggressive lesions demanding more radical treatment with resection of the segment and subsequent bone graft. Decompression is also indicated for

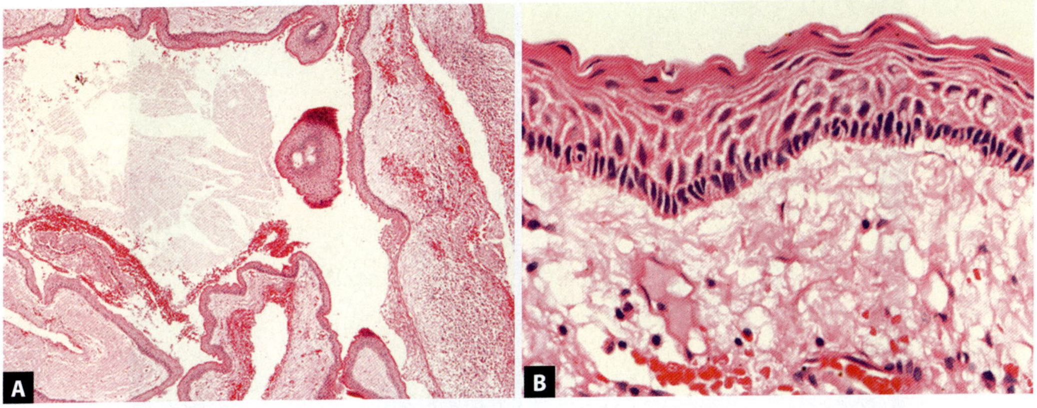

Figs 5.13A and B: Odontogenic keratocyst. (A) Stratified squamous parakeratinized epithelium with a corrugated surface; (B) Typical basal palisading; hyperchromatism

larger lesions allowing shrinkage of the cyst with peripheral bone formation and removal of the cyst later on with simple enucleation. Recurrence rates may vary from 5 to 60 percent according to the literature due to various reasons, more realistic recurrence rate appears to be around 30 percent.

Box 5.4: Odontogenic keratocyst

Key features helpful in diagnosis

- Presents as a multilocular or unilocular radiolucency.
- May mimic ameloblastoma when presents as large multilocular lesions.
- Majority of the patients are in 2nd and 3rd decades.
- Lining epithelium is parakeratinized stratified squamous and shows basal palisading.
- Cyst wall is uninflamed and may contain satellite cysts.
- Cyst may be associated with nevoid basal cell carcinoma syndrome.
- Behavior is more aggressive than other odontogenic cysts.

Nevoid Basal Cell Carcinoma Syndrome

Nevoid basal cell carcinoma syndrome (NBCCS) is an autosomal dominant disease which shows multisystem manifestations as a result of mutations in *PTCH* gene mapped in chromosome 9q22.3-q31. In order to diagnose the syndrome there should be at least two major criteria or one major and two minor criteria.

Major criteria include:

- More than two basal cell carcinomas (BCC) or one in patients younger than 20 years
- Histologically proven odontogenic keratocyst
- Three or more palmar or plantar pits
- Calcification of falx cerebri
- Bifid ribs
- First degree relative with the syndrome.

Minor criteria include:

- Macrocephaly
- Congenital abnormalities such as cleft lip or palate, frontal bossing, coarse facies, hypertelorism
- Skeletal deformities such as syndactyly
- Ovarian fibroma
- Radiologic abnormalities such as bridging of sella turcica, vertebral abnormalities (spina bifida occulta).

Basal cell carcinoma syndrome (BCCS) are found in more than 90 percent of the patients (**Figs 5.14A and B**) who are over 40 years and 75 to 80 percent of them present with OKCs. In addition to BCC a minority may develop other tumors such as medulloblastoma, meningioma, cardiac fibroma and fetal rhabdomyoma. Except for aggressive BCCs which can bring about a fatal outcome, most others are not life threatening. OKCs are treated in the same way as nonsyndromic cysts. Regular follow-up is

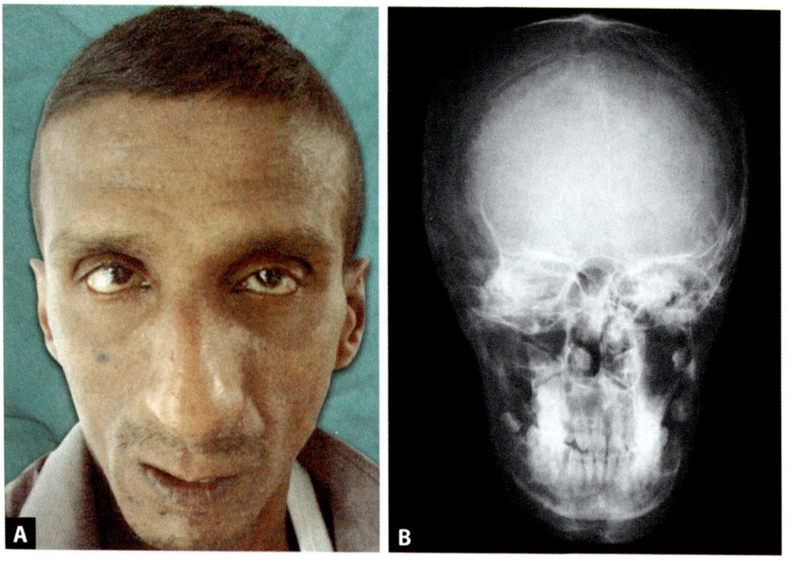

Figs 5.14A and B: Nevoid basal cell carcinoma syndrome. Characteristic facial appearance with hypertelorism and slightly prognathic mandible. *Note:* (A) The small BCC; (B) calcification of falx cerebri

mandatory to identify new lesions which may arise during the course of the disease.

Orthokeratinized Odontogenic Cyst

Orthokeratinized odontogenic cyst (OOC) has been recognized as a new entity in the recent past. It was classified as the orthokeratinized variant of OKC. However, due to histopathological as well as behavioral differences it is justifiable to label this as a separate entity. Approximately, up to 15 percent of keratinizing cysts in jaw bones are OCCs.

Clinical and Radiological Features

Clinical and radiological features are mostly similar to that of OKC. However, there is a significant male predominance to the disease (2:1). The majority of them occur in the angle of the mandible and simulate dentigerous cysts. Although many of those present as unilocular radiolucencies, some have multilocularity.

Histopathology

Histopathological features are different from OKC. Lining is stratified squmous with marked orthokeratin on the surface showing a very prominent granular cell layer (**Fig. 5.15**). The epithelium is much thinner than OKC in some cases mimicking the appearance of dermoid/epidermoid cyst. The characteristic corrugated surface and basal palisading seen in OKC is not present.

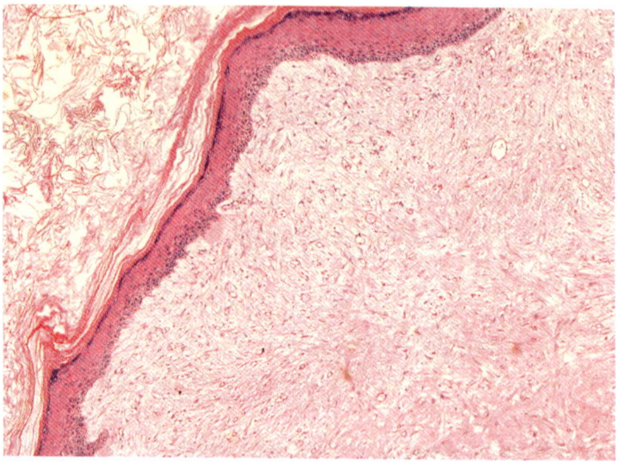

Fig. 5.15: Orthokeratinized odontogenic cyst. Lining epithelium is composed of markedly orthokeratinized straitified squamous epithelium and basal palisading is not present

Treatment

This is much less aggressive in behavior compared to OKC and needs only enucleation and surface curettage. The recurrence rate of approximately 2 percent is justifiable evidence to suggest that OCC is a separate entity.

Gingival Cyst of Newborn

Historically two types of gingival cysts are described in infants under the names of Epstein's pearls and Bohn's nodules. The former is of developmental non odontogenic in origin and the latter is odontogenic in origin. Bohn's nodules arise from remnants of dental lamina known as glands of Serres. Epstein pearls may arise as a result of epithelial inclusions at the line of fusion of nasal processes and palatine shelves. It has also been suggested that they may arise due to abortive glandular differentiation leading to formation of small cysts.

Clinical Features

Bohn's nodules occur on alveolus of infants who usually are less than 3 months (**Fig. 5.16A**). Although these lesions are very common ranging from 50 to 94 percent according to different studies, the need to perform a biopsy is unlikely as they undergo spontaneous involution. Clinically they appear as small white nodules.

Epstein pearls are also known as midpalatal raphae cysts and occur in relation to midpalatine raphae (**Fig. 5.16B**). Radiological changes are not evident as these are present within the soft tissue.

Histopathology

Histopathologically both lesions share similar appearances. They are small circular structures lined by thin parakeratinized stratified squamous epithelium. Lumen is filled with keratin. However, there is no basal palisading which helps to differentiate them from odontogenic keratocyst.

Treatment

Treatment is not indicated as these lesions undergo spontaneous involution. It may be necessary to squeeze out the contents to enhance the process of involution.

Gingival Cyst of Adults

Gingival cyst of adults (GCA) is a soft tissue lesion present on the gingival mucosa with minimal radiological changes. Various theories have been put forward regarding the pathogenesis,

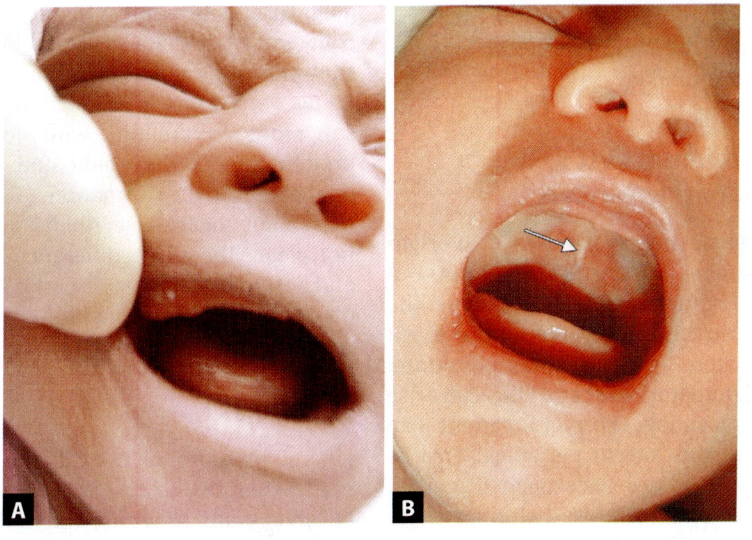

Figs 5.16A and B: Gingival cyst of newborn. (A) Bohn's nodules on the maxillary alveolus; (B) Epstein pearls on the midpalatal region (*Courtesy:* Dr Dilip George)

including its origin from epithelial rests of dental lamina, cystic degeneration of surface epithelial projections and traumatic implantation of surface epithelium. Recent evidence suggests that it arises from junctional epithelium which is a derivative of reduced enamel epithelium.

Clinical and Radiological Features

Gingival cyst of adults (GCA) accounts for 0.06 to 0.08 percent of odontogenic cysts. This is mostly diagnosed in the 5th to 6th decade. Females are affected more than males (2:1). Mandibular lesions are more common and the preferred site appear to be attached gingiva on the buccal or labial surface in relation to canine to premolar area. Patients usually present with slow growing well circumscribed pink or bluish swellings and most lesions are less than 1 cm in diameter. Related teeth are vital. Swelling is fluctuant as there is no overlying bone.

Histopathology

Histopathologically most of the cyst wall is uninflamed except towards the junctional epithelium. Lining epithelium is thin stratified squamous non keratinized consisting of 2 to 4 cell layers. Frequently epithelial cells are either flat or cuboidal simulating the appearance of reduced enamel epithelium. Localized areas of epithelial thickening are seen in some cases.

Treatment is by simple surgical excision and recurrence is unlikely.

Lateral Periodontal Cyst and Botryoid Odontogenic Cyst

Both these lesions are developmental in origin with considerable similarities in terms of location, histology and radiological features. The term lateral periodontal cyst (LPC) implies that it occurs on the lateral aspect of the periodontium. However, inflammatory LPC and OKC can arise in the same location. Botryoid variant can extend beyond this site to periapical area as well. Three possibilities have been discussed with regards to pathogenesis, including origin from reduced enamel epithelium, remnants of dental lamina and cell rests of Malassez. Reduced enamel epithelium theory suggests that it arises as a dentigerous cyst on the lateral side of the tooth with expansion of the follicle and subsequent eruption of the tooth.

Clinical and Radiological Features

Both entities are uncommon and LPC accounts for about 0.5 to 0.7 percent of the odontogenic cysts. Botryoid type is even rarer. Fifth and sixth decades of life show the highest frequency. The majority of the cases are reported from incisor, canine and premolar areas of the mandible.

Lateral periodontal cyst (LPC) is usually diagnosed on routine radiographs as most of them are without any symptoms. Pain is a feature in occasional cases. The clinical appearance simulates gingival cysts of adults to some extent as some cases may be fluctuant. Those who have botryoid variant can present with a significant swelling compared to LPC.

Radiologically most lesions are less than 1 cm in diameter and presents in between mid-radicular area of two roots. Associated root resorption is unlikely. The botryoid type is usually multilocular but some cases are unilocular. However, they grow to a much larger size than the LPC and can extend into periapical area.

Histopathology

Diagnosis of LPC should be reached by excluding gingival cyst of adult, inflammatory LPC and collateral type of OKC. Histopathologically LPC shows an uninflamed cyst wall and characteristic lining composed of nonkeratinized stratified squamous epithelium with focal areas of proliferation of the epithelium giving rise to epithelial plaque formation (**Fig. 5.17**). The reason for localized epithelial proliferation is not clear. The main difference between LPC and botryoid odontogenic cyst is the multicystic nature of the latter and the cystic spaces are separated by thin fibrous septae.

Treatment

Lateral periodontal cyst (LPC) is treated by enucleation of the cyst without sacrificing the adjacent tooth. However, botryoid cysts in some patients give rise to recurrence after simple enucleation. Therefore, regular follow-up is indicated.

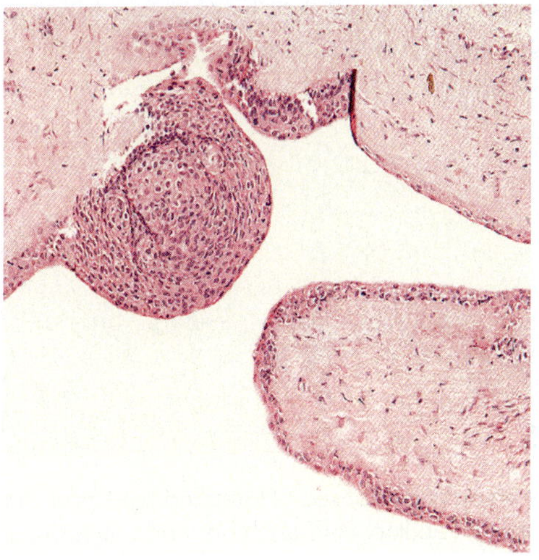

Fig. 5.17: Lateral periodontal cyst/Botryoid cyst. The cyst is lined by stratified squamous nonkeratinized epithelium with prominent epithelial plaque formation. The cyst wall is uninflamed

Glandular Odontogenic Cyst (Sialo-odontogenic Cyst)

The sialo-odontogenic cyst was first described in 1987 by Padayachee and Van Wyk. A year later Gardner et al, introduced the term glandular odontogenic cyst (GOC). This is an aggressive lesion compared to other odontogenic cysts except OKC. It shares histological similarities with LPC, botryoid cyst and low grade central muco epidermoid carcinoma, hence the accurate diagnosis is a must. Although, there was a controversy about the origin of the lesion, it is accepted that the cyst is of odontogenic origin. The main confusion was based on the glandular differentiation in the cystic epithelium. It shows the pluripotential nature of odontogenic epithelium than anything else. Moreover, a few cases have been reported with hyaline bodies which is claimed to be a secretory product of odontogenic epithelium providing evidence for odontogenic nature.

Clinical and Radiological Features

Glandular odontogenic cyst (GOC) is an uncommon lesion comprising of 0.17 to 0.2 percent of odontogenic cysts. Peak incidence of the cyst is in the 6th decade. There is a slight male preponderance. The anterior mandible is the frequently reported site of occurrence. Pain is a feature in some patients.

Glandular odontogenic cyst (GOC) presents as a multilocular or unilocular radiolucency with well defined borders in most cases. However, features supporting aggressive behavior such as perforation of cortical plates, root resorption and displacement have also been reported.

Histopathology

The cyst lining is composed of non keratinized stratified squamous epithelium of varying thickness. Superficial layer of the lining epithelium shows either cuboidal or columnar cells with cilia (**Figs 5.18A and B**). Epithelial plaque formation is seen similar to that of LPC and botryoid cyst. Because of the presence of pseudoglandular spaces containing PAS and mucicarmine positive material and microcysts within the epithelium, low grade central mucoepidermoid carcinoma should be excluded. Goblet cells are also found on the upper layers of the epithelium. The cyst wall is usually uninflamed as the cyst is of developmental in origin.

Box 5.5: Glandular odontogenic cyst

Key features helpful in diagnosis

- Most patients are in 6th decade of life.
- Anterior mandible is the most common site.
- Presents as a unilocular or multilocular radiolucency with resorption and displacement of adjacent teeth.
- Lining epithelium is non keratinized stratified squamous with surface cells showing columnar appearance with cilia.
- Mucoepidermoid carcinoma should be excluded as pseudoglandular differentiation and goblet cells are frequently present.

Treatment

Small unilocular lesions are treated by enucleation and surface curettage. Large multilocular lesions need marginal or segmental jaw resection. Marsupialization is recommended for larger lesions in order to preserve adjacent vital structures. However, a second surgery should be followed with enucleation and curettage of the bony cavity. Recurrence rates have been

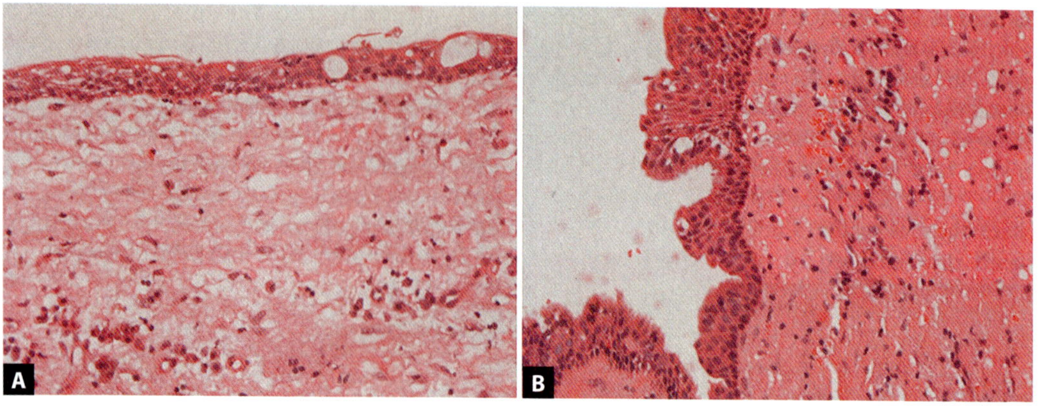

Figs 5.18A and B: Glandular odontogenic cyst. (A) Cyst lining is composed of stratified squamous non-keratinized epithelium with a few pseudoglandular spaces; (B) Papillary configurations and cilia formation

reported up to 55 percent confirming the aggressive nature of the cyst. Regular follow-up is mandatory.

Malignant Transformation in Odontogenic Cysts

Malignant transformation of odontogenic cysts is a rare phenomenon. Most of the reported cases have shown malignant changes into squamous cell carcinoma. However, rarely mucoepidermoid carcinoma arising in relation to dentigerous cyst has been reported. According to the literature malignant change may vary from 0.13 to 2 percent. Sixth and seventh decades are to accountable for most cases and it appears that the lower figure is more realistic. Male to female ratio appears to be 2:1 and the mandible is affected four times more commonly than the maxilla. Malignant transformation is seen in odontogenic keratocyst, radicular cyst, dentigerous cyst, lateral periodontal cyst and residual cyst. It is known that most intraosseous carcinomas of jaw bones arise from cystic lesions. In order to confirm the diagnosis a few possibilities such as arising from surface epithelium, metastatic deposit and cystic degeneration of a solid epithelial tumor should be excluded. Evidence of epithelial dysplasia in the cystic epithelium and transition of dysplastic cystic epithelium to squamous cell carcinoma can be identified in a majority of the cases.

NONODONTOGENIC CYSTS

Nasopalatine Cyst (Incisive Canal Cyst)

Nasopalatine duct cyst (NPC) arises within the nasopalatine canal or soft tissue of the palate at the opening of the canal. NPC is by far the most common nonodontogenic cyst in jaw bones accounting for more than 75 percent. Overall 10 percent of all cysts in jaw bones are of this type. The current literature reveals that the entity median palatine cyst is a posteriorly placed NPC. Exact pathogenesis of NPC is not known. Out of the theories put forward by various people relating to different structures, cystic degeneration of the remnants of the nasopalatine duct appears to be the most reasonable.

Clinical and Radiological Features

The most common age group to be affected is 3rd to 6th decade of life. There is a marked male predilection (2.5:1). The majority of patients present with a swelling of the midline of the anterior palate. Some complain of swelling of the mid anterior labial sulcus. If the lesion is larger, it is visible from both sides together with lifting of the anterior nasal floor. Displacement of two upper central incisors may present. Positive vitality testing is helpful in excluding the possibility of a radicular cyst.

Smaller lesions are usually diagnosed during routine radiological examination. When interpreting a radiograph for NPC, reference should always be made to a possible anatomical variation of a larger incisive fossa in order to avoid over diagnosis leading to unnecessary treatment. NPC is a round to oval radiololucency in between roots of upper central incisors (**Fig. 5.19**). Intact lamina dura with positive vitality further enhance the accuracy of clinical diagnosis.

Histopathology

Microscopically, lining epithelium is nonkeratinized stratified squamous in over 70 percent of the cases. However, it is very frequent to have various other types of epithelium, at least in part of the lining including, pseudostratified columnar, cuboidal or rarely simple columnar type (**Fig. 5.20**). Goblet cells are also seen in some cases. Although NPC is developmental in origin inflammatory cells are present in the cyst wall of most cases as a secondary phenomenon. Another characteristic feature is the presence of neurovascular bundle within the capsule. Mucous glands are also present in up to 30 percent of the cases.

Treatment

Treatment is by enucleation. Some lesions are biopsied before enucleation as clinical diagnosis

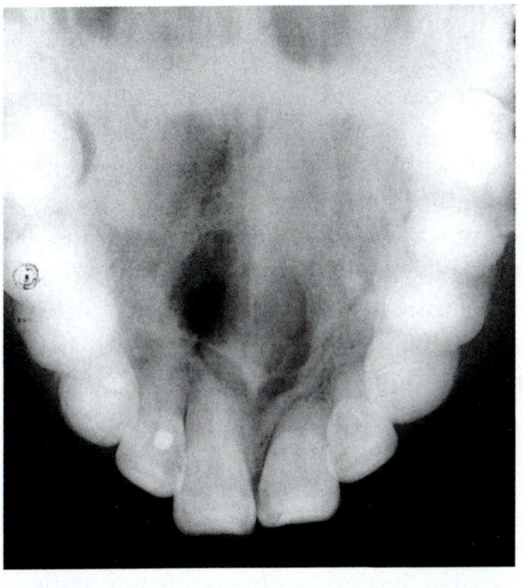

Fig. 5.19: Nasopalatine cyst. Well-defined radiolucency in between the roots of upper central incisors extending into palate (*Courtesy:* Dr Jimmy Makdissi)

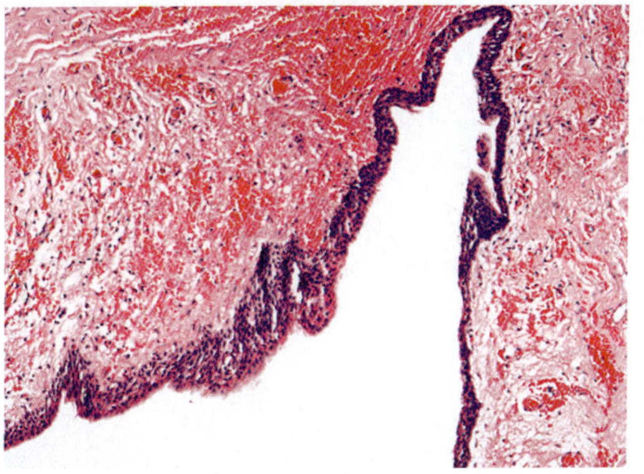

Fig. 5.20: Nasopalatine cyst. Lining epithelium is comprised of stratified squamous in areas and pseudostratified columnar ciliated in others

may not be confirmatory. Once complete enucleation is achieved recurrence is unlikely.

Nasolabial Cyst

Nasolabial cyst (NLC) is a rare developmental cyst in the soft tissues of the nasolabial fold. Bilateral cysts are present up to 10 percent. Pathogenesis of the cyst is attributed to two theories. One of them is the fissural cyst concept relating it to development from epithelial remnants from the line of fusion of maxillary, lateral nasal and medial nasal processes. But this is unlikely as fissural theory has almost been abandoned now. Most likely the origin is from epithelial remnants of the lower part of nasolacrimal duct.

Clinical and Radiological Features

The nasolabial cyst has a marked female predilection unlike other cystic lesions (3.5:1). Fourth and fifth decades of life show the highest frequency. Swelling of upper lip lateral to the midline with elevation of alar of the nose is the characteristic clinical presentation. Some lesions can grow-up to a reasonable size causing nasal obstruction and difficulty in wearing upper denture. Rupture of the cyst results in a discharging sinus either into oral or nasal cavity.

Radiological features are not very prominent unlike other intra bony cysts. Saucerization of alveolus is usually seen above the apices of

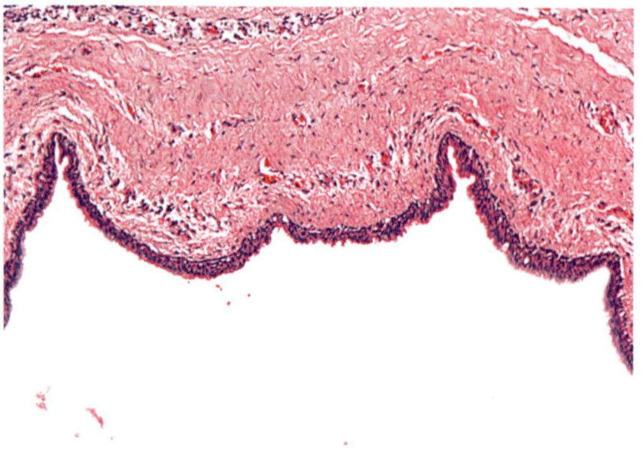

Fig. 5.21: Nasolabial cyst. Fibrous cyst wall is lined by pseudostratified columnar epithelium with some areas containing cilia

upper incisor teeth as a radiolucency. There can be changes in the nasal aperture.

Histopathology

Lining epithelium of NLC is usually pseudostratified columnar mostly without any cilia. Presence of cilia though is a feature in some cases. Goblet cells can be found in abundance in some cases. Rare cases may show cuboidal or flat squamous epithelium focally. The cyst wall contains inflammatory cells as a secondary phenomenon (**Fig. 5.21**).

Treatment

Treatment is by enucleation of the cyst from an intra oral approach. If the lesion extends into the nasal side, it is advisable to excise the affected part of the nasal mucosa. Recurrence is unlikely.

Aneurysmal Bone Cyst

Aneurysmal bone cyst (ABC) is a non-epithelialized cyst that rarely occurs in jaw bones. Definite pathogenesis of the cyst is not known. Trauma, vascular malformation and bleeding into a pre-existing lesion have been considered as possible mechanisms. Presence of ABC within fibro-cemento-osseous lesions such as cemento ossifying fibroma and fibrous dysplasia is well documented. Central giant cell granuloma and giant cell tumor can also be associated with ABC. In contrast most ABCs especially in extragnathic skeleton occur without a pre-existing lesion.

Clinical and Radiological Features

Aneurysmal bone cyst represents approximately 0.5 percent of cysts in jaw bones and jaw lesions account for 2 percent of all ABCs. Long bones and vertebral column are the common sites for the lesion. There is no significant gender difference. The posterior mandible is the most common site in jaw bones (**Figs 5.22A and B**). The lesion is frequently seen in young people especially in the 2nd decade of life. Usual presentation is a rapidly growing swelling with most patients complaining of pain. Because of the faster growth, cortical perforation or "egg-shell crackling" can be present.

Most lesions present as multilocular lesions whereas a minority shows a unilocular radiolucency. Marked cortical expansion is a feature with some presenting with cortical perforation. There is ballooning expansion of the affected bone. This should be included in the differential diagnosis of multilocular radiolucency in the angle of the mandible with other lesions described under OKC. Reactive bone formation can give rise to radio-opacities within the radiolucency in some cases.

Histopathology

Ameurysmal bone cyst (ABC) does not have a cyst lining. However, there is a pseudolining in some cases with giant cells and granulation tissue (**Fig. 5.23**). Large vascular spaces are present within the cyst wall. Extravasated blood and hemosiderin pigment is present. Some areas of the lesion are very similar to giant cell granuloma. Osteoid and woven bone formation is a feature. Especially, solid type ABCs can mimic the appearances of fibro cemento osseous lesions.

Treatment

Treatment is by enucleation and curettage. Bleeding is to be expected during surgery. Some aggressive lesions with significant bone loss need segmental surgery and reconstruction. Recurrence has been reported from 8 to 44 percent in different studies.

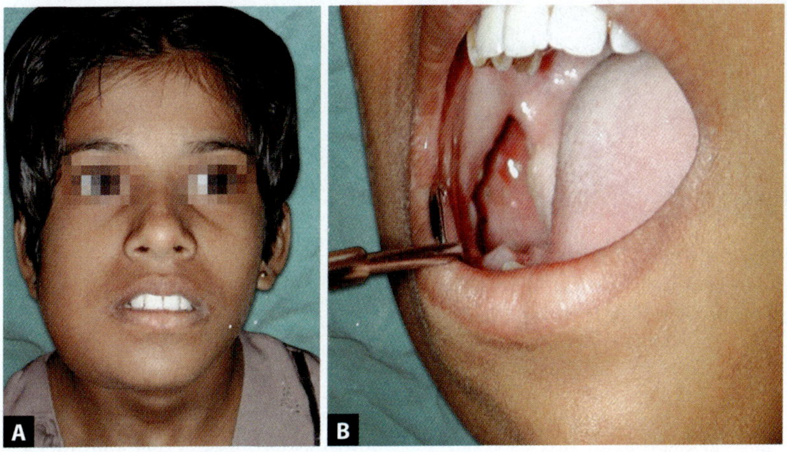

Figs 5.22A and B: Aneurysmal bone cyst. (A) Young girl with a large swelling of the right posterior body of the mandible; (B) Cystic cavity (*Courtesy:* Dr DK Dias)

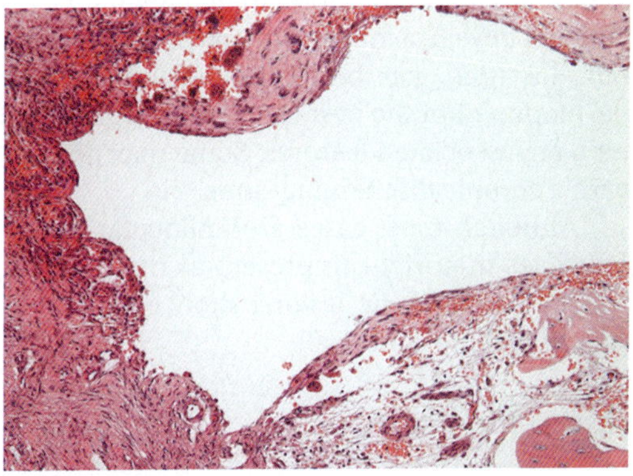

Fig. 5.23: Aneurysmal bone cyst. Pseudolining of granulation tissue and giant cells. Cyst wall is markedly vascular

Solitary Bone Cyst (Simple Bone Cyst, Traumatic Bone Cyst, Hemorrhagic Bone Cyst, Unicameral Bone Cyst)

Solitary bone cyst (SBC) is a rare cystic lesion in jaw bones. It usually presents in long bones. Although pathogenesis of this lesion is uncertain, the most likely cause appears to be trauma leading to intramedullary hemorrhage. It is suggested that failure to organize the hematoma leads to cyst formation. The reason for this failure is not clear. Prevalence of SBC is 0.5 to 1 percent according to literature. Rarely this lesion is associated with fibrocemento-osseous lesions.

Clinical and Radiological Features

The majority of SBCs are diagnosed in the 2nd decade of life. There is no significant gender difference. Over 90 percent of the reported cases are from mandible. Swelling can be the presenting feature in some. History of a trauma can be elicited in most patients.

Identification of SBC is usually accidental in routine radiographs (**Fig. 5.24**). Unilocular radiolucency with well defined borders is common and scalloping is frequently observed in relation to the upper border in between roots. Occasional cases may show root resorption. Presence of bony septae gives rise to multilocular appearance in a minority of lesions.

Histopathology

Solitary bone cyst (SBC) is a nonepithelial cyst. The amount of tissue received for diagnostic purposes can be very small. Fibrous and granulation tissue with admixed fibrin and multinucleate giant cells are present (**Fig. 5.25**). Red blood cells and hemosiderin pigment are also seen.

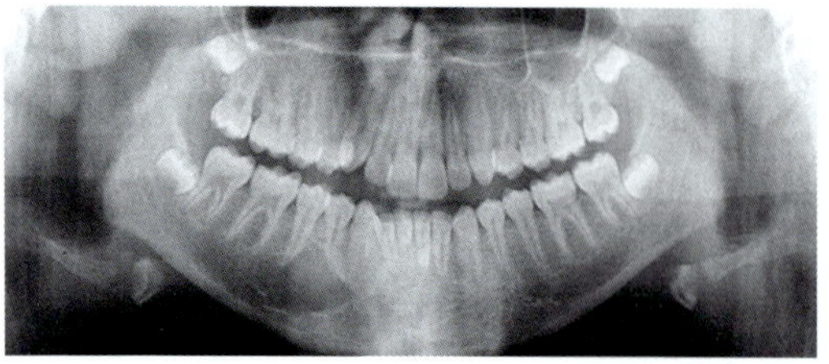

Fig. 5.24: Solitary bone cyst. Unilocular radiolucency with well-defined and well corticated margins in the right body of the mandible (*Courtesy:* Dr Jimmy Makdissi)

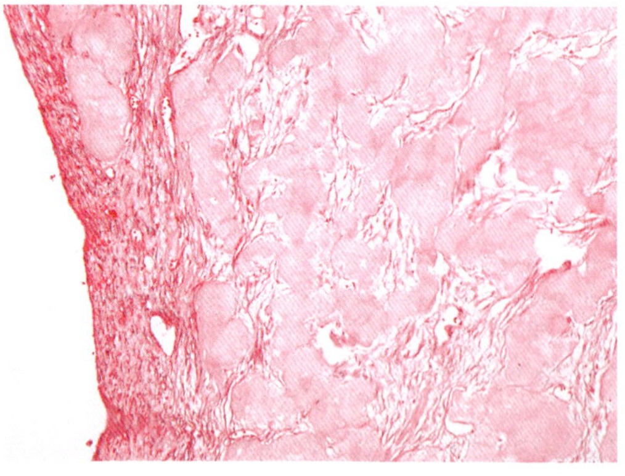

Fig. 5.25: Solitary bone cyst. There is no lining epithelium and the cyst wall contains fibrous and granulation tissue with fibrin deposits

Treatment

Treatment is usually by curettage. The cyst cavity is empty compared to other cystic lesions. Recurrence is very unusual.

Surgical Ciliated Cyst of the Maxilla (Postsurgical Maxillary Cyst)

This rare cyst occurs subsequent to a surgical procedure in the maxilla. In most patients it appears to be the Caldwell-Luc operation to gain access to antral cavity. It shows a higher prevalence in Japan compared to rest of the world. Entrapment of antral epithelium in the healing bony wound is suggested as the possible pathogenesis.

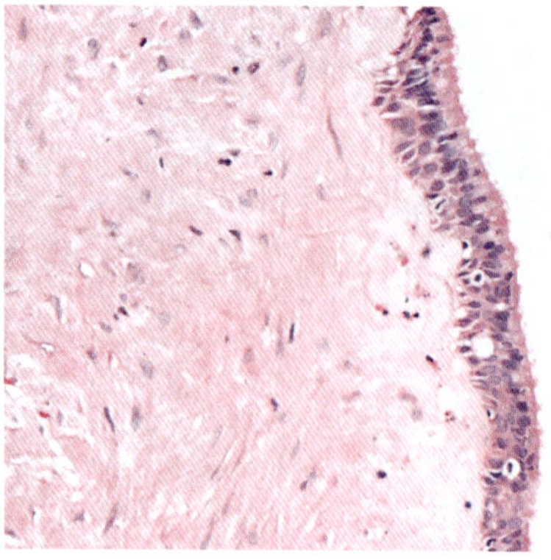

Fig. 5.26: Surgical ciliated cyst of the maxilla. Non-inflamed fibrous cyst wall is lined by pseudostratified columnar ciliated epithelium

Clinical and Radiological Features

The highest incidence is in 5th and 6th decades. Males are affected more than females (2:1). Patients reveal a history of maxillary surgery but the time gap between the surgery and development of the cyst can vary. Swelling and pain are associated features. Some may present with a chronic discharging sinus.

Although most cases are unilocular radiolucencies minority can present as multilocular lesions. Large cystic lesions show evidence of thinning of the sinus wall.

Histopathology

The cyst is lined by pseudostratified columnar ciliated epithelium (**Fig. 5.26**). Squamous metaplasia is seen in some. The cyst wall shows features of inflammation in varying intensities.

Treatment

Enucleation of the cyst is the usual treatment. However, larger lesions may benefit by marsupialization before enucleation.

Oral Lymphoepithelial Cyst

Oral lymphoepithelial cyst (OLC) is a rare soft tissue lesion of the oral mucosa with exact histopathological similarities to cervical lymphoepithelial cyst. Pathogenesis of OLC is attributed to several mechanisms. Some cases may arise as a result of epithelial inclusions within lymphoid tissue whilst others arise due to cystic dilatation of minor salivary gland ducts or tonsillar crypts following obstruction.

The floor of the mouth and lateral border of the tongue appear to be the sites for more than 95 percent of the cases. Slight male predilection is evident. Although, OLC occurs at any age, 3rd decade is the most common.

Histopathologically, the cyst is lined by a thin stratified squamous epithelium which is usually parakeratinized (**Fig. 5.27**). Occasional cases may be orthokeratinzed. Pseudostratified columnar ciliated epithelium with goblet cells can be found in a minority. The most characteristic feature is the presence of lymphoid tissue with proper germinal centers in some OLC. Except in rare cases lymphoid infiltrate is found below the epithelium in the entire cyst.

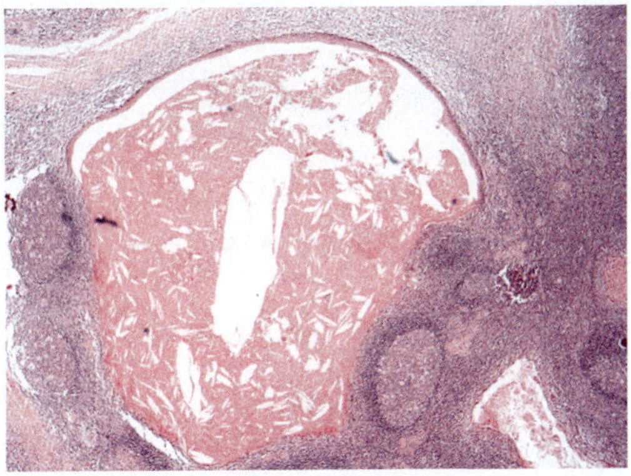

Fig. 5.27: Oral lymphoepithelial cyst. The cyst is lined by thin parakeratinized stratified squamous epithelium. *Note:* The lymphoid tissue with germinal centers in close proximity to the epithelium

Treatment

Treatment of OLC is by enucleation. After complete removal of the lesion it should not recur.

Cervical Lymphoepithelial Cyst (Branchial Cleft Cyst)

Cervical lymphoepithelial cyst (CLC) arises as a developmental anomaly from the second branchial arch in 90 percent of the cases. Rarely, it arises from the 1st and 3rd arch. Developmental anomalies arising from branchial arches present as sinuses, fistulae, cysts or combinations of above. The cyst arises most likely as a result of incomplete obliteration of branchial cleft with entrapment of epithelial remnants.

Most patients present in 3rd and 4th decade of life as a swelling along the anterior border of sternocleidomastoid in the upper neck. It is a fluctuant swelling ranging from 2 to 10 cm in diameter. Bilateral presentation has rarely been reported.

Histopathological features of OLC and CLC are very much similar (**Fig. 5.27**). Recurrence is unlikely once surgically removed. Although malignant transformation of the cystic epithelium has been reported, it is exceptionally rare.

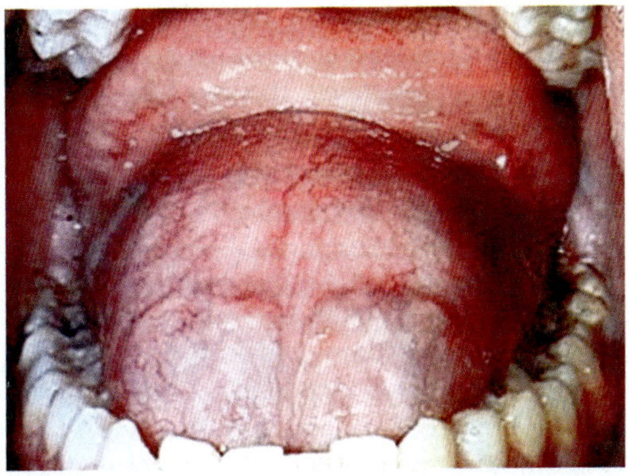

Fig. 5.28: Dermoid cyst. Typical presentation of dermoid cyst in the floor of the mouth

Dermoid and Epidermoid Cyst

The dermoid and epidermoid cyst in the oral mucosa appears to represent a simpler version of a teratoma. Although by definition a teratoma should have tissues from all three germ layers, these lesions have tissues mostly from ectoderm. It should be noted that the more common type of epidermoid cyst that we see in the skin is a different entity and arises from the infundibulum of the hair follicle. A sebaceous cyst is the common synonym that has been used over the years incorrectly for epidermoid cyst of the skin.

The most common intraoral location for dermoid/epidermoid cyst is the midline of the floor of the mouth (**Fig. 5.28**). It rarely occurs in other sites such as the tongue. When the cyst occurs in the floor of the mouth it can arise either above or below the geniohyoid muscle giving rise to intraoral or extraoral swelling

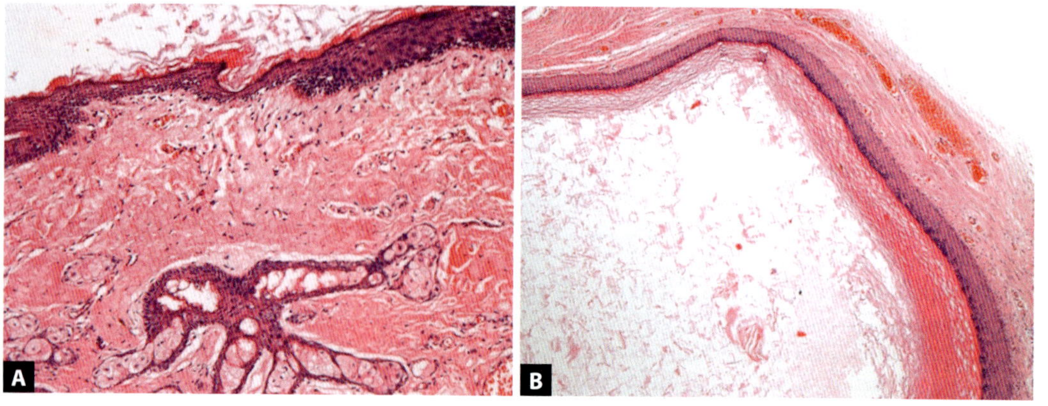

Figs 5.29A and B: Dermoid cyst/epidermoid cyst. Both lesions are lined by orthokeratinized epithelium. Dermoid cyst contains sebaceous glands in the cyst wall

respectively. Intraoral swelling lifts the tongue upwards and extraoral swelling gives rise to double chin appearance. This is a slow growing painless swelling. Most cases are diagnosed in children and some cysts are present from birth.

Histopathology

The cyst is lined by stratified squamous orthokeratinized epithelium which is very similar to the epidermis (**Figs 5.29A and B**). The only difference between a dermoid and an epidermoid is the presence of skin appendages in the former. The cystic cavity is filled with keratin. Some lesions may have a range of other tissues and epithelia and they probably are choristomal cysts described under a different name below.

Treatment is by surgical excision and recurrence is uncommon. Exceptionally rarely malignant transformation into squamous cell carcinoma has been reported.

Thyroglossal Duct Cyst

The third week of embryonic life shows evidence of the developing thyroid gland as a proliferation of endodermal cells in the area later in the development known as foramen cecum. Then the thyroid anlage descends to the neck below the thyroid cartilage. An epithelial tract (thyroglossal duct) is formed along this line and maintains its attachment to tongue. By the 10th week of development the duct disintegrates leaving epithelial residues which later turn into thyroglossal duct cyst in some people.

Approximately 70 percent of the developmental cysts in the neck are of this type. Intraoral lesions are rare and amount up to 2 percent of the cases. Most cases are diagnosed in the 1st and 2nd decade of life. The cyst usually presents as a midline swelling of the neck in any location from foramen cecum to suprasternal notch. Majority of these lesions occur below the hyoid bone. A painless, slow growing, fluctuant swelling is the usual presentation. Difficulty in speaking and breathing has been reported in rare cases. Lateral presentation is exceedingly rare.

Histologically, the cyst is lined by pseudostratified columnar epithelium with cilia in some cases. Some areas can have stratified squamous epithelium. Lesions which are close to the oral cavity tend to have frequent squamous epithelium. The cyst wall contains thyroid tissue in up to 50 percent of the cases. The amount of thyroid tissue present may vary and serial sections are necessary to identify this feature in some lesions (**Fig. 5.30**).

Treatment is by surgical excision. However, it is advisable to remove the entire tract together with the cyst in order to avoid possible recurrence. The accepted surgical technique is known as Sistrunk procedure where cyst is removed together with muscle surrounding the tract and midline segment of the hyoid bone.

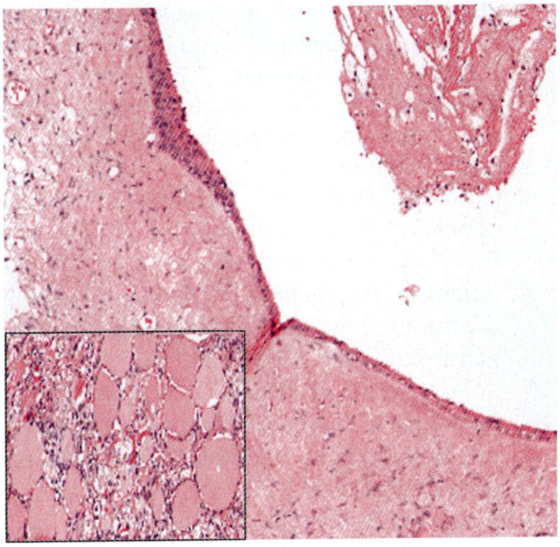

Fig. 5.30: Thyroglossal duct cyst. The cyst lining is composed of stratified squamous and respiratory type epithelium. Inset shows thyroid tissue from another part of the cystic lesion

Developmental Cysts of Foregut Origin (Gastrointestinal Choristomal Cysts, Heterotopic Gastrointestinal Cysts, Oral Alimentary Tract Cyst, Foregut Duplication Cyst)

Cysts of foregut origin occur in the neck as well as in the oral cavity. The most common site in the oral cavity is the tongue and is known as a lingual foregut cyst by some. This is essentially presence of tissue foreign to a particular site. Therefore the term gastrointestinal choristoma or choristomal cyst may be more appropriate. The majority of these cases especially in the tongue are seen in infants and children except for a few cases reported in adults. There is a male predilection. Usual presentation is a swelling of the mid dorsal surface of the tongue without surface mucosal changes. Cases have also been reported from the ventral surface and also from the floor of the mouth.

Histopathologically, the cyst lining shows a marked diversity. It can be gastric, intestinal, respiratory or stratified squamous epithelium (**Fig. 5.31**). According to the author's experience, the majority of lesions have a combination of different types in the same cyst. It is very rare to have only a single type of epithelium.

Treatment is by simple surgical excision.

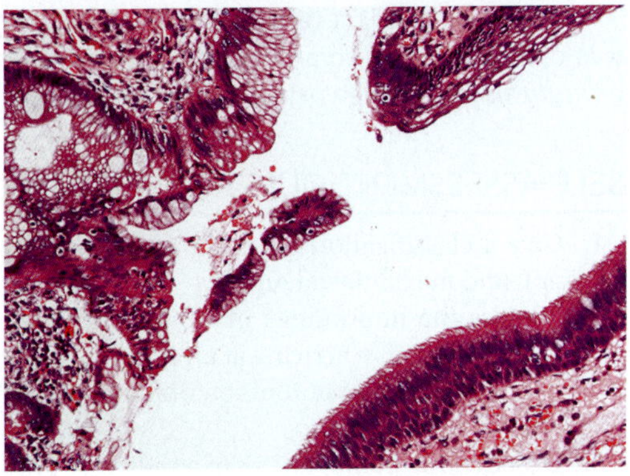

Fig. 5.31: Developmental cysts of foregut origin. *Note:* The presence of gastric, respiratory and stratified squamous epithelium in the same cyst

Cystic Hygroma

Cystic hygroma is a cavernous type of lymphangioma. Although this can occur in any anatomic site of the body, the neck is the most preferred site. Classically they present in the posterior triangle of the neck. Eighty to ninety percent of the lesions are diagnosed before the age of 2 years. There is no sex predilection. The lesion is a multilobulated painless mass with a bluish color.

Histopathologically, the lesion is composed of dilated lymphatic spaces lined by endothelial cells.

Treatment is by complete surgical excision. There is a significant possibility of recurrence.

Parasitic Cysts

Parasitic cysts are exceedingly rare lesions in the oral mucosa. Hydatid cyst and cysticercosis have been reported from the oral cavity. Although cysticercosis caused by *Taenia solium* is a common parasitic infection around the world, oral lesions are very rare. This disease is caused by the larval form of cysticercus cellulosae of the pig tapeworm *Taenia solium*. The most common intraoral location is the tongue as it prefers vascular organs. Management of these patients should be carried out by the relevant medical experts as involvement of other organs and lesions in the brain can be a common presentation.

A hydatid cyst is a rare human disease and it is caused by the larval form of *Echinococcus granulosus* (Dog tapeworm).

SELF-ASSESSMENT QUESTIONS

1. Give a classification for cystic lesions of the oral and maxillofacial region.
2. Discuss the importance of clinicopathological correlation in arriving at an accurate diagnosis of a cystic lesion of the oral and maxillofacial region.
3. Describe the pathogenesis of a radicular cyst.
4. Describe how a cyst expands using radicular cysts and odontogenic keratocyst as examples.
5. Compare and contrast radicular cyst, dentigerous cyst and odontogenic keratocyst.
6. Describe the pathogenesis of dentigerous cyst.
7. Describe the reasons for and against for classifying odontogenic keratocyst as a neoplastic lesion (keratocystic odontogenic tumor).
8. Describe the advantages of marsupialization as a treatment option for cystic lesions.
9. Describe the pathogenesis, histological and radiological features of developmental non-odontogenic cysts.
10. List the nonepithelial cysts in the oral and maxillofacial region and comment on their etiopathogenesis and management.

SUGGESTED READING

1. Barreto DC, Gomez RS, Bale AE, Boson WI, De Marco L. *PTCH* gene mutations in odontogenic keratocysts. J Dental Research. 2000;79:1418-22.
2. Carter LC, Carney YL, Perez-Pudlewski D. Lateral periodontal cyst; multifactorial analysis of a previously unreported series. Oral Surg Oral Med Oral Pathol. 1996;81:210-6.
3. Chaudhry AP, Yamane GM, Scharlock SE, SunderRaj M, Jain R. A clinico-pathological study of intraoral lymphoepithelial cysts. J Oral Med. 1984;39:79-84.
4. Cohen MM. Naevoid basal cell carcinoma syndrome; molecular biology and new hypothesis. Int J Oral Maxillofac Surg. 1999;28:216-33.
5. Craig GT. The paradental cyst. A specific inflammatory odontogenic cyst. Br Dent J. 1976;141:9-14.
6. David VC, O'Connell JE. Nasolabial cyst. Clin Otolaryngol Allied Sci. 1986;11:5-8.
7. Gardner DG, Kessler HP, Morency R, Schaffner DL. The glandular odontogenic cyst: an apparent entity. J Oral Pathol. 1988;17:359-66.
8. Gurol M, Burkes EJ, Jacoway J. Botryoid odontogenic cyst; analysis of 33 cases. J Periodontal. 1995;66:1069-73.
9. Jorgenson RJ, Shapiro SD, Salinas CF, Levin LS. Intraoral findings and anomalies in neonates. Pediatrics. 1982;69:577-82.
10. Kaffe I, Naor H, Calderon S, Buchner A. Radiological and clinical features of aneurysmal bone cyst of the jaws. Dentomaxillofac Radiol. 1999;28:167-72.
11. Katz AD, Hachigian M. Thyroglossal duct cysts; a thirty year experience with emphasis on occurrence in older patients. Am J Surg. 1988;155:741-4.
12. King RC, Smith BR, Burk JL. Dermoid cyst in the floor of the mouth. Review of the literature and case reports. Oral Surg Oral Med Oral Pathol. 1994;78:567-76.
13. Lin LM, Huang GT, Rosenberg PA. Proliferation of epithelial cell rests, formation of apical cysts, and regression of apical cysts after periapical wound healing. J Endod. 2007;33:908-16.
14. Lin LM, Ricucci D, Lin J, Rosenberg PA. Nonsurgical root canal therapy of large cyst-like inflammatory periapical lesions and inflammatory apical cysts. J Endod. 2009;35:607-15.
15. Li TJ, Kitano M, Chen XM, Itoh T, Kawashima K, Sugihara K, Nozoe E, Mimura T. Orthokeratinized odontogenic cyst: a clinicopathological and immunocytochemical study of 15 cases. Histopathology. 1998;32:242-51.
16. Mass EW, Kaplan I, Hirshberg A. A clinical and histopathological study of radicular cysts associated with primary molars. J Oral Pathol Med. 1995;24:458-61.
17. Mervyn Shear, Paul M Speight. Cyst of the oral and maxillofacial regions. 2007, Blackwell Munksgaard, Oxford.
18. Nair PNR. New perspectives on radicular cyst: do they heal? Inter Endod. 1998;31:155-60.
19. Nxumalo TN, Shear M. Gingival cyst in adults. I Oral Pathol Med. 1992;21:309-13.
20. Saito Y, Hoshina Y, Nagamine T, Nakajima T, Suzuki M, Hayashi T. Simple bone cyst.

A clinical and histopathologic study of fifteen cases. Oral Surg Oral Med Oral Pathol. 1992;74:487-91.
21. Swanson KS, Kaugars GE, Gunsolley JC. Nasopalatine duct cyst: an analysis of 334 cases. J Oral maxillofac Surg. 1991;49:268-71.
22. Van der Waal I, Rauhamaa R, Van der Kwast WA, Snow GB. Squamous cell carcinoma arising in the lining of odontogenic cysts; Report of 5 cases. Int J Oral Surg. 1985;14:146-52.
23. Williams TP, Connor Jr FA. Surgical management of the odontogenic keratocyst: aggressive approach. J Oral Maxillofac Surg. 1994;52:964-6.
24. Woolgar JA, Rippin JW, Brown RM. A comparative study histologic study of odontogenic keratocyst in basal cell nevus syndrome and non syndrome patients. J Oral Pathol. 1987;16:75-80.

Chapter

6

Odontogenic Tumors

Vinay Hazarey, WM Tilakaratne

Chapter Outline

INTRODUCTION

Odontogenic tumors are a rare group of neoplasms. A thorough knowledge is necessary to evaluate and predict their occurrence, clinical features, radiological features, histopathology and pathogenesis, biological behavior and treatment options. Odontogenic tumors show a spectrum of pathological entities arising from abnormal odontogenesis. The correct interplay of dental tissues leads to normal tooth development. However, variations during any developmental stage lead to malformations, developmental anomalies, hamartomas and neoplasms.

The development of a normal tooth depends upon inductive influences exerted by one tissue on another. It has long been believed that the main inductive effect is exerted by the odontogenic epithelium on adjacent mesodermal tissues. This results in formation of dental papilla and later appearance of odontoblasts on its surface. When dentine formation starts, the final functional maturation of ameloblasts takes place and enamel is deposited on the dentine surface in the crown area. Therefore, dentine does not form in the absence of odontogenic epithelium and enamel normally does not form unless some dentine has already been laid down. From these considerations it can be suggested that variations in the degree of induction exerted by the odontogenic epithelium may result in a marked variation in the pattern of tumors developed from these tissues. It is not suggested that each pattern necessarily indicates a distinct and separate type of tumor—rather, there is continuum of interactions leading to spectrum of odontogenic tumors.

Odontogenic tumors are neoplasms originating from dental tissues or their formative elements. They are classified on the basis of inductive potential of odontogenic tissues. As the different dental tissues exhibit a mutual interdependence, classification helps in understanding the biological behavior and growth potential of these lesions.

Thoma and Goldman in 1946 suggested that odontogenic tumors should be divided into tumors of ectodermal, mesodermal, and mixed origin. This classification forms the nucleus of the classification adopted by the

▪ Table 6.1
WHO histological classification of odontogenic tumors

BENIGN TUMORS

Odontogenic epithelium with mature, fibrous stroma without odontogenic ectomesenchyme
- Ameloblastoma, solid/multicystic type
- Ameloblastoma, extraosseous/peripheral type
- Ameloblastoma, desmoplastic type
- Ameloblastoma, unicystic type
- Squamous odontogenic tumor
- Calcifying epithelial odontogenic tumor
- Adenomatoid odontogenic tumor
- Keratocystic odontogenic tumor

Odontogenic epithelium with odontogenic ectomesenchyme, with or without hard tissue formation
- Ameloblastic fibroma
- Ameloblastic fibrodentinoma
- Ameloblastic fibro-odontoma
- Odontoma, complex type
- Odontoma, compound type
- Odontoameloblastoma
- Calcifying cystic odontogenic tumor
- Dentinogenic ghost cell tumor

Mesenchyme and/or odontogenic ectome-senchyme with or without odontogenic epithelium
- Odontogenic fibroma
- Odontogenic myxoma/myxofibroma
- Cementoblastoma

MALIGNANT TUMORS

Odontogenic carcinomas
- Metastasizing (malignant) ameloblastoma
- Ameloblastic carcinoma—primary type
- Ameloblastic carcinoma—secondary type (dedifferentiated), intraosseous
- Ameloblastic carcinoma—secondary type (dedifferentiated)
- Peripheral
- Primary intraosseous squamous cell carcinoma—solid type
- Primary intraosseous squamous cell carcinoma derived from keratocystic odontogenic tumor
- Primary intraosseous squamous cell carcinoma derived from odontogenic cysts
- Clear cell odontogenic carcinoma
- Ghost cell odontogenic carcinoma

Odontogenic sarcomas
- Ameloblastic fibrosarcoma
- Ameloblastic fibrodentino–and fibro-odonto-sarcoma

American Academy of Oral Pathologists in 1950. Pindborg et al in 1970 suggested classification for WHO Histological Typing of Odontogenic Tumors, Jaw cysts and Allied Lesions. The WHO in 2005 revised this classification and introduced a range of new entities with a better understanding of pluripotential nature of the odontogenic epithelium.

WHO histological classifiation of odontogenic with benign and malignant tumors are depicted in **Table 6.1**.

AMELOBLASTOMA

Ameloblastoma is the second most common tumor amongst odontogenic tumors. The WHO defines it as a locally invasive neoplasm of epithelial odontogenic origin without any inductive changes in the connective tissue. It can occur at either intraosseous (central) or extraosseous (peripheral) location. Intraosseous neoplasms are usually aggressive in clinical behavior and often locally invasive. These neoplasms can invade the soft and hard tissues of jaws. Prior to it being called an ameloblastoma by Ivy and Churchill in 1930, it was called an adamantinoma. The Greek term adamantinoma envisages a tumor containing hard tissues. There is no evidence of any hard tissues, since there is no induction. Adamantinomas are tumors of long bones and should not be confused with an odontogenic neoplasm, ameloblastoma. The first case of ameloblastoma was described by Cusack in 1827. The first case of ameloblastoma developing in dentigerous cyst was reported by Cahn.

Solid/Multicystic Type

Clinical Features

In the early stages, it is asymptomatic and may be diagnosed upon routine radiographic examination. It may present as a variably sized swelling of the jaw (**Fig. 6.1A**). Usually the swelling is slow growing and may take a few years to cause facial disfigurement. Thinning and expansion of buccal and lingual cortical plates may occur, often presenting clinically as eggshell crackling. Complete destruction of either cortical plates may present as a firm, or fluctuant swelling. Displacement and mobility of adjoining teeth can occur. An untreated ameloblastoma can cause unsightly disfigurement of the face and pathological fracture (**Fig. 6.1B**). A tooth or teeth may be clinically missing as ameloblastoma may be associated with an impacted tooth, giving it dentigerous cyst-like features. Pain and facial disfigurement are features of advanced tumors. Ameloblastomas are more common in the mandible (80%) than in the maxilla (20%).

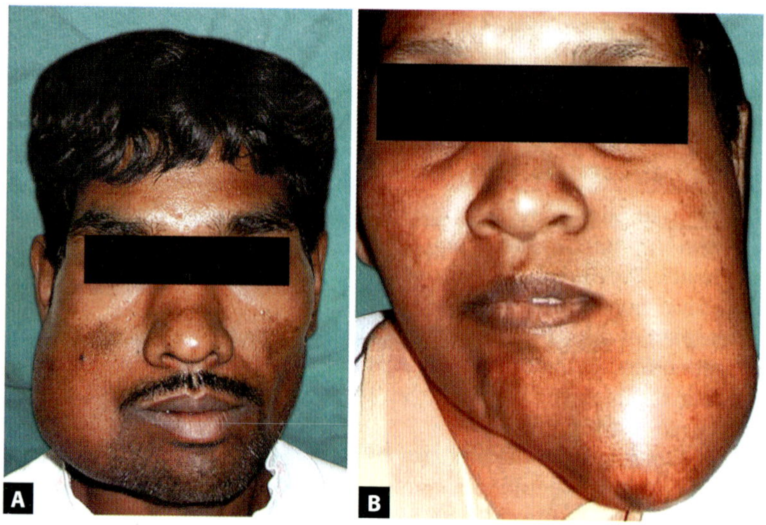

Figs 6.1A and B: Ameloblastoma. (A) Slow growing tumor at the right angle of the mandible; (B) A long standing tumor with marked disfigurement of the face

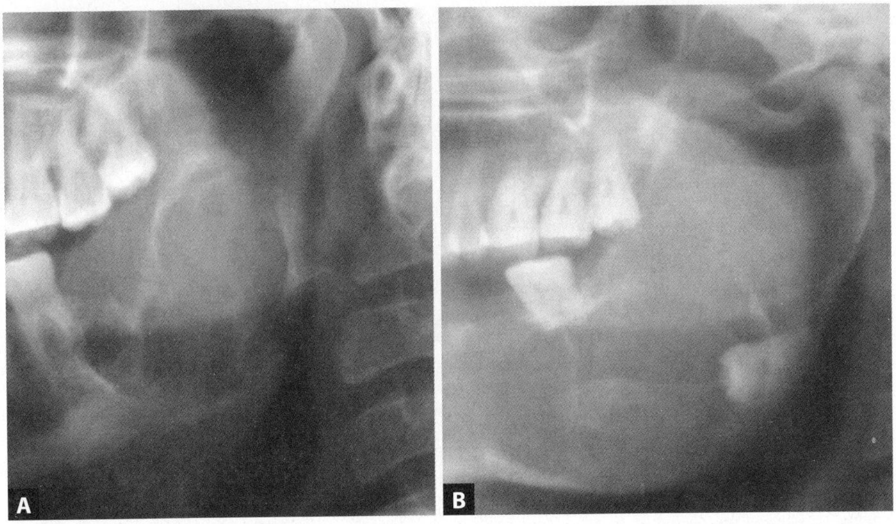

Figs 6.2A and B: Ameloblastoma. (A) Multilocular radiolucency is the most common radiological presentation; (B) Some cases mimic the appearance of dentigerous cyst

Approximately 60 percent are located in the ramus and body of the mandible, 30 percent in the premolar-molar area and 10 percent in the anterior mandible. Maxillary lesions located in the premolar area cause palatal and buccal expansion.

The distribution amongst males and females is almost equal. The average age of patients reporting to clinics is in between the 3rd and 4th decade, often with a history of 3 to 4 years duration. However, the age range varies from 4 to 92 years. The mean age of patients at the time of diagnosis is 35.9 years.

Radiological Features

Radiographically, it presents more commonly as a multilocular radiolucency (multicystic) (**Fig. 6.2A**) and less commonly as a unilocular radiolucency. The periphery is well-defined and often corticated and scalloped. Multilocular lesions show numerous coarse curved septa dividing the internal structure into multiple compartments giving it a honeycomb (smaller locules of uniform size) or soap bubble (larger locules of variable size) appearance. Unilocular lesions are similar to odontogenic cysts and are often difficult to distinguish from a dentigerous cyst when associated with an impacted or unerupted tooth (**Fig 6.2B**). Resorption of the roots and displacement of involved teeth are common. However, desmoplastic ameloblastoma resembles fibro-osseous lesions and presents as a mixed radiodense lesion.

Histopathological Features

The WHO defines an ameloblastoma as a neoplasm without inductive changes in the connective tissue. The epithelial proliferations can give rise to two main histopathological types defined as follicular and plexiform.

In the follicular subtype, the tumor epithelium is arranged into follicles which possess a peripheral layer of tall columnar cells resembling preameloblasts or internal dental epithelium. These cells show hyperchromatism and reversed polarity of the nuclei. The central part of these follicles shows resemblance to stellate reticulum (**Fig. 6.3A**). As the center of the follicles undergoes metaplastic change, the follicular variant is qualitatively described as acanthomatous, granular cell or basal cell subtypes.

The acanthomatous variant shows extensive squamous metaplasia and keratin formation within the follicle (**Fig. 6.3B**). In Granular cell variant, transformation of stellate reticulum

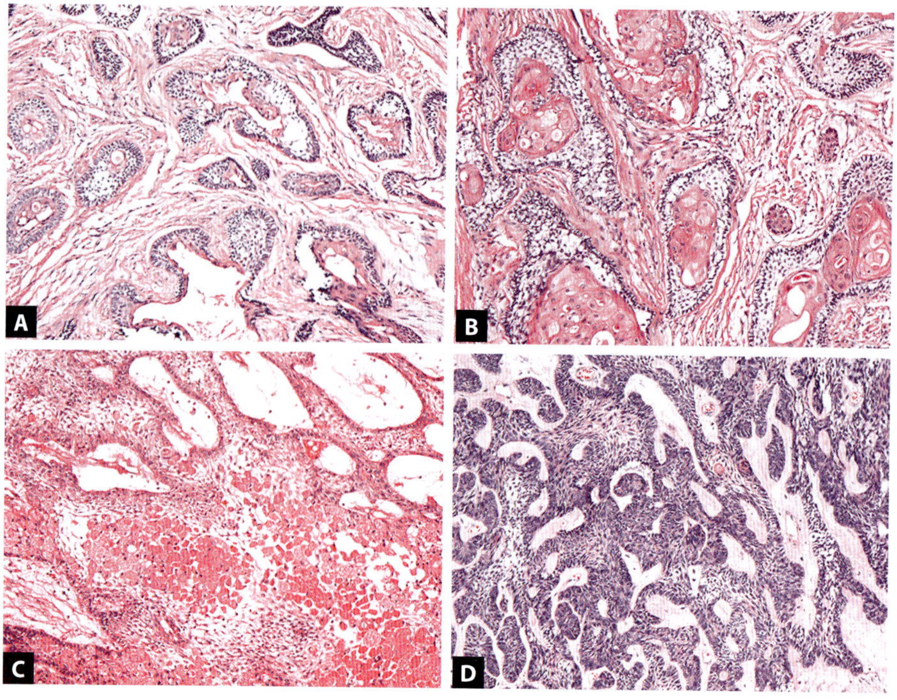

Figs 6.3A to D: Ameloblastoma solid/multicystic type. (A) Follicular type showing numerous follicular structures with peripheral ameloblast-like cells and central stellate reticulum cells; (B) Central cells show squamous metaplasia in acanthomatous type; (C) Granular cell changes in granular cell ameloblastoma; (D) Plexifom type with odontogenic epithelium arranging into a branching pattern

cells to granular cells is seen (**Fig. 6.3C**). The granules are large, round and PAS positive. These acidophilic granules are similar ultrastructurally and histochemically to lysosomes.

The Plexiform variant is characterized by a branching network of odontogenic epithelium (**Fig. 6.3D**). The peripheral cells of these strands are not as columnar as in the follicular variant and stellate reticulum is very scanty. It is suggested that follicular and plexiform nomenclature has no clinical significance.

Pathogenesis

Ameloblastomas may arise from the basal layer of dental lamina, remnants of Hertwig's root sheath or epithelial cell rest of Malassez. Basal layers of oral epithelium and cell rests of Serres are also thought to be important in the pathogenesis of peripheral ameloblastomas. Mutation in genes during odontogenesis is responsible for neoplasia. The fos-oncogene and tumor-necrosis-factor-receptor-1 are the most over-expressed genes. Some genes including sonic Hedgehog (SHH), cadherins 12 and 13 and transforming growth factor β1 (TGF-β1) are under-expressed according to different studies.

Treatment

Surgical excision is the treatment of choice. Segmental osteotomies are usually adequate for unicystic ameloblastomas. However, large lesions may require a hemimandibulectomy or maxillectomy. Enucleation as a treatment for any form of ameloblastoma is controversial. Tumors are radio-resistant. Ameloblastoma is an aggressive neoplasm known for recurrences, especially if inadequately excised. Inadequate excision is responsible for high rates of recurrence. The malignant potential exists for intraosseous ameloblastoma and these malignant counterparts are known and classified as malignant ameloblastomas. The recurrence rate is 33 percent. Peripheral (extraosseous) lesions are nonaggressive and the recurrence is rare. Regular follow-up is essential to identify early recurrence.

Extraosseous/Peripheral Type

The extraosseous/peripheral ameloblastoma is the extraosseous counterpart of the intraosseous solid/multicystic ameloblastoma. Syn-onyms are soft tissue ameloblastoma, ameloblastoma of mucosal origin and ameloblastoma of the gingiva. It may arise from odontogenic epithelial remnants within the gingival lamina propria or from the basal cell layer of the gingival epithelium. Peripheral ameloblastoma accounts for 1.3 to 10 percent of all ameloblastomas.

Clinical Features

Although, it occurs at any age from 9 and 92 years, most are reported from 5th to 7th decade and the mean age is significantly higher than for the intraosseous counterpart. The male:female ratio is 1.9:1 with the mandible affected more than the maxilla. It appears as a painless, firm and exophytic growth with a smooth, pebbly or papillary surface. Rarely, the intraosseous ameloblastoma may extend to the gingival tissues and merge with the gingival epithelium, creating an exophytic peripheral ameloblastoma like lesion.

Radiological Features

Apart from a superficial erosion or depression (saucerization or cupping) of the bone crest due to pressure resorption, there is rarely any significant bone involvement.

Histopathological Features

A peripheral ameloblastoma consists of odontogenic epithelium with the same histomorphological cell types and patterns similar to solid/multicystic ameloblastoma. Some lesions are located entirely within the connective tissue of the gingiva, showing no continuity with the surface epithelium, whereas others seem to fuse with, or originate from the mucosal epithelium. Squamous cells in the acanthomatous areas of the peripheral ameloblastoma may show ghost cell formation and in some parts of the tumor islands, vacuolated or clear cells occur in discrete clusters. Basal cell metaplasia is a common feature. The stroma is made up of mature, fibrous connective tissue (**Fig. 6.4A**).

Peripheral odontogenic fibroma, peripheral variant of squamous odontogenic tumor and odontogenic gingival epithelial hamartoma (OGEH) mimic the appearance of peripheral ameloblastoma. Some lesions are histologically

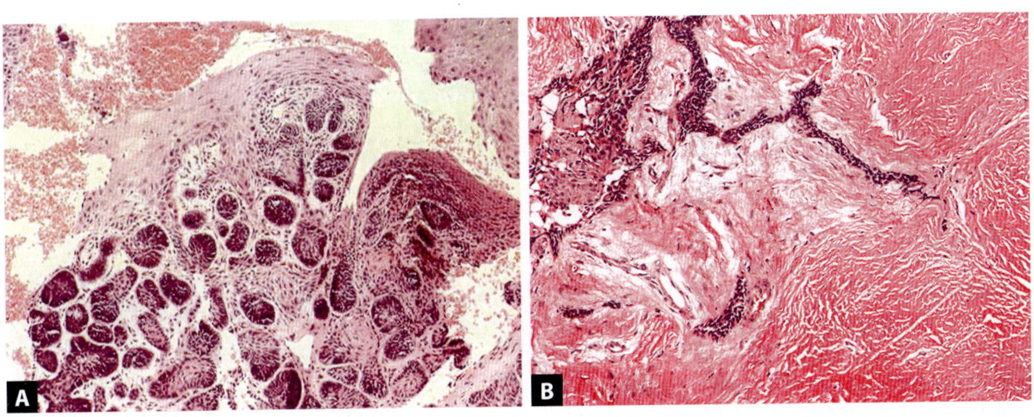

Figs 6.4A and B: (A) Peripheral ameloblastoma composed of basaloid islands of odontogenic epithelium below the surface epithelium; (B) Desmoplastic ameloblastoma shows strands of ameloblast-like cells arranged in a dense and hyalinized fibrous stroma

very similar to basal cell carcinoma. The present view is that peripheral ameloblastoma and OGEH represent the same lesion.

Desmoplastic Type

Desmoplastic ameloblastoma is a distinct variant of the ameloblastoma with 150 cases reported in the literature. It is described as "ameloblastoma with pronounced desmoplasia" by Eversole in 1984. The mean age of desmoplastic ameloblastoma is 42.9 years. This variant of ameloblastoma is common in the anterior region of jaws with slight preponderance to the maxilla. Three distinct radiologic variants have been described:

- Unilocular containing varying amount of radiopaque material
- Multilocular containing varying amount of radiopaque masses
- Mixed pattern mostly mimicking the appearances of fibro-osseous lesions.

Histopathologically, it shows collagenous mature connective tissue stroma in which odontogenic islands are compressed or squeezed by the stromal tissue, giving rise to stretched out tail-like islands (**Fig. 6.4B**). The lesional tissue shows a combination of fibro-osseous and odontogenic architecture. The desmoplastic variant has a relatively low recurrence potential. Central stellate reticulum-like cells are often scanty in the epithelial proliferation and the cells making up the periphery of the strands and cords often are flattened or cuboidal rather than tall and columnar in appearance. Reversed polarity of nuclei and subnuclear vacuole formation may be difficult to recognize. Marked immunoexpression of TGF-β has been observed and may explain the significant desmoplasia in the tumor.

Unicystic Type

The unicystic variant is common in the younger age group and has a relatively low recurrence rate. Unicystic ameloblastomas are commonly associated with impacted teeth. Two main histopathological variations are identified: in the subtype referred to as luminal type, a relatively innocuous epithelial lining at least in part, shows cuboidal or columnar basal cells with hyperchromatic nuclei, nuclear palisading with reversed polarity, cytoplasmic vacuolation with intercellular spacing and subepithelial hyalinization (**Fig. 6.5A**). These histopathological criteria are described by Vicker and Gorlin (1970). Sometimes, a cyst lining similar to the luminal type with a nodule projecting into lumen of the cyst is evident. The nodule comprises odontogenic epithelium with a plexiform pattern resembling that seen in the plexiform ameloblastoma (Intraluminal type). The name plexiform unicystic ameloblastoma has been used for these lesions. The second variety is referred to as a mural ameloblastoma showing part of the wall of the cyst infiltrated by typical plexiform or rarely follicular ameloblastoma (**Fig. 6.5B**).

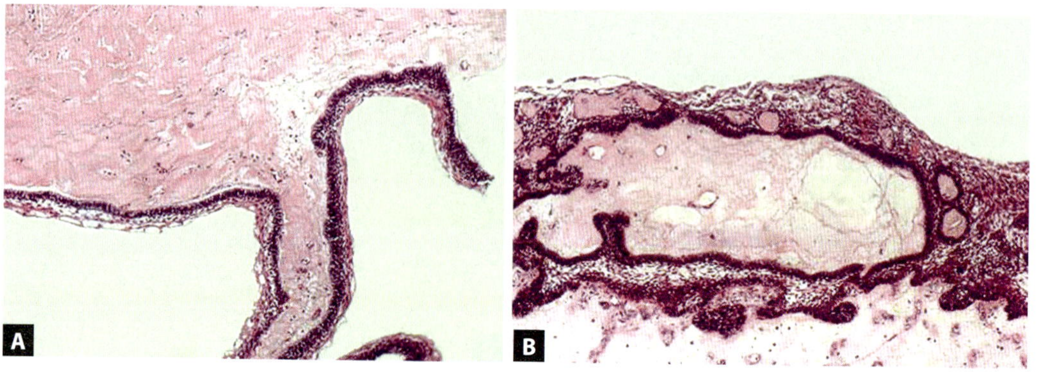

Figs 6.5A and B: Unicystic ameloblastoma. (A) Luminal type is composed of odontogenic epithelium with peripheral basal cells showing reversed polarity and surface stellate reticulum-like cells; (B) The epithelium proliferates into cyst wall in mural type

The luminal and intraluminal variants are treated conservatively with enucleation and curettage. However, the mural variant needs to be treated in a similar way to solid multicystic ameloblastomas. According to some, enucleation may not be appropriate to treat any type of ameloblastoma. The histopathological diagnosis of a unicystic ameloblastoma is exceptionally important as various subtypes have different treatment options and prognosis. Serial sectioning of the biopsy is mandatory to exclude the presence of conventional ameloblastomas. Unicystic ameloblastomas have lower recurrence rates of 10 to 20 percent.

Box 6.1: Ameloblastoma—key features helpful in diagnosis

- Second most common benign odontogenic tumor
- Occur equally in men and women, most commonly in 3rd and 4th decades of life
- Slow growing locally aggressive neoplasm causing facial asymmetry, expansion of the jaw bones and displacement of the teeth
- More often multilocular radiolucency and less often unilocular cyst-like radiolucency
- Histologically, tumor cells resemble ameloblast-like cells in the odontogenic apparatus.

SQUAMOUS ODONTOGENIC TUMOR

Pullon et al in 1975 first described a particular odontogenic tumor located in the periodontium as squamous odontogenic tumor (SOT). It is defined as a benign, but locally infiltrative neoplasm consisting of islands of well-differentiated squamous epithelium in a fibrous stroma. The epithelial islands occasionally show foci of central cystic degeneration. It may arise from epithelial rests of Malassez located in the periodontal ligament. Peripheral SOTs may originate in gingival surface epithelium as a "dropping off" phenomenon, or from remnants of dental lamina. Some consider that SOT may have a hamartomatous nature.

Clinical Features

The age range is between 8 to 74 years with a mean age of 38.7 years. Males are affected more than females (1.4:1). Squamous odontogenic tumor usually occurs intraosseously and probably develops in the periodontal ligament between the roots of vital erupted permanent teeth. The mandible is affected more than the maxilla. Mobility of teeth and moderate pain are possible indicators of an underlying tumor. A rare peripheral variant is also seen. SOTs in the maxilla are more aggressive than in the mandible.

Radiological Features

Squamous odontogenic tumor shows a well-defined unilocular and triangular radiolucency between the roots of adjacent teeth. Extensive lesions may have a multilocular pattern, involving the mandible or maxillary sinuses. The peripheral variant of SOT may reveal some saucerization of underlying bone which is explained as a pressure phenomenon rather than a result of neoplastic infiltration.

Histopathological Features

Histologically, SOT is composed of islands of well-differentiated squamous epithelium in a fibrous stroma (**Fig. 6.6**). Individual islands reveal a peripheral layer of cuboidal or even flat epithelial cells. Islands may undergo microcysts formation and individual cell keratinization. Some islands may contain calcified material. Mitotic activity of tumor cells is not increased.

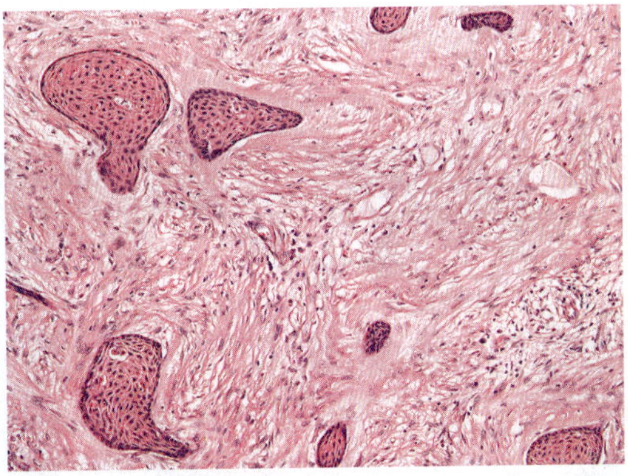

Fig. 6.6: Squamous odontogenic tumor. Islands of benign squamous epithelium arranged in a fibrous stoma

These islands are surrounded by mature connective tissue with little or no inflammatory response. SOT may be confused with other conditions including ameloblastoma and rarely squamous cell carcinoma. Histopathological misinterpretation may thus lead to over treatment or under treatment.

Treatment

Conservative surgical procedures such as enucleation, curettage or local excision are the accepted modalities of treatment. However, tumors in the maxilla need radical treatment because of aggressive potential of SOTs in this location. Recurrences are rare in mandibular lesions.

Box 6.2: Squamous odontogenic tumor

Key features helpful in diagnosis

- Rare odontogenic tumor
- Its location between roots of vital teeth suggests origin from epithelial rests of Malassez located in the periodontal ligament
- Males are affected more commonly than females
- Average age of occurrence is 38 years.
- Mandible more commonly affected than maxilla
- Clinically manifests as mobility of teeth, swelling and moderate pain
- Radiographically presents as well-defined unilocular and triangular radiolucency between the roots of adjacent teeth
- Histopathology shows islands of well-differentiated squamous epithelium in a fibrous stroma.

CALCIFYING EPITHELIAL ODONTOGENIC TUMOR

Calcifying epithelial odontogenic tumor (CEOT) is an uncommon, benign, odontogenic neoplasm. The calcifying epithelial odontogenic tumor was first introduced into the scientific literature almost 50 years ago by Jens Pindborg. CEOT is a locally invasive epithelial odontogenic neoplasm, and is characterized by the presence of amyloid material that may become calcified. Commonly it is called Pindborg's tumor. Odontogenic epithelium is evidently the origin of this tumor but the particular cell remains unknown. The original hypothesis by Pindborg was that the tumor arises from the stratum intermedium of the enamel organ still remains the most likely cause. Its reduced invasiveness, compared to ameloblastoma may be explained by the reduced invasive potential and reduced activity of the stratum intermedium compared to the growth potential of the dental lamina.

Clinical Features

Calcifying epithelial odontogenic tumor (CEOT) accounts for approximately 1 percent of all odontogenic tumors occurring in patients between 20 and 60 years of age, with a mean around 40 years. There is no gender predilection. Most cases are intraosseous; approximately 6 percent arise in extraosseous locations. Intraosseous tumors affect the mandible more often than the maxilla with a ratio of 2:1. There is usually a predilection for the premolar/molar region (**Fig. 6.7A**). It presents as a hard, painless slow-growing lesion. Uncommon

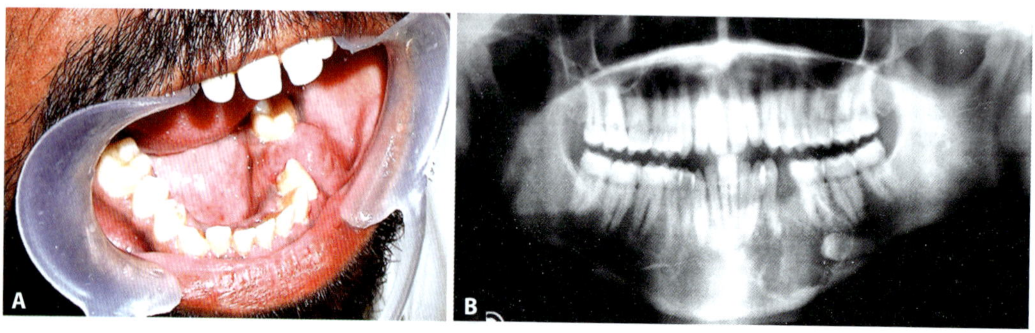

Figs 6.7A and B: Calcifying epithelial odontogenic tumor. (A) Usually presents as a swelling in the posterior mandible; (B) Radiologically, it shows a lesion with mixed radiodensity

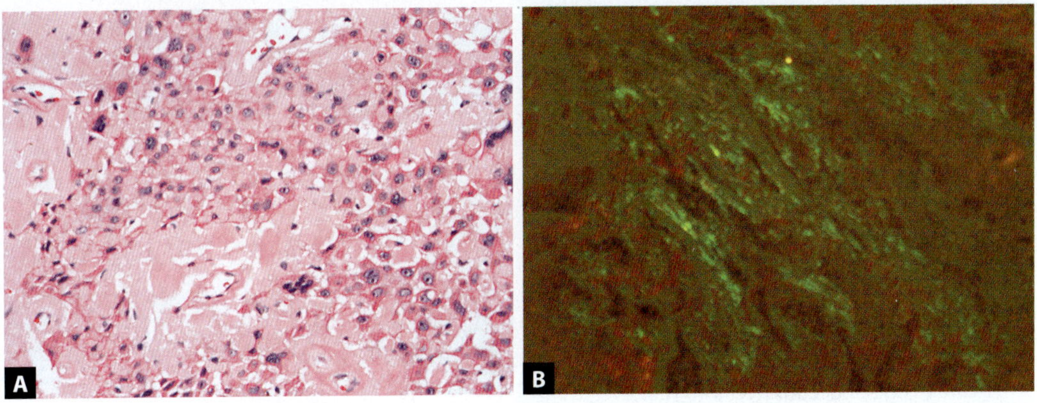

Figs 6.8A and B: Calcifying epithelial odontogenic tumor. (A) Epithelial component consists of sheets of polygonal cells that often have distinct intercellular bridges and the stroma contains amyloid; (B) Amyloid showing apple green birefringence with polarized microscope after staining with congo red

peripheral variant of Pindborg's tumor presents clinically as a nodular mass on gingival mucosa, frequently in an anterior location.

Radiological Features

An early tumor may be completely radiolucent. As the tumor matures most lesions become mixed radiolucent-radiopaque lesions. Moreover, the radiographic picture shows a spectrum ranging from a unilocular to a multilocular radiolucency (**Fig. 6.7B**). This is frequently associated with the crown of an impacted tooth often a mandibular third molar, or may appear in place of a tooth.

In some, the radioopacity is so complete that it resembles a bone tumor. In almost all cases, the radiographic border between tumor and surrounding bone appears to be well-defined and circumscribed. CEOT as a radiolucency resembles the presentation of other radiolucent jaw lesions, such as dentigerous cyst, odonto-genic keratocyst, ameloblastoma, and odontogenic myxoma. The mixed radiolucent-radiopaque lesion suggests a calcifying odontogenic cyst, ameloblastic fibro-odontoma and even desmoplastic ameloblastoma. Sometimes, the radiographic picture resembles tumors in bone such as ossifying fibroma, osteoblastoma, or even osteosarcoma if the lesion shows diffuse margins.

Histopathological Features

The CEOTs are unencapsulated and infiltrating tumors. The characteristic epithelial component consists of sheets and islands of polygonal cells that often have distinct intercellular bridges (**Fig. 6.8A**). The nuclei are centrally located and often have a prominent nucleolus. The nuclei may be pleomorphic, hyperchromatic, and bizarre in appearance. Binucleated cells may be frequent. Although multinucleated giant cells may be observed, increased numbers and/or abnormal mitotic figures are distinctly uncommon and if present would be a cause for concern. Clear cells are sometimes present. Rounded, pale eosinophilic masses may be found within the sheets of tumor cells and can undergo calcification, often in the form of Liesegang rings. The surrounding tissue may also contain large clumps of homogeneous eosinophilic material. The eosinophilic material stains positive for amyloid with Congo red, crystal violet, and Thioflavine T. When exposed to a polarized microscope positive areas demonstrate apple green birefringence (**Fig. 6.8B**).

Treatment

The CEOT is a locally invasive tumor. Small tumors may be enucleated, but larger ones require local resection. An overall recurrence rate of about 14 percent has been reported. A relatively higher recurrence rate of 22 percent has been noted for the clear cell variant. Long-term follow-up is recommended.

Box 6.3: Calcifying epithelial odontogenic tumor

Key features helpful in diagnosis
- Accounts for less than 1 percent of all odontogenic tumors
- No gender predilection
- Average age of occurrence is 40 years
- Mandible twice more commonly affected than maxilla
- Clinically manifests as a hard, painless slow-growing swelling
- Radiographically presents as a well-defined unilocular or multilocular radiolucency
- Histopathologically shows sheets and islands of polygonal cells with prominent intercellular bridges and pleomorphic hyperchromatic nuclei
- Liesegang rings and amyloid-like material is also evident.

ADENOMATOID ODONTOGENIC TUMOR

Adenomatoid odontogenic tumor (AOT) is a benign lesion with a slow but progressive growth. It occurs in both intraosseous and peripheral forms. Bernier and Tiecke introduced the term adenoameloblastoma. In 1961, Gorlin et al introduced the term ameloblastic adenomatoid tumor. In 1968, Abrams et al. suggested the term odontogenic adenomatoid tumor. Philipsen and Birn proposed the name adenomatoid odontogenic tumor in 1969. AOT accounts for 2 to 7 percent of all odontogenic tumors.

The long-term debate as to whether AOT is an anomalous developmental hamartomatous growth or a true benign neoplasm has not been settled. Meanwhile, investigators who prefer to consider AOT to be a hamartoma point to the limited size of most cases (attributed to its minimal growth potential) and to the lack of recurrence to support their belief. Those who prefer to consider AOT to be a nonaggressive noninvasive benign neoplasm presumably believe that the limited size of most cases stems

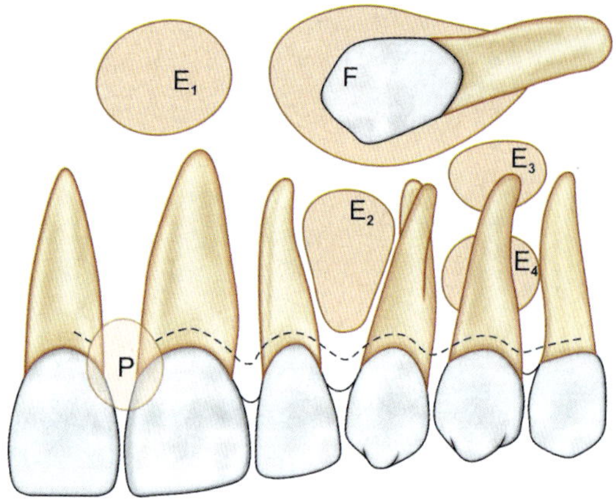

Fig. 6.9: Adenomatoid odontogenic tumor. It presents in varying associations in relation to teeth. (F: Follicular, E_1, E_2, E_3, E_4: Extrafollicular)

from the fact that most are detected early (often on a routine dental radiograph) and removed before the slow-growing tumor reaches a clinically noticeable size. Depending on the location, AOT has been classified into follicular and extra-follicular variants (**Fig. 6.9**).

Immunohistochemical studies revealed differences between the duct- and nonduct-forming cells; the nonduct-forming columnar cells expressed amelogenin reactivity, whereas the duct-forming cells showed no reactivity to amelogenin or the other enamel matrix protein (enamelin and sheathlin) antibodies. The tumor cells immediately adjacent to the droplets also demonstrate cytoplasmic positivity to the enamel protein, sheathlin. These findings provide additional support for the odontogenic origin of AOT and indicate that some of the epithelial tumor cells display features that are consistent with neoplastic (pre)ameloblasts in a state of arrested development, yet they apparently are metabolically active enough to produce basement membrane and enamel matrix proteins.

Clinical Features

The age range varies between 3 and 82 years. More than two-thirds are diagnosed in the second decade of life and 90 percent are found before the age of 30. The male:female ratio is 1:1.9. AOT almost exclusively occurs intraosseously with a preference for the maxilla over the mandible with a ratio of 2.1:1. The rare peripheral type occurs almost exclusively in the anterior maxillary gingiva. Intraosseous AOTs may be found in association with unerupted permanent teeth (follicular type), in particular the four canines that account for 60 percent with the maxillary canines alone accounting for 40 percent. Most AOTs are asymptomatic. When growth of the intraosseous variant causes cortical expansion, it may present as a palpable bony-hard swelling with or without slight pain (**Fig. 6.10A**). The intraosseous AOTs may cause displacement of neighbouring teeth. The peripheral variant presents as an epulis-like lesion of the gingiva.

Radiological Features

The intraosseous, follicular AOT shows a well-defined, unilocular radiolucency around the crown and often part of the root of an unerupted permanent tooth, mimicking a dentigerous cyst. If not associated with an unerupted tooth (extrafollicular type), AOT presents as a unilocular radiolucent lesion (**Fig. 6.10B**). In two thirds of the intraosseous variant, the radiolucency shows discrete radiopaque foci towards the periphery. AOT that appears without radiographic evidence of calcification is most suggestive of the more common dentigerous cyst. The peripheral variant may disclose erosion (saucerization) of the alveolar bone crest.

Histopathological Features

The most striking pattern is that of variably sized solid nodules of cuboidal or columnar cells of odontogenic epithelium forming nests or rosette-like structures with minimal stromal connective tissue. Between the epithelial cells and in the center of the rosette-like configurations, eosinophilic amorphous material is present (**Fig. 6.11**). Conspicuous within the cellular areas are appearance of tubular or duct-like appearance. The duct-like spaces are lined by a single row of columnar epithelial cells, with the nuclei polarized away from the luminal surface. The lumen may be empty or contain eosinophilic material or cellular debris. These nodules may contain pools of amorphous amyloid-like material and globular masses of calcified substances. Melanin pigmentation of both lesional tissue and stroma cells has been described. Occurrence of a hyaline, dysplastic material or calcified osteodentin may be found in AOTs. CEOT-like areas are occasionally found in AOTs.

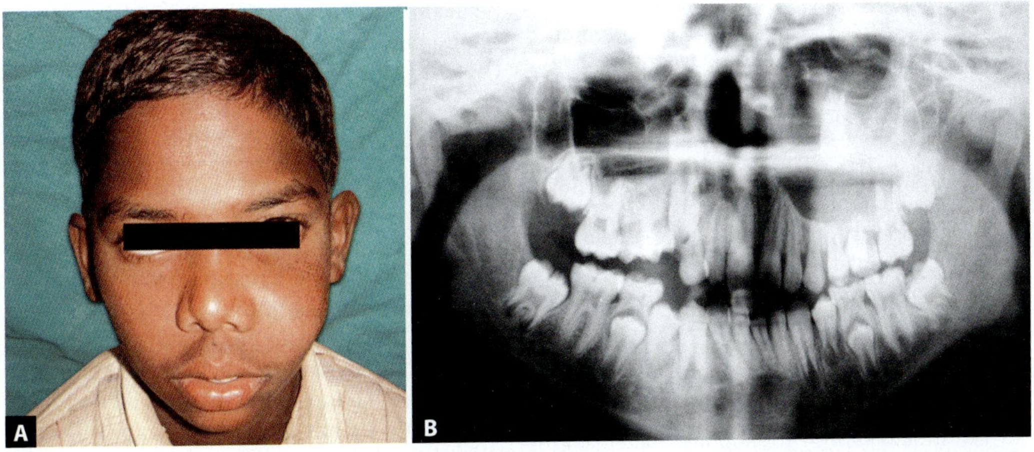

Figs 6.10A and B: Adenomatoid odontogenic tumor. (A) Usually present as a bony hard swelling in relation to maxillary canine; (B) Radiographically a unilocular radiolucency mimicking the appearance of a dentigerous cyst

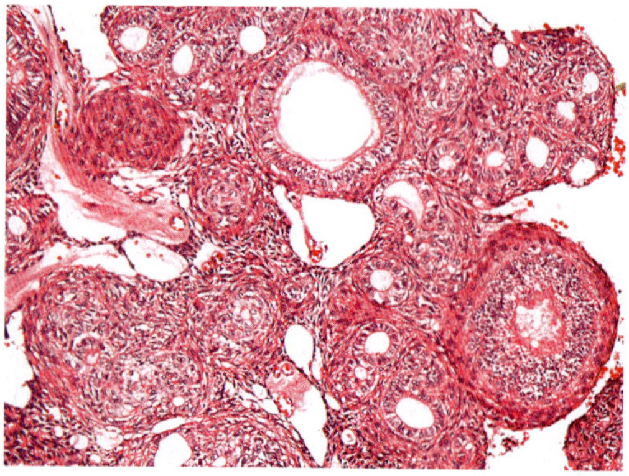

Fig. 6.11: Adenomatoid odontogenic tumor. Odontogenic epithelium forming nests or rosette-like structures with frequent duct like structures

Treatment

Although there may be expansion of the alveolar bone overlying central lesions, the cortex is almost invariably intact. Because of the uniformly benign biological behavior of nearly all typical AOTs and the consistent presence of a well-developed fibrous capsule, conservative complete surgical excision usually accomplished by enucleation and curettage is the treatment of choice.

Recurrences are extremely rare.

Box 6.4: Adenomatoid odontogenic tumor

Key features helpful in diagnosis

- Accounts for 2 to 7 percent of all odontogenic tumors
- Average age of occurrence is second decade of life
- Maxilla twice more commonly affected than mandible
- Often associated with impacted teeth especially canines
- Radiographically presents as well-defined unilocular radiolucency often associated with crown of an impacted tooth. Two-third of the cases show discrete calcific foci
- Histologically shows variably sized solid nodules of cuboidal or columnar cells of odontogenic epithelium forming nests or rosette-like structures with eosinophilic "material" in the center and interspersed with structures of tubular or duct-like appearance.

KERATOCYSTIC ODONTOGENIC TUMOR

Odontogenic keratocyst (OKC) has been one of the most controversial pathological entities of the maxillofacial region since Philipsen first described it in 1956. The WHO's recent classification of head and neck tumors reclassified keratocyst as a benign neoplasm recommending the term "keratocystic odontogenic tumor" (KCOT). The former orthokeratinized variant of the OKC is at present not recognized as being part of the spectrum of a KCOT. Multiple OKCs are indicative of the presence of nevoid basal cell carcinoma syndrome (NBCCs). In the earlier literature, OKC was described as a cholesteatoma by Hauer in 1926 and Kostecka in 1929. The term 'odontogenic keratocyst' was introduced by Philipsen in 1956, and subsequently in a paper by Pindborg and Hansen (1963), the designation 'keratocyst' was used to describe any jaw cyst in which keratin was formed to a large extent. It was believed that this cyst arises from primordial odontogenic epithelium that led to the term 'primordial cyst' Shear (1960); Shear and Altini (1976); Pindborg et al (1971). The term 'primordial cyst' has now fallen into disuse. A benign unicystic or multicystic, intraosseous tumor of odontogenic origin, with a characteristic lining of parakeratinized stratified squamous epithelium and potentially aggressive, infiltrative behavior. It may be solitary or multiple. The frequency of OKC has been reported to vary from 3 to 11 percent of odontogenic cysts (*see* Chapter 5 on Cysts of the Oral and Maxillofacial Region).

AMELOBLASTIC FIBROMA

Ameloblastic fibroma (AF) is a locally aggressive neoplasm arising from enamel organ and odontogenic mesenchyme of the primitive dental pulp. In 1891, Kruse first described cystic tumors of the mandible, which are known today as ameloblastic fibromas. AF consists of odontogenic ectomesenchyme resembling the dental papilla and epithelial strands and nests resembling dental lamina and enamel organ. Dental hard tissues are not present. If there is dentine formation, the lesion is referred to as ameloblastic fibrodentinoma (AFD). AF is a rare odontogenic tumor. The relative frequency of AF ranges from 1.5 to 4.5 percent. Ameloblastic fibroma has the same histogenesis as odontoma. It arises from odontogenic epithelium of the enamel organ and odontogenic mesenchyme of the primitive dental pulp. It too, represents an aborted attempt at tooth formation, but it occurs prior to any enamel or dentine formation. Intermediate in this spectrum of aborted tooth formation attempts is the ameloblastic fibro-odontoma, which actually forms some dentine and enamel, but much less organized than in odontoma.

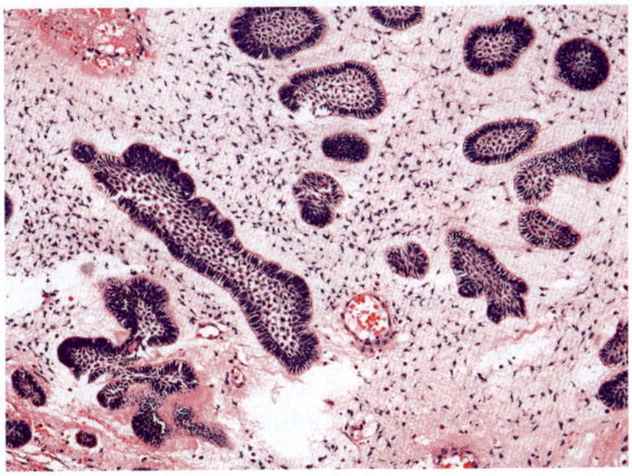

Fig. 6.12: Ameloblastic fibroma. Islands and strands of neoplastic odontogenic epithelium are arranged in a hypercellular stroma

Clinical Features

Most cases of AF present as a painless swelling or are discovered due to disturbances of tooth eruption. It usually grows to a certain size, sometimes large, then ceases to grow and does not extend beyond its own capsule. Less commonly, it exhibits continued slow growth. The mean age is 14.8 years. It is essentially a tumor that occurs in children and teenagers. There is no sex predilection. The mandibular molar area is the preferred site, but the tumor may occur in any location.

Radiological Features

Radiographically, the tumor presents as a well demarcated radiolucency, often in connection with a malpositioned tooth. It may be either unilocular or multilocular, and may be associated with the crown of an impacted tooth and mimic a dentigerous cyst. Due to the age of occurrence, the mass frequently displaces developing teeth. It may also resorb roots and displace the inferior alveolar canal.

Histopathological Features

The epithelial component of AF consists of branching and anastomosing epithelial strands that form knots of varying size. These have a peripheral rim of columnar cells similar to the inner enamel epithelium that embraces a loosely arranged spindle-shaped epithelium identical to stellate reticulum (**Fig. 6.12**). The epithelial strands lie in a myxoid and cell-rich stroma with stellate-shaped fibroblasts with long slender cytoplasmic extensions resembling embryonic tooth pulp. The amount of epithelium may vary. The epithelial component resembles ameloblastoma. In contrast to the follicular type of ameloblastoma, these follicular islands in AF seldom demonstrate microcyst formation. The odontogenic epithelial cells are strongly positive for cytokeratin and immature dental papilla like mesenchymal tissue, especially around the dental lamina-like odontogenic epithelium, is positive for tenascin. Vimentin staining is observed in some areas of dental papilla-like cells and in the basement membrane of the epithelium. These findings suggest that AF develops at the early stage of tooth formation. Histological features similar to AF, may be observed in the hyperplastic dental follicle.

Treatment

Ameloblastic fibroma usually requires only local excision and curettage as it is an encapsulated mass that is readily removed. The tumor usually does not invade the neurovascular bundle or even the inferior alveolar canal. Therefore, nerve preservation is usually achieved. Most ameloblastic fibromas are sufficiently large and destructive and strongly suggest need of resection rather than enucleation and curettage. Recurrence may occur but this does not justify initial aggressive treatment. The reappearance of a tumor may represent renewed growth of the residual tumor rather than true recurrence. Such recurrent lesions should be treated more aggressively. AF rarely transforms into an ameloblastic fibrosarcoma.

Box 6.5: Ameloblastic fibroma

Key features helpful in diagnosis

- Essentially occurs in children and teenagers
- Presents as either unilocular or multilocular well-demarcated radiolucency, often in connection with a malpositioned tooth
- Branching and anastomosing epithelial strands in a myxoid stroma resembling embryonic tooth pulp
- Represents an aborted attempt at tooth formation, prior to any enamel or dentine formation.

AMELOBLASTIC FIBRO-ODONTOMA

Ameloblastic fibro-odontoma (AFO) is a tumor which has intermediate features between an ameloblastic fibroma and an odontome. It represents a limited proliferation of odontogenic epithelium of the enamel organ and odontogenic mesenchyme of the primitive dental pulp. This proliferation comprises the soft tissue recapitulation of the dental follicle, which then produces some enamel but mostly dentine.

Ameloblastic fibro-odontoma may be a hamartoma representing an aberrant or aborted attempt at tooth formation. This aborted attempt at tooth formation or aberrancy occurs during the formation of enamel and dentine. This is in contrast to ameloblastic fibroma, in which the aborted attempt occurs before hard tissues are formed. In an odontome the aborted attempt occurs during the formation of enamel and dentine. Therefore, all three lesions share some features of developmental disturbances of tooth formation. However, ameloblastic fibroma shows more features of a true neoplasm.

Clinical Features

The AFO is less common than AF. The mean age is between 8 to 12 years. There is no gender or site predilection. AFO presents as an asymptomatic jaw expansion that may resorb tooth roots, displace developing teeth and inferior alveolar canal.

Radiological Features

Radiographically, AFO exhibits a well-circumscribed unilocular or multilocular radiolucency with varying levels of radio-opacity depending on the extent of mineralization. AFO is often associated with an unerupted tooth.

Histopathological Features

The AFO is composed of soft and hard tissues. These circumscribed tumors combine the histological features of ameloblastic fibroma and odontoma. Thus, in addition to the presence of dental papilla-like tissue with epithelial strands and islands, as seen in the ameloblastic fibroma, there is inductive change with formation of dentine and enamel (**Fig. 6.13**). Occasionally, tumors may show inductive changes limited to formation of dentine. These have been called ameloblastic fibro-dentinomas but they merely represent a minor variation of an ameloblastic fibro-odontoma.

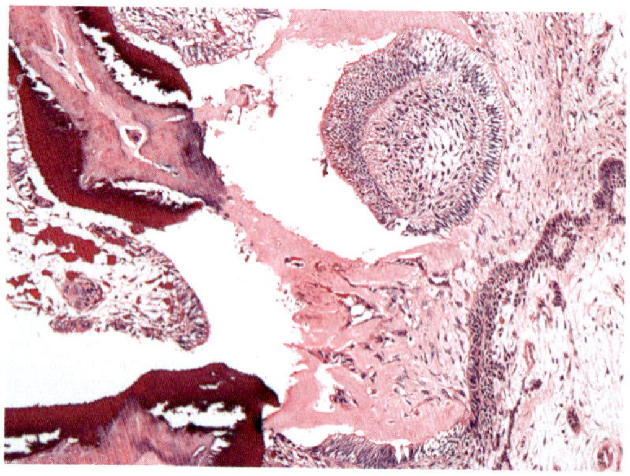

Fig. 6.13: Ameloblastic fibro-odontoma. There is evidence of inductive changes with dentine and enamel formation in addition to the features of ameloblastic fibroma

Box 6.6: Ameloblastic fibro-odontoma

Key features helpful in diagnosis

- AFO shows features of both neoplasm and hamartoma.
- Represents an aborted attempt at tooth formation or aberrancy occurs during the formation of enamel and dentine.
- Essentially occurs in children and teenagers.
- Presents as either unilocular or multilocular well-demarcated radiolucency, often in connection with a malpositioned tooth.
- Shows presence of dental papilla-like tissue with epithelial strands and islands along with inductive changes with the formation of dentine and enamel.

ODONTOMAS

Odontomas are the most common types of odontogenic tumors. Odontomas are considered to be developmental anomalies (hamartomas) rather than true neoplasms. Broca first coined the term "odontome" in 1866. He defined it as a tumor formed by an overgrowth of complete dental tissue. This term was expanded over time to include many odontogenic tumors or cysts. In a landmark paper, Thoma and Goldman narrowed the term "odontoma" to include tumors that were composed of well-differentiated tooth structure. Shafer and Gorlin defined odontoma as a tumor that has developed and differentiated enough to produce enamel and dentine.

The origin of odontoma is unknown. Several theories have been proposed, including trauma and infection. It seems that these conditions are more likely to result in a hypoplastic tooth germ rather than an odontoma. Odontomas have been associated with dilacerated roots in the anterior maxilla. This association could represent the dual result of trauma. As tooth formation occurs early in life and odontomas have been found in unusual locations such as the inner ear, nasopharynx, palate, and soft tissues of the jaw indicating that pathogenesis is likely to involve an embryologic disturbance.

Odontomas are actually mixed odontogenic hamartomas. They arise from both the odontogenic epithelium, which produce enamel, and the odontogenic mesenchyme producing dentine via odontoblast differentiation. As they are composed of both cell types and form products of both cell types, they have previously been termed "composite" odontomas. This nomenclature has been abandoned since it is assumed that they are composites of two tooth forming cell lines, as are all teeth. Odontomas represent an attempt to duplicate tooth formation but in a distorted fashion.

Odontomas are most likely hamartomas of aborted tooth formation, of which there are two general types. One type, which forms multiple small tooth-like structures, is called the compound odontoma. The other type forms an amorphous calcified mass and is called the complex odontoma.

Odontoma, complex type (OC) is a tumor-like malformation (hamartoma) composed of hap hazardly arranged enamel, dentine and sometimes cementum.

Clinical Features

Compound odontomas occur more often anterior to the mental foramen with a predilection to the maxilla whereas, complex odontomas occur posterior to the mental foramen with increased frequency in the mandible. There is no sex predilection. Most occur in children and young adults. It is doubtful whether new odontomas arise after the age of 25 years.

Odontomas usually form hard, painless masses and are small rarely exceeding the diameter of the associated impacted tooth. Most lesions are discovered as incidental radiographic findings. However, they can be associated with significant signs and symptoms. The most common symptom is an impacted permanent tooth or a retained deciduous tooth. In one study, Budnick found that 61 percent of odontomas were associated with impacted teeth. Swelling was the second most common complaint (**Fig. 6.14A**).

Radiological Features

The compound odontoma presents as a radiopaque mass in which the outline of miniature teeth may be noticed. The complex

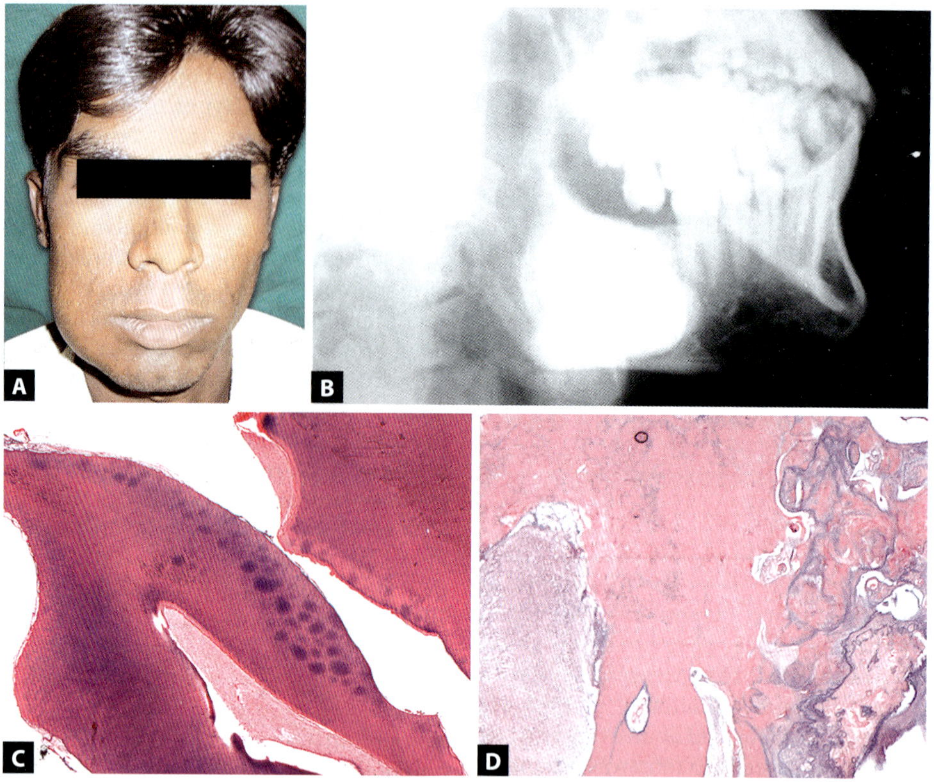

Figs 6.14A to D: Odontoma. (A) Swelling of the right side angle of the mandible; (B) Uniformly radiopaque lesion representing a complex odontome; (C) Histologically compound odontome shows tooth like structures; (D) Complex odontome is composed of irregularly arranged dental hard tissue, mostly dentine

odontoma will present as a dense amorphous and irregularly shaped mass (**Fig. 6.14B**). In both a well-demarcated border, with adjacent bone can usually be seen. An odontoma in its early stage of formation, when calcification of its distorted dentine is incomplete appears as a mixed radiodense lesion but has a well-demarcated border with bone.

Both compound, as well as complex odontomas if superimposed over roots, may also suggest the appearance of cementoblastoma or, if not discovered until after the age of 30 years, periapical cemento-osseous dysplasia and early florid cemento-osseous dysplasia. In addition, complex odontomas bear a radiographic resemblance to osteoblastoma, ossifying fibroma, and even lingual tori or osteomas that are projected over the mid mandible and therefore appear as a central lesion. Ameloblastic fibro-odontoma also mimics the appearance of an immature odontoma radiologically.

Histopathological Features

Odontomas are composed essentially of mature dental tissues namely enamel, dentine, cementum and pulp. They are arranged in discrete tooth-like structures (compound odontoma) (**Fig. 6.14C**) or as unstructured sheets of dental hard tissue (complex odontoma) (**Fig. 6.14D**). In addition, components of the enamel organ may be present. The bulk of the tumor usually consists of dentine that is normal in appearance. Cementum may be cellular or acellular, and enamel may be mature or consist only of matrix. Occasionally, epithelial ghost cell keratinization may be seen with a fibrous capsule and a small amount of supporting fibrous tissue, or possibly a dentigerous cyst may arise from compound odontoma.

Treatment

Conservative surgical excision is the treatment of choice for odontomas, results in little or no chance of recurrence. Complications of odontoma include infection, malocclusion, delayed eruption or noneruption of adjacent teeth and cyst formation.

Box 6.7: Odontomas

Key features helpful in diagnosis

- Occurs in children and young adults
- Compound odontoma has predilection for anterior maxilla and complex odontoma for posterior part of the mandible.
- Presents as a mixed radiopaque lesion with well-demarcated border.
- Mature dental tissues, enamel, dentine, cementum, and pulp tissue may be arranged in discrete tooth like structures (compound odontoma) or as unstructured sheets (complex odontoma).

CALCIFYING CYSTIC ODONTOGENIC TUMOR

The calcifying odontogenic cyst (COC) was first described as a distinct clinical entity by Gorlin and his colleagues in 1962. Gold (1963) chose a similar, but not identical term for the lesion, namely 'Keratinizing and calcifying odontogenic tumor'. The so-called calcifying odontogenic cyst represents a heterogeneous group of lesions that exhibits a variety of clinicopathologic and behavioural features. Because of this diversity, there has been confusion and disagreement on the terminology and classification of these lesions. The 1992 WHO classification includes this cyst and all its variants in the category of odontogenic tumors. Fejerskov and Krogh suggested the term 'calcifying ghost cell odontogenic tumor' and Freedman and his associates suggested the name 'cystic calcifying odontogenic tumor'. It is a rare, well circumscribed solid or cystic lesion derived from odontogenic epithelium and ectomesenchyme.

It has become obvious that calcifying cystic odontogenic tumor (CCOT) has a spectrum with one end as a cystic lesion and the other presenting as a more solid tumor. Praetorius et al in 1981 classified COCs into two entities, a cyst (type 1) and a neoplasm (type 2). Type 1 was further subclassified as type 1A (simple unicystic), type 1B (odontome producing), and type 1C (ameloblastomatous), and the term dentinogenic ghost cell tumor was proposed for the type 2 lesion (neoplasm). In the 2005 WHO classification dentinogenic ghost cell tumor is a separate entity.

Clinical Features

Swelling is the most frequent complaint and occurs in about half of the reported cases, only rarely has there been pain. Intraosseous lesions may produce a bony expansion and may be fairly extensive. Lingual expansion may sometimes be observed. Occasionally, the CCOT may perforate the cortical plate and extend into the soft tissues. CCOT is predominantly an intraosseous lesion, although 13 to 30 percent of cases have appeared as peripheral (extraosseous). Both the intraosseous and extraosseous forms occur in equal frequency in the mandible and maxilla.

About 65 percent of cases were found in the incisor and canine region. The mean age is 33 years and most cases are diagnosed in the second and third decade of life. CCOTs that are associated with odontomas tend to occur in younger patients, with a mean age of 17 years. The peripheral lesions on the gingiva, present as painless swelling or nodule, which may resemble fibrous epulis or peripheral giant cell granuloma.

Radiological Features

Calcifying cystic odontogenic tumor is an expansile lesion and sometimes discovered on routine radiographic examination. It is usually unilocular with a well-defined radiolucency. Radiopaque structures within the lesion either irregular calcification, or tooth-like densities may be seen. Radiological differential diagnose

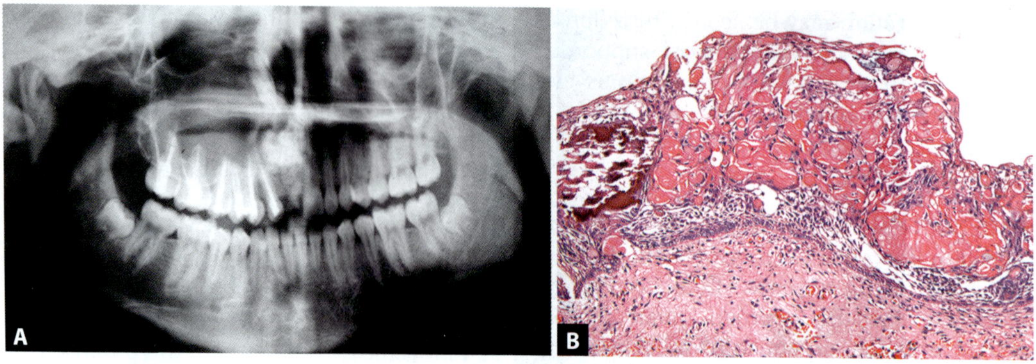

Figs 6.15A and B: Calcifying cystic odontogenic tumor. (A) Radiologically, it presents as a lesion of mixed radiodensity. Note the lesion in the anterior maxilla; (B) Histologically, the tumor is characterized by the presence of ghost cells, calcification and the basal layer showing cells similar to ameloblasts with reversed polarity

include tumors with mixed radiodensity (**Fig. 6.15A**).

Histopathological Features

The epithelial lining has characteristic odontogenic features with a prominent basal layer consisting of palisaded columnar or cuboidal cells and hyperchromatic nuclei which are polarized away from the basement membrane (**Fig. 6.15B**). The epithelium may be regular 6 to 8 cells thick over part of its length and be continuous with parts that may be very thin and others that are considerably thickened. Budding from the basal layer into the adjacent connective tissue and epithelial proliferations into the lumen are frequently seen. Multiple daughter cysts may be present within the fibrous wall and a foreign-body reaction to herniated ghost cells may be conspicuous. Melanin deposits are sometimes present in the epithelial lining. The most remarkable feature of the CCOT is the presence of ghost cells which are found in groups, particularly in the thicker areas of the epithelial lining. The spinous cells in such situations may be widely separated by intercellular oedema and the epithelium around the ghost cells is often convoluted.

The ghost cells or shadow cells are enlarged, ballooned, ovoid or elongated epithelial cells. They are eosinophilic and although the cell outlines are usually well defined, they may sometimes be blurred so that groups of them appear fused. A few ghost cells may contain nuclear remnants but these are in various stages of degeneration and in the majority all traces of chromatin have disappeared leaving only a faint outline of the original nucleus. The ghost cells represent an abnormal type of keratinization and have an affinity for calcification.

Atubular dentinoid (dysplastic dentine) is often found in the wall close to the epithelial lining and often in relation to the epithelial proliferations. It is frequently described as being found, particularly in contact with masses of ghost cells, then the tumor is better described as a dentinogenic ghost cell tumor. Calcification within ghost cells is common.

The cells are positive for cytokeratins and involucrine which is characteristic of terminal differentiation of keratinocytes. Some ghost cells in the linings of COCs are strongly stained with amelogenin, a protein that is unique to enamel matrix. Therefore, the presence of ghost cells in jaw tumors represents evidence of ameloblastic differentiation.

Treatment

Calcifying cystic odontogenic tumor is treated by surgical enucleation or local excision. In the presence of a complex odontome, conservative removal is still adequate. An ameloblastoma or one of its variants with foci of ghost cells must be treated as a conventional ameloblastoma rather than CCOT.

Box 6.8: Calcifying cystic odontogenic tumor

Key features helpful in diagnosis
- Majority of patients in 2nd and 3rd decades
- Usually presents as a unilocular radiolucency with radiopaque foci
- Most remarkable feature is the presence of ghost cells
- Atubular dentinoid (dysplastic dentine) is often found in contact with masses of ghost cells.

DENTINOGENIC GHOST CELL TUMOR

Dentinogenic ghost cell tumor (DGCT) was considered a solid variant of the calcifying odontogenic cyst in the past. DGCT is a locally invasive neoplasm characterized by ameloblastoma-like islands of epithelial cells in a mature connective tissue stroma. Aberrant keratinization may be found in the form of ghost cells in association with varying amounts of dysplastic dentine.

Clinical Features

Dentinogenic ghost cell tumor (DGCT) occurs as an intraosseous and less commonly as an extraosseous variant. The age range is from the second to the ninth decade. DGCT is somewhat more common in men than in women. It may occur in any tooth-bearing area of the jaws (**Fig. 6.16A**). The extraosseous variant shows a predilection for the anterior part of the jaws, while the intraosseous variant most often affects the canine to first molar region. The tumor is usually asymptomatic. The extraosseous variant presents as sessile, sometimes pedunculated, exophytic nodule of the gingival or alveolar mucosa. There may be bony expansion and in some cases resorption of cortical bone with extension into soft tissues. Adjacent teeth may be displaced and mobile.

Radiological Features

Radiographs of extraosseous DGCT show saucerization of the underlying bone in about 20 percent of the cases. Teeth in the affected area may be displaced. Radiographs of intraosseous DGCT show a radiolucent to mixed radiolucent/radiopaque appearance depending on the amount of calcification. The borders are usually well-demarcated. Most are unilocular. Resorption of adjacent teeth is a common finding.

Histopathological Features

There is no difference between the microscopic features of the intra- and extraosseous variants. Sheets and rounded islands of odontogenic epithelium are seen in a mature connective tissue. The epithelium of the tumor islands resembles that of an ameloblastoma, mitoses

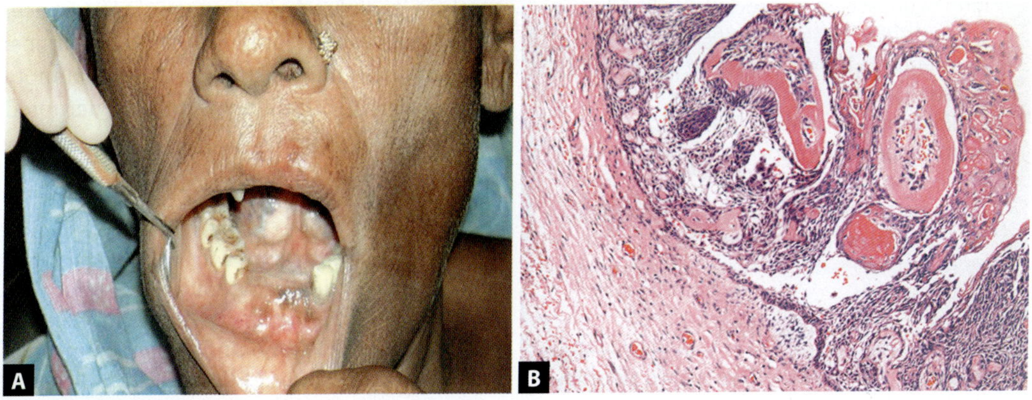

Figs 6.16A and B: Dentinogenic ghost cell tumor. (A) A large lesion in the anterior mandible; (B) In addition to the features of CCOT. *Note:* Presence of dentine

are not seen. Small cysts may form in the epithelial islands. A characteristic feature is the transformation of epithelial cells into ghost cells. Individual, as well as large islands of ghost cells, may be seen. Where basal layer cells are transformed into ghost cells the basement membrane disappears. When ghost cells extrude into the fibrous connective tissue a foreign body reaction can be seen. Some ghost cells undergo calcification. DGCT forms dysplastic dentine in small amounts (**Fig. 6.16B**) where ghost cells can become trapped. DGCT can be distinguished from an ameloblastoma by the presence of large numbers of ghost cells and dysplastic dentine but it may be difficult to distinguish from a multicystic calcifying cystic odontogenic tumor (CCOT). Malignant transformation of a DGCT into an odontogenic ghost cell carcinoma occurs rarely.

Treatment

Intraosseous DGCT may require wide local resection, particularly if the tumor is radiologically ill-defined. Recurrences have been reported in some intraosseous cases, and malignant transformation has been documented.

Box 6.9: Dentinogenic ghost cell tumor

Key features helpful in diagnosis

- A locally invasive neoplasm characterized by ameloblastoma-like islands of epithelial cells in a mature connective tissue stroma
- Aberrant keratinization may be found in the form of ghost cells in association with varying amounts of dysplastic dentine
- Age range is from the second to the ninth decade
- Radiolucent to mixed radiolucent/radiopaque appearance depending on the amount of calcification
- A characteristic feature is the transformation of epithelial cells into ghost cells.

ODONTOGENIC FIBROMA

Odontogenic fibroma (OF) is a rare neoplasm characterized by varying amounts of odontogenic epithelial rests in a mature, fibrous stroma. This has been a controversial diagnosis. At present the term OF is applied to two histological types of lesions namely the epithelium-poor type (formerly termed simple type) and the epithelium—rich type (formerly termed complex or WHO-type). Solid fibrous masses associated with crowns of unerrupted teeth consisting of hyperplastic dental follicles have been misdiagnosed as OF in the past. It has been suggested that the epithelium-poor type of OF derives from the dental follicle whereas the epithelium-rich type arises from the periodontal ligament.

Clinical Features

Odontogenic fibroma appears to occur more frequently in children and young adults, although a few cases have been reported in older persons. Female predilection has been noted with a ratio of 2.2:1. It has a preponderance for occurrence in the mandible, with most lesions found in the mandibular molar/premolar area. Topographically, two variants can be distinguished; an intraosseous or central type and an extraosseous or peripheral type. It presents as a slow growing, progressive but painless swelling, often with cortical expansion (**Fig. 6.17A**).

Radiological Features

It appears as a unilocular radiolucent area with well defined, often sclerotic borders. Rarely, the occurrence of calcified material may produce a mixed radiolucent/radiopaque appearance. Larger lesions show scalloping of the margins. Adjacent teeth may be displaced. Some tumors are associated with the crown of an unerupted tooth.

Histopathological Features

Despite the controversy, two histological types have been described: the epithelium-poor type and the epithelium-rich type. The epithelium-poor type of OF is a noninfiltrating connective tissue lesion resembling a dental follicle. It shows minimal cells with dispersed delicate collagen fibers. Fibromyxoid quality is evident due to

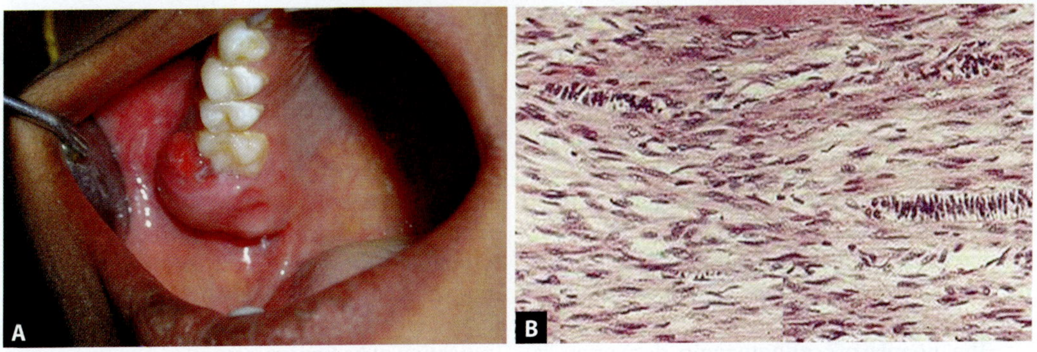

Figs 6.17A and B: Odontogenic fibroma. (A) Clinical appearance of a lesion; (B) The tumor is composed of fibrous stroma containing inactive stands of odontogenic epithelium

the presence of ground substances. Remnants of occasional inactive-looking odontogenic epithelium appear as small irregular islands and cords (**Fig. 6.17B**). Calcifications are seen occasionally. The epithelium-rich type of OF is composed of cellular, fibroblastic connective tissue interwoven with less cellular and often vascular areas. Islands or strands of inactive-looking odontogenic epithelium are very frequently observed. This type shows foci of calcified material considered to be metaplastically produced dysplastic cementum/osteoid/dentine.

The rarity of the central odontogenic fibroma excludes it from most differential diagnosis lists. Most presentations suggest the more common radiolucent odontogenic cysts and tumors such as odontogenic keratocyst, ameloblastoma, or odontogenic myxoma as well as ameloblastic fibroma. In younger individuals, the presentation also suggests central giant cell granuloma.

Treatment

Odontogenic fibromas can be treated by enucleation and curettage. They readily separate from their bony crypt and show no evidence of bony infiltration. Recurrence rate is considered low.

Box 6.10: Odontogenic fibroma

Key features helpful in diagnosis

- Occurs in children and young adults
- Female predilection
- Presents as a slow growing progressive swelling
- Appears as a unilocular radiolucency with well-defined sclerotic borders
- Epithelium-poor type resembles a dental follicle and epithelium-rich type is cellular.

ODONTOGENIC MYXOMA

Odontogenic myxoma (OM) is a benign neoplasm arising from odontogenic mesenchymal tissue with similar growth characteristics, clinical and radiographic presentation to those of ameloblastoma. It shows infiltrative growth but does not metastasize. Myxomas of jaws, by contrast, show a close structural resemblance to dental mesenchyme, occasionally contains epithelial rests, affect the tooth-bearing areas of the jaws and a tooth is frequently absent. In 1947, Thoma and Goldman first described myxomas of the jaws. Since then OM has been a subject of continuous scientific debate and has been discussed avidly. OM is an intraosseous neoplasm characterized by stellate and spindle-shaped cells embedded in an abundant myxoid or mucoid extracellular matrix. When a relatively greater amount of collagen is evident, the term myxofibroma may be used. Evidence which support odontogenic origin has been perpetuated by almost exclusive occurrence in the tooth-bearing areas of the jaws, frequent occurrence in young individuals and association with an unerupted tooth or a developmentally absent tooth, histologic resemblance to dental mesenchyme, especially the dental papilla; and the occasional presence of sparse amounts of odontogenic epithelium.

The neoplasm's odontogenic derivation is believed to originate from the primitive mesenchymal portion of the developing tooth germ (dental follicle, dental papilla, periodontal ligament) as an inductive effect of nests of odontogenic epithelium on mesenchymal tissue or as a direct myxomatous change of fibrous tissue in an odontogenic fibroma. While myxomas do occur in long bones, these are rare and are thought to arise from pluripotential mesenchymal stem cells. The jaws also contain a small population of nonodontogenic pluripotential mesenchymal stem cells that may give rise to a myxoma. However, the much greater incidence of myxomas in the jaws parallels the much greater amount of primitive mesenchyme associated with 20 primary and 32 permanent tooth formations, increasing the likelihood of a myxoma. Though unproven, myxomas in the jaws are thought to originate from odontogenic mesenchyme rather than from somatic mesenchyme and are thus termed OMs.

The frequency of OM varies in different parts of the world between 3 to 20 percent of all odontogenic tumors. In most studies, OM is the third most frequent odontogenic tumor (after odontoma and ameloblastoma).

Clinical Features

Small OMs are asymptomatic. Large OMs cause painless expansion. Cortical perforation may occur when the tumor is large. The age range varies from 1 to 73 years, with a mean age of 30 years. The majority is diagnosed in the 2nd to 4th decades. Cases in individuals younger than 15 years are common, in contrast to the rarity of ameloblastomas in that age group. OM is slightly more common in females.

Two-thirds of OMs are located in the mandible. The myxoma differs from the ameloblastoma in site preference. While ameloblastoma is much more commonly seen in the third molar areas, particularly in the mandible, odontogenic myxoma is evenly distributed throughout the jaws. Tooth displacement and root resorption may be seen. Some cases show displacement of the inferior alveolar canal, indicative of its benign nature.

Radiological Features

The radiographic features of OM are variable, ranging from small unilocular lesions to large multilocular neoplasms, which often displace teeth or, less frequently, resorb roots. The multilocular trabecular pattern has been described as honey comb, soap bubble, tennis racket, spider web and stepladder pattern (fine residual bony trabeculae arranged at right angles to one another) in appearance (**Fig. 6.18A**). Most multilocular myxomas are greater than 4.0 cm whilst unilocular myxomas tend to be smaller. The borders of the tumor are usually well-defined and corticated but can be poorly defined or diffuse. Larger OMs may present with periosteal reactions. Only 5 percent of myxomas are associated with unerupted teeth.

CT may reveal fine bony septae and allows for anatomic delineation. Advanced imaging studies such as CT and MRI should be used to clearly define tumor margins and to identify the true extent of the myxoma before surgery is performed. The radiographic differential diagnosis due to multilocular radiolucency strongly suggests an ameloblastoma or keratocystic odontogenic tumor. If the individual is younger than 15 years, the possibility of an ameloblastic fibroma increases. Other multilocular radiolucent lesions include central giant cell granuloma (increasingly likely in individuals between 5 and 15 years of age) and central hemangiomas (cavernous or arteriovenous types), which may also present as "honeycombed" radiolucencies.

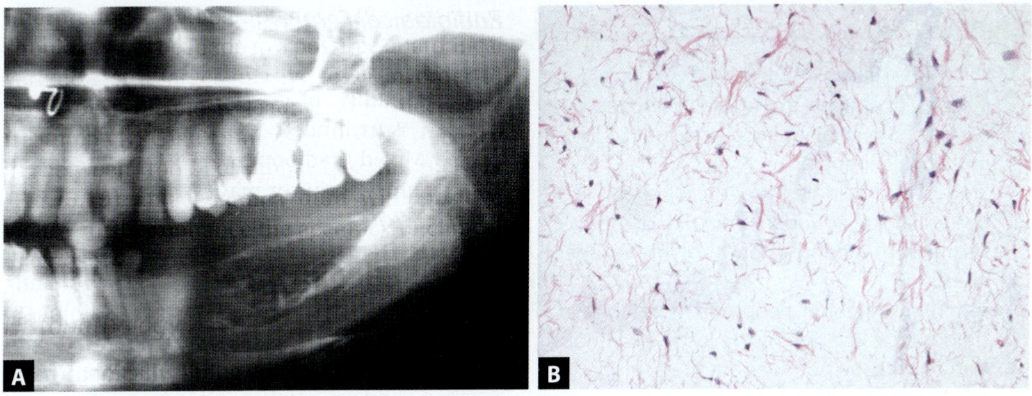

Figs 6.18A and B: Odontogenic myxoma. (A) Radiographically it presents as a multilocular radiolucency; (B) Note the marked myxoid stroma and cells with long cytoplasmic processes

Histopathological Features

Odontogenic myxoma is usually a well delineated, nonencapsulated gray-white to tan-yellow mass that can be rubbery, soft, or gelatinous in texture. The margins usually are ill defined in gelatinous specimens. On the cut surface, it is typically glistening, translucent, homogeneous and depending on the amount of collagen present, fine white bands of collagen may be visible macroscopically. OM is characterized by randomly oriented stellate, spindle-shaped and round cells with long, fine, anastomosing pale or slightly eosinophilic cytoplasmic processes extending from the centrally placed nucleus (**Fig. 6.18B**). Cells are evenly dispersed in an abundant mucoid or myxoid stroma that contains only a few fine collagen fibres. Binucleated cells, mild pleomorphism and mitotic figures may occur. Rests of odontogenic epithelium are not obvious in most lesions and are not required for establishing the final diagnosis. Some OMs may permeate into the marrow spaces in a pseudomalignant pattern. OMs are unencapsulated and extend to surrounding bone by expansion rather than cellular growth, possibly as a result of the large content of hyaluronic acid. Some OMs have a tendency to produce collagen fibres and are designated myxofibroma. There is no evidence that more collagenous variants behave differently.

Odontogenic myxoma is strikingly similar microscopically to myxoid, enlarged or 'hyperplastic' dental follicle and the dental papilla of a developing tooth. Misdiagnosis of these entities should be avoided by correlation with the clinical and radiographic features. The clinical differential diagnosis is essentially similar to that of ameloblastoma. The microscopic differential diagnosis should also include myxoid nerve sheath tumors, chondromyxoid fibroma, low-grade myxoid fibrosarcoma and other myxoid sarcomas.

Treatment

Curative treatment of an odontogenic myxoma is accomplished by resection with 1.0 to 1.5 cm bony margins. Recurrence is expected with enucleation and curettage procedures but may not be clinically detected for 5 years or more. Seeding of tumor cells can occur because of the loose gelatinous consistency of the tumor, resulting in unresectable recurrences. Therefore, enucleation and curettage is not advised. Recurrence rates from various studies average about 25 percent but in spite of this, the prognosis is good. Recurrence usually follows incomplete removal within two years but may occur much later.

Box 6.11: Odontogenic myxoma

Key features helpful in diagnosis
- Majority of patients in the 2nd to 4th decades
- Ranges from small unilocular lesions to large multilocular neoplasms
- Stellate and spindle shaped cells evenly dispersed in an abundant mucoid or myxoid stroma with varying amounts of fine collagen fibers
- Although a benign neoplasm, it exhibits insidious local invasion by the loose, gelatinous nature of tissue but does not metastasize.

BENIGN CEMENTOBLASTOMA

Benign cementoblastoma (BC) is characterized by proliferation of cementoblasts forming disorganized cementum around the apical one half of a tooth root. Described initially in 1930 by Norberg, CB is a rare tumor of mesenchymal odontogenic origin consisting of cementum tissue with functional cementoblasts. CB accounts for 0.2 percent and 6.2 percent of odontogenic tumors. True cementoma is a synonym for BC.

Cementoblastomas are odontogenic tumors and are derived from ectomesenchymal cells of the periodontium, including cementoblasts. It is thought to evolve in three stages. The first stage is characterized by periapical osteolysis, followed by a cementoblastic stage and then inactive stage of maturation and calcification. BC is considered a neoplasm with unlimited growth potential. Its etiology is unknown and trauma does not seem to play a role.

Clinical Features

The most common finding is a painful swelling at the buccal and lingual/palatal aspect of alveolar ridges. Vitality of involved tooth remains intact. Lower-lip paresthesia or a pathological fracture of the mandible is rarely reported. The age ranges from 8 to 44 years. There is no distinct gender predilection. The majority of CBs are located in the mandible, particularly related to the permanent first molar. Association with a primary tooth is exceptionally rare.

Radiological Features

Radiographically, the tumor is well-defined and is mainly of a radiopaque or mixed-density, surrounded by a thin radiolucent zone. Mixed radioopque-radiolucent lesion may be amorphous or may have a wheel-spoke pattern. Root resorption, loss of root outline and obliteration of the periodontal ligament space are common findings. The distinguishing feature of a CB is its peripheral radiolucent margin to adjacent bone and its obliteration of one half of the root. These features distinguish it from other radiopaque lesions that may become superimposed over tooth roots, such as osteoblastoma, ossifying fibroma and odontoma. These features also distinguish a small CB from hypercementosis and focal bone sclerosis, so called condensing osteitis.

Histopathological Features

Benign cementoblastoma has a thin fibrous capsule that is usually continuous with the periodontal membrane. The tumor consists of sheets of cementum-like material continuous with the root. It consists of dense masses of acellular cementum-like material in a fibrous, sometimes rather vascular stroma that may contain multinucleated cells (**Fig. 6.19**). Tumor mass blends with the root showing simultaneous root resorption. Invasion of the root canal is common. Proliferating cementum is lined

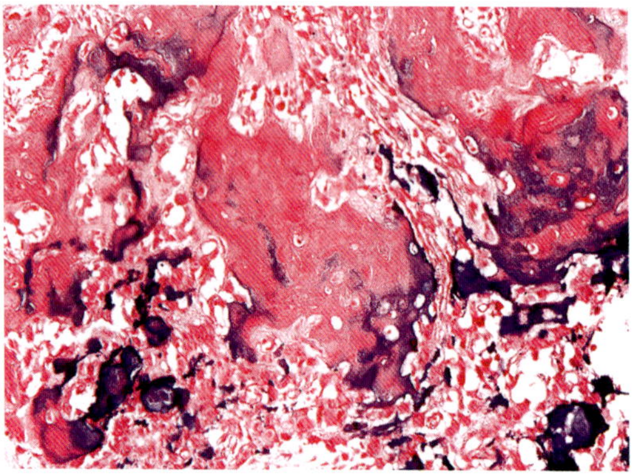

Fig. 6.19: Cementoblastoma. Irregularly arranged cementum in a fibrovascular stroma

by numerous plump cells. Cementoclasts may also be present, and reversal lines are prominent. Some of the cemental material may be uncalcified, particularly at the periphery of the mass. Tumor cementum is often arranged perpendicular to the capsule. The fibrous stroma is highly vascular. In the more mature parts of the tumor, basophilic reversal lines may produce a pattern similar to Paget's disease of bone.

Treatment

Treatment of choice is early surgical removal due to its capacity for persistent growth, expansion and involvement of adjacent structures. The tumor is readily enucleated and it usually does not recur. Because of its capsule, apparently bulbous mass is readily separated from the surrounding bone. In case of incomplete removal, together with the associated tooth, recurrence is not uncommon.

Box 6.12: Benign cementoblastoma

Key features helpful in diagnosis

- Tumor with proliferation of cementoblasts forming disorganized cementum.
- Presents in 2nd decade.
- Radiopaque or mixed-density, surrounded by a thin radiolucent zone.
- Dense masses of acellular cementum-like material in a fibrous stroma.

MALIGNANT AMELOBLASTOMA (METASTASIZING AMELOBLASTOMA)

Ameloblastoma is considered as a benign tumor that can be locally invasive and shows high recurrence rate depending on initial type of treatment. Ameloblastomas rarely metastasize or undergo malignant transformation. This malignant behavior is present in less than 2 percent of ameloblastomas. Emura first described metastasis of ameloblastoma to cervical lymph nodes. In 1932 Vorzimar and Perla described metastasis to lungs. Malignant ameloblastoma (MA) is an ameloblastoma that metastasizes in spite of a benign histologic appearance. In the WHO classification (2005) it is included under odontogenic carcinomas. Origin of MA is most likely to be the same as that of nonmalignant ameloblastoma, however precise mechanism by which slow growing cytologically none malignat tumor spreads to distant location is not clear. MA is usually preceded by multiple local recurrences of primary tumor hence, it is suggested that possible mechanism of metastasis may be related to local recurrence which increases aggressiveness or malignant behavior of the tumor and also spillage or implantation of tumor cells in blood or lymphatic during surgical intervention. Metastasis occurs through blood vessels, lymphatics or by aspiration.

Clinical Features

Malignant ameloblastoma do not show any specific clinical features distinct from conventional ameloblastoma. There is predilection for occurrence of tumor in the mandible than maxilla (7.6:1). Mean age of occurrence is 34 years and male to female ratio is 1.2:1. Common signs and symptoms are swelling of jaw, pain, delayed tooth eruption, ulceration and tooth mobility. Factors which may contribute for metastasis are duration of tumor, extend and size of tumor and initial type of surgery. Most common sites of metastasis are lungs (75%), bone (25%), cervical lymph node (18%), liver (11%), brain (10%), other nodes, spleen and kidney (3.5%). The time lapse from diagnosis to metastasis appears to be 9 to 10 years.

Radiological Features

Radiological features are similar to conventional ameloblastoma. CT and MRI are useful in accurate evaluation of the extension of tumor.

Histopathological Features

The histopathological features are indistinguishable from conventional ameloblastoma. MA does not show cytological atypia or mitotic activity. It is the clinical behavior which determines its malignant status (**Fig. 6.20**).

Treatment

Adequate initial surgical treatment of primary neoplasm plays the most important role in prevention of postoperative metastasis. Radical resection and primary reconstruction is the most

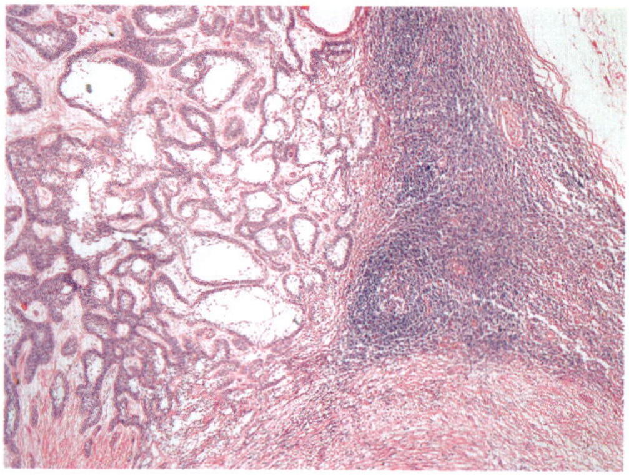

Fig. 6.20: Malignant ameloblastoma. Cytologically benign follicles of ameloblastoma in a lymph node

accepted therapeutic modality. Neck dissection for cervical lymph nodes and lobectomy of lung metastasis is done with preservation of lung function.

Box 6.13: Malignant ameloblastoma

Key features helpful in diagnosis

- Majority of patients are in 3rd and 4th decade
- Radiologic features are similar to conventional ameloblastoma
- Histopathological features are indistinguishable from conventional ameloblastoma
- Does not show cytological atypia or mitotic activity.

AMELOBLASTIC CARCINOMA

Ameloblastic carcinoma (AC) is the malignant epithelial odontogenic tumor that histologically retain the features of ameloblastic differentiation and exhibits cytological features of malignancy. The term AC was introduced by Shafer in 1974 and WHO (2005) recognises different subtypes. They are ameloblastic carcinoma (a) primary type, ameloblastic carcinoma (b) secondary type (dedifferentiated) intraosseous and ameloblastic carcinoma—secondary type (dedifferentiated) peripheral. AC may arise in a pre-existing benign ameloblastoma. The term "dedifferentiated ameloblastoma" has been applied when morphologic features of typical ameloblastoma are noted in some areas.

Clinical Features

Ameloblastic carcinomas are twice more common than malignant ameloblastoma. There is a predilection for occurrence in the mandible over maxilla. The mean age of occurrence is in the range of 15 to 84 years. It is more common in males with male-to-female ratio of 1.4:1. Common signs and symptoms are, swelling, pain, trismus, dysphonia, rapid growth and paresthesia.

Radiological Features

The radiologic features show ill-defined large multilocular radiolucency, perforation of cortical plates, extension into neighboring tissue and occasionally foci of calcification.

Histopathological Features

Ameloblastic carcinoma shows odontogenic epithelial cells arranged in the form of islands, cords and sheets with infiltrative pattern within the stroma of mature fibrous tissue. Island and cords show outer layer of tall columnar to cuboidal ameloblast like cells. The central cells are stellate reticulum like in appearance and hypercellular without an orderly pattern. The epithelial cells show characteristics features of malignancy such as nuclear hyperchromatism, mild pleomorphism, and increased mitotic activity with occasional abnormal forms (**Fig. 6.21**). Mitotic figures may attain a count of 2 to 5 per high-power field. In some cases individual cell keratinization and keratin formation may be seen. Necrosis and dystrophic calcifications may also be observed. Rare cases of AC may reveal clear cell differentiation. Aneuploidy has been found to be more frequently present in the ameloblastic carcinoma and may be used as a strong predictor of malignant potential of a questionable lesion.

Treatment

The treatment of choice is radical surgery with neck dissection. Local recurrences and

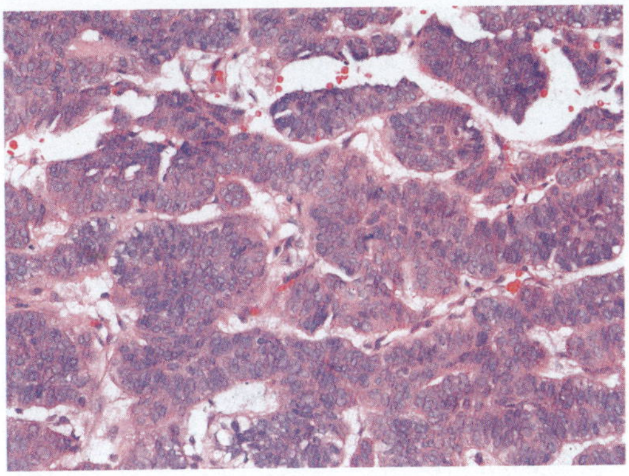

Fig. 6.21: Ameloblastic carcinoma. Strands of ameloblastic epithelium showing cytological atypia with mitotic figures

metastasis to the neck and lung seem to be common.

> **Box 6.14: Ameloblastic carcinoma**
>
> **Key features helpful in diagnosis**
>
> - Presents as a large ill-defined multilocular radiolucency
> - Histologically retains the features of ameloblastic differentiation but exhibits cytological features of malignancy
> - Demonstrates greater cytologic atypia and mitotic activity.

PRIMARY INTRAOSSEOUS SQUAMOUS CELL CARCINOMA

Primary intraosseous squamous cell carcinoma (PIOSCC) is a central jaw carcinoma derived from odontogenic epithelial remnants. Central squamous cell carcinoma of the jaw was first described by Loos in 1913. Pindborg et al suggested the term primary intraosseous carcinoma, which was accepted by the World Health Organisation (WHO) classification in 1992. In the WHO classification (2005), it is included under odontogenic carcinomas and subcategories include primary intraosseous squamous cell carcinoma—solid type, primary intraosseous squamous cell carcinoma derived from keratocystic odontogenic tumor and primary intraosseous squamous cell carcinoma derived from odontogenic cysts.

Solid Type

Clinical Features

The male:female ratio approaches 2:1 with a mean age of 55 years, although cases have been encountered during infancy. PIOSCC is more often found in the body and posterior mandible than the maxilla. Maxillary cases are most frequently seen in the anterior segment. Most cases are asymptomatic and are discovered incidentally during the course of routine dental radiographs. Persistent pain and swelling of the jaw seems to be an important presenting symptom of PIOSCC. Other symptoms that may be observed are perineural invasion of the inferior alveolar nerve causing paresthesia of the lip. It spreads both regionally and distantly.

Radiological Features

Radiographically, PIOSCCs are osteolytic. The margins of the radiolucency are often irregular, diffuse, ill defined and noncorticated. Larger extensive lesions may show cortical bone expansion and destruction.

Histopathological Features

The PIOSCC is characterized by islands of neoplastic squamous epithelium with the features of squamous cell carcinoma. The PIOSCC may reveal a distinct odontogenic pattern with basal-type cells forming alveoli or arranged in to plexiform pattern with palisading of the peripheral cells. Keratinization is not marked. In order to arrive at the diagnosis, the possibility of metastatic squamous cell carcinoma has to be excluded.

Derived from Keratocystic Odontogenic Tumor

When a squamous cell carcinoma arises within the jaw bones without connection to the oral mucosa in the presence of a keratocystic odontogenic tumor (KCOT) is termed as Primary intraosseous squamous cell carcinoma derived from keratocystic odontogenic tumor. Although the epithelium of the KCOT seems to have a higher mitotic activity than that of other odontogenic cysts, there is little evidence that the KCOT is associated with malignant change more often than any other type of odontogenic cyst.

Clinical Features

Most of these lesions are encountered in older patients, 40 years and above, with male predilection. The mandible is involved much more frequently than the maxilla. Early lesions are generally insidious, usually presenting as a benign odontogenic cyst and the diagnosis of carcinoma is only made after microscopic examination. In others, symptoms such as pain, swelling, loosening of teeth, nonhealing extraction sockets, and paresthesia are common.

Radiological Features

Radiographically, early lesions are often indistinguishable from any odontogenic cyst. In some, the margins of the radiolucent defect appear irregular and ragged. Late lesions are obviously destructive. A multilocular appearance with cortical destruction and frequent soft tissue extension characterizes these late-stage neoplasms.

Histopathological Features

Histopathologically, it shows a well differentiated squamous cell carcinoma with recognizable KCOT. Epithelial dysplasia of varying degrees is often present. The main differential diagnosis should include squamous odontogenic tumor, central high-grade mucoepidermoid carcinoma and metastatic lesions.

Treatment

The treatment of choice for the PIOSCCs ex KCOT is radical surgery with or without neck dissection. Due to the small number of cases of PIOSCCs ex KCOTs, no relevant information on recurrence rate, frequency of metastasis, or prognosis are available. Long-term follow-up, as with patients with oral cancer, is mandatory.

Derived from Odontogenic Cyst Lining

This is defined as a squamous cell carcinoma arising within the jaws without connection to the oral mucosa, and in the presence of an odontogenic cyst other than keratocystic odontogenic tumor.

Clinical Features

In a series of 28 patients the mean age was 56 years and age ranges from 4 to 90 years. Male-to-female ratio is almost 2:1. Ratio of mandibular to maxillary lesions is 3:1. Clinical symptoms are nonspecific and include pain and swelling.

Radiological Features

The radiographic features may mimic any type of odontogenic cyst. PIOSCCs ex odontogenic cysts are nonspecific and are characterized by a radiolucency surrounded by a relatively well defined radiopaque border.

Treatment

Odontogenic cysts with PIOSCCs can not be differentiated clinically and radiographically from conventional cysts, most of them are enucleated at first stage surgery. After the histopathologic diagnosis has been established the treatment of choice for the PIOSCCs ex odontogenic cyst is radical surgery.

CLEAR CELL ODONTOGENIC CARCINOMA

Clear cell odontogenic tumor (CCOT), first described as a separate entity by Hansen et al and later by Waldron et al in 1985, and is an unusual intraosseous tumor histologically characterized by odontogenic epithelial cells with clear vacuolated cytoplasm. Since all the cases showed locally aggressive behavior, but no evidence of lymph node or distant metastasis, they considered CCOT to be a benign, locally aggressive lesion. In the past it was called clear cell ameloblastoma and clear cell odontogenic tumor and was considered a benign tumor in the previous WHO classification of 1992. Additional cases of CCOT, which were published later, also confirmed the tumor's potential to metastasize. As a result, the tumor is now considered to be a malignant neoplasm, and the name has been changed to clear cell odontogenic carcinoma (CCOC).

Clinical Features

Clear cell odontogenic tumor tends to occur in older adults; the mean age at diagnosis is approximately 60 years and ranges from 17 to 89 years. The tumor has a strong female predilection. The male:female ratio is 1:1.6. The most frequently affected site is the mandible, and the maxillary:mandibular ratio is 1:7.7 with the posterior region of the mandible consisting of 90 percent of the cases. The CCOC usually causes swelling of the jaws, loosening of teeth and associated pain in some patients.

Radiological Features

Radiographically, CCOC appears as a poorly delineated unilocular or multilocular radiolucent lesion with prominent bone destruction. Root resorption and root divergence is present in a majority of cases.

Histopathological Features

The majority of tumors show biphasic pattern. A classic case of CCOC demonstrates budding and branching cords, islands and sheets of neoplastic polygonal epithelial cells. Lesional cells exhibit central to eccentric small dark uniform nuclei and there is little evidence of nuclear pleomorphism or mitotic activity. The cells exhibit abundant pale cytoplasm with clear cells showing distinct cell borders. Cords of dark-staining basaloid cells with scanty eosinophilic cytoplasm may also be seen. Tumor islands display peripheral ameloblastomatous palisaded columnar cells (**Fig. 6.22**). However, no evidence of central stellate reticulum, squamous differentiation or cystic change is observed. Some tumors contain (monophasic pattern) islands of entirely clear cells. Many of the tumor cells contain abundant delicate and coarse diastase degradable PAS-positive granules, which are negative for mucin and amyloid. Cytokeratin 19 and EMA immunostaining pattern together with histopathological features may help in the final diagnosis of CCOC.

Since clear cells are frequently seen in other neoplasms in the oral and maxillofacial region, it is important to rule out lesions such as salivary gland tumors, melanotic tumors, metastatic renal cell carcinoma and clear cell variant of calcifying epithelial odontogenic tumor.

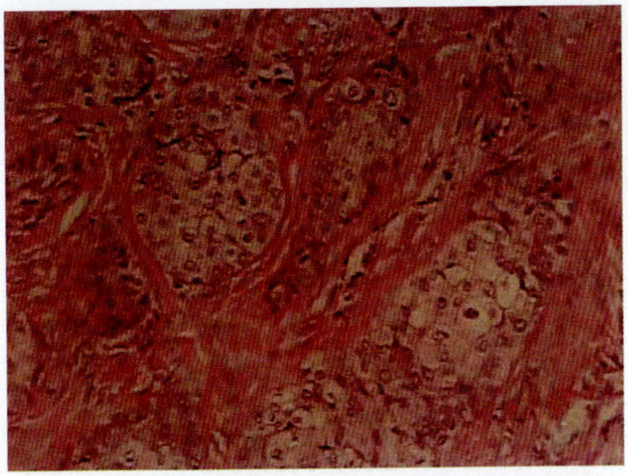

Fig. 6.22: Clear cell odontogenic carcinoma. Islands of clear cells with some islands showing peripheral palisading and reversed polarity of basal cells

Treatment

The CCOC exhibits an aggressive growth pattern and frequently recurs. The tumor can metastasize to regional lymph nodes and lungs, as well as to bone. Therefore radical resection with tumor-free margins is the treatment of choice, and long-term follow-up is mandatory. Adjuvant radiotherapy is a rational option for tumors that have eroded cortical bone.

Box 6.15: Clear cell odontogenic carcinoma

Key features helpful in diagnosis

- Presents as poorly delineated unilocular or multilocular radiolucent lesion with prominent bone destruction
- Occurs in older adults
- Female predilection
- Composed of cells showing uniform nuclei and clear cytoplasm
- Demonstrates an aggressive clinical course, with invasion of contiguous structures and a tendency to recur.

GHOST CELL ODONTOGENIC CARCINOMA

Ghost cell odontogenic carcinoma (GCOC) is a malignant odontogenic epithelial tumor with features of calcifying cystic odontogenic tumor and/or dentinogenic ghost cell tumor. Synonyms are calcifying ghost cell odontogenic carcinoma, malignant epithelial odontogenic ghost cell tumor, carcinoma arising in a calcifying odontogenic tumor, malignant calcifying odontogenic cyst, malignant calcifying ghost cell odontogenic tumor and dentinogenic ghost cell ameloblastoma.

Clinical Features

The tumor is rare and it occurs more commonly in Asians than other races. There is a predilection for occurrence in the maxilla than mandible (2:1). The mean age of occurrence at the time of diagnosis is 37 years ranging from 13 to 73 years. Male-to-female ratio is 2.6:1. Common symptoms are swelling of jaws with paresthesia, displacement of roots and root resorption. Large lesions in the maxilla often destroy the sinus wall and involve nasal and orbital cavities and extend to adjacent structures. Biological behavior of the tumor is variable from slowly growing locally invasive tumor to highly aggressive rapidly growing tumor. It shows expansile multiloculated to poorly demarcated radiolucency with radiopaque material.

Histopathological Features

A malignant neoplasm generally characterized by two types of epithelial cells. The malignant component of some tumors is found in nests, strands, and islands of varying size dominated by small, round, undifferentiated basaloid cells with hyperchromatic nuclei, frequent mitoses, and cytologic atypia. Masses of ghost cells, some of which may show dystrophic calcification, often intermingle with small basaloid cells. Small deposits of dentinoid in close association with ghost cells may or may not be present. In some tumors, the epithelial component is formed predominantly by large cells with vesicular nuclei admixed with few cells showing squamous differentiation. Areas of necrosis with an acute and chronic inflammatory cell infiltrate are frequent findings. In addition to the malignant epithelial component, one may find a typical, simple unicystic type of calcifying odontogenic cyst. The cyst is lined by stratified epithelium that has a distinct basal cell layer of columnar cells overlaid by a loose, stellate reticulum-like epithelium of variable thickness. Foci of ghost cells are scattered within the epithelial lining. Nests of tumor cells invade and destroy the surrounding bone, skeletal muscle, and connective tissue. The stroma consists of a mature, fibrous connective tissue which may occasionally show desmoplasia.

Treatment

The treatment of the tumor is by initial radical surgery combined with radiation therapy. The biologic behavior of GCOC appears to be unpredictable. Some cases have been associated with long-term survival following definitive surgery. However, others show poor clinical outcomes with locally recurrent disease or metastases.

Box 6.16: Ghost cell odontogenic carcinoma

Key features helpful in diagnosis

- Ameloblastic carcinoma with ghost cell keratinization
- Presents as an expansile multiloculated to poorly demarcated radiolucency mixed with radiopaque material
- Variable biologic behavior.

AMELOBLASTIC FIBROSARCOMA

Ameloblastic fibrosarcoma (AFS) is an odontogenic tumor with a benign epithelial and a malignant ectomesenchymal component. It is regarded as the malignant counterpart of the ameloblastic fibroma.

Clinical Features

There is a wide age range (3–89 years) with a mean age of 27.5 years at diagnosis. Patients with AFS derived from a pre-existing AF have a mean age of 33 years. Sixty-three percent of reported cases have occurred in males and 37 percent in females. The mandible is the most commonly affected site (78%), followed by the maxilla (20%). In both jaws the posterior region is the site of predilection. Pain and swelling are the most common findings. Ulceration and bleeding, as well as paresthesia of the lower lip have also been reported. Involvement of cervical and submandibular lymph nodes in cases of AFS seems to be uncommon.

Radiological Features

Radiographically, radiolucency with irregular and indistinct margin is characteristic. Large radiolucencies with a multilocular appearance and gross expansion and thinning of the cortical bone may be seen. In cases where radio-opacities are observed within radiolucent areas, diagnosis of ameloblastic fibrodentinosarcoma or ameloblastic fibro-odontosarcoma is likely.

Histopathological Features

The histologic pattern of AFS resembles ameloblastic fibroma in which the epithelial tissue is benign but the connective tissue component is malignant. The malignant ectomesenchymal component consistently takes up more than 70 percent of the tumor area compared to 30 percent by odontogenic epithelium. The epithelium is composed of budding and branching cords of small polygonal epithelial cells admixed with islands and knots. Larger islands have peripheral columnar cells with hyperchromatic nuclei. The mesenchymal component of the neoplasms shows a marked increase in cellularity. A hypercellular connective tissue stroma displaying mitotically active cells surrounds the epithelial component. Recurrent tumors tend to show greater stromal cellularity and mitotic rate.

Treatment

Radical extensive surgery, usually partial or total mandibulectomy or maxillectomy is the treatment of choice. In some cases post surgical radiotherapy or adjuvant chemotherapy should be considered. Metastasis seems to be rare in AFSs. Out of 49 AFS cases, there was only one case with histologic documentation of metastasis to lymph nodes. Due to the fact that, metastasis is rare in AFS survival seems to be good.

AMELOBLASTIC FIBRODENTINOSARCOMA AND FIBRO-ODONTOSARCOMA

Ameloblastic fibrodentinosarcoma (AFDS) and fibro-odontosarcoma (AFOS) are exceedingly rare malignant odontogenic sarcomas. The WHO classification of 1992 differentiated between odontogenic sarcomas without dental hard tissues (ameloblastic fibrosarcomas) and those revealing evidence of dentinoid (ameloblastic fibrodentinosarcoma) or dentinoid plus enameloid fibro-odontosarcoma.

Clinical and Radiological Features

Pain and swelling are frequently associated with the lesions. Oral mucosal ulceration and or bleeding were usually related to occlusal trauma. Mobility of teeth and tissue proliferation through extraction sockets were noted in some cases. Radiographically, AFDS and AFOS have to be differentiated from ameloblastic fibrosarcoma by the presence of radiopaque foci in an otherwise radiolucent lesion.

Histopathological Features

Both AFDS and AFOS consist of epithelial and ectomesenchymal component, including dentinoid, some of which may be dysplastic. However AFOS shows enameloid in addition to dentinoid material. The epithelial component consists of follicles and strands of odontogenic epithelium as observed in ameloblastic fibromas. Intraepithelial and stromal microcysts may form. Some epithelial islands may show ghost cells representative of a presence of intracellular keratinization. The malignant ectomesenchymal component shows increased cellularity, pleomorphism, hyperchromatism and increased mitotic activity, as in ameloblastic fibrosarcomas.

Box 6.17: Ameloblastic fibrodentinosarcoma and fibro-odontosarcoma

Key features helpful in diagnosis
- Exceedingly rare
- Pain, swelling, ulceration, bleeding, mobility of teeth
- Radiographically, presence of radiopaque foci in an otherwise radiolucent lesion
- Histological picture resembles ameloblastic fibroma except the presence of cytological atypia.

Treatment

The treatment of choice for both AFDS and AFOS is radical surgery.

SELF-ASSESSMENT QUESTIONS

1. Give a classification for odontogenic tumors.
2. Discuss the behavior of the different types of ameloblastoma in relation to histopathology.
3. Comment on the statement "Odontome is a hamartoma".
4. Comment on the statement "Ameloblastic fibroma, ameloblastic fibro-odontoma and odontoma may be a spectrum of a same disease".
5. Explain the justification of odontogenic keratocyst being regarded as an odontogenic tumor.
6. Describe the clinicopathological findings of adenomatoid odontogenic tumor.
7. Discuss the differential diagnosis of a multilocular radiolucency at the angle of the mandible.
8. Describe the options available for the treatment of an ameloblastoma.
9. Write an account of odontogenic tumors with ghost cell differentiation.
10. What is the difference between malignant ameloblastoma and ameloblastic carcinoma?

SUGGESTED READING

1. Braunshtein E, Vered M, Taicher S, Buchner. A. Clear cell odontogenic carcinoma and clear cell ameloblastoma: a new case and comparative analysis of the literature. J Oral Maxillofac Surg. 2003;61(5):1004-10.
2. Chirapathomsakul D, Sastravaha P, Jansisyanont PA. Review of odontogenic keratocysts and the behavior of recurrences. Oral Surg Oral Med Oral Pathol Oral Radiol Endod. 2006;101:5-9.
3. Eversole LR, Duffey DC, Powell NB. Clear cell odontogenic carcinoma. A clinocpathologic analysis. Arch otolaryngol Head Neck Surg. 1995;121:685-9.
4. Ling Lin Y, Dean K White. Textbook of Odontogenic Tumors: Reichart squamous odontogenic tumor: Oral and Maxillofacial Surgery Clinics of North America. 2004;16: 355-7.
5. Marx, Stern. Oral and Maxillofacial Pathology: a Rationale for Diagnosis and Treatment Ilinos; Quintessence Publishing; 2003.
6. Okada H, Yamamoto H, Tilakaratne WM. Odontogenic Tumors in Sri Lanka: Analysis of 226. Cases J Oral Maxillofac Surg. 2007;65: 875-82.
7. Shear M. The aggressive nature of the odontogenic keratocyst: is it a benign cystic neoplasm? Part 1. Clinical and early experimental evidence of aggressive behavior. Oral Oncology. 2002;38:219-26.
8. Shear M. The aggressive nature of the odontogenic keratocyst: is it a benign cystic neoplasm? Part 2. Proliferation and genetic studies. Oral Oncology. 2002;38:323-31.
9. Siriwardena BS, Tennakoon TM, Tilakaratne WM. Relative frequency of odontogenic tumors in Sri Lanka: Analysis of 1677 cases. Pathol Res Pract. 2012;208(4):225-30.
10. Siriwardena BSMS, Tilakaratne WM, Rajapaksha. Clear cell odontogenic car-cinoma—a case report and review of literature. Int. J Oral Maxillofac Surg. 2004;33: 512-4.
11. Thosaporn W, Iamaroon A, Pongsiriwet S. A comparative study of epithelial cell proliferation between the odontogenic keratocyst, orthokeratinized odontogenic cyst, dentigerous cyst, and ameloblastoma. Oral Diseases. 2004;10:22-6.
12. World Health Organization Classification of Tumors Pathology and Genetics of Head and Neck Tumors Lyon; IARC Press; 2005.

Chapter 7

Fibrocemento-osseous Lesions and Related Conditions

WM Tilakaratne

Chapter Outline

INTRODUCTION

Fibrocemento-osseous lesions are a very diverse group of lesions of jaw bones. The disease categories vary from developmental, reactive, dysplastic to neoplastic processes. Characteristic features of all the diseases in this category is the replacement of bone by fibrous tissue and subsequent mineralization in this form of bone, cementum or just calcification. Many lesions contain an admixture of these hard tissue components. Further, there are controversies in relation to their classification, diagnosis, and management of these lesions. The definitive diagnosis should be reached with the correlation of clinical findings, histopathological features and radiological/ imaging analysis because of the histological similarities among the different lesions in the group. Diagnosis is important as treatment modalities are different for these conditions and more importantly some lesions in the group may not need any treatment once the diagnosis is established. It should be stressed that in the absence of clinical and radiological information a pathologist should only offer the diagnosis as consistent with a fibrocemento-osseous lesion for a given biopsy. The above approach avoids the possibility of inappropriate treatment for some of the lesions in the group.

CLASSIFICATION

Cemento-osseous Dysplasias

Nonhereditary

- Periapical cemental dysplasia
- Focal cemento-osseous dysplasia
- Florid cemento-osseous dysplasia.

Hereditary

Familial gigantiform cementoma.

Fibrocemento-osseous Neoplasms

- Conventional cemento-ossifying fibroma
- Juvenile aggressive cemento-ossifying fibroma.

Fibrous Dysplasia

- Monoostotic fibrous dysplasia
- Polyostotic fibrous dysplasia
- Polyostotic fibrous dysplasia with endocrinopathy (McCune-Albright syndrome)
- Polyostotic fibrous dysplasia with pigmentation (Jaffe-Lichtenstein syndrome)
- Craniofacial fibrous dysplasia.

CEMENTO-OSSEOUS DYSPLASIAS

Periapical Cemental Dysplasia (Periapical Cemento-osseous Dysplasia)

Periapical cemental dysplasia (PCD) is a reactive fibrocemento-osseous lesion described by Stafne in 1934. Since 1992, the WHO recognized this as a fibrocemento-osseous lesion. This entity was previously described under many different names such as fibrocementoma, periapical osteofibroma, local osteofibroma, periapical fibrous dysplasia, periapical cementifying dysplasia and multiple cementomas. Although aetiology of the condition is unknown, it appears to originate from elements of the periodontal ligament. It is considered as a reactive process.

Clinical and Radiological Features

The clinical features of PCD are well-established and remarkably constant. There is a marked predilection for females (14:1) and blacks. The lesions are most often detected in patients over the age of 30 and are rare before the age of 20. The most common presentation is a middle age female with multiple periapical radiolucencies in relation to lower anterior teeth. The affected teeth are vital. A single tooth may be affected but multiple lesions are often the norm. The affected teeth are invariably asymptomatic.

Initial presentation of PCD is usually a circumscribed radiolucency in relation to the periapical region. With time it shows increasing amounts of calcification resulting in a progressive pattern that successively evolves from radiolucent to mixed density, to radiopaque (**Figs 7.1A and B**). The mature lesions show a radiopaque lesion with a radiolucent rim at the periphery. Rarely in some

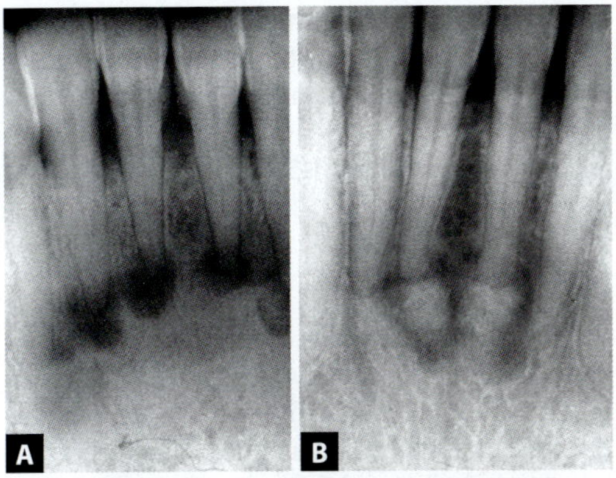

Figs 7.1A and B: Periapical cemental dysplasia. Multiple radiolucencies in the periapical area of lower anterior teeth. Mature lesions are more radiopaque (*Courtesy:* Professor Jos Hille)

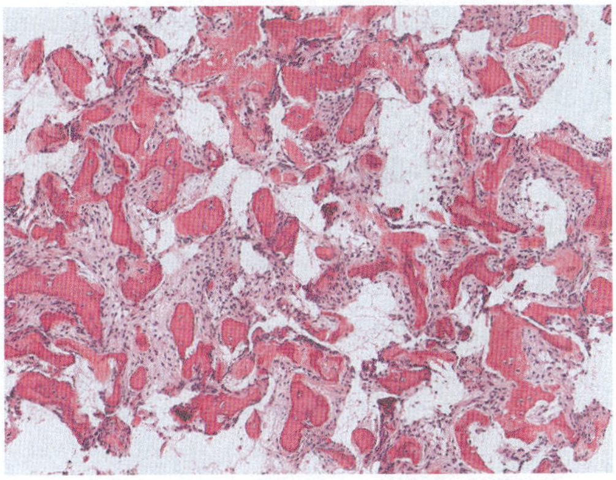

Fig. 7.2: Periapical cemental dysplasia. Thin irregular trabeculae of bone and cementum-like areas in a loosely arranged fibrous stroma

lesions, calcification is not always predictable and in fact they regress, some stay unchanged and some resolve. The size of the lesion usually does not exceed 0.5 cm. However, rare lesions may reach a diameter of 1.0 to 1.5 cm. Depending on the age of the lesion they can be divided in to three phases and histopathological features of these stages are correlated with the radiological findings. The early stage is the radiolucent phase or the osteolytic stage, followed by mixed radiodense lesion and finally the radiopaque stage representing a mature lesion.

Histopathological Features

Histopathological features are not pathognomonic for PCD as other reactive dysplasias share similar features. However, three radiological stages are correlated with histopathology. Stage 1 or the osteolytic stage shows cellular fibrous tissue containing frequent small blood vessels. The lesion is usually unencapsulated and hard tissue formation is not evident. When it matures into a lesion with a mixed radiodensity, evidence of hard tissue formation begins to appear, ranging from dysplastic bone, trabeculae of woven bone and foci of cementum-like tissue (**Fig. 7.2**). Finally, the bulk of the lesion is replaced by hard tissue with less fibrous and vascular tissue components and the lesion becomes radiopaque.

Differential Diagnosis

When a patient presents with classical clinical and radiological features, the clinician may not have any difficulty in arriving at the diagnosis, even without histopathological features unlike other reactive/dysplastic cemento-osseous dysplasias. If the lesion is a single lesion it may mimic the appearances of various other lesions depending on the stage. Periapical granuloma is the nearest differential diagnosis at the radiolucent stage. The affected tooth in PCD is usually vital, unlike in the case of periapical granuloma. Mature lesions and lesions with mixed radiodensity should be differentiated from entities such as condensing osteitis and focal sclerosing osteomyelitis. As rare cases may grow up to 1.5 cm in size and when present as a single lesion, differential diagnosis should include odontogenic tumors with hard tissue formation. Histologically most of the diseases in fibrocemento-osseous lesions have similar histology. However, focal cemento-osseous dysplasia (FCOD) and florid cemento-osseous dysplasia are the nearest differential diagnosis. FCOD is strikingly vascular compared to two other cemental dysplasias.

Treatment and Prognosis

Periapical cemental dysplasia (PCD) is a self-limiting condition and very rarely enlarges to a clinically palpable lesion. Exceptionally rare cases have been reported to have paresthesia or anaesthesia due to impinging on the mental nerve. Practically treatment is not indicated except taking follow-up radiographs in 6 to 12 months intervals.

Box 7.1: Periapical cemental dysplasia

Key features helpful in diagnosis

- Predilection for middle-aged black females
- One or more (0.5 cm or less) circumscribed lesions in periapical areas of vital lower anterior teeth. Painless and accidental findings in radiographs
- Radiographic appearances may vary from radiolucent, mixed density to radiopaque
- Histologically, cellular fibrous tissue with woven bone, cementum-like areas and calcifications.

Focal Cemento-osseous Dysplasia

Focal cemento-osseous dysplasia (FCOD) often presents as an asymptomatic, focal and circumscribed lesion in tooth bearing areas. FCOD may represent the most common fibrocemento-osseous lesion of jaw bones. This lesion has previously been described by various names such as osseous dysplasia, reaction of bone to injury and localized fibro-osseous cemental lesion. The present name of FCOD was introduced by Tormich and Summerlin in 1989. It is known that some of these lesions have been diagnozed as cemento-ossifying fibroma in the past leading to over treatment, especially if the lesion is diagnosed without adequate clinical and radiological details.

Clinical and Radiological Features

Focal cemento-osseous dysplasia (FCOD) shows a high female predilection of 8:1. The condition predominantly occurs in the 4th and 5th decades with an average age of 38. Because of the fact that the lesion is painless and non-expansile, it is usually discovered during routine radiographic examination. Seventy percent of the cases occur in the tooth-bearing areas, especially in the posterior mandible, although many occur in edentulous areas where a tooth was previously extracted.

Radiographically, they are usually well circumscribed with or without a sclerotic border and may be radiolucent, mixed radiodense or radiopaque in appearance (**Fig. 7.3**). Most lesions are less than 1.5 cm in diameter and rarely exceed 2.0 cm.

Histopathological Features

Focal cemento-osseous dysplasia (FCOD) is comprised of connective tissue stroma containing loose collagen fibers with sinusoidal-like vascular spaces adjacent to thick irregular bony trabeculae and irregular shaped cementoid calcifications (**Fig. 7.4**). Free hemorrhage

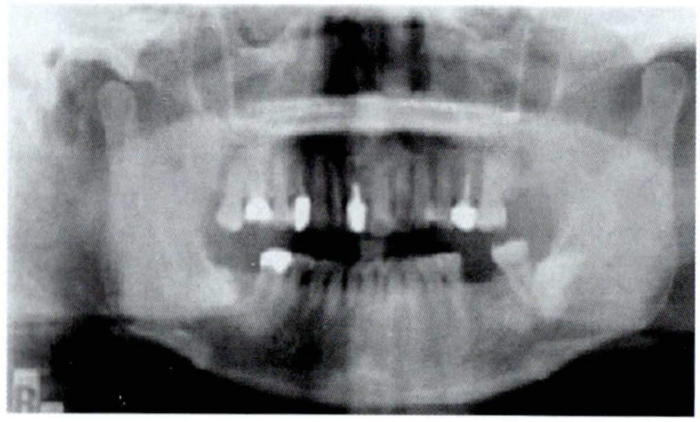

Fig. 7.3: Focal cemento-osseous dysplasia. Late stage of FCOD in the edentulous left lower molar area showing radiopaque lesion (*Courtesy:* Dr RD Jayasinghe)

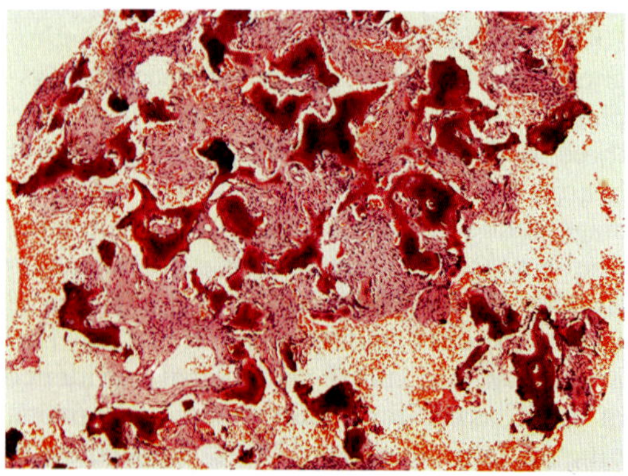

Fig. 7.4: Focal cemento-osseous dysplasia. Thin irregular bony-trabeculae and cementum-like tissue arranged in between cellular fibrous-tissue. The lesion is significantly vascular

is interspersed throughout the lesion. Increased vascularity in the lesion is obvious as macroscopic features also show brown hemorrhagic fragments. Presence of simple bone cysts is a feature in some cases.

Differential Diagnosis

The main clinical, radiographic, and microscopic differential diagnosis of FCOD appears to be cemento-ossifying fibroma (COF). Although PCD shows similar features to FCOD in occasional cases, proper clinicopathological correlation allows the clinician to come to a definitive diagnosis. The differentiation between FCOD and COF is important as the two lesions are totally different in terms of pathogenesis and behavior. Both lesions are more common in the posterior mandible although a significant number of COFs occur in the maxilla. Both tend to be circumscribed and can be radiolucent, mixed radiodense, or radiopaque. Displacement, root resorption, cortical expansion and characteristically expansion of the inferior border of the mandible may present in COF unlike in FCOD. A notable difference between the two lesions is the intraoperative findings. Ossifying fibroma tends to shell out as a solid mass, whereas FCOD is adherent to surrounding bone, and as a result, is removed in gritty, hemorrhagic tissue fragments. In FCOD, lesional tissue tends to blend with the cortex and medullary bone in contrast to the encapsulation evident in COF. As mentioned previously, FCOD is composed of loose collagen fibers with sinusoidal-like vascularity adjacent to thick irregular bony trabeculae and uneven cementoid calcifications whereas COF shows a hypovascular, uniformly cellular, often storiform stroma with intermixed dense collagen. The calcified components are often thin, separate, bony trabeculae with osteoblastic rimming and calcifications/cementum-like areas. The definitive diagnosis should be reached with clinico-pathological correlation.

Treatment and Prognosis

Focal cemento-osseous dysplasia (FCOD) does not need treatment once the diagnosis is established. The lesions typically persist without remarkable change and sometimes regress. However, occasional cases have subsequently developed into florid cemento-osseous dysplasia (FLCOD). Progression from a solitary to multiple site involvement supports the theory of FCOD as being part of a spectrum of a single disease process.

Box 7.2: Focal cemento-osseous dysplasia

Key features helpful in diagnosis

- Painless, nonexpansile, usual location is posterior part of the mandible
- Most often presents as a circumscribed radiolucency with opacities, less than 1.5 cm in diameter
- Difficult to remove surgically, resulting in small hemorrhagic gritty fragments in the biopsy
- Thick curvilinear trabeculae of woven and/or lamellar bone and/or oval calcifications in a more loosely arranged fibrous stroma than in cemento-ossifying fibroma
- Sinusoid-like vascular spaces adjacent to bony trabeculae and free hemorrhage.

Florid Cemento-osseous Dysplasia

Florid cemento-osseous dysplasia (FLCOD) presents as multiple masses of cemento-osseous tissue in tooth bearing areas of jaw bones, frequently affecting the posterior regions. FLCOD has been recognized under many names including multiple enostosis, chronic diffuse sclerosing osteomyelitis/osteitis, gigantiform cementoma and sclerotic cemental masses. The current term florid cemento-osseous dysplasia was introduced by Melrose et al in 1976.

Clinical and Radiological Features

Florid cemento-osseous dysplasia commonly occurs in middle age females. The majority of the patients are in the fourth and fifth decades with a mean age of 42 years. It shows bilateral symmetrical involvement in most cases. However, it is not unusual to find cases with extensive involvement of all four posterior quadrants of jaws. Many patients are partially or totally edentulous when the condition is first discovered. Until the lesions expand to a noticeable size, the diagnosis may be an accidental finding in radiographs.

Radiographically, it shows all the phases described previously under PCD. Lesions start as variably well demarcated and corticated radiolucencies with patchy sclerosis developing within them with time. In mature lesions the margin is diffuse and poorly defined. The most common radiographic presentation is multiple confluent sclerotic lobular masses admixed with less well-defined areas of a mixed radiodense pattern in different sites (**Figs 7.5A and B**). Well-defined radiolucent areas representing simple bone cysts are a frequent finding. The above feature is usually seen in mature lesions with the bulk of the lesion showing radiopaque areas. Cortical expansion may be a feature when simple bone cysts become larger. In rare cases, radiopaque lesions may mimic the appearances of Paget's disease. It is not uncommon to observe fusion of lesional tissue with roots of adjacent teeth.

Histopathological Features

Histopathological features described are invariably in cases of late stage as the lesions are not diagnosed until they grow into a reasonable size. Most of the biopsy specimens of FLCOD show benign fibro-osseous tissue containing bone which ranges from woven bone to densely sclerotic lamellar bone and large areas of cementum-like calcifications (**Figs 7.6A and B**). They contain prominent pagetoid reversal and resting lines. Marrow spaces are also replaced by lesional tissue. When a lesion progresses into the final radiopaque stage, individual trabeculae fuse and form lobular masses of mostly acellular cemento-osseous material. Inflammatory cells are absent unless there is secondary infection. Solitary bone cyst formation is more frequent in FLCOD than in other types of cemento-osseous dysplasias.

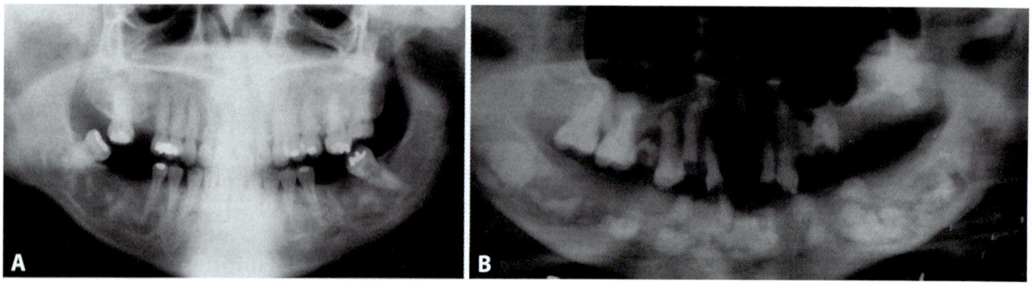

Figs 7.5A and B: (A) Early lesions showing multiple radiolucencies and scattered radiopacities within; (B) An advanced case with numerous radiopaque lesions (*Courtesy:* Professor Jos Hille)

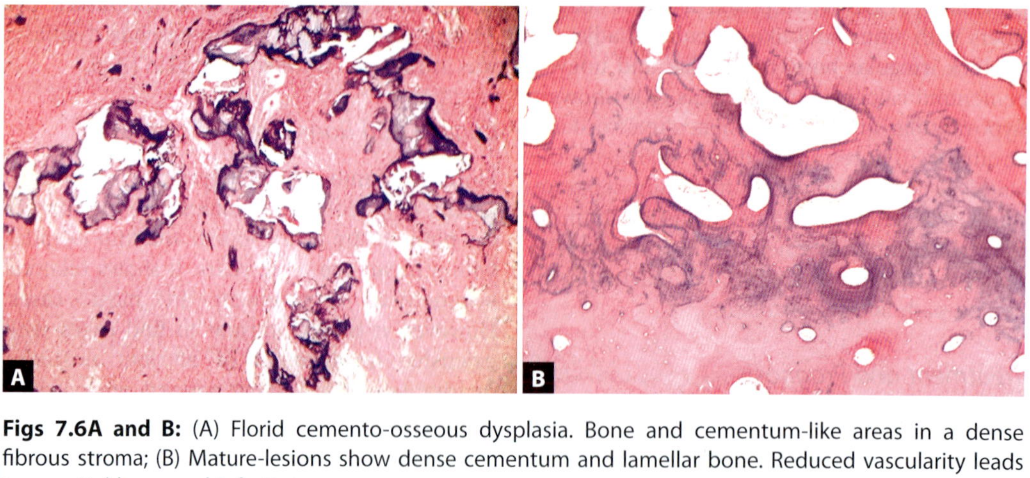

Figs 7.6A and B: (A) Florid cemento-osseous dysplasia. Bone and cementum-like areas in a dense fibrous stroma; (B) Mature-lesions show dense cementum and lamellar bone. Reduced vascularity leads to nonvital bone and infection

Differential Diagnosis

Differential diagnosis is a challenge only in focal forms of fibrocemento-osseous dysplasias as the clinical and radiological features are distinct in the florid form. However, mature lesions may mimic the appearances of Paget's disease radiographically. Serum alkaline phosphatise is markedly raised in Paget's and it is very unusual for the disease to be restricted only to jaw bones. FLCOD and chronic diffuse sclerosing osteomyelitis (CDSO) are frequently confused with each other partly because of the terms that have been used synonymously for both in the past. CDSO is a primary inflammatory/ infective condition in the mandible mostly in patients with chronic periodontal disease. It is characterized by repeated episodes of mild swelling and pain. Histological features may mimic the appearances of FLCOD with secondary infection. It is unusual to find the classic multiple site and at times symmetrical involvement seen in FLCOD.

Treatment and Prognosis

Treatment is usually not indicated unless infection supervenes leading to osteomyelitis. Therefore, asymptomatic patients should be kept under regular follow-up and clear instructions should be given to prevent secondary infection. This includes good oral hygiene measures in order to prevent periodontal disease and tooth loss. Further, in asymptomatic patients, surgical intervention for diagnostic purposes is not recommended as altered osseous tissue is very susceptible to infection. Management of the symptomatic patient is more problematic mainly due to the nature of hard tissue which has less blood supply and may be surrounded by dead bone. Symptoms usually appear due to extraction of teeth, biopsy procedures and exposure of sclerotic masses as a result of continuous alveolar atrophy under a denture. It is evident that even antibiotics and/or surgical excision of the sclerotic bone are not always successful in controlling the complications of infection. However, removal of dead bone and antibiotic treatment may enhance healing. When simple bone cysts arise within the lesion biopsy is indicated for the diagnosis, and removal of the cyst and curettage of the surrounding area assist in healing.

Box 7.3: Florid cemento-osseous dysplasia

Key features helpful in diagnosis

- Predilection for middle-aged black females
- Involvement of two or more jaw quadrants
- Radiographic features are multiple confluent lobular sclerotic masses in tooth-bearing areas
- Initially, proliferation of cellular fibrous tissue with trabeculae of woven bone and oval calcifications
- Late-stage lesions show acellular, avascular and sclerotic bony masses
- Superimposed infection lead to osteomyelitis.

Familial Gigantiform Cementoma (Familial Florid Cemento-osseous Dysplasia)

This is a rare hereditary condition with radiographic and histological features almost identical to FLCOD. In some cases these may grow at an alarmingly high rate causing visible jaw deformity and various abnormalities of teeth eruption including impaction, malposition and malocclusion.

Clinical features, diagnosis, differential diagnosis and treatment are very similar to that of FLCOD except the few differences highlighted in the key features helpful in diagnosis. Surgical reduction is indicated in cases growing fast leading to disfigurement.

Box 7.4: Familial gigantiform cementoma

Key features helpful in diagnosis

- Autosomal dominant inheritance with variable expressivity
- Multiple quadrant involvement of radiopaque lesions similar to FLCOD
- Absence of gender and racial predilection
- Onset at a younger age compared to other cemento-osseous dysplasias
- Histopathological features are identical to FLCOD.

FIBROUS DYSPLASIA

Historically, fibrous dysplasia (FD) is identified as a developmental and tumor-like fibrocemento-osseous lesion of unknown etiology, characterised by replacement of normal bone by proliferating cellular fibrous tissue with subsequent mineralization. FD is subdivided into monostotic FD, polyostotic FD, craniofacial FD and FD with associated syndromes such as polyostotic FD with endocrinopathy (McCune-Albright syndrome) and polyostotic FD with pigmentation (Jaffe-Lichtenstein syndrome). Recently, etiology of FD took a new turn when Cohen and Howell described that somatic mutation in the *GNAS 1* (guanine nucleotide-binding protein, α stimulating activity polypeptide 1) gene causing different types of FD depending on the time of mutation. The mutation appears to be a sporadic postzygotic mutation. When mutation occurs in an undifferentiated stem cell in early embryonic life that mutation express in osteoblasts, melanocytes and endocrine cells causing polyostotic FD with pigmentation and endocrinopathy or McCune-Albright syndrome. If the mutation takes place at a later stage after migration and differentiation of skeletal progenitor cells, FD appears in multiple bones causing polyostotic FD. When mutation takes place postnatally, mutated cells are restricted to a single site and the resultant FD appears in one bone, referred to as monostotic FD.

Box 7.5: Fibrous dysplasia

Key features helpful in diagnosis

- Onset is usually in the 1st and 2nd decades, slowly growing painless swelling.
- Commonly in the maxilla with some involvement of adjacent bones.
- Radiographically it shows ground-glass appearance with ill defined borders.
- Trabeculae of woven bone with minimal or occasional osteoblastic rimming in a background of cellular fibrous stroma blending into surrounding bone.
- Mature lesions show woven or rarely lamellar bone formation parallel to each other.

Monostotic Fibrous Dysplasia and Craniofacial Fibrous Dysplasia

The monostotic form accounts for 80 to 85 percent of cases of FD. Although the term "monostotic" can be readily applied to cases of FD affecting the mandible alone (**Fig. 7.7A**), this is generally not so for FD affecting the maxilla or other facial bones. When the maxilla is affected, disease process can extend into zygoma, sphenoid and palatine bone, etc (**Fig. 7.7B**). Therefore, the term craniofacial dysplasia is preferred for such cases (**Fig. 7.8B**). Common patterns of contiguous involvement include maxilla-zygoma sphenoid-frontal-

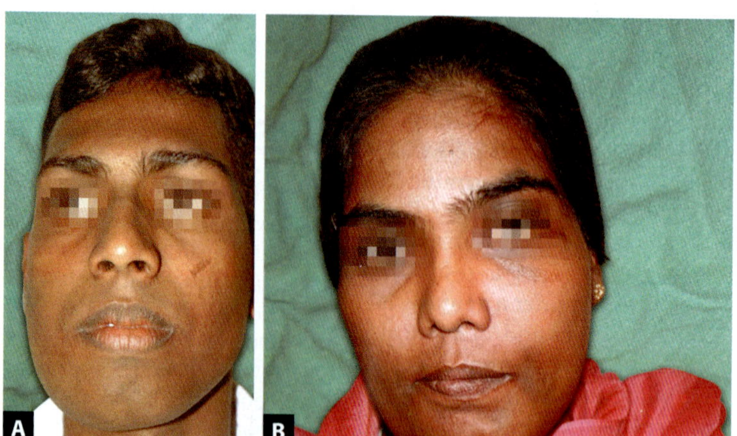

Figs 7.7A and B: Fibrous dysplasia. (A) Young male patient with both maxillary and mandibular expansion; (B) In a female showing involvement of maxilla and zygoma (*Courtesy:* Dr T Sabesan)

nasal bones and frontal-sphenoid-temporal-zygoma bones. Although multiple bones are affected the lesional distribution is restricted to contiguous bones within a defined anatomical area which is not a typical feature in polyostotic form of the disease. Therefore, it is justifiable to use the term craniofacial FD for lesions of this nature. Clinically, craniofacial FD presents as a painless enlargement of the affected bone, most often during the first and second decades of life. Maxilla affects much more frequently than the mandible when craniofacial FD occurs in the jaws and the maxillary sinus is commonly involved. There is no significant gender predilection. Lesion usually presents as a painless slow growing bony lump. Occasional cases may show rapid growth. Early lesions are radiolucent, although with time typically the lesion starts to show ground-glass appearance (**Fig. 7.8A**) with indistinct borders that blend into the surrounding uninvolved bone. Mandibular lesions often present with bucco-lingual expansion and involvement of the lower border. Inferior dental canal may displace superiorly. Narrowing of periodontal spaces may be a feature in some cases. Maxillary lesions usually cause obliteration of the sinus and/or displacement of the sinus floor superiorly. Increase density of bones of the skull base has also been described in craniofacial FD (**Fig. 7.8B**).

Polyostotic Fibrous Dysplasia; Polyostotic Fibrous Dysplasia with Endocrinopathy (McCune-Albright Syndrome); Polyostotic Fibrous Dysplasia with Pigmentation (Jaffe-Lichtenstein Syndrome)

Polyostotic FD is characterized by the involvement of multiple bones. The disease starts earlier than the monostotic form. Most cases start to show features in the first decade of life. Although the skull bones, including mandible and maxilla may be involved in polyostotic form, the features are dominated by the involvement of long bones. Pathological fractures of affected long bones have been described as a frequent finding unlike in jaw bones.

Clinical and Radiological Features

The majority of polyostotic and syndromic forms are easily diagnosed on clinical and radiological investigations alone. Three percent of the polyostotic form has endocrinopathies, precocious puberty and *Café-au-lait* type pigmentation. The above combination is defined as McCune-Albright syndrome. *Café-au-lait* spots are prominent macules on the trunk and thighs with markedly irregular

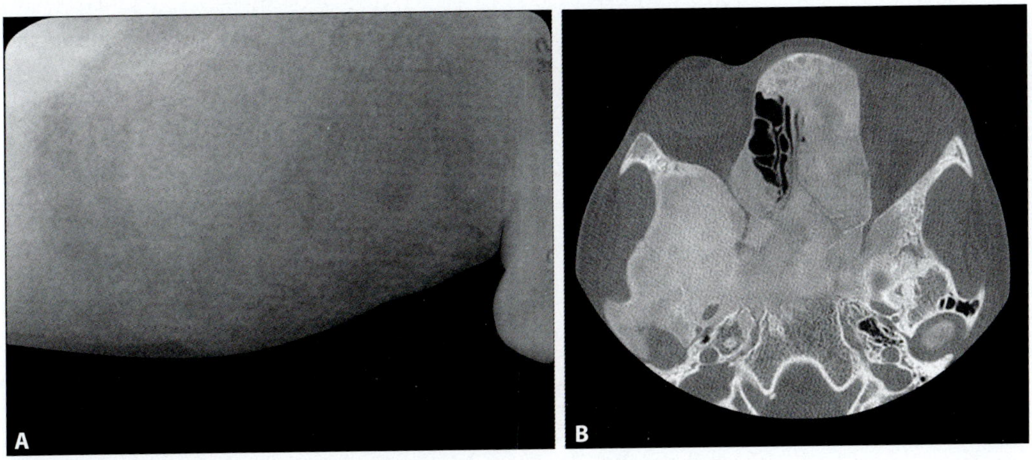

Figs 7.8A and B: Fibrous dysplasia. (A) Characteristic "ground glass" appearance in a periapical radiograph; (B) CT shows involvement of multiple cranial bones in a case of craniofacial fibrous dysplasia (*Courtesy:* Dr RD Jayasinghe and Dr Jimmy Makdissi)

borders. Sexual precocity is the most common endocrine manifestation in syndromic patients and menstruation and other secondary sexual characteristics appear in the first year of life. Jaffe-Lichtenstein syndrome is a combination of skin pigmentation with polyostotic FD without endocrine abnormalities.

Radiological examination reveals a marked variation in the number of bones involved, ranging from a few, to 75 percent of the skeleton, in rare cases. The margins of extragnathic FD appear well defined compared to jaw lesions which are mostly poorly-defined. Radiological features change with the maturation of the lesion similar to other fibrocemento-osseous lesions. Early lesions may be radiolucent with gradual transition to ground glass appearance and mature lesions are mostly radiopaque.

Histopathological Features

Histopathological features vary with the age of the lesion similar to radiological features. Hematoxylin and eosin sections show mostly loose fibrous tissue and the arrangement may vary from lesion-to-lesion, or at times within the lesion, ranging from whorled, fascicular or random configuration. Mitotic activity in fibroblasts is a rare event although it may be observed in rapidly growing lesions. Hard tissue formation starts to appear with the continuation of the disease process and the irregular trabeculae of mostly woven bone without a prominent osteoblastic rim is characteristic. Rimming may be evident focally in some cases. Bony trabeculae do not join each other especially in early lesions giving the characteristic appearance (**Fig. 7.9A**). Although different sites share similar histopathological features, jaw lesions may have some differences. Features such as marked ossification, lamellar maturation, very variable size and shape of bony trabeculae, cementum-like mineralization can lead to a broad differential diagnosis with other cemento-osseous conditions of jaw bones. In older lesions with lamellar maturation, together with reversal and resting lines, is indicative of normal bone turn over. Mature lesions after many years show parallel arrangement of bony trabeculae which can be either woven or more often lamellar bone (**Fig. 7.9B**). Cystic degeneration appears to be a rare event in jaw lesions of FD.

Differential Diagnosis

Diagnosis of FD is usually by clinicopathological correlation as it can be confused with other cemento-osseous lesions as well as lesions forming reactive-bone. The latter consists of periosteal reactions in osteomyelitis, lesions of hyperparathyroidism, giant cell granuloma and low grade osteosarcoma. The above problem is common when the biopsy is taken from

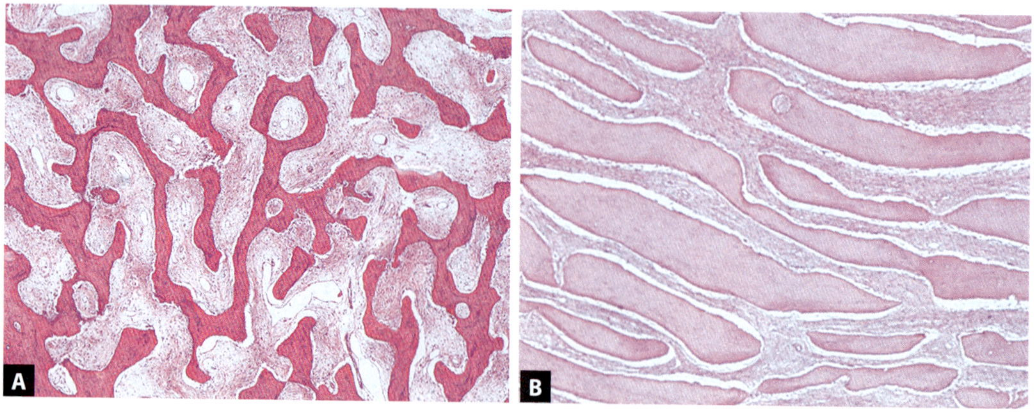

Figs 7.9A and B: Fibrous dysplasia. (A) Irregular bony trabeculae in a fibrocellular stroma is characteristic in early lesions; (B) A mature lesion shows prominent parallel arrangement of bone with lamellar differentiation

the periphery of a slow growing lesion. It is important to remember that cortical expansion due to periosteal reaction is very common in children and adolescents due to low grade chronic osteomyelitis of dental origin. Therefore, diagnosis of such cases with a superficial biopsy should be avoided. The most difficult practical differential diagnosis histologically would be FD and other cemento-osseous lesions. These have been discussed under different entities. It should be emphasised that the importance of clinical and radiological features aid the interpretation of histopathology to arrive at the definitive diagnosis. Differentiation of cemento-ossifying fibroma (COF) from FD is very necessary as the two disease entities should be treated differently, as the former is a neoplastic process. If the biopsy is taken with the intact capsule of COF, differentiating it from FD is straightforward. However, if the biopsy is from the central part of the lesion it may show similar features. Looking for features such as osteoblastic rimming in COF and blending of lesional tissue with surrounding normal bone in FD may be helpful, in addition to radiological features and clinical features. Though rare, intramedullary and parosteal osteosarcoma, with the help of cytological features, should be differentiated from FD.

Treatment and Prognosis

Management of FD is a clinical challenge to surgeons, at least in some cases. Single mandibular lesions may be surgically resected without much of a problem. More complex maxillary lesions, especially true craniofacial FD can pose significant problems in management and patients may need several surgeries at different stages. Regrowth can be expected in 25 to 50 percent of the cases following contouring procedures. Although growth of most lesions stops when skeletal maturation is reached, some cases show late reactivation. Medical treatment for FD has been tried by some centers with variable results. Bisphosphonates appear to work well for children rather than for adult patients as osteonecrosis is a common complication of the drug in adults. It has been reported that bisphosphonates reduce bone pain and bone turn over in these patients.

Although rare, sarcomas can arise in craniofacial FD, usually osteosarcoma or fibrosarcoma. Most have occurred in patients who had received radiation therapy. The above treatment option is contraindicated for FD because of the known risk. A few examples have been reported in the literature of spontaneous malignant transformation.

CEMENTO-OSSIFYING FIBROMA

Cemento-ossifying fibroma (COF) is the true neoplastic disease in the category of fibrocemento-osseous lesions. This is classified under bone related lesions in the WHO classification of odontogenic tumors in 2005 together with fibrous dysplasia and osseous dysplasias. COF is defined as a well demarcated lesion composed of fibrocellular tissue and mineralized tissue of varying appearances. In addition to the conventional type of COF, WHO recognizes juvenile COF as a separate entity presenting in two different ways, namely juvenile trabecular ossifying fibroma (JTOF) and juvenile psammomatoid ossifying fibroma (JPOF).

Conventional Cemento-ossifying Fibroma

Ossifying fibroma and cementifying fibroma are now considered to be one and the same lesion. Both these lesions frequently contain bone and cementum-like tissue. Techniques which have been used to differentiate bone and cementum in these lesions yielded inconclusive results. It is accepted that most pathologists find it difficult to differentiate bone and cementum when it is not fully formed by conventional histopathological methods. Therefore, the term cemento-ossifying fibroma is accepted as the appropriate term.

Clinical and Radiological Features

Cemento-ossifying fibroma (COF) commonly occurs in young to middle aged adults. The majority of the patients are in third and fourth decades. There is a striking female predilection. The most common site of involvement is the posterior mandible accounting for 80 percent of the cases. The maxillary posterior region appears to be the next most common site. Usual presentation is a slowly growing, painless and expansile bony hard lump (**Fig. 7.10**). Although the majority of COFs are a few centimeters in diameter, cases have been reported expanding more than 10 centimeters under the label of giant COF. The tumors usually do not perforate the cortex.

Radiologically, COF is a well demarcated round or oval, mostly unilocular lesion (**Figs 7.11A and B**) with extremely rare cases showing multilocularity. The features depend on the age of the lesion similar to other fibrocemento-osseous lesions. Early lesions are radiolucent. When hard tissue formation begins the tumor tends to show mixed radio density. However, towards the later stages the whole lesion may appear radiopaque. Adjacent teeth may be displaced and resorption of roots is seen in some examples.

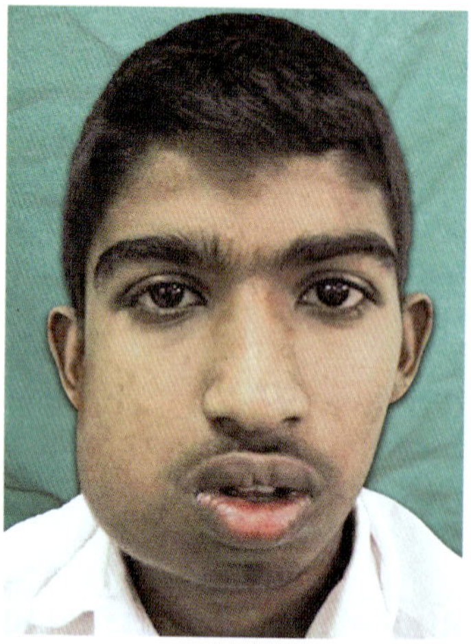

Fig. 7.10: Cemento-ossifying fibroma presenting as a bony hard swelling in the posterior body of the mandible in a young adult

Histopathological Features

A well demarcated margin is identifiable at the edges of the excision (**Fig. 7.12A**). The lesional tissue ranges from fibrocellular tissue to densely sclerotic tissue. The majority of COFs consist of dense fibrous connective tissue with varying degrees of cellularity. It is frequently hypercellular with numerous fibroblasts which have a storiform pattern, whorled pattern or rarely random arrangement. An occasional multinucleated giant cell may be seen. The stromal vascularity is not marked. The calcified components consist of thin separate trabeculae of woven bone that may be lined by osteoblasts (**Fig. 7.12B**). Lamellar bone can be present but is not a constant finding. Cementum-like deposits of cellular or acellular spherules may also be present, either alone, or in combination with the bony trabecular component. Both bony and cementum-like areas fuse into thick

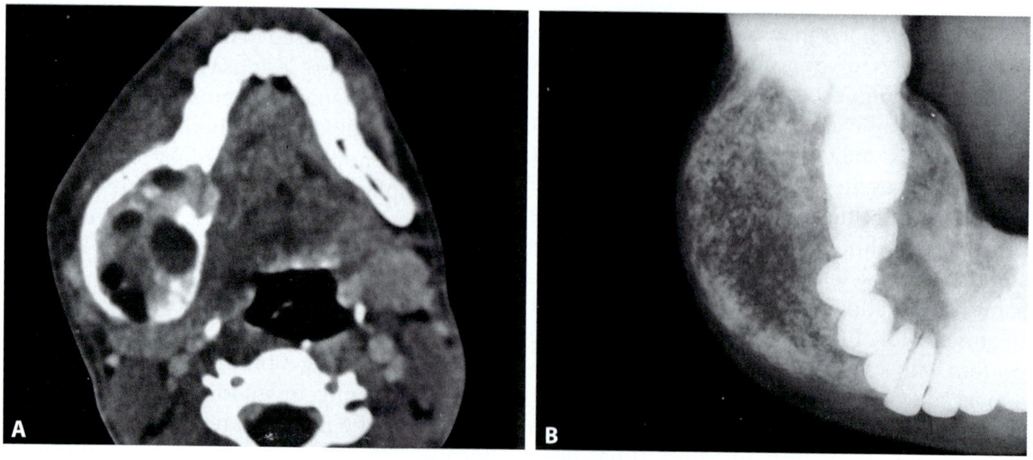

Figs 7.11A and B: Cemento-ossifying fibroma. (A) CT image showing a well circumscribed lesion in the body of the mandible; (B) Radiographic view of a COF with mixed radiodensity and displaced teeth

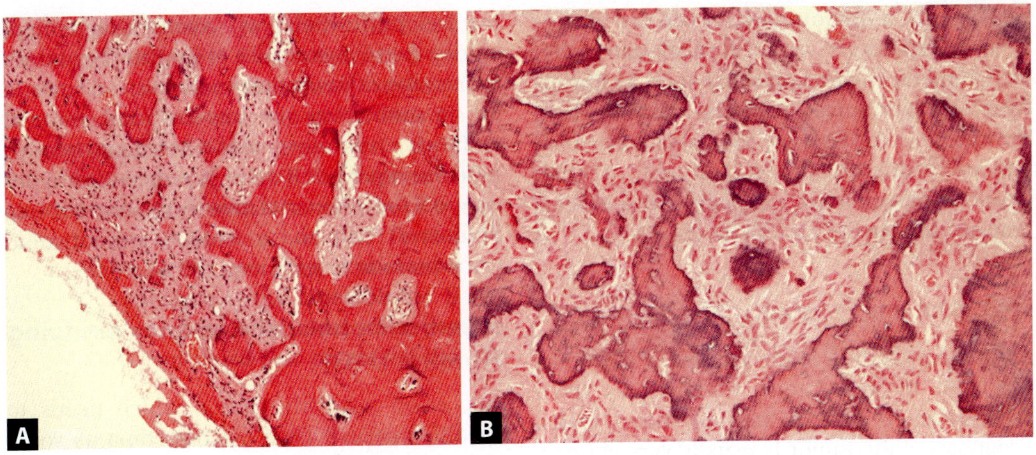

Figs 7.12A and B: Cemento-ossifying fibroma. (A) Capsule around the tumor help in differentiating COF from other lesions of the group; (B) Bone, cementum-like areas and calcifications in a fibrocellular stroma. Osteoblastic rimming is evident focally

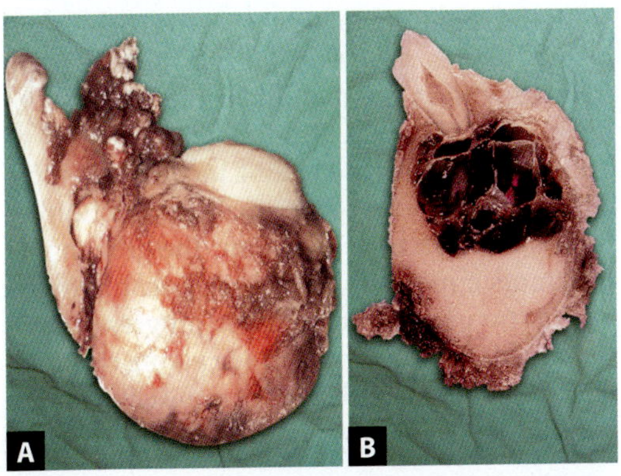

Figs 7.13A and B: Cemento-ossifying fibroma. (A) Macroscopic appearance of a COF; (B) Cystic changes within the tumor

bony islands in mature lesions. Sclerotic lesions are susceptible to osteomyelitis. Large tumors may develop aneurysmal bone cysts within the lesion, but it is not a common feature unlike in some other fibrocemento-osseous lesions (**Figs 7.13A and B**).

Differential Diagnosis

Although differentiation of this lesion from other lesions should be achieved with the clinicopathological correlation similar to other fibrocemento-osseous conditions, histological and radiological demonstration of encapsulation or at least good demarcation lead to the diagnosis of COF. Radiological differential diagnosis of COF includes demarcated lesions with mixed radiodensity such as focal cemento-osseous dysplasia, calcifying epithelial odontogenic tumor, adenomatoid odontogenic tumor, ameloblastic fibro-odontoma and complex odontoma, etc. However, early tumors which are radiolucent may mimic various other tumors which present as unilocular radiolucencies.

Radiologically, it is not difficult to differentiate COF from other cemento-osseous lesions as most of the conditions of the latter do not have demarcated margins.

Histopathological differential diagnosis is more challenging as the features of COF are identical to some other fibrocemento-osseous lesions. The histopathological distinction of FCOD and COF is quite difficult, if not impossible. Because of the histopathological overlap between these two lesions, large number of FCODs has been misdiagnosed as COF, when the diagnosis is arrived without proper clinicopathological correlation. Macroscopic features in the biopsy are sometimes helpful as FCOD is usually received as multiple haemorrhagic fragments. The above differentiation is mandatory as two entities have completely different treatment options and more importantly the two lesions behave differently as well. Although other fibrocemento-osseous lesions such as fibrous dysplasia, periapical cemental dysplasia and florid cemento-osseous dysplasia have very similar histopathological features to COF, proper assessment of radiological and clinical features lead to the correct diagnosis.

Treatment and Prognosis

Simple enucleation is the treatment of choice for most tumors. Larger tumors may need reconstruction of the area by bone grafts. Prognosis of the tumor is usually very good as the tumor is significantly separated from the surrounding tissue. Therefore, recurrence is not a common event. Malignant transformation has not been reported.

Box 7.6: Conventional cemento-ossifying fibroma

Key features helpful in diagnosis

- Slow growing solitary lesion
- Majority in the mandible
- Radiographically, a well demarcated lesion with smooth, often sclerotic borders
- During surgery it "Shells out" from surrounding bone
- Cellular fibrous stroma, often with storiform pattern, cellularity varies depending on the age of the lesion
- Histologically, irregular bone trabeculae, some with osteoblastic rimming
- Cementum-like areas or globular calcifications may present.

Juvenile Aggressive Cemento-ossifying Fibroma

It is known that a subset of COFs which occur in young patients tend to have a different behavior. Many believe that these lesions are unique because of their reported tendency to occur in children and adolescents, complex histologic features, and purported tendency for locally aggressive growth. Controversy exists as not all juvenile types exhibit locally aggressive behavior and not all lesions reported in this group have the same histopathological features. Further, there is no general agreement among pathologists with regard to the proper terminology, histopathologic features, or criteria for separating these lesions from conventional ossifying fibromas. WHO recognizes two different types of COFs under aggressive types namely, juvenile trabecular cemento-ossifying fibroma (JTOF) and juvenile psammomatoid cemento-ossifying fibroma (JPOF).

Juvenile Trabecular Cemento-ossifying Fibroma (JTOF)

This is an aggressive lesion which needs to be differentiated from osteosarcoma as some histopathological features are suspicious of malignancy.

Clinical and Radiological Features

Age of presentation may vary from 2 to 25 years with the majority of cases being diagnosed before 15 years of age. Maxilla affects more frequently than the mandible. There is a slight male predominance. Symptoms are related to the site of involvement and include swelling, epistaxis, proptosis, exophthalmos, and diplopia. Pain is a rare presentation. The growth rate of tumors appears to have a relationship to the age of the patient. Some cases progress slowly but others, particularly those in young children, often grow very rapidly alarming the clinicians to suspect a malignancy (**Fig. 7.14**). Radiologically,

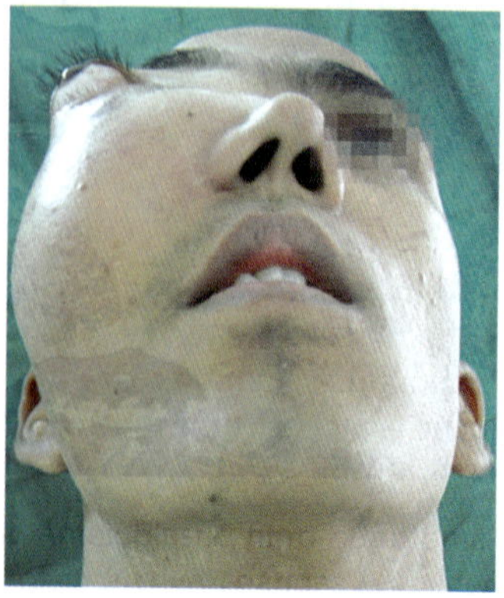

Fig. 7.14: Juvenile trabecular cemento-ossifying fibroma. Rapidly growing lesion of juvenile aggressive COF affecting the maxilla of a young patient (*Courtesy:* Dr Kumara Ekanayake)

a tumor shows a well-defined unilocular or rarely multilocular radiolucent lesion that may contain fine specks of radio-opacities.

Box 7.7: Juvenile trabecular cemento-ossifying fibroma

Key features helpful in diagnosis

- Mean age of occurrence is 12 years
- Either jaw is affected but with slight maxillary predominance
- Well demarcated radiographically; radiolucent with small opacities
- Highly cellular fibrous stroma with ribbons and strands of cellular osteoid with prominent osteoblastic rimming
- Remains with woven bone throughout
- Variable presence of myxoid areas with cystic degeneration.

Histopathological Features

Histologically lesions are uniform and show highly cellular fibrous stroma with ribbons and strands of cellular osteoid with numerous osteoblasts on their surface (**Fig. 7.15**). Osteoclasts may also be prominent in relation to osteoid. Irrespective of the age of the lesion lamellar differentiation of woven bone is not present. Precaution should be taken to differentiate this from osteosarcoma especially with narrow osteoid rims and mitoses are frequent. Focal areas show myxoid and cystic degeneration. Hemorrhage may be a feature in some tumors. Differential diagnosis from other fibrocemento-osseous lesions is not a challenge on the basis of the arrangement of strands of osteoid. Some lesions may resemble fibrous dysplasia but blending with adjacent tissue is not a feature of JTOF. Lesions with increased cellularity and mitoses should be differentiated from osteosarcoma.

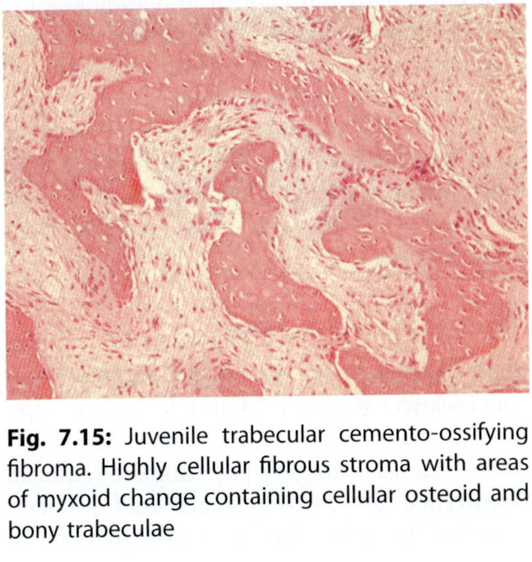

Fig. 7.15: Juvenile trabecular cemento-ossifying fibroma. Highly cellular fibrous stroma with areas of myxoid change containing cellular osteoid and bony trabeculae

Treatment and Prognosis

Excision of the lesion is the treatment of choice. These tumors have a tendency for local recurrence with reported rates ranging from 25 to 58 percent. However, radical surgery does not appear to be appropriate because recurrences may be managed by local excision. Although some lesions have a very aggressive course, malignant transformation has not been reported.

Juvenile Psammomatoid Cemento-Ossifying Fibroma (JPOF)

Juvenile psammomatoid cemento-ossifying fibroma is the other aggressive type of COF. This is a lesion which occurs predominantly in orbit and paranasal sinuses than jaw bones.

Clinical and Radiological Features

This is a progressively growing lesion. The age of occurrence ranges from 7 to 60 years. Facial asymmetry is usually present at the time of diagnosis. Other symptoms may include exophthalmos, bulbar displacement, proptosis, impaired vision, nasal obstruction, periorbital pain, headache, and sinusitis especially if orbit and sinuses are affected. Out of the two jaws, maxillary lesions are predominant and only 10 percent of the jaw tumors appears to be in the mandible. Males are affected twice as often as females.

Radiographically, most of the tumors are well demarcated and range from completely radiolucent to spotty mixed radiodensity. Mixed-density lesions with areas of definite loculations are typical in cases involving the cranial vault. Clouding or obliteration of the sinuses resembling sinusitis may be a feature in tumors affecting paranasal sinuses.

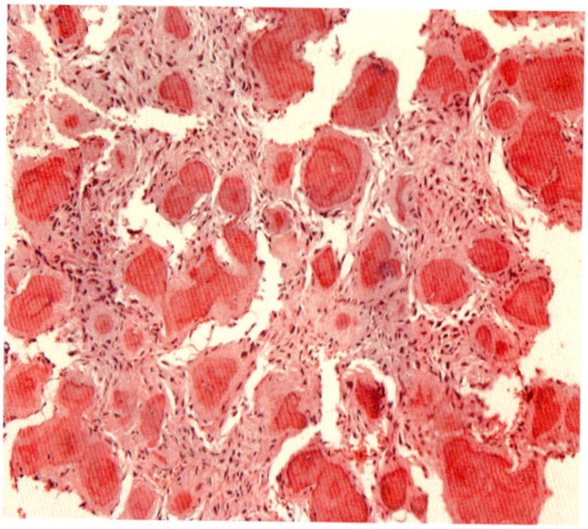

Fig. 7.16: Juvenile psammomatoid cemento-ossifying fibroma. Characteristic psammomatous type calcifications arranged in a richly cellular fibrous stroma

Histopathological Features

Microscopically, the tumor is characterized by a fibrovascular stroma containing small ossicles resembling psammoma bodies (**Fig. 7.16**). The number and size of calcified bodies increase with age. The above structures tend to contain reversal lines in mature lesions. Hypercellularity of the lesion is a prominent feature and whorled pattern is more evident in less mineralized lesions. Some lesions are predominantly myxoid with very less amount of fibrocemento-osseous tissue. These myxoid areas may undergo cystic change with edema, hemorrhage and clusters of multinucleated giant cells mimicking the appearance of an aneurysmal bone cyst. Mitotic figures may be seen, but are never prominent. Some lesions may be difficult to separate from conventional COF histologically. However, extremely cellular stroma with closely packed ossicles and myxoid areas with hemorrhage, multinucleated giant cells, and cystic degeneration are not typically seen in conventional COF.

Differential Diagnosis

Differentiation of COF from other fibrocemento-osseous lesions should be achieved with clinico-pathological correlation. FCOD appears to be the nearest differential diagnosis out of fibrocemento-osseous dysplasias. In the absence of proper clinical and radiological features, FCOD can be misdiagnosed as COF. As the former has been described recently, it is accepted that most of the lesions of FCOD have been misdiagnosed as COF in the past. At the time of the surgery, early lesions of FCOD can be very vascular and removed in pieces unlike COF that tends to shell out as a single mass. The size of the lesion and especially the histopathological features are also helpful in differentiating the two lesions. COF shows a capsule and separation from normal tissue. This feature helps to a greater extent in differentiating COF from fibrous dysplasia. Presence of osteoblastic rim around bony trabeculae is a feature in COF but usually absent in fibrous dysplasia.

Histopathologically, the dilemma of how to distinguish conventional COF from juvenile forms (JTOF and JPOF) still exists. Although, there are histopathological features present in aggressive forms, such as the extremely cellular stroma, spherical ossicles, and garlandlike strands of cellular osteoid, may be quite variable from one tumor to another, from field-to-field within the same tumor, and may even be observed focally in conventional COF. Moreover, the myxoid tissue, cystic degeneration, and aneurysmal bone cyst like areas characteristic of some juvenile forms may simply be reactive changes and may not be specific. Although the histopathological characteristics, when combined with the clinical and radiographic features, may sometimes be sufficient to permit distinction of juvenile forms from conventional COF, many cases lead to challenges in diagnosis. Sometimes the diagnosis of juvenile forms is more dependent on age, location, and behavior than histopathology. However, care should be taken to distinguish between JTOF from osteosarcoma.

Treatment and Prognosis

JPOF appears to be best managed by conservative excision although lesions that involve the orbit or cranial vault may need rather extensive surgery for complete removal. Recurrence rates of 20 to 56 percent have been reported. Patients who are under 10 years of age show much higher recurrences of up to 90 percent in some series. A second curettage appears to be curative in most cases. Multiple recurrences have been reported in patients less than 5 years of age.

Box 7.8: Juvenile psammomatoid cemento-ossifying fibroma

Key features helpful in diagnosis

- Majority of the cases occurs in childhood or adolescence, some cases may occur in adults
- Common sites to be involved are orbit and paranasal sinuses than jaws
- Well demarcated mixed density with loculated radiolucent areas or obliteration of sinus
- Variable cellularity often with whorled pattern containing closely packed calcified bodies resembling psammoma bodies
- Definite myxoid component is evident in most cases.

RELATED CONDITIONS

Cherubism

Cherubism is an autosomal dominant disease with a high degree of penetrance and variable expressivity. There is almost 100 percent penetrance in males and 70 percent in females. The disease produces a characteristic facial profile with painless symmetrical expansion of the mandible. The name cherubism is related to the similar appearance of affected individuals to little angels or cherubs in Renaissance paintings. Genetic mutations that take place in the disease have been identified as *SH3BP2* gene located in chromosome 4.

Clinical and Radiological Features

The disease usually starts during the age of 3 to 5 years in a large number of patients and rarely affects as early as the first year of life. Diagnosis is usually made a few years after the onset of the disease and starts regressing after puberty in most cases. The characteristic appearance of chubby cheeks is due to bilateral symmetrical enlargement of the mandible (**Figs 7.17A and B**). Another feature frequently reported is the upward look of eyes (eyes to heaven appearance) due to the involvement of the

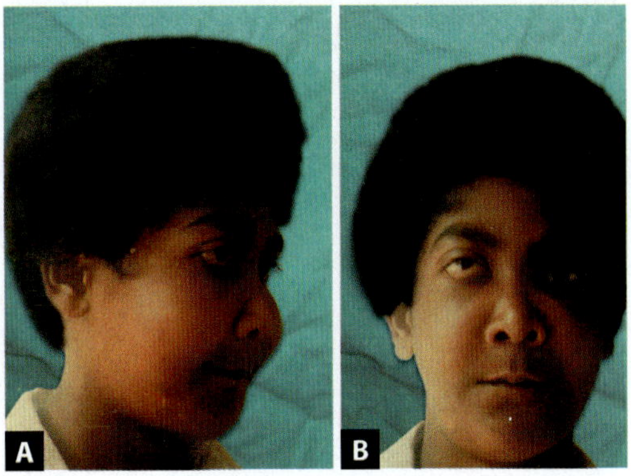

Figs 7.17A and B: Cherubism. Characteristic appearance of a patient with chubby cheeks and upward eyes (*Courtesy:* Dr AMO Peries)

orbital floor and the infraorbital rim. Maxillary involvement is much less common than the mandible. Failure in eruption of teeth, malocclusions, missing teeth and V-shaped palate are some of the other associated features.

Radiographically, bilateral symmetrical and multilocular radiolucent lesions with sclerotic and well defined margins are characteristic of cherubism. In addition, root resorption, displacement of teeth and agenesis of some teeth may be present.

Histopathological Features

Histopathological features are similar to giant cell granuloma and Brown tumor of hyperparathyroidism. The main feature is the presence of osteoclast like giant cells in a fibrovascular stroma. Shape of the fibroblasts may range from plump to spindle. Hemosiderin laden macrophages are common. Perivascular cuffing of capillaries by collagen and eosinophilic deposits is a useful diagnostic feature (**Fig. 7.18**).

Treatment and Prognosis

Since most cases undergo involution after puberty follow-up is essential and almost all the facial features return back to normal by fourth decade. Surgical intervention is indicated for severe cases and early surgical intervention has shown good results.

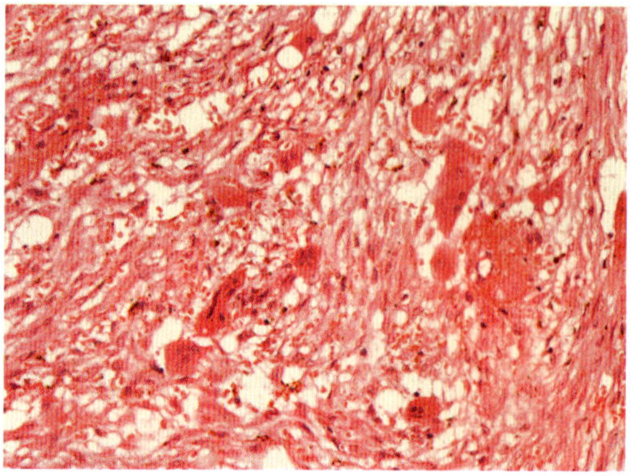

Fig. 7.18: Cherubism. Fibrous stroma containing multinucleate giant cells, hemosiderin pigments are evident focally. Perivascular cuffing is shown in a single blood vessel

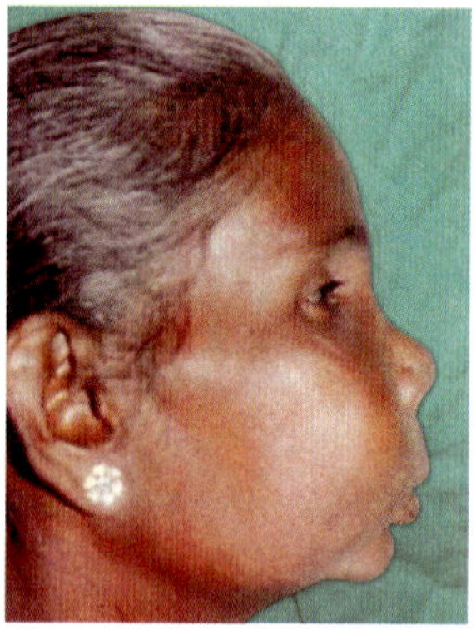

Fig. 7.19: Paget's disease. Maxillary and other facial bone involvement in a patient with Paget's disease

Paget's Disease

Paget's disease or osteitis deformans is characterised by impaired and abnormal bone remodelling as a result of an imbalance in bone deposition and resorption. Although Sir James Paget described the disease as a chronic inflammatory disease, the exact etiology is not known up to date. The disease can either affect a single bone (monostotic form) or more frequently multiple bones (polyostotic form). Recent evidence shows a genetic predisposition of the disease and up to 30 percent of the patients have a positive family history. One such locus has been identified in chromosome 18q-21-22. Although viral etiology has been suggested over the years due to identification of paramyxovirus particles in osteoclasts, existence of a cause and effect relationship has not been established.

Clinical Features

Patients are usually more than 40 years of age with a male predilection. The prevalence shows a wide regional variation and people from Europe and America are prone to develop the disease much more frequently than Asians and Africans. The exact incidence is difficult to predict as a large number of cases are identified only during the postmortem examination. Involvement of the skull is common resulting in increase in head size and shape, leading to frequent presenting compliant of increased hat size. At the same time, involvement of various foramina may lead to compression of multiple cranial nerves leading to paralysis and loss of hearing and sight. Involvement of weight bearing bones may result in a bowing deformity. The maxilla is more commonly affected than the mandible (**Fig. 7.19**). Gradual increase in the size of jaw bones lead to spacing of teeth and dentures may become tight. Jaw involvement predisposes the patients to develop osteomyelitis of the maxilla which is an uncommon site in a healthy individual.

Radiological Features

Radiological features of the disease vary according to the stage of the disease. The early osteoclastic phase shows diffuse radiolucency. A circumscribed area of radiolucency in the skull in the early stage of the disease is defined as osteoporosis circumscripta. Radiological features of Paget's disease show similarities to various stages of fibrous dysplasia. When the disease is advanced, the radiological features are more sclerotic giving rise to "cotton wool appearance" (**Fig. 7.20**). Radiographs of jaw bones reveal hypercementosis, loss of lamina dura in some patients and ankylosis of teeth in advanced cases.

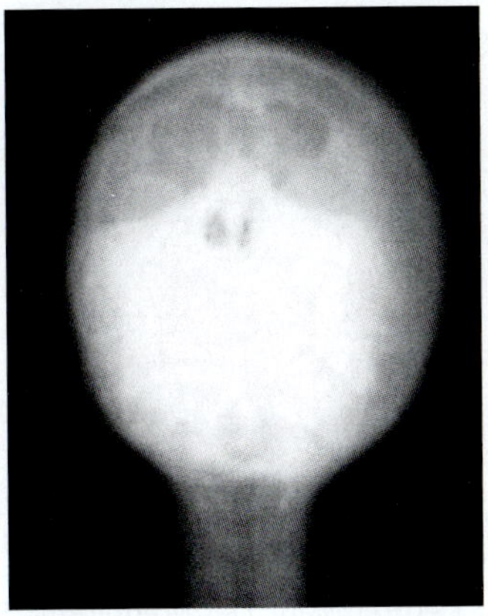

Fig. 7.20: Paget's disease. Radiographic features of the patient in Figure 7.19. Note the involvement of facial bones containing extremely sclerotic bone and peripheries are similar to "cotton wool" appearance

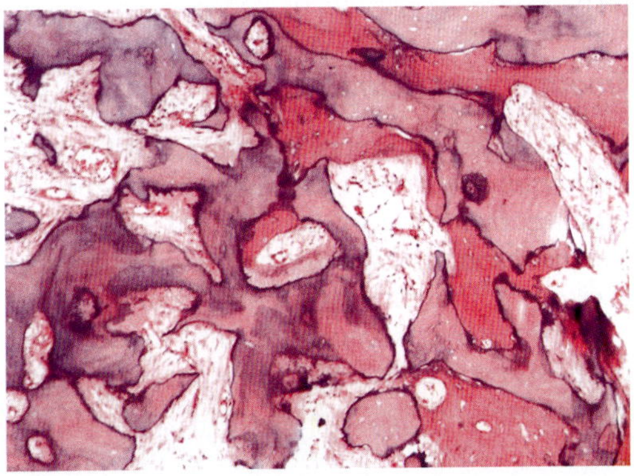

Fig. 7.21: Paget's disease. Irregular trabeculae of bone with prominent resting and reversal lines

Histopathological Features

As the hallmark of the disease is imbalance between bone formation and deposition, active phases of starting bone formation is revealed by the presence of numerous resting and reversal lines. Characteristic mosaic appearance is produced due to the same reason. The osteoclastic phase is characterised by numerous osteoclasts surrounding bony trabeculae (**Fig. 7.21**). Fibrous tissue, which is present at this phase, appears to be highly vascular. When the disease is in the sclerotic phase, osteoblasts predominate and the woven bone matures to lamellar bone with very little osteoclastic activity. Biopsy is not indicated in most cases for the diagnosis. Biopsy procedures in late cases in jaw bones may predispose the patient to osteomyelitis.

Treatment and Prognosis

Diagnosis of the disease is not challenging as most of the clinical and radiographic features are characteristic. Serological tests show markedly increased alkaline phosphatase levels with normal calcium and phosphorous levels. Markers of bone resorption may be identified in urine. N-telopeptides, C-telopeptides and pyridinoline cross-link assays are useful in this context. Treatment is required only in symptomatic cases. Bone pain can be controlled by simple analgesics such as aspirin. In order to reduce the bone turn over parathyroid hormone antagonists, namely calcitonin and biphosphonates have been recommended. Development of osteosarcoma with a poor prognosis has been reported in 1 percent of the patients with Paget's disease.

Central Giant Cell Granuloma

Central giant cell granuloma (CGCG) is a lesion which occurs centrally inside the mandible and maxilla. The behavior of this lesion is not uniform as some lesions behave in an aggressive way. The term "reparative granuloma" used in the past has become obsolete. A more aggressive entity known as giant cell tumor is a true neoplastic lesion unlike giant cell granuloma. However, giant cell lesion found in hyperparathyroidism is known as Brown tumor and is histopathologically identical to CGCG.

Clinical Features

The lesion is commonly found in the 10 to 30 years old age group with a female predilection. Anterior mandible and maxilla are the most common sites for occurrence and 75 percent of the cases have been reported in the mandible crossing the midline. The majority of these lesions are asymptomatic and are found in

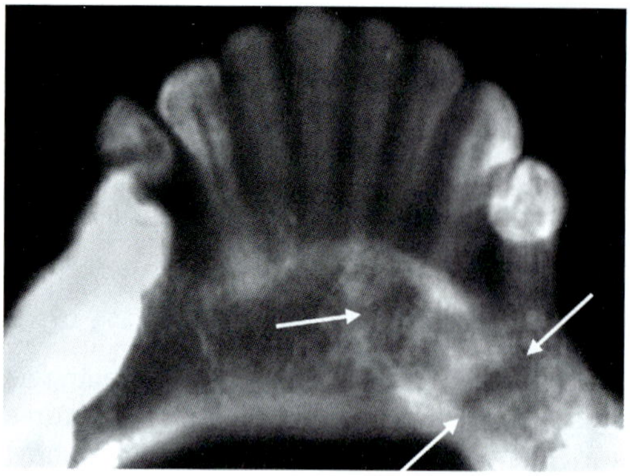

Fig. 7.22: Central giant cell granuloma. Multilocular radiolucency from canine to first molar area in the mandible

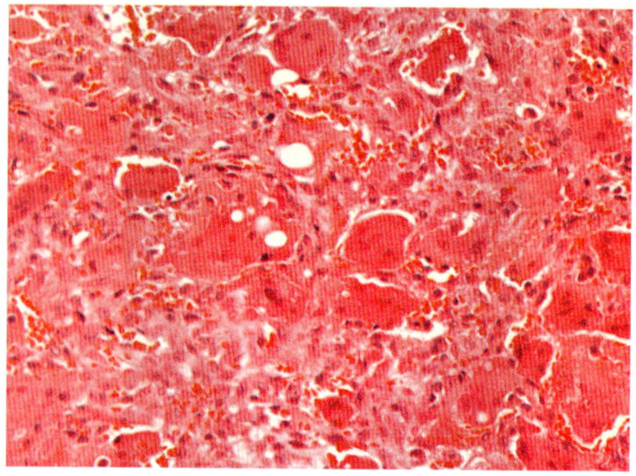

Fig. 7.23: Central giant cell granuloma. Frequent giant cells of varying size and mononuclear cells in a background of fibrovascular tissue. Note the marked vascularity

radiological investigations. However, less numbers of patients may present with pain, paresthesia and cortical perforation.

Radiological Features

Central giant cell granuloma (CGCG) presents as either unilocular or multilocular radiolucent lesion (**Fig. 7.22**). The defect is usually well delineated but cortication of margins is not a common finding. Aggressive lesions show resorption of roots. When they are multilocular, the appearances are similar to other multilocular lesions such as ameloblastoma. Differentiation between Brown tumor of hyperparathyroidism and CGCG is not possible unless other associated features such as loss of lamina dura and generalized "ground glass appearance is present in the former".

Histopathological Features

The lesion is composed of giant cells in a background of mononuclear cells and fibrous tissue (**Fig. 7.23**). Less aggressive forms show giant cells arranged into nodules and separated by thick fibrous tissue septae. Foci of osteoid and woven bone are also present. The lesion can be vascular and hemosiderin pigments are common. More aggressive forms show an increased amount of mononuclear cells and giant cells with less fibrous tissue. In addition, bone formation may be lacking in aggressive forms.

Treatment and Prognosis

The accepted treatment for most CGCGs is by curettage. Recurrence rates have been reported ranging from 11 to 50 percent. Recurrent lesions respond either to recurettage or surgical excision. Different treatment modalities such as corticosteroids, calcitonin and interferon-α have shown variable results for aggressive lesions.

Osteopetrosis (Marble Bone Disease, Albers-Schonberg Disease)

Osteopetrosis is a generalized hereditary condition in which bone becomes denser than normal due to defective bone resorption combined with continuous bone formation and endochondral ossification. The disease starts at birth or in early infancy is known as infantile form and inherited as autosomal recessive trait whereas the adult form is less severe and inherited as an autosomal dominant trait.

Clinical Features

The most of the clinical features in the disease are due to lack of bone resorption and continuous bone formation resulting in reduced marrow spaces leading to normocytic anemia. Patients present with hepatosplenomegally as a result of extramedullary hematopoiesis. Increased susceptibility to infection is a common feature and patients may present to clinics with osteomyelitis. Facial deformities appear in the form of a broad face, hypertelorism, frontal bossing and snub nose common in the infantile type. Narrowing and obliteration of bony foramina of the skull base lead to deafness and blindness. Pathological fractures of bones are not unusual in these patients. About 40 percent of the patients with the adult form are asymptomatic and diagnosis may result after routine radiological examinations for other diseases.

Radiological Features

There is generalized increase in bone density and obliteration of normal architecture leading to radiopacity of the whole skeleton. Sinuses are either obliterated or reduced in size. Unerupted teeth are a feature in the severe form. Pathological fractures may present in radiographs.

Histopathological Features

The bone is dense and sclerotic with marrow spaces either obliterated or replaced by fibrous tissue. Globular amorphous bone deposition in the marrow spaces is a feature. Although there are numerous osteoclasts, function may not be evident as Howship's lacunae are missing.

Treatment and Prognosis

Prognosis depends on the type of disease, as the majority of infantile types succumb to the disease in the first decade. The adult form has a long survival. Bone marrow transplantation is necessary to restore the hematopoietic function. Oral calcitriol combined with a calcium-free diet has provided improvement for some patients. In addition, supportive therapy such as blood transfusions and antibiotics may be necessary and osteomyelitis of the jaw bones have successfully been treated with resection of the affected part with antibiotics and hyperbaric oxygen.

Other Conditions

Chronic sclerosing osteomyelitis is presented in Chapter 4 and aneurysmal bone cyst and solitary bone cyst in Chapter 5.

SELF-ASSESSMENT QUESTIONS

1. Give a classification for fibrocemento-osseous lesions of jaw bones.
2. Discuss the importance of clinicopathological correlation in the diagnosis of fibrocemento-osseous lesions.
3. Discuss the radiological differential diagnosis of fibrocemento-osseous lesions.
4. Discuss the management of fibrocemento-osseous lesions.
5. Compare and contrast focal cemento-osseous dysplasia and cemento-ossifying fibroma.
6. Describe the different clinical presentations of fibrous dysplasia.
7. Using the knowledge of histopathology describe the changing pattern of radiological features of fibrocemento-osseous lesions.
8. Cemento-ossifying fibroma is a tumor with diverse histopathology and behavior. Discuss the statement critically.
9. Compare and contrast lesions presenting with giant cells as a main component.
10. What are the dental implications of patients with Paget's disease and osteopetrosis?

SUGGESTED READING

1. Chapurlat RD. Medical therapy in adults with fibrous dysplasia of bone. J Bone Miner Res. 2007;21:114-9.
2. Collins MT. Spectrum and natural history of fibrous dysplasia of bone. J Bone Miner Res. 2006;21:99-104.
3. Lan Su, Weathers DR, Waldron CA. Distinguishing features of focal cemento-osseous dysplasias and cemento-ossifying fibromas. Oral Surg Oral Med Oral Pathol. 1997;84:301-9.
4. MacDonald-Jankowiski DS, Fibro-osseous lesions of the face and jaws. Clinical Radiology. 2004;59:11-25.
5. Panda N, Parida PK, Sharma R, Bapuraj JR. A clinicoradiologic analysis of symptomatic craniofacial fibro-osseous lesions. Otolaryngol Head and Neck Surg. 2007;136:928-33.

6. Slootweg PJ. Maxillofacial fibro-osseous lesions; classification and differential diagnosis. Semin Diagn Pathol. 1996;13:104-12.
7. Summerlin DJ, Tormich CE. Focal cemento-osseous dysplasia: clinicopathologic study. Oral Surg Oral Med Oral Pathol. 1994;78: 611-20.
8. Waldron CA. Fibrocemento-osseous lesions of the jaws. J Oral Maxillofac Surg. 1984; 43:249-62.
9. Williams HK, Mangham C, Speight P. Juvenile aggressive ossifying fibroma. An analysis of eight cases and a comparison with other fibro osseous lesions. J Oral Pathol Med. 2000;29:13-18.

Chapter 8

Soft Tissue and Bone Tumors

KA Moutasim, GJ Thomas

Chapter Outline

INTRODUCTION

Most oral soft-tissue masses are reactive lesions, representing a localized hyperplastic inflammatory response to chronic trauma or inflammation. These lesions result from the proliferation of normal connective tissue elements, particularly fibrous and vascular tissue, and usually contain a variable infiltrate of inflammatory cells. Although a number of pathological conditions is distinguished, often according to clinical or pathological features, they all represent variations of the same pathogenic process. In addition to inflammatory and reactive lesions, there are over 200 types of soft tissue tumors with many variant patterns. Soft tissue tumors can be challenging for establishing a diagnosis and the clinical presentations could be very similar.

SOFT TISSUE TUMORS AND TUMOR-LIKE LESIONS

The most common soft tissue tumors encountered in the oral cavity are reactive lesions, e.g. epulides and fibroepithelial polyps.

REACTIVE LESIONS

Epulides

Epulides are common swellings that present clinically on the gingiva ('Epulis' is Greek for 'on the gum'). These are hyperplastic lesions associated with trauma and chronic irritation (commonly due to subgingival calculus deposits), arising most commonly on the anterior interdental gingivae. They are more common in women. Clinically, an epulis may be sessile or pedunculated (supported by a stalk) (**Fig. 8.1A**). Color and consistency will vary depending on the vascularity and the degree of fibrous proliferation within the lesion. Most epulides are either fibrous or vascular (pyogenic granuloma).

Fibrous Epulis

A 'fibrous epulis' has a firm texture, and similar color to that of the adjacent gingivae.

Histopathology

Fibrous epulides are usually composed of bundles of mature, cellular fibrous tissue covered by hyperplastic stratified squamous epithelium. The surface epithelium may be ulcerated, and a mild-to-moderate inflammatory infiltrate is often present. Foci of metaplastic bone formation are commonly found within the fibrous tissue (**Fig. 8.1B**).

Pyogenic Granuloma

When an epulis presents with a significant vascular component, it is termed a pyogenic granuloma. Clinically, this presents as a soft,

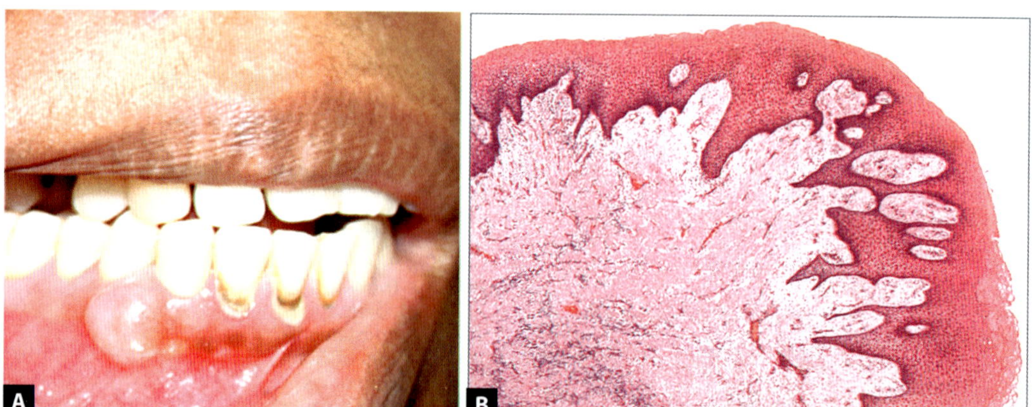

Figs 8.1A and B: Fibrous epulis. (A) Clinical appearance; (B) Histopathologically, it is composed of mature fibrous tissue covered by hyperplastic stratified squamous epithelium (*Clinical Picture Courtesy*: Dr T Sabesan)

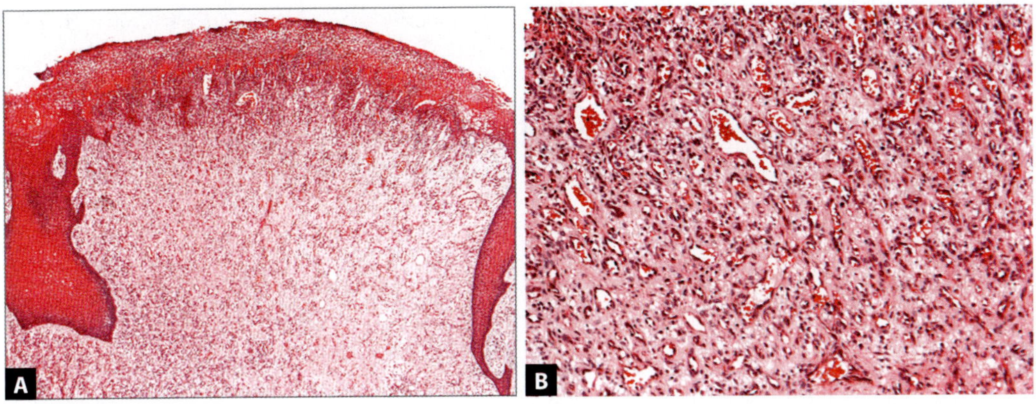

Figs 8.2A and B: Pyogenic granuloma. The surface is ulcerated, beneath which are proliferating endothelial cells forming small vascular spaces containing red blood cells

purple-red lump, which may hemorrhage spontaneously. These lesions may present on sites other than the gingivae, including the buccal and labial mucosae. The 'pregnancy epulis' is simply a pyogenic granuloma presenting during pregnancy. As to be expected, it is most common in woman of childbearing age, most arising during the first trimester of pregnancy.

Histopathology

Pyogenic granuloma and pregnancy epulis are commonly ulcerated, and characterized by sheets of proliferating endothelial cells, which form capillary spaces of variable size. These are supported by a loose, edematous fibrous stroma, with an inflammatory infiltrate usually present (**Figs 8.2A and B**).

Peripheral Giant Cell Granuloma (Giant Cell Epulis)

The peripheral giant cell granuloma originates from the periodontal membrane, and is a relatively frequent reactive lesion found on the gingiva or alveolar ridge. It occurs over a wide age range, though it is more common between the 5th and 6th decades, and shows a slight female predominance. Clinically, the lesion often has a red, brown or bluish color, is commonly ulcerated and located interdentally. Radiographs are essential to exclude a central giant cell granuloma which, if the cortical bone is perforated, could present similarly. For central lesions, hyperparathyroidism must be excluded.

Histopathology

Histologically, the lesion is characterized by the presence of focal aggregates of variably-sized, osteoclast-like multinucleate giant cells, set in a vascular stroma of plump mononuclear cells. Extravasated red blood cells and hemosiderin deposition are often present (**Figs 8.3A and B**).

Management

Epulides are generally managed by surgical excision under local anesthetic. It is best to defer treatment of a pregnancy epulis until after delivery, since lesions may regress spontaneously. Notably, some pregnancy epulides have a tendency for recurrence, particularly if excised during the most vascular phase.

FIBROUS LESIONS

Fibroepithelial Polyp

These are common, hyperplastic lesions that present as pale, firm swellings varying in size from a few millimeters to a centimeter or so, and may be pedunculated or sessile. Trauma is thought to be involved in the pathogenesis, and as such these lesions commonly present on the

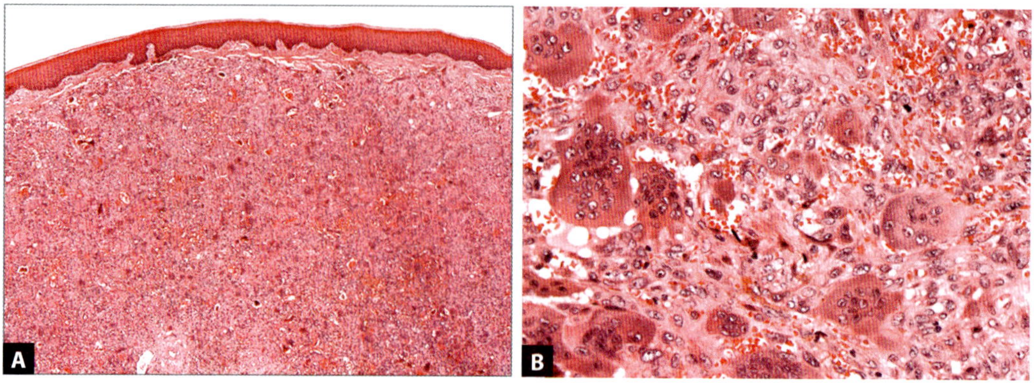

Figs 8.3A and B: Giant cell epulis (giant cell granuloma) composed of focal aggregates of multinucleated giant cells admixed with mononuclear cells in a vascular stroma

buccal mucosa along the occlusal line. When fibroepithelial polyps arise on the hard palate under the fitting surfaces of dental prostheses they become flattened and leaf-like, and are sometimes referred to as 'leaf fibroma'.

Histopathology

Fibroepithelial polyps are composed of bundles of mature collagen containing scattered fibroblasts. Inflammation is usually mild or absent. The overlying surface epithelium is of variable thickness and usually hyperkeratinized (**Fig. 8.4**).

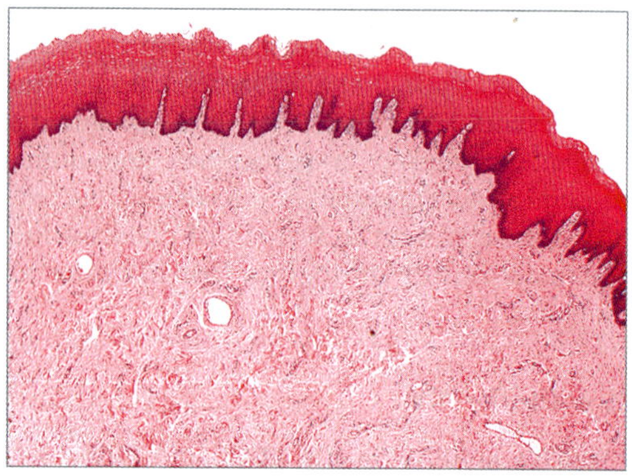

Fig. 8.4: Fibroepithelial polyp. The lesion is covered by keratinized acanthotic stratified squamous epithelium

Denture-induced Fibroepithelial Hyperplasia

These are hyperplastic mucosal overgrowths associated with ill-fitting dental prostheses, particularly lower dentures. They present as firm, leaf-like swellings usually on the labial and vestibular sulci embracing the denture flanges. Females are affected more commonly than males. Often, the patient will have been wearing an ill-fitting denture for a number of years before presentation and will generally have been asymptomatic.

Histopathology

The microscopic appearance is the same as a fibroepithelial polyp; bundles of mature collagen interspersed with scattered fibroblasts and covered by variably hyperplastic and hyperkeratinized stratified squamous epithelium.

Management

Fibroepithelial hyperplasias are generally excised under local anesthetic with removal of the underlying cause of chronic trauma (smoothing sharp tooth cusps, trimming overextended dentures or fitting new dentures) to prevent recurrence.

Papillary Hyperplasia of the Palate

This condition presents on the hard palate, usually seen in middle-age to elderly female patients, almost invariably under an ill-fitting upper denture. The exact etiology is unknown, but it is thought that the chronic trauma from a rocking denture predisposes to the condition, and also potentiates the growth of fungal microorganisms. Clinically, there are multiple pin-point projections on the anterior hard palate vault, giving a cobblestone or pebbled appearance to the palate. Occasionally, the hyperplasia may also extent onto the edentulous ridges. There is frequently an overall erythematous appearance, particularly when *Candida* is present.

Histopathology

The mucosa is composed of multiple papillary projections consisting of proliferating fibrous and granulation tissue covered by hyperplastic stratified squamous epithelium. A chronic inflammatory infiltrate is frequently present (**Fig. 8.5**). The degree of epithelial hyperplasia may be marked, producing a pseudoepitheliomatous appearance, with deep, branching rete processes that may mimic the invasive appearance of squamous cell carcinoma. However, cellular atypia is not a feature of this disease and it has no malignant potential.

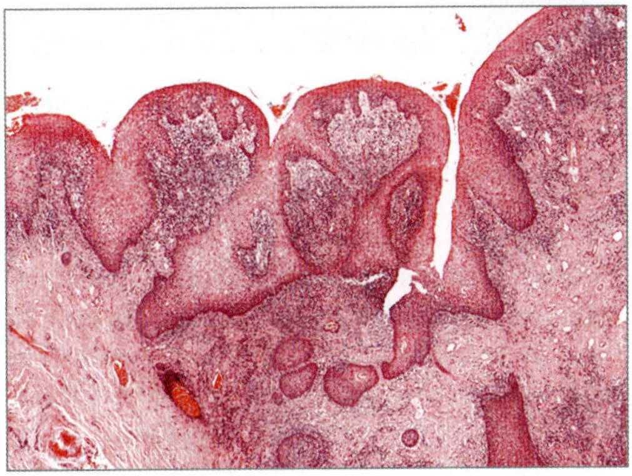

Fig. 8.5: Papillary hyperplasia. There are multiple papillary projections consisting of proliferating fibrous and granulation tissue covered by hyperplastic stratified squamous epithelium. A chronic inflammatory infiltrate is present

Management

The patient should be advised to remove the dental appliance at night and to practice appropriate oral and denture hygiene. Topical antifungal therapy is used to treat underlying candidal infection. Surgical excision of papillary tissue and the fabrication of new dental prostheses can then be carried out.

Squamous Papilloma

Squamous papilloma is a local, human papilloma virus (HPV)-induced epithelial hyperplasia, presenting clinically as a solitary, usually pedunculated nodule, which is white with a papillary surface (**Fig. 8.6A**). HPV-6 and HPV-11 are most commonly associated (found in around 50-68% of papillomas). Although squamous papillomas can occur at any age, they are more common in patients aged 30 to 50 years.

Histopathology

The lesion is composed of hyperplastic stratified squamous epithelium, forming finger-like projections which are hyperkeratinized (giving the lesion a white appearance). The epithelium surrounds cores of vascular fibrous tissue, and there is sometimes a mild infiltrate of chronic inflammatory cells in the stroma (**Fig. 8.6B**). Superficial keratinocytes may have a koilocytic appearance similar to other HPV-induced lesions (a koilocyte is a keratinocyte with a pyknotic nucleus surrounded by a clear zone). Lesions most commonly have a stalk but can be sessile. It is important to remember that a number of different oral lesions have a papillary or verruciform appearance.

Management

Squamous papillomas are treated by conservative excision and recurrence is unlikely. Although associated with HPV infection, the lesions appear to have low infectivity and are not contagious.

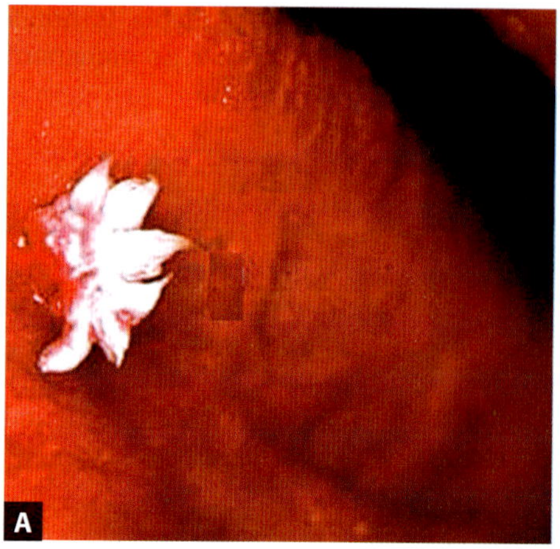

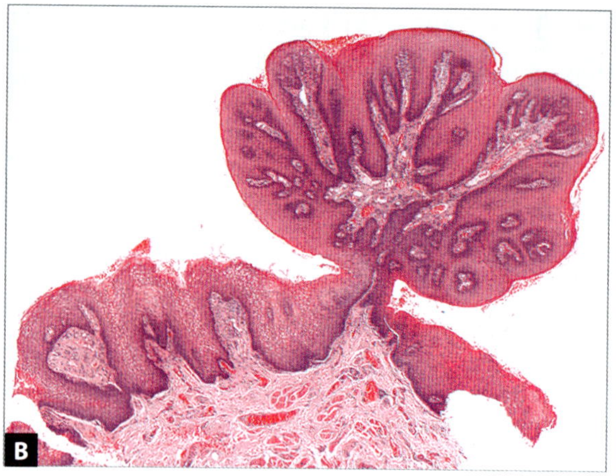

Figs 8.6A and B: Squamous cell papilloma. (A) An exophytic, papillary and whitish lesion is the characteristic presentation; (B) Histopathologically it shows hyperplastic stratified squamous epithelium, forming finger-like projections (*Courtesy*: Dr AM Attygalla)

Focal Epithelial Hyperplasia (Heck's Disease)

Heck's disease (focal epithelial hyperplasia) is a condition with a strong genetic predisposition that was originally described in Native Americans and Inuits of Greenland. It is now known to exist in numerous ethnic groups and populations, and to be associated with HPV-13 infection (and possibly HPV-32). Since transmission is by casual contact, it is not uncommon for multiple family members to be affected, particularly children. Clinically, Heck's disease most commonly presents as multiple raised plaques on the labial and buccal mucosae, and tongue. Occasionally, lesions may impart a 'cobblestoned' appearance to the mucosa, in which case Crohn's disease or orofacial granulomatosis should be considered in the differential diagnosis.

Histopathology

The lesions are composed of markedly acanthotic stratified squamous epithelium which has widened rete processes, producing a sessile, exophytic growth pattern. The epithelial surface may be hyperkeratinized, but it lacks the striking papillary pattern seen in squamous papilloma. Mitosoid bodies (keratinocytes with collapsed nuclei resembling mitoses) may be seen in the suprabasal epithelial layers (**Fig. 8.7**). Presence of HPV can be demonstrated with immunohistochemistry (**Fig. 8.8**).

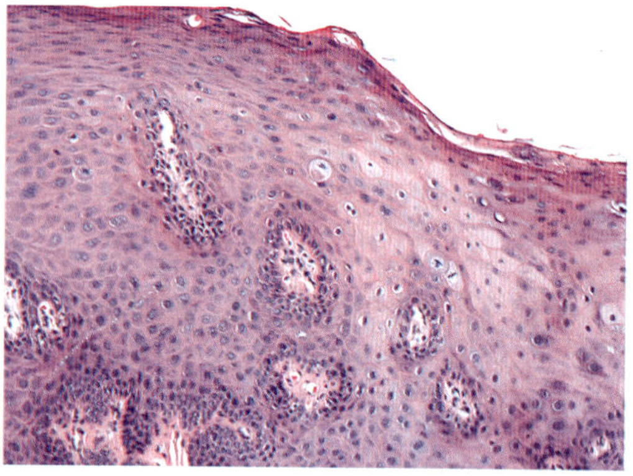

Fig. 8.7: Focal epithelial hyperplasia (Heck's disease). Hyperplastic epithelium containing virally damaged cells and mitosoid bodies (*Courtesy*: Dr B Almeda)

Management

In many cases, intervention is unnecessary and lesions regress spontaneously. Some lesions are managed by conservative excision.

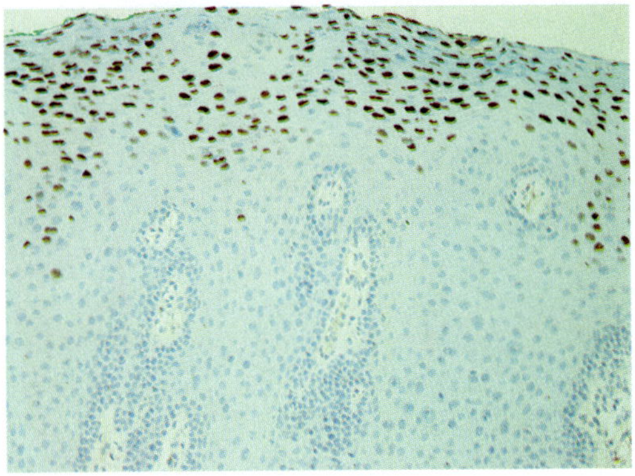

Fig. 8.8. Immunohistochemical stain for HPV showing strong positivity in surface cells in Heck's disease (*Courtesy*: Dr B Almeda)

Nodular Fasciitis

Although there is some evidence that nodular fasciitis contains clonal chromosomal abnormalities, this is regarded as a reactive lesion. Although self-limiting and benign, it often presents as a rapidly growing mass with sometimes alarming histological appearances, and can be mistaken for a malignant process. It usually occurs in the superficial fascia, commonly on the angle of the mandible or the zygomatic prominence, but may also affect intraoral sites, particularly the buccal mucosa and lips. Children and young adults are most commonly affected, with no particular gender predilection. Trauma is often implicated in the etiopathogenesis. Cranial fasciitis, a particular form of nodular fasciitis, is seen in infants and involves the soft tissue of the scalp. Nodular fasciitis may also show prominent intravascular growth (intravascular fasciitis).

Histopathology

Histologically, nodular fasciitis consists of haphazardly arranged fibroblasts within a mucoid or myxoid connective tissue. The fibroblasts are plump and large, and resemble those of granulation tissue, with pleomorphic cells sometimes seen. Mitoses are common, reflecting the rapid growth of the lesion, but abnormal mitotic forms are not present. There is usually a mild-to-moderate infiltrate of chronic inflammatory cells, and extravasated erythrocytes.

Management

Nodular fasciitis, despite its worrying clinical presentation and pathological appearances, is a self-limiting lesion that is treated by simple surgical excision. Spontaneous regression without treatment has also been reported. Larger lesions, particularly if situated deeply within tissues, may need a wider excision. Recurrence rates are low, and reported to range from 1 to 6 percent.

VASCULAR LESIONS

Pyogenic Granuloma

Most pyogenic granulomas arise on the gingiva (see under epulides), but they can also arise at other intraoral sites including the lips, buccal mucosa and tongue. The clinical and histological appearances are, however, the same.

NEURAL LESIONS

Traumatic Neuroma

Traumatic neuromas can occur at any age, and result from the reactive proliferation of a damaged nerve as a result of trauma or surgery. The lesion presents as a small, smooth, submucosal nodule, which in some cases, may be extremely painful on pressure. Sites most commonly affected within the mouth are the tongue, lower lip, and alveolar mucosa close to the mental foramen.

Histopathology

The lesion is poorly circumscribed, and is characterized by numerous haphazardly arranged, proliferating nerve fibers embedded within fibrovascular tissue (**Fig. 8.9**).

Management

Traumatic neuroma is treated by simple surgical excision. The lesion occasionally recurs.

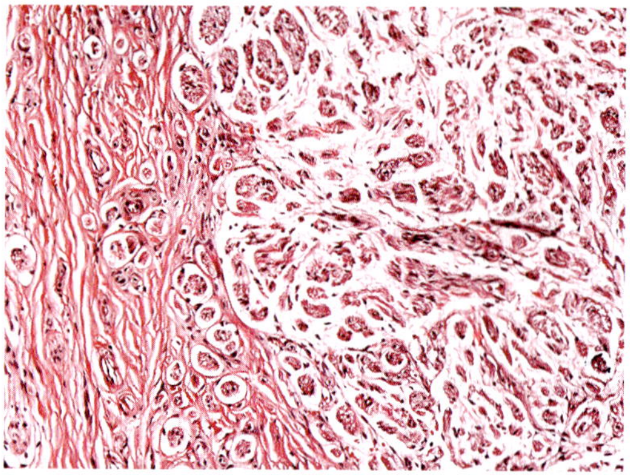

Fig. 8.9: Traumatic neuroma consisting of numerous proliferating nerve fascicles and fibrous tissue

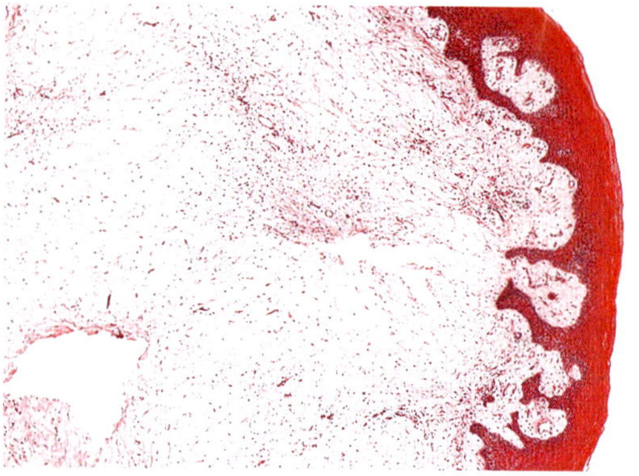

Fig. 8.10: Oral focal mucinosis consisting of a nodule of loose myxoid connective tissue covered by stratified squamous epithelium

OTHER REACTIVE LESIONS

Oral Focal Mucinosis

Oral focal mucinosis is an uncommon lesion, and is probably due to overproduction of hyaluronic acid by fibroblasts. The lesion primarily occurs in young adults, and has a female predilection. The sites most commonly affected are the gingiva and hard palate, with the lesion presenting as a soft, sessile nodule with normal or pale surface color.

Histopathology

The lesion is composed of an unencapsulated area of loose myxoid or 'mucinous' connective tissue. This contains mild-to-moderate fibroblast numbers which sometimes have delicate fibrillar processes. The overlying epithelium may be atrophic or hyperplastic (**Fig. 8.10**).

Management

Treatment is by surgical excision. Lesions do not recur.

Verruciform Xanthoma

The verruciform xanthoma occurs generally in middle aged and older patients. It has a female predilection. The sites most commonly affected are the alveolar mucosa and gingiva. The lesion has a similar clinical appearance to a viral papilloma, presenting as a soft, slightly raised, sessile nodule with a papillary surface.

Histopathology

Histologically, a verruciform xanthoma has a papillary surface, which is usually hyperkeratinized. The diagnostic feature of the lesion is found within the connective tissue papillae between the epithelial rete processes, which are packed with foamy histiocytes or xanthoma cells (**Figs 8.11A and B**).

Management

Treatment is by surgical excision, and recurrence is rare.

BENIGN AND MALIGNANT TUMORS

Benign neural and vascular tumors are relatively common in the oral cavity, but intraoral soft tissue sarcomas are rare. The lesions all present similarly, either as superficial nodules or deep-seated masses. Benign tumors are usually freely mobile, whereas sarcomas infiltrate into adjacent structures and are fixed. Features such as rapid growth, pain and ulceration are more likely to be found in malignant tumors. For all spindle cell and pleomorphic sarcomas, it is

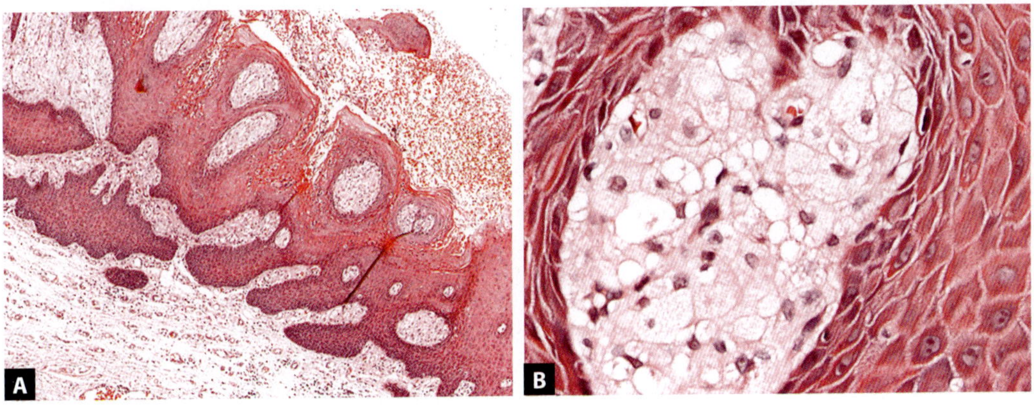

Figs 8.11A and B: Verruciform xanthoma. The lesion has a papillary, hyperkeratinized surface. The diagnostic feature of the lesion is found within the connective tissue papillae between the epithelial rete processes which are packed with foamy histiocytes or xanthoma cells

important to exclude the possibility of spindle cell (poorly differentiated) squamous cell carcinoma and melanoma, which occur more frequently within the oral and maxillofacial region. Immunochemistry plays an essential role in the diagnosis of soft tissue tumors (**Table 8.1**) with genetic analysis also being increasingly important.

▪ Table 8.1
Immunological markers helpful to differentiate cell lineages

Cell/tissue type	*Immunochemical marker*
Myofibroblast	Smooth muscle actin (SMA)
Epithelial	Cytokeratins
Skeletal muscle	Desmin, myoglobin, myo-D1
Smooth muscle	SMA, Calponin
Endothelial (vascular)	CD31, CD34, factor VIII-related antigen
Neural	S100, Leu7, myelin basic protein
Melanocyte	S100, HMB45, Melan A, tyrosinase
Hematolymphoid (lymphocytes, etc.)	CD45

FIBROUS TUMORS

Myofibroma/Myofibromatosis

Solitary and multicentric myofibromas (myofibromatosis) are benign tumors composed of myofibroblasts (contractile, smooth muscle-like fibroblasts), with a predilection for the soft tissues of the head and neck. Solitary lesions are more common than multicentric disease, and although these tumors can occur at any age, most (~ 90%) occur in children aged 2 and under, representing the most common fibrous proliferation in childhood. It should be, noted, however, that oral lesions tend to present in children and adolescents, rather than infants, and are usually solitary, with the tongue most commonly affected. Myofibromatosis involving the oral cavity is extremely rare. Superficial lesions present as painless, firm, exophytic nodule on the skin or the oral mucosa, whereas deeper tumors form palpable masses.

Histopathology

Myofibromas are generally well-circumscribed spindle cell tumors composed of cellular areas which alternate with fascicular or hyalinized areas, producing a nodular appearance (**Fig. 8.12**). The tumor cells are positive for smooth muscle actin (SMA), but negative for desmin.

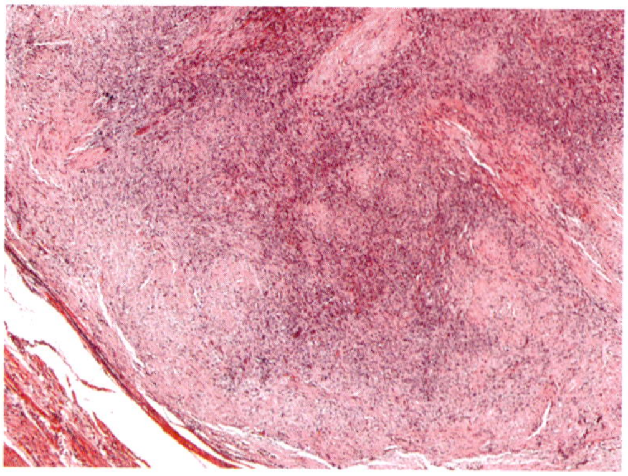

Fig. 8.12: Myofibroma. A spindle cell lesion with a vaguely nodular appearance. The margin of the tumor is well demarcated

Management

Local surgical excision is curative; but recurrences may occur.

Myofibrosarcoma

Myofibrosarcomas are relatively rare. They can occur at any age, but low-grade tumors have a predilection for the head and neck (up to 30% of cases), particularly affecting the tongue, face and neck. Such low-grade tumors are usually slow-growing, arising in the deep soft tissues and also intraosseously.

Histopathology

Tumors usually infiltrate into adjacent tissues, and are most commonly composed of fascicles or broad sheets of spindle cells, similar in appearance to fibrosarcoma. Some tumors are focally myxoid, giving a nodular-fasciitis-like appearance. Although the tumor cells are relatively uniform, nuclear atypia is present, but may be only focal. Mitotic activity is variable. Most low-grade myofibrosarcomas are immunoreactive for SMA and desmin. High grade (pleomorphic) myofibrosarcoma tends to affect the extremities, and histologically has the same appearance as malignant fibrous histiocytoma, but contains SMA-positive cells.

Management

Low-grade myofibrosarcomas are prone to recurrence (recurrence rate is around 27%), but rarely metastasize. Tumors should be treated by complete, but conservative, excision.

Fibromatosis (Desmoid Tumor, Aggressive Fibromatosis)

Fibromatosis is a fibroblastic proliferation of cells arising from the musculoaponeurotic tissues of the body. Although fibromatosis does not metastasise, it is a locally aggressive tumor that is currently classified as a tumor of borderline malignancy. Fibromatosis is relatively rare, with around 10 to 15 percent of cases affecting the head and neck, and may be seen in association with Gardner's syndrome. It occurs primarily in children and young adults, with no gender predilection. Clinically, the lesions are painless, deep-seated and show slow, progressive growth and infiltration into adjacent structures. Fibromatosis usually develops adjacent to the mandible.

Histopathology

The tumor consists of long, sweeping fascicles of uniform, spindle cells, which infiltrate into adjacent tissues. The tumor cells are arranged around numerous small, dilated blood vessels, and cellularity may vary from region to region. Around 90 percent of cases show nuclear positivity for beta-catenin, which may be helpful in the differential diagnosis of these lesions.

Management

Fibromatosis is treated by surgical excision, including a thin margin or normal tissue. In the head and neck, this is often difficult, if not impossible, due to the anatomical complexity of the region. The difficulty in obtaining clear surgical margins is reflected in the relatively high recurrence rates of head and neck fibromatoses (reported as 25–50% in larger series).

Fibrosarcoma

Before the advent of advanced immunohistochemical and genetic diagnostic techniques, fibrosarcomas were regarded as one of the most common soft tissue malignancies. It is now evident that many of the tumors originally thought to be fibrosarcomas were spindle-cell malignancies of other types. The term 'fibrosarcoma' is now used to define a fascicular spindle cell malignancy that is negative for all other connective tissue markers. This tumor usually affects the soft tissues of the lower extremities, and is relatively rare in the head and neck region, and may be associated with previous radiotherapy. Fibrosarcoma tends to occur in middle aged adults, presenting as a deep-seated soft tissue mass.

Histopathology

Fibrosarcomas are diffusively infiltrative tumors composed of long, interlacing fascicles of atypical, mitotically-active fibroblasts. Fibrosarcoma is a diagnosis of exclusion, with tumor cells showing negative immunoreactivity for markers such as cytokeratin, S-100, desmin, CD34, CD99. Limited tumor expression of SMA may be seen, making distinction from myofibrosarcoma somewhat arbitrary.

Management

Fibrosarcomas are treated by wide local excision, with more radical surgery required for poorly differentiated lesions. Metastasis is uncommon, and usually a late event. The overall 5-year survival rate for head and neck fibrosarcoma is 20 to 35 percent.

Fibrous Histiocytoma

This tumor is also called a dermatofibroma when occurring in the skin, but is rare in the oral cavity. It occurs predominantly in the vestibule and buccal mucosa, usually in middle aged or older patients, presenting as an asymptomatic mass. Tumor cells show fibroblastic and histiocytic features, and this varied microscopic appearance has lead to the use of numerous diagnostic terms (xanthogranuloma, dermatofibroma).

Histopathology

The tumor is usually poorly demarcated. As with other fibroblastic tumors, plump spindled fibroblasts are present, commonly arranged in a storiform (irregular and whorled) pattern. Additionally, rounded histiocyte-like cells are present which may contain lipid (foamy histiocytes) or sometimes form multinucleate giant cells. The cells are arranged in a fibrous stroma. Nuclear atypia is absent, and immunohistochemical markers are generally negative, but SMA may be positive.

Management

Fibrous histiocytomas are treated by surgical excision, with recurrence rates reported at 5 to 10 percent. Recurrence is higher in more deeply-seated lesions.

Malignant Fibrous Histiocytoma (Undifferentiated Pleomorphic Sarcoma, Pleomorphic Fibrosarcoma)

Malignant fibrous histiocytoma (MFH) is one of the less common sarcomas affecting the head and neck region, usually occurring in older adults (50-70 years), and similar to other sarcomas, presenting as a deep-seated soft tissue mass. MFH is a malignant fibroblastic mesenchymal tumor, and is not derived from histiocytes as originally believed. It has been suggested that this lesion does not exist as a separate entity, but represents the pleomorphic progression of various other sarcoma types. However, it is clear that many pleomorphic sarcomas lack specific histological or immunochemical differentiation features. Thus, similar to fibrosarcoma, MFH is also a diagnosis of exclusion.

Histopathology

Malignant fibrous histiocytoma has a wide spectrum of appearances, and is generally divided into five different types: pleomorphic-storiform, myxoid, inflammatory, giant-cell and angiomatoid. Most MFHs are of the pleomorphic-storiform type, and consist of a storiform proliferation of bizarre, pleomorphic spindle to epithelioid cells showing high-grade features, including necrosis and abnormal mitotic forms. Multinucleated giant cells may be present, and in sufficient numbers to categorize the tumor as a giant cell variant. Tumors may also contain inflammatory or myxoid areas, and areas of vascular proliferation—thus the five different tumor subtypes.

Management

Malignant fibrous histiocytoma is treated by radical surgical resection, with or without chemoradiotherapy. Recurrence is common, and occurs in at least 40 percent of lesions, with a similar number metastasizing. Five-year survival is around 30 percent.

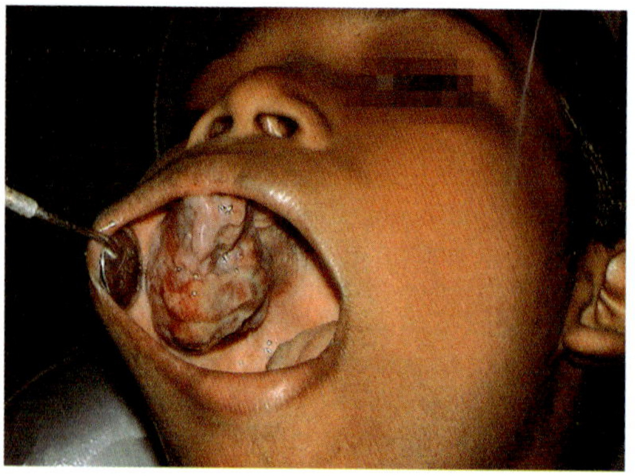

Fig. 8.13: Hemangioma: A large hemangioma of the right buccal mucosa (*Courtesy*: Dr AM Attygalla)

VASCULAR TUMORS

Hemangioma

Although widely referred to as tumors, hemangiomas represent abnormal hamartomatous proliferations of vascular tissue rather than true neoplasms. They are particularly common in the head and neck, and can present at any age, but often during childhood and adolescence. They most frequently affect the lips, tongue, labial and buccal mucosae. Clinically, they can be flat or raised with an occasionally lobulated surface, and are mostly solitary although multiple lesions can occur. Their color ranges from red to bluish/purple, and the lesions typically blanch under pressure (**Fig. 8.13**). Trauma can precipitate hemorrhage, but otherwise patients are asymptomatic, unless the lesions are part of an angiomatous syndrome (e.g. Sturge-Weber syndrome).

Histopathology

Hemangiomas are abnormal proliferations of endothelial cells, and can be broadly classified into capillary, cavernous and mixed types depending on the size of the vascular spaces formed. These spaces are generally filled with red blood cells, which can occasionally thrombosis (**Fig. 8.14A**).

Management

Special investigations (ultrasonography, MRI) should be undertaken to study the lesion and associated possible feeder vessels. Surgical incision into a suspected hemangioma should be avoided. Oral hemangiomas are usually excised, but can be treated with cryosurgery, laser ablation or intralesional injection of corticosteroids or sclerosing agents.

Sturge-Weber Syndrome (Encephalotrigeminal Angiomatosis)

This condition is characterized by venous malformations involving the leptomeninges over the cerebral cortex causing neurological symptoms, in combination with hemangiomas over branches of the trigeminal nerve, presenting as the characteristic 'Port-wine stain.' Hemangiomas may also present intraorally. Neurological symptoms can present as convulsions, learning disabilities and hemiparesis on the contralateral side of the lesion. 'Port-wine' facial hemangiomas may also be present in isolation.

Lymphangioma

Like hemangiomas, these represent hamartomatous malformations of the lymphatic system, presenting most commonly during infancy or early childhood. They arise most commonly on the tongue, where they cause macroglossia, but can affect any part of the oral cavity. Lymphangiomas often have a characteristic papillary, multinodular surface. Cystic hygromas are lymphangiomas that affect the developing lymphatics in the neck and can

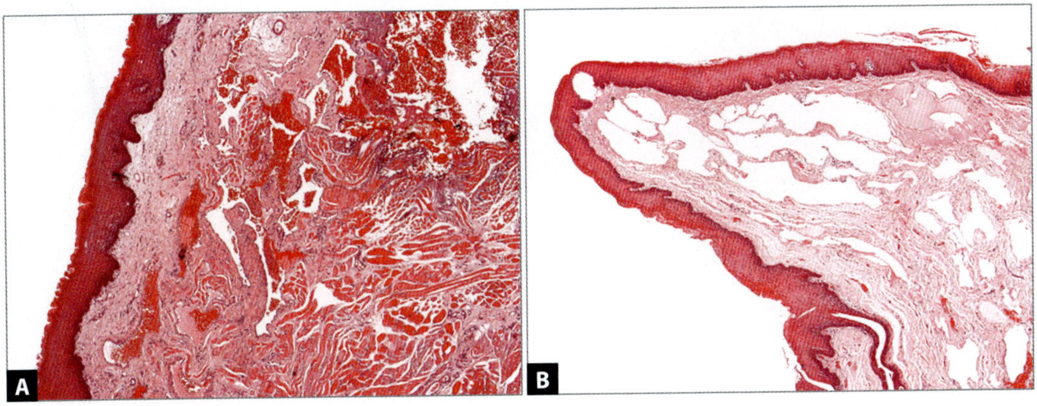

Figs 8.14A and B: (A) Hemangioma; (B) Lymphangioma. The connective tissue contains numerous irregular and dilated endothelial-lined spaces filled with red blood cells or lymph respectively

cause gross enlargement on the affected side. They can be potentially life-threatening, if they involve vital structures.

Histopathology

On microscopy, lymphangiomas appear as thin-walled endothelial-lined spaces filled with clear fluid (lymph), with occasional lymphocytes or scanty red blood cells. Like hemangiomas, they can be classified as cavernous or capillary, depending on the size of the spaces. The prominent lymphatic vessels in lymphangiomas are characteristically in direct apposition to the overlying epithelium (**Fig. 8.14B**).

Management

Many lymphangiomas undergo spontaneous regression. Progressive lesions can be amenable to surgical excision. Other options include sclerosing agents and intralesional corticosteroid therapy.

Angiosarcoma

Angiosarcoma is a rare malignancy of endothelial cell origin. More than half of all angiosarcomas are found in the head and neck region, most commonly on the scalp. It is rare in the oral cavity but when occurring, may present intraosseously, or as a submucosal mass. Clinically, angiosarcoma usually affects older individuals (>65 years), and presents as a rapidly-growing red or purplish submucosal mass, which is fixed to underlying tissues, that may ulcerate and bleed spontaneously.

Histopathology

The histopathological appearances vary greatly. Well-differentiated tumors may be composed of atypical endothelial cells forming obvious vascular channels, but there may be little evidence of vasoformation in poorly differentiated lesions. Tumors are immunoreactive for vascular markers including CD31, CD34 and factor VIII-related antigen.

Management

Angiosarcomas are usually treated by wide local excision with radiotherapy sometimes used for multifocal lesions. The overall survival rate is poor (5-year survival rate 10–15%), with 50 percent of patients dying within 15 months.

Kaposi's Sarcoma

Kaposi's sarcoma (KS) is a vascular tumor of lymphatic endothelial origin, associated with HHV-8 infection. KS can be classified into four different clinical subtypes: classic/sporadic, endemic African/lymphadenopathic,

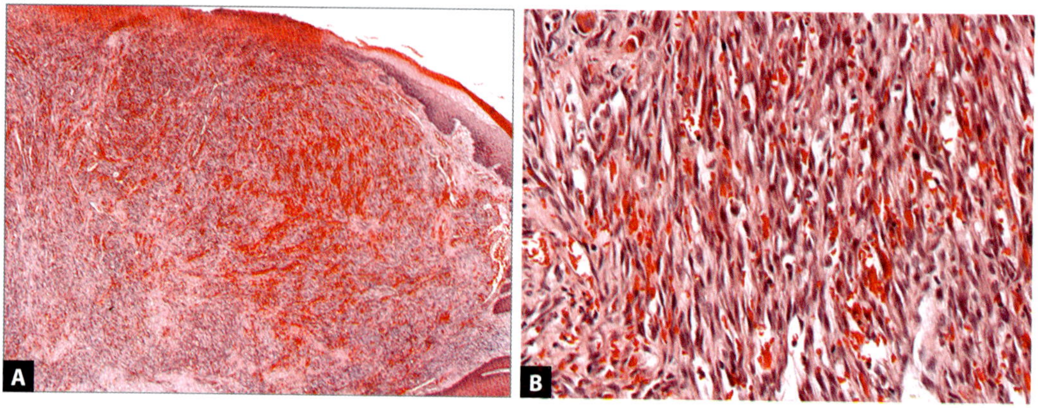

Figs 8.15A and B: Kaposi sarcoma. Advanced lesions are composed of fascicles of elongated, uniform spindle cells separated by slit-like vascular spaces

AIDS-associated, and iatrogenic/transplant-associated. In non-endemic areas, most cases of head and neck KS are associated with immunosuppression, particularly HIV infection. AIDS-associated KS is the most aggressive form of the disease, found in around 10 percent of patients with AIDS. It occurs at a much younger age than the classic form, most frequently in the 4th decade of life. The clinical appearance varies according to stage, with earlier lesions appearing as a flat red-to-blue patch. Later lesions appear as a purplish-red plaque or nodule, which may be ulcerated.

Histopathology

Advanced lesions are composed of fascicles of elongated, uniform spindle cells separated by slit-like vascular spaces (**Figs 8.15A and B**). The tumor contains extravasated erythrocytes and chronic inflammatory cells. The tumor cells are positive for HHV-8, and usually positive for vascular markers (CD31, CD34).

Management

Radiation and/or chemotherapy are the treatments of choice, with the use of surgery generally limited to diagnostic biopsy. Chemotherapeutics include azidothymidine, vincristine and vinblastine. Antiretroviral therapy also has helped in managing proliferating KS lesions.

NEURAL TUMORS

Granular Cell Tumor

The granular cell tumor is an uncommon benign neoplasm of neural origin. The granular cells were thought to be of primitive striated muscle origin; hence the term "granular cell myoblastoma" was originally used to describe these tumors. It is now evident that the granular cells are of nerve sheath origin, and are most likely to be Schwann cells. Granular cell tumor has a female predilection, and may occur at any age, but most commonly presents in the 4th decade of life. The head and neck is a favored site for this tumor, typically presenting on the tongue. However, any site in the oral cavity may be affected. Clinically, the lesion presents as a painless, firm, polypoid mass with an intact surface epithelium. It can grow up to 5 cm in size, and usually has a slightly yellowish surface. Multiple lesions may occasionally occur.

The congenital gingival granular cell tumor (congenital epulis) is a related lesion that presents as a polypoid mass in the newborn, most commonly on the maxillary alveolar ridge. It can be pedunculated or sessile; and is more common in girls than boys.

Histopathology

The granular cell tumor is typically unencapsulated, and composed of uniform sheets of

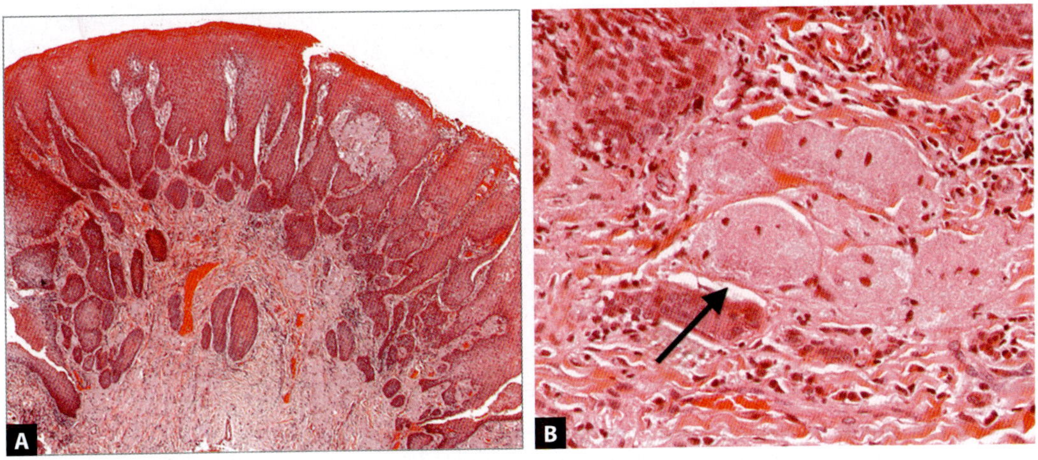

Figs 8.16A and B: Granular cell tumor. The epithelium overlying the tumor is hyperplastic giving a pseudoepitheliomatous appearance which could be mistaken for a squamous cell carcinoma. The tumor cells (arrow) are in the deeper tissue showing large, and polyhedral shape with abundant granular cytoplasm

eosinophilic cells with an abundant granular cytoplasm. The cells generally have a plump, polyhedral morphology, with small, bland nuclei (**Figs 8.16A and B**). The overlying epithelium invariably displays pseudoepitheliomatous hyperplasia, which can result in the misdiagnosis of this lesion as a squamous cell carcinoma if the granular cells are overlooked or if the biopsy is superficial. Ultrastructurally, the cellular granules appear to be comprised of phagolysosomes. Immunohistochemically, granular cell tumors are positive for the S-100 protein, confirming their neural origin.

Management

Surgical excision under local anesthetic is the treatment of choice. Recurrence is uncommon.

Neurofibroma

Neurofibroma is a benign neoplasm of the nerve sheath that can present as a solitary tumor or as multiple lesions in the neurofibromatosis syndrome (von Recklinghausen's disease), associated with mutations or abnormalities of the NF-1 gene. Solitary neurofibromas can occur at any age but is more common in teenagers and young adults; usually presenting as a slowly-growing, asymptomatic mass. The favored sites intraorally are the tongue and buccal mucosa.

Neurofibromas may occur as part of the generalized syndrome of neurofibromatosis (usually neurofibromatosis type 1, also called von Recklinghausen neurofibromatosis). NF type 1 is inherited as an autosomal dominant trait, and is characterized by multiple neurofibromas which occur anywhere in the body, including the oral cavity. Oral involvement is seen in around 70 percent of cases. In addition to neurofibromas, the syndrome also presents with Café-au-lait cutaneous pigmentation (which may precede the neural lesions), neurological symptoms and bone abnormalities. Notably, the neurofibromas in neurofibromatosis can undergo malignant transformation in around 10 percent of cases, although this is uncommon in oral lesions. Malignant transformation is exceptionally rare in solitary neurofibromas.

Histopathology

Neurofibromas are unencapsulated but well-demarcated tumors containing a variety of spindle cells, including Schwann cells and fibroblasts in a myxoid stroma, which can contain mast cells and lymphocytes (**Fig. 8.17A**). The plexiform neurofibroma has characteristic pathological

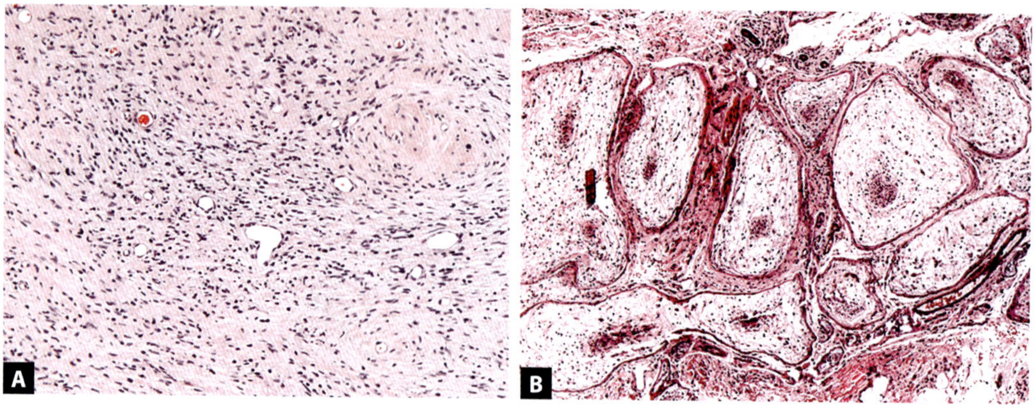

Figs 8.17A and B: (A) Neurofibroma composed of a variety of spindle cells, including Schwann cells and fibroblasts in a myxoid stroma; (B) The plexiform neurofibroma has a multinodular appearance

features, and is found almost exclusively in patients with NF-1. Grossly, the multinodular or fusiform enlargement of the involved nerve leads to a 'bag of worms' appearance. Histologically, there is tortuous expansion of the nerve, with increased endoneural matrix and separation of nerve fascicles, combined with a proliferation of Schwann cells, fibroblasts and axons in a collagen-rich matrix (**Fig. 8.17B**). Immunohistochemistry for S-100 is helpful in establishing diagnosis. Marked cytologic and nuclear atypia should alert to the possibility of malignant transformation.

Management

Simple surgical excision of a solitary neurofibroma is curative. Whilst surgical excision of the multiple lesions in neurofibromatosis is often helpful, more extensive disease may render surgery difficult. Malignant transformation to a neurosarcoma is a sign of poor prognosis.

Schwannoma (Neurilemmoma)

Schwannoma is a common benign tumor of the Schwann cells of the nerve sheath (neurilemma), and up to 45 percent of all schwannomas affect the head and neck region. It can occur at any age (usually between 25–55 years), and has no particular gender predilection. The head and neck is a favored site for schwannomas; and when they arise in the oral cavity, the tongue is the most common site. The clinical presentation is usually that of an asymptomatic, slow-growing solitary nodule.

Histopathology

Unlike neurofibromas, schwannomas are encapsulated tumors with a biphasic growth pattern; the "Antoni A" pattern typically shows palisaded spindle cells, with parallel elongated nuclei, with "Antoni B" areas consisting of more haphazardly arranged spindle cells within a myxoid stroma. Palisadal areas contain prominent eosinophilic areas referred to as Verocay bodies (**Fig. 8.18**). S-100 protein is positive on immunohistochemistry.

Management

Surgical excision is curative; with recurrence unlikely.

Neuromas of the MEN Syndrome

The multiple endocrine neoplasia (MEN) syndromes are characterized by tumors of at least two endocrine glands. They are inherited in an autosomal dominant manner. MEN Type III (also known as MEN Type IIb) is characterized by medullary thyroid carcinoma, adrenal pheochromocytoma and multiple mucosal neuromas, which may involve the oral cavity. Mutation of the oncogene RET underlies the

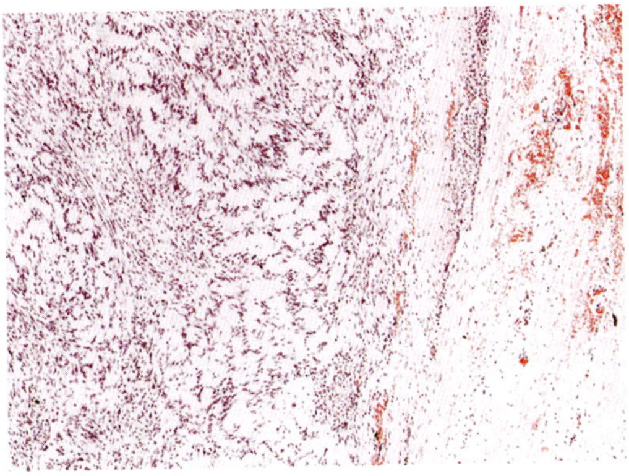

Fig. 8.18: Schwannoma showing characteristic a "Antoni A" pattern of palisaded spindle cells, with parallel elongated nuclei (Verocay body)

development of MEN Type III. Clinically, the mucosal neuromas in MEN Type III are small, multiple nodules that appear in childhood. Intraorally, the sites of predilection are the tongue, lips and buccal mucosa.

Histopathology

Microscopically, mucosal neuromas typically present as enlarged, tortuous nerve bundles in a myxoid stroma. Immunohistochemistry for S-100 is positive.

Management

The neuromas themselves are treated by simple surgical excision. However, in an undiagnosed individual, the onset of multiple neuromas is highly suggestive of MEN Type III and should alert the clinician to arrange for appropriate endocrine investigations for the other components of the syndrome.

Malignant Peripheral Nerve Sheath Tumor

Also referred to as malignant schwannoma or neurofibrosarcoma, the malignant peripheral nerve sheath tumor (MPNST) is a rare malignancy that is believed to be of Schwann cell origin. Intraorally, the sites most commonly affected are the tongue and soft palate. MPNSTs may arise *de novo*, or from malignant transformation of neurofibromas (particularly type 1 NF). Adults in the 3rd to 5th decade of life are most commonly affected. Whilst there is no particular gender predilection in *de novo* MPNSTs, those that arise on a background of type 1 NF seem to be more common in men, typically a decade or so earlier than in non-syndrome patients. Clinically, MPNSTs are usually slow-growing, and may present with pain or paresthesia, or with muscle atrophy and weakness.

Histopathology

The spindle cell arrangement can closely resemble that of fibrosarcomas, and as such differentiation on histological grounds may be difficult. The cells may have a wavy nuclear outline, and cellular and nuclear atypia is commonly pronounced, with high mitotic activity. The fascicles of cells are usually less organized than in fibrosarcoma. Immunohistochemistry usually reveals patchy positivity for S-100 protein. Other markers of nerve sheath differentiation such as Leu-7 and myelin basic protein are also useful.

Management

The MPNSTs are resistant to chemotherapy and radiotherapy, and wide surgical excision is the treatment of choice. Recurrences are common, and distant metastasis occurs in at least 50 percent of cases. Tumors associated with NF-1 behave more aggressively. Prognosis is dependent on the overall clinical, radiological and histological features at diagnosis, with a 5-year survival of 40 to 75 percent.

ADIPOSE TUMORS

Lipoma

Lipomas are benign neoplasms of fat cells. In the oral cavity, they most commonly arise on the buccal mucosa, tongue and floor of the mouth. Clinically, they present as a slow growing, asymptomatic soft mass, with an intact epithelial surface (**Fig. 8.19A**). On microscopy, the tumor presents as lobules of mature adipocytes separated by fine connective tissue (**Fig. 8.19B**). Simple surgical excision is curative with minimal likelihood of recurrence.

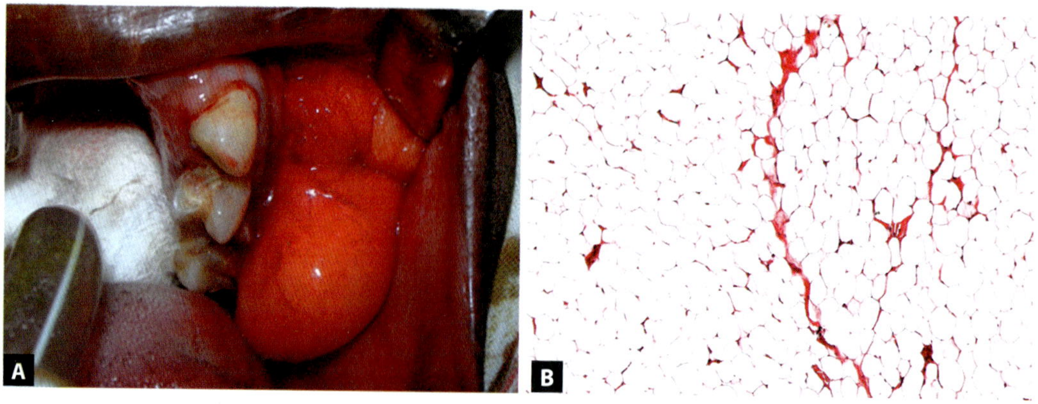

Figs 8.19A and B: Lipoma. (A) Circumscribed and yellowish lesion on the buccal mucosa; (B) Consisting of mature adipocytes separated by delicate connective tissue septa (*Courtesy*: Dr AM Attygalla)

Liposarcomas

Liposarcomas are rarely seen in the head and neck. They tend to present in middle age, most commonly affecting the tongue and buccal mucosa intraorally. Because of their tendency to grow slowly, they may be mistaken for a benign process. Several histological subtypes are recognized. The most common type affecting the head and neck is the well-differentiated (lipoma-like) variant. Histologically, this resembles a lipoma but is not encapsulated, shows greater variation in the size and shape of adipocytes, and contains scattered lipoblasts. Wide local excision is the treatment of choice, with post-operative radiotherapy considered if excision is incomplete or surgical margins are close. Recurrence is common, with 5-year survival rate for well-differentiated liposarcomas reported to be 85 to 100 percent (67% for all subtypes).

Muscle Tumors

Smooth muscle neoplasms are generally rare in the oral cavity. When they arise, they most commonly affect the tongue, hard palate and buccal mucosa, and are usually derived from vascular smooth muscle. They can present in any age group.

Leiomyomas

Leiomyomas are benign neoplasms that present clinically as generally asymptomatic, slow-growing masses. Histologically, they present as interlacing fascicles of spindle cells with elongated, cigar-shaped nuclei. The tumors are strongly immunoreactive for smooth muscle actin, and show variable desmin positivity. Leiomyomas are treated by conservative excision. Recurrence is rare.

Leiomyosarcomas

Leiomyosarcomas are malignant neoplasms that are exceedingly rare in the oral cavity. Although well-differentiated lesions resemble leiomyoma, atypical spindle cells can be found, and the tumors are more commonly composed of interlacing fascicles of pleomorphic, mitotically active spindle cells (**Fig. 8.20**). As with leiomyomas, immunohistochemistry for muscle markers, particularly smooth muscle actin, is helpful to distinguish them from other spindle cell malignancies. Treatment is by radical excision, sometimes with adjuvant chemotherapy or radiotherapy. The 5-year survival is 35 to 50 percent.

Rhabdomyomas

Rhabdomyomas are rare benign neoplasms of striated muscle, with a predilection for the head and neck. They are generally categorized into three subtypes: fetal, juvenile and adult. They are most frequent in the 5th to 6th decade of life, most commonly affecting the floor of the mouth, tongue and soft palate.

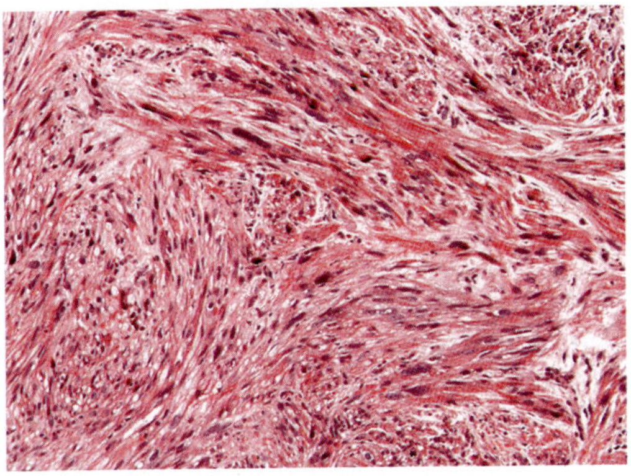

Fig. 8.20: Leiomyosarcoma. A malignant spindle cell tumor showing marked nuclear pleomorphism. Immunochemistry is required to distinguish this from other malignant spindle cell tumors

Histopathology

Adult rhabdomyomas characteristically are composed of large polygonal cells with abundant eosinophilic cytoplasms, closely resembling mature skeletal muscle cells. Indeed, cross-striations may be present (**Figs 8.21A and B**). Rhabdomyomas are positive for desmin, myoglobin and muscle-specific actin on immunohistochemistry.

Management

Treatment is by conservative excision. Recurrence is reported, but rare.

Rhabdomyosarcomas

Rhabdomyosarcomas are one of the most common soft tissue sarcomas of children and young adults. They are malignant tumors of skeletal muscles, generally divided into three types: embryonal (including botryoid), alveolar and pleomorphic. Around two-thirds of rhabdomyosarcomas arise in the head and neck, where they present as a rapidly growing mass. The embryonal subtype forms the majority of head and neck lesions. In the oral cavity, the tongue and soft palate are the most commonly affected sites. Botryoid rhabdomyosarcomas present as grape-like polypoid growths, which may cause obstruction.

Histopathology

The histological appearances vary according to subtype: embryonal rhabdomyosarcomas are composed of primitive mesenchymal cells of varying form (round, spindle and 'strap' cells). The strap cells are more differentiated, with brightly eosinophilic cytoplasm and cross-striations. Alveolar rhabdomyosarcoma (ARMS) is composed of nests of primitive round cells which are discohesive, producing a pseudoglandular appearance. ARMS are almost invariably associated with one of two chromosomal translocations: t(2;13) (q35;q14) found in around 80 percent of cases, or t(1;13) (p36;q14) in around 20 percent of cases. Pleomorphic rhabdomyosarcoma is composed

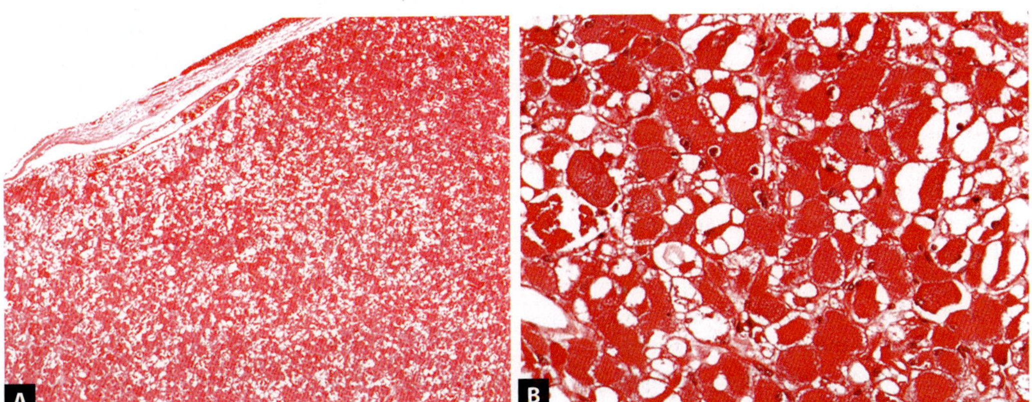

Figs 8.21A and B: Rhabdomyoma. The tumor is well-circumscribed and composed of large, eosinophilic polyhedral cells, with spider cells seen in places

of anaplastic, round to, —spindled tumor cells, showing high-grade features including frequent mitoses and necrosis. Immunochemical analysis for markers of skeletal muscle (desmin, myogenin, muscle-specific actin), as well as genetic analysis, are required for accurate diagnosis.

Management

The treatment regime consists of radical surgery followed by chemotherapy (usually a combination of vincristine, dactinomycin and cyclophosphamide). Postoperative radiotherapy may be used if complete surgical excision is not possible. The prognosis of rhabdomyosarcomas depends on the subtype with 5-year survivals of 66 percent (embryonal), 50 percent (alveolar) and < 30 percent (pleomorphic). Survival for botryoid subtypes is nearly 90 percent.

BONE TUMORS AND TUMOR-LIKE LESIONS

Tori and Exostoses

The term exostosis is used clinically to describe bony protuberances and outgrowths of mature bone. The precise name given to an exostosis is usually in reference to its site of occurrence. Thus, torus mandibularis and torus palatinus are bony exostoses that arise in the mandible and the palate, respectively. These are entirely benign lesions, which are generally asymptomatic. The etiology is unknown but some studies have demonstrated a possible autosomal dominant mode of inheritance in some patients.

Torus palatinus presents clinically as a nodular, bony mass in the midline of the hard palate. It is more common in females than males, and usually presents in young adulthood. Torus mandibularis usually arises on the lingual surface of the mandible in the premolar area, above the mylohyoid ridge. It is almost always bilateral. Bony exostoses may present in other sites in the oral cavity; for example on the posterior maxillary buccal alveolar ridge, where they are often multiple.

Histology

Exostoses are typically composed of dense lamellar bone with small marrow spaces filled with fibrofatty tissue.

Management

Tori and exostoses are generally asymptomatic, and thus require no treatment unless the overlying mucosa is frequently traumatized, or if the lesions interfere with dental prostheses. In these instances, surgical excision is the treatment of choice, with recurrence generally rare.

Osteoma

Osteomas are benign neoplasms of bone. They consist of mature bone of either the compact or cancellous type. Periosteal osteomas arise on the outer surface of bone, whilst endosteal osteomas are within the bone. The etiology is relatively unknown, but it is thought that previous trauma or infection may contribute to the pathogenesis. Although osteomas present frequently in the head and neck, particularly the paranasal sinuses, they are rarer in the jaws. Clinically, an osteoma presents as a slow-growing, solitary hard mass, more commonly in the mandible than the maxilla. Multiple osteomas occur as part of Gardner's syndrome.

Gardner's Syndrome

Gardner's syndrome is a rare autosomal dominant familiar disorder characterized by multiple osteomas of the jaws (particularly the mandible), intestinal polyps and epidermoid cysts. Dental anomalies such as multiple supernumerary and impacted teeth and odontomes may also be present. The polyps arise most commonly in the colon and have a high-risk of malignant transformation to adenocarcinoma.

Histopathology

Osteomas are broadly classified into two types. The compact type consists of mature, dense lamellar bone with few marrow spaces, similar in appearance to exostoses. The cancellous type consists of lamellar trabeculae with fibrofatty marrow.

Management

Surgical excision of an osteoma is curative. The presence of multiple osteomas raises the possibility of Gardner's syndrome, especially since they may precede the onset of the other features of the syndrome.

Osteochondroma

Osteochondromas consist of a mixture of cartilage and bone. Whether or not they are a true neoplastic process or merely representative of aberrant cartilage growth on a bony surface is unknown. In the head and neck, osteochondromas have been reported in the jaws (particularly the mandibular condyle), as well as in the sinuses and skull bones.

Histopathology

On microscopy, the osteochondroma consists of chondrocytes forming a cartilaginous cap on top of, and in direct contact with the medullary cavity of a bony stalk.

Osteoblastoma

Osteoblastomas present rarely in the mandible or the maxilla. Osteoblastomas are twice as common in men, than women and the majority are diagnosed before the age of 30. Dull, occasionally severe pain often accompanies the lesion, which usually presents as a localized swelling. Radiographically, the lesions are well-circumscribed with an occasionally sclerosed margin and a mixed radiolucent and radio-paque center.

Histopathology

Osteoblastomas are composed of thin, irregular bone trabeculae in a fibrous, highly vascular stroma. Osteoblasts line the trabeculae, with numerous osteoclasts also present. The cortical bone is intact, and nuclei are generally bland with no atypia; which help distinguish this tumor from osteosarcoma.

Management

Surgical excision or curettage is curative.

Soft tissue tumors with any odontogenic origin, e.g. Cemento-ossifying fibromas are covered in Chapter 7.

Osteosarcoma

Osteosarcoma refers to a heterogenous group of malignant bone tumors that have histopathological evidence of osteogenic differentiation, but differ in their location, clinical behavior and pathological appearance. The most commonly occurring conventional (or classical) osteosarcoma, arises within the bone and can be subdivided into osteoblastic, chondroblastic and fibroblastic variants depending on the predominant cell type and matrix formed (bone, cartilage or fibrous). Conventional osteosarcoma needs to be distinguished from the centrally occurring low-grade intramedullary osteosarcoma and the subperiostially occurring parosteal osteosarcoma; both have better prognosis. There are also several other histological variants.

Osteosarcoma most often affects appendicular bones and is relatively rare in the jaws, with the mandible more commonly affected. Elsewhere in the body, osteosarcomas present during childhood and adolescence, but in the jaws they tend to present later in the 3rd and 4th decades of life. Osteosarcomas of the jaw can arise *de novo* or on the background of a pre-existing condition, such as Paget's disease or as a complication of radiotherapy. Syndromes associated with an increased risk of osteosarcoma include hereditary retinoblastoma and Li-Fraumeni syndrome.

Osteosarcomas present as painful swellings associated with tooth displacement, mobility and loss (**Fig. 8.22A**). Paresthesia may also be present, particularly when the inferior alveolar nerve is affected. Maxillary osteosarcomas may be associated with nasal obstruction, sinus symptoms and visual disturbances.

Radiographic features of osteosarcoma are variable. Early lesions present with symmetrically widened periodontal ligament spaces and localized bone resorption around involved dental structures. Foci of radiolucency or

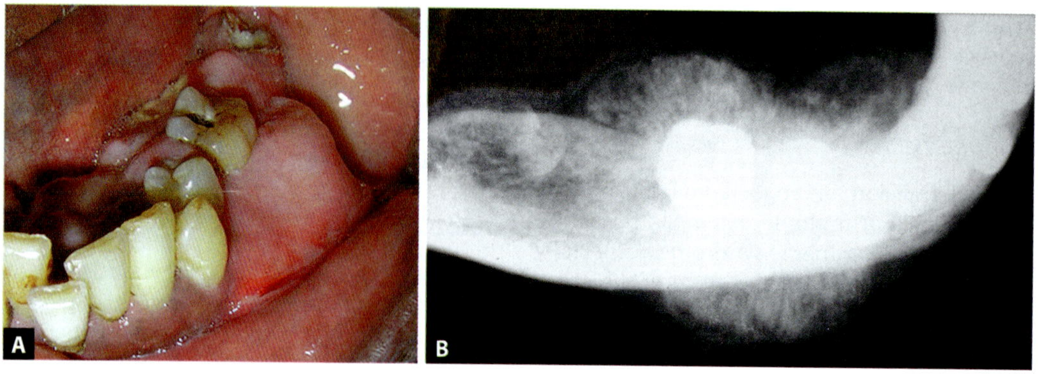

Figs 8.22A and B: Osteosarcoma. (A) Mandibular lesion showing involvement of both buccal and lingual plates; (B) Radiograph shows characteristic sun-ray appearance (*Courtesy*: Dr AM Attygalla)

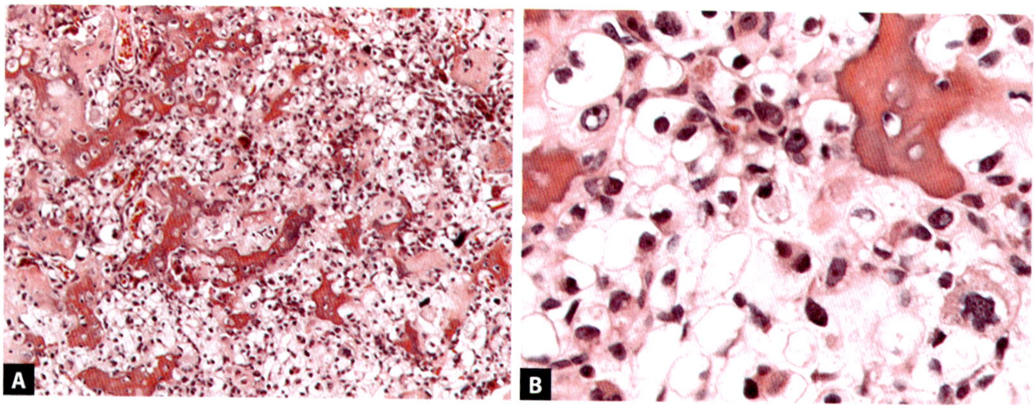

Figs 8.23A and B: Osteosarcoma (osteoblastic subtype) consisting of pleomorphic, osteoid-forming osteoblasts

radio-opacity may be present, depending on the degree of calcification within the tumor. Advanced tumors exhibit an irregular, moth-eaten radiographic appearance with ragged radio-opacities. The classic "sun-ray" appearance of osteosarcomas is seen when tumorous bone formation radiates outward from the affected periosteum, but this is not a diagnostic feature (**Fig. 8.22B**).

Histopathology

Most jaw tumors are of the classical type. Tumors are composed of a sarcomatous stroma containing malignant osteoblasts, which give rise to osteoid, the unmineralized precursor of bone. Malignant osteoblasts have a variable appearance and may appear spindled, epithelioid, polygonal or round. Tumors often have a heterogeneous appearance with osteoblastic, chondroblastic and fibroblastic elements all present, and tumors arbitrarily designated as osteoblastic, chondroblastic or fibroblastic depending on the predominant type of extracellular matrix present (**Figs 8.23A and B**).

Management

Osteosarcomas of the jaws behave differently to those of long bones; the major complication is local recurrence, with metastasis often a late stage event. Surgery is therefore the main treatment for osteosarcoma, with wide, *en bloc* resection recommended. This may be combined

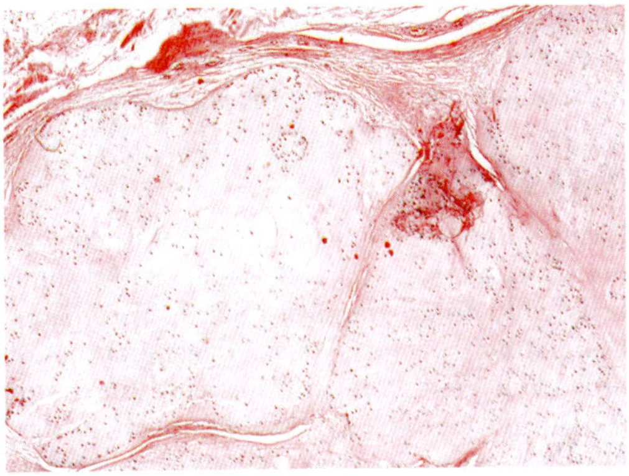

Fig. 8.24: Chondroma consisting of well-defined lobules of mature cartilage

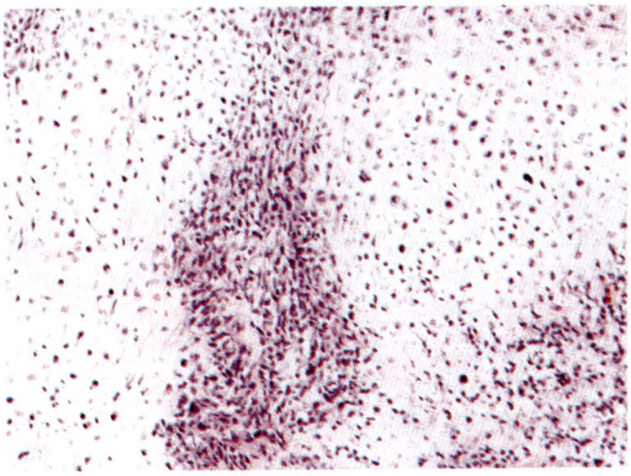

Fig. 8.25: Chondrosarcoma consisting of pleomorphic chondrocytes forming a myxochondroid matrix

with neoadjuvant or adjuvant chemotherapy. The role of chemotherapy is currently unclear in jaw tumors, but patients with high-grade tumors may benefit. Adjuvant radiotherapy is advocated for tumors which have been incompletely excised. The 5-year survival rate is around 60 to 80 percent.

CARTILAGE-FORMING TUMORS

Chondroma

Chondromas are benign tumors of cartilage that present rarely in the head and neck. In the jaws, they tend to favor the anterior maxilla and the coronoid and condylar processes of the mandible. They are mostly diagnosed in the 5th decade of life. They present as radiolucencies on radiography, with occasional foci of radio-opacity within.

Histopathology

Chondromas consist of bland, well-lobulated mature hyaline cartilage (**Fig. 8.24**). The chondrocytes show no atypical features and nuclei are well-defined. Chondromas can be difficult to distinguish from well-differentiated chondrosarcomas, and as such all chondromas should be viewed with a high index of suspicion.

Management

Surgical excision is the treatment of choice, with minimal likelihood of recurrence. A recurring chondroma should alert to revisiting the original diagnosis.

Chondrosarcoma

Chondrosarcomas are malignancies of cartilage origin. Similar to osteosarcomas, they are a heterogeneous group of tumors. Clinical behavior is variable; over 90 percent are low-to-intermediate grade tumors, which grow slowly and have a low incidence of metastasis. Though generally rare in the jaws, they are most common in the anterior maxilla, followed by the mandibular condyle and coronoid processes. They tend to present in adulthood and middle age, and have no particular gender predilection. There is a 25 to 30 percent risk of chondrosarcoma developing in Ollier's disease and Maffucci's syndrome. The clinical presentation is that of a painful swelling with associated tooth mobility and paresthesia. Metastasis is uncommon. Radiographic features are variable, usually presenting as an ill-defined, mottled radiolucency.

Histopathology

Chondrosarcomas usually contain hyaline-type cartilage containing chondrocytes that have enlarged nuclei (**Fig 8.25**). Chondosarcomas are usually hypercellular, and the degree of cellularity increases with tumor grade. High-grade lesions contain pleomorphic cells with large, atypical nuclei. The finding of mitotic activity in any cartilage lesion is suggestive of malignancy. However, mitoses are not invariably present even in high-grade tumors.

Management

Chondrosarcomas tend to recur and wide surgical resection to achieve clear margins is required, particularly since chondrosarcoma infiltrates between normal bone trabeculae. Tumors are generally radioresistant, although proton beam therapy has been successfully used. Prognosis depends primarily on adequate excision with reported five-year survival rates of 43 to 95 percent.

OTHER TUMORS OF BONE

Hemangiomas

Intrabony hemangiomas, like soft tissue hemangiomas, are hamartomatous proli-ferations of blood vessels. When they arise in the jaws, they present most commonly in the posterior mandible. The female to male ratio is 2:1, and they are normally detected in the first two decades of life. They present as firm, slowly growing, expansile alveolar lesions. Gingival bleeding from associated teeth is an occasional feature, in addition to pain and tooth mobility. Radiographic examination reveals a multilocular swelling with a characteristic soap-bubble appearance and resorption of roots within the lesion.

Ewing's Sarcoma

Ewing's sarcoma is a poorly differentiated neuroectodermal tumor closely related to the primitive neuroectodermal tumor (PNET). Less than 3 percent of Ewing's sarcomas arise in the maxillofacial region, most commonly the mandibular ramus. They have a slight male predilection and generally present in adolescents and young adults, with 90 percent occurring in patients under 30 years of age. The clinical presentation is that of a painful mass that may be associated with mucosal ulceration, loosening of teeth and facial deformity. Systemic symptoms include leukocytosis and elevated temperature. Radiographic features showing irregular, moth-eaten radio-opacities are generally non-specific, and can mimic an infective process. Periosteal reaction can result in an onion-skin radiographic appearance.

Histopathology

Ewing's sarcoma is composed of sheets of uniform, densely packed small round blue cells with finely granular nuclear chromatin. Geographic necrosis and degeneration of individual cells is frequently present. The tumor cells are positive for CD99 by immunochemistry. FISH is used to demonstrate the characteristic chromosomal translocation t(11;22)(q24;q12) resulting in the fusion of the EWS and FLI-1 genes, which is found in more than 90 percent of cases.

Management

Treatment is by wide surgical resection with neoadjuvant multi-agent chemotherapy. Chemotherapeutic agents include vincristine, doxorubicin, etoposide, cyclophosphamide and ifosfamide. Five-year survival rates have improved to over 65 percent.

Langerhans Cell Histiocytosis

Formerly known as Histiocytosis X, Langerhans cell histiocytosis is a rare spectrum of diseases characterized by a monoclonal proliferation of bone marrow-derived Langerhans cells. It can present in isolation, or in disseminated, multi-organ form. The term "histiocytosis X" was used previously to encompass eosinophilic granuloma (solitary disease), Hand-Schüller-Christian syndrome (triad of skull defects, exophthalmus and diabetes insipidus) and Letterer-Siwe syndrome (systemic disease with fever, otitis media, hepatosplenomegaly, lymphadenopathy, bone and cutaneous lesions). Many cases do not fit into these rigid categories, and a more useful categorization incorporates unifocal disease, multifocal unisystem disease and multifocal multisystem disease.

Langerhans cell histiocytosis presents mostly in the 2nd or 3rd decade of life, and has a male predilection. It has a tendency to favor the skull bones, but can present in any bone. Mucosal and cutaneous involvement in the head and neck are common. Mucosal swelling, ulceration and loose teeth are common symptoms when it presents in the oral cavity. Radiographic appearance shows solitary or multiple osteolytic lesions, with loss of alveolar bone (with involved teeth appearing to "float in space") and occasionally, severe destruction of the jaw bones. However, radiographic appearance can also be relatively inconspicuous, with minimal, periapical bone loss mimicking inflammatory dental lesions.

Histopathology

On microscopy, Langerhans cell histiocytosis is characterized by the proliferation of Langerhans cells with characteristic reniform nuclei and indented nuclear membranes, arranged in sheets or clusters (**Fig. 8.26**). An inflammatory infiltrate composed mainly of eosinophils, lymphocytes and polymorphonuclear leukocytes is also usually present. Multinuclear giant cells may occasionally be seen. Electron microscopy of Langerhans cells shows characteristic rod-shaped granules (Birbeck bodies) within the cytoplasm. Langerhans cells are positive for S-100 protein and CD1a antigen on immunohistochemistry.

Management

Treatment varies depending on the location and extent of disease. Solitary lesions are generally managed by curettage and low-dose radiation therapy, and usually have a good prognosis. Involved teeth are sacrificed at surgery. Long-term follow-up to monitor for recurrent or additional disease is essential. Multifocal disease generally requires more aggressive treatment, with corticosteroids, chemotherapy and immunosuppressive therapy frequently used in addition to surgery. Acute, disseminated disease generally has a poor prognosis.

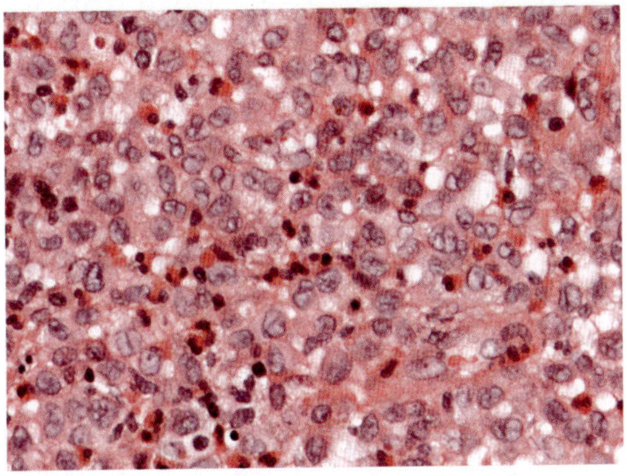

Fig. 8.26: Langerhans cell histiocytosis composed of Langerhans cells with characteristic reniform nuclei and indented nuclear membranes, arranged in sheets or clusters. An inflammatory infiltrate of eosinophils is present

Myeloma

Myeloma is a plasma cell dyscrasia that generally presents as a disseminated disease affecting multiple bones (multiple myeloma), although it may also occur as a solitary lesion (plasmacytoma). It is characterized by the neoplastic expansion of a clone of immunoglobulin-producing plasma cells, and in most patients by the presence of monoclonal gammaglobulins in the serum (most commonly IgG). Multiple myeloma most commonly affects the skull, vertebrae, sternum, ribs and pelvic bones. Around 14 percent of patients have oral involvement, and it is most commonly diagnosed in the 5th to 6th decade of life. The radiographic appearance of multiple myeloma shows multiple, well-demarcated, punched-out radiolucencies producing the so-called 'pepper-pot' skull appearance. By definition, bone marrow aspiration must show at least 10 percent plasma cells to fulfil the diagnostic criteria of myeloma. In addition to high levels of immunoglobulin in serum, immunoglobulin fragments can also pass in urine (Bence-Jones protein).

The disease symptoms present as organs are infiltrated by malignant plasma cells. Thus, bone pain and pathological fractures can be seen. Anemia, thrombocytopenia and leukopenia as a result of bone marrow infiltration can lead to bleeding problems and susceptibility to infections. Hypercalcemia and renal failure are possible sequelae of advanced disease.

Myeloma presents more commonly in the mandible than the maxilla. Pain, paresthesia and loosening of involved teeth may present, in addition to mucosal swellings and intraoral ulceration may occur. Myeloma is frequently complicated by amyloidosis (Chapter 17).

Solitary plasmacytoma and extramedullary plasmacytoma (arising outside the bone) are rare, but they mostly arise in the head and neck region. They can present as swellings in the oral cavity. Immunohistochemical analysis shows heavy and light chain positivity.

Histopathology

Myeloma is composed of sheets of neoplastic plasma cells with minimal supporting stroma. Cell morphology can be strikingly similar to normal plasma cells. Immunohistochemical stains for plasma cell markers (CD138) and also kappa (κ) and lambda (λ) immunoglobulin light chains to confirm antibody restriction (i.e. monoclonality), should be undertaken when a diagnosis of myeloma is suspected.

Management

The management of myeloma is dependent on symptoms, and is by chemotherapy. Bone marrow transplantation is an option in selected cases. Due to the chronic, progressive nature of the disease, careful monitoring is essential.

Metastatic Tumors

An estimated 1 percent of neoplasms are thought to metastasize to the jaws, the majority of those presenting in mandible. The most common neoplasms that spread to the jaws are breast, lung, prostate, colorectal and renal carcinomas. The primary mode of metastasis to the jaws is via the hematogenous route, with most patients being middle-aged and female. Clinically, the angle and body of the mandible are most frequently affected, with swelling, pain, paresthesia and tooth mobility all being potential symptoms. Radiographic appearance can be variable and nonspecific, with some metastases presenting as irregular, moth-eaten radiolucencies, and others exhibiting an osteoblastic appearance.

Histopathology

Metastatic tumor deposits can show great variability histologically, dependent on their tissue of origin. Immunohistochemical analysis is often helpful in determining the site of the primary tumor.

Management

Further investigations to determine the extent of metastatic disease is important. Often, jaw metastasis is representative of more disseminated disease and thus the prognosis is generally poor.

SELF-ASSESSMENT QUESTIONS

1. List the common reactive connective tissue lesions that occur in the oral cavity.
2. How does a reactive lesion differ from a neoplastic one?
3. Discuss the role of radiographs in the diagnosis of a giant cell epulis (giant cell granuloma)?
4. List the common benign tumors affecting the oral cavity.
5. What are the clinical symptoms and signs that are more likely to be found in malignant tumors?
6. Describe two hamartomatous "vascular tumors" occurring in the head and neck.
7. Name and describe two syndromes that may be associated with oral neural tumors.
8. Describe the clinical presentation, histopathology and management of two hematological malignancies that can affect the jaws.
9. How do osteosarcomas of the oral cavity differ from osteosarcomas of the axial skeleton?
10. List the most common metastatic cancers of the jaws and describe the clinical and radiographic features of such tumors.

SUGGESTED READING

1. Bennett JH, Thomas G, Evans AW, Speight PM. Osteosarcoma of the jaws: a 30-year retrospective review. Oral Surg Oral Med Oral Pathol. 2000;90: 323-333.
2. Fletcher CDM. Distinctive soft tissue tumors of the head and neck. Mod Pathol. 2002;15:324–30
3. Jordan RC, Regezi AJ. Oral spindle cell neoplasms: a review of 307 cases. Oral Surg Oral Med Oral Path Oral Radiol Endod. 2003;95:717-24.
4. Mendenhall WM, Fernandes R, Werning JW, Vaysberg M, Malyapa RS, Mendenhall

NP. Head and neck osteosarcoma. Am J Otolaryngol. 2010 [Epub ahead of print]
5. Nowparast B, Howell FV, Rick GM. Verruciform xanthoma: a clinicopathologic review and report of fifty-four cases. Oral Surg Oral Med Oral Pathol. 1981;51:619-25.
6. Peters E, Cohen M, Altini M, Murray J. Rhabdomyosarcoma of the oral and paraoral region. Cancer. 1989;63:963-6.
7. The Pathology and Genetics of Head and Neck Tumors (World Health Organisation Classification of Tumors). Barnes L, Eveson JW, Reichart P, Sidransky D (Eds). IARC Press. 2005.
8. Vered M, Allon I, Buchner A, Dayan D. Clinicopathologic correlations of myofibroblastic tumors of the oral cavity. I. Nodular fasciitis. J Oral Pathol Med. 2007;34:426-35.
9. Vered M, Allon I, Buchner A, Dayan D. Clinicopathologic correlations of myofibroblastic tumors of the oral cavity. II. Myofibroma and myofibromatosis of the oral soft tissues. J Oral Pathol Med. 2007;36:304-14.
10. Wright BA, Jackson D. Neural tumors of the oral cavity: a review of the spectrum of benign and malignant oral tumors of the oral cavity and jaws. Oral Surg Oral Med Oral Pathol. 1980;49:509-22.

Chapter 9

Diseases of the Maxillary Antrum

Philip McLoughlin

Chapter Outline

INTRODUCTION

The maxillary sinus is found in the body of the maxilla which lies directly above the oral cavity. The size of the sinuses varies and right and left may even be different in the same skull. As it has a close relationship to the mouth many of the disorders affecting the maxillary sinus may manifest in the oral cavity and *vice versa.*

GROWTH AND ANATOMY OF THE MAXILLARY SINUSES

The maxillary sinus is the first paranasal sinus to form. At around the 70th day of gestation a small ridge develops just above the inferior turbinate bone. Shortly after an evagination starts just above this ridge and enlarges laterally from the nasal cavity. At birth a rudimentary sinus is present measuring approximately 7 × 4 × 4 mm with its longest dimension in the anteroposterior axis. From birth the growth rate of the maxillary sinus is estimated to be 2 mm vertically and 3 mm anteroposteriorly each year. At the end of the first year of life the lateral margin of the sinus extends under the medial portion of the orbit. By the 9th year the lateral sinus margin extends to the malar bone and the lateral growth ceases by the 15th year. By 8 years of age the maxillary sinus floor is at the level of the nasal floor. There is, however, some variation in growth after this time. If the sinus continues a downward growth pattern it reaches the plane of the hard palate by 12 years of age. The final downward growth of the sinus, however, does not cease until the third molar has erupted. In 20 percent of adults the most dependent part of the maxillary sinus is above the nasal cavity floor, 15 percent of it lies at the same level as the nasal floor and below the level of the nasal floor in 65 percent of adults. Growth anomalies occur in about 10 percent of people, usually in the form of hypoplasia. Hypoplasia of the maxillary sinus results from trauma, infection, surgical intervention or irradiation during the development of the bone. Underdevelopment is also a feature of second branchial arch anomalies as in Treacher Collins syndrome and mandibulofacial dysostosis. In thalassemia major, the demand for bone marrow is so great that the maxillary sinus often fails to pneumatise.

The maxillary sinus lies within the body of the maxilla, the most superior point being directly beneath the orbital apex. The anterior sinus wall is the facial surface of the maxilla with the infraorbital foramen perforating this about 1cm below the orbital rim. The floor of the sinus is lowest near the second premolar and first molar teeth and usually lies 3 to 5 mm below the nasal floor. Occasionally tooth roots of premolar, and less commonly canine teeth, project into the antrum. Sometimes there is dehiscent bone over the tooth roots such that they are separated from the main sinus cavity by sinus mucosa only. The maxillary sinus ostia is located high on the medial wall, drainage is through the ethmoid infundibulum and then into the nasal fossa. This path of drainage is necessarily aided and accomplished by intact ciliary action of cilia located in the maxillary sinus lining epithelium (**Box 9.1**).

Box 9.1: Anatomy and physiology

Key features helpful in diagnosis

- The maxillary sinus is closely related to dental roots and the orbit and its contents
- In the majority of adults the most dependent part of the sinus is below the nasal floor
- Ciliary action is necessary for normal sinus drainage
- Hypoplasia is a common abnormality

ACUTE AND CHRONIC MAXILLARY SINUSITIS

Sinusitis is a common disease in the oral and maxillofacial region. In order to understand the disease, thorough knowledge about anatomy of the maxillary sinus and other paranasal sinuses are exceptionally important.

Etiological factors

Maxillary sinusitis has over a dozen described etiologies, ranging from the well-known IgE mediated hay fever affecting sinus mucosa, to the involvement in systemic diseases such as cystic fibrosis and Wegener's granulomatosis. However, over 90 percent of established maxillary sinusitis is of infective origin and the pathology and pathogenesis is remarkably similar irrespective of the causative agent. Although unremitting sinusitis may raise the question of a more sinister underlying pathology.

A variety of infective agents can affect the sinonasal mucosa, causing acute or chronic inflammation with, or without secondary polyp formation. A large number of tissue neutrophils is a good lead to this possibility.

The most commonly implicated viruses are rhinoviruses, parainfluenza and influenza viruses, adenoviruses and respiratory syncytial virus. The onset of mucopurulent discharge means that secondary bacterial infection has occurred as a result of obstruction of the sinus ostium by swollen nasal mucosa. Decreasing sinus aeration results in lower oxygen availability, and an alteration of the normal resident flora culminating in acute bacterial sinusitis. Clinically, this manifests as facial pain centerd over the maxilla, worsened by stooping. If left unchecked the infection can spread becoming a pansinusitis with more paranasal sinuses involved and rarely, lead to secondary intracranial involvement.

Clinicopathological and radiological features

In cases of noncomplicated viral infections, maxillary sinus imaging is usually normal or shows minimal sinus mucosal thickening. In overt bacterial colonization with pyogenic strains, mucosal thickening with a fluid level may be evident (**Figs 9.1A and B**). Plain radiography is non-specific under these circumstances and computerized tomography is the standard investigation (**Figs 9.2A and B**). Direct sinus puncture will produce the best bacterial cultures. The most commonly implicated pathogens are *Streptococcus pneumoniae, Haemophilus influenzae, and* alpha-hemolytic streptococci, with less commonly *Staphylococcus aureus* and *Pseudomonas* strains being isolated. In cases of chronic sinusitis with persistent low sinus, oxygen availability anaerobes predominate including *peptostreptococci, Bacteroides spp.,* and *fusobacteria.* It is estimated that 10 to 20 percent of maxillary sinus infections are secondary to dental infection or secondary to tooth extraction.

As acute bacterial sinusitis results from sinus ostial obstruction, it presents as an isolated event rather than a generalized process, so the most common picture is a unilateral sinusitis rather than a pansinusitis. Even when both maxillary antra are involved one side is generally more severely affected, asymmetry being the hallmark of bacterial disease. On the other hand, pansinusitis is usually found in patients with an allergic sinusitis, because the allergic process is a systemic rather than truly local event.

Chronic sinusitis results from either persistent acute inflammation **(Fig. 9.3)** or repeated bouts of acute sinusitis. Up to one third of patients with acute sinusitis go on to develop the chronic form of the disease. Such chronic disease results in an atrophic, sclerosing, or hypertrophied polypoid mucosa, although

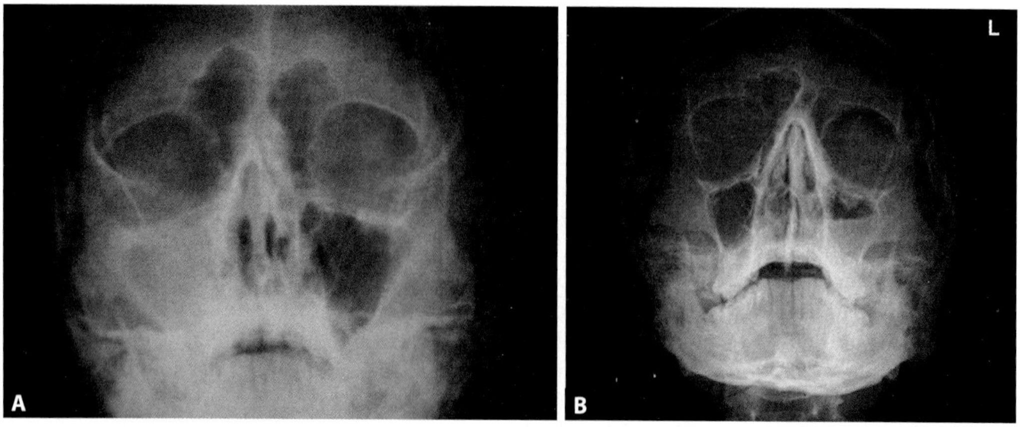

Figs 9.1A and B: (A) Occipitomental plain radiograph of a patient with mucosal thickening in acute right maxillary sinusitis; (B) Fluid level in right maxillary sinus. (*Courtesy:* Dr Jimmy Makdissi)

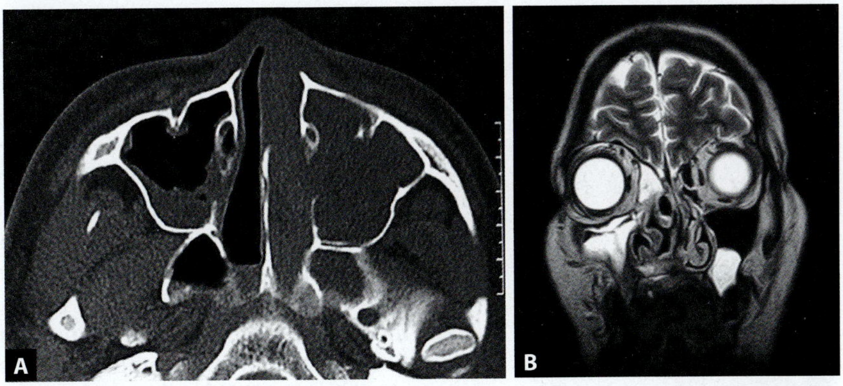

Figs 9.2A and B: (A) Axial CT cut showing profound left maxillary sinusitis, but with involvement of the right side in addition. Opacity of the sphenoid sinuses implies a pansinusitis; (B) MRI appearance of right maxillary sinusitis

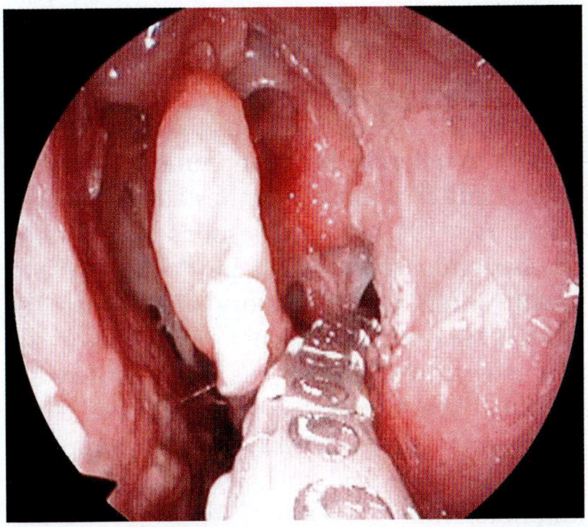

Fig. 9.3: Endoscopic nasal view showing inflamed and thickened nasal and sinus mucosa, the sinus ostium is being surgically widened for improved drainage

these varied changes may coexist. Ciliary function in chronically inflamed and scarred mucosa becomes less than optimal rendering it vulnerable to further infection, the reinfection cycle so often seen in this condition. Reactive bone is found in the chronically inflamed sinus wall being the periosteal reaction to inflammation, thick sclerotic new bone may be the result consolidating the ostial blockage.

Occasionally, the chronically inflamed mucosa develops a papillary hyperplasia, resulting in the so titled papillary hyperplastic sinusitis, which can be confused histologically with a low grade intestinal type adenocarcinoma, both may show a lining of a single layer of columnar epithelium with goblet cells and the low grade adenocarcinoma often displays very little pleomorphism. Close clinical and pathological correlation is advised. The history of sinusitis, lack of tumor mass and chronically inflamed lamina propria indicate hyperplastic maxillary sinusitis rather than the malignant alternative.

Treatment

Acute bacterial sinusitis usually resolves with an appropriate course of an antibiotic. The insidious chronic disease more often dictates surgical intervention.

Open approaches to the maxillary sinus were first described in the early 1700s. The wellknown Caldwell-Luc operation (**Fig. 9.4**) was first described in the United States by George Walter Caldwell in 1893 and then by Henri Luc of France in 1897. Subsequent advances in the understanding of the physiologic drainage pattern of the maxillary sinus led to intranasal middle meatus antrostomy in the late 1960s and the early 1970s. Functional endoscopic sinus surgery (FESS) is based on the surgical approach performed by Messerklinger and Wigand in Europe via the ostiomeatal complex. FESS has become the standard surgical treatment for chronic maxillary sinusitis, with external approaches being used as an adjunct in more complicated cases or in tumor management (**Box 9.2**).

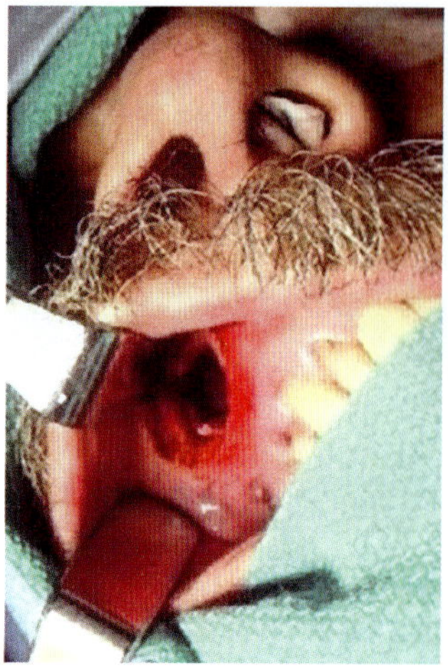

Fig. 9.4: Intraoperative photograph showing the traditional Caldwell-Luc access to the maxillary sinus

Box 9.2: Acute and chronic sinusitis

Key features helpful in diagnosis

- The most common etiology in acute sinusitis is bacterial infection.
- Plain radiographic imaging may be unhelpful and CT should be used
- Chronic sinusitis results from prolonged osteomeatal blockage and compromised ciliary action
- Surgical treatment is usually performed using a functional endoscopic technique

FUNGAL INFECTIONS OF THE MAXILLARY SINUSES

Aspergillosis

Clinical and Pathological Features

Seven pathogenic species are generally implicated, of these *Aspergillus fumigatus* accounts for 90 percent of cases, the remainder attributable to *A. niger* and *A. flavus. A. flavus* is particularly prevalent in the Middle-East and especially parts of Saudi Arabia. Aspergillosis infection of the maxillary sinuses is indeed a global infection, occurring worldwide and at any age. It is a filamentous fungus found naturally in soil and dried grass and decaying food.

Aspergillosis of the maxillary sinus is considered to occur in three identifiable forms:

i. Noninvasive; either as an aspergilloma or allergic in type.
ii. Semi-invasive; being locally destructive without true invasion.
iii. Invasive; representing true fungal tissue invasion which can be either nonfulminant or fulminant in nature.

Noninvasive aspergillosis results in the formation of an aspergilloma (fungus ball) which behaves and mimics chronic sinusitis, indeed suspicion should be aroused of aspergillosis in a refractory case of maxillary sinus infection. The characteristic feature is a gray/brown exudate within the maxillary sinus cavity. Calcification, visible as deposits on radiographs may occur. Histological sections show the presence of numerous large branching and septate fungal hyphae **(Figs 9.5A and B)**.

Allergic *Aspergillus* sinusitis is similar in nature to allergic bronchopulmonary aspergillosis and is a mixed manifestation of a type I and type III immune responses generated by *Aspergillus* antigens. It particularly affects young adults with a history of asthma. The sinus is filled with thick mucus as well as crystal like structures known as Charcot-Leydun crystals. The diagnosis in each case is by microscopy and treatment with an appropriate course of antifungal such as ketoconazole or amphotericin.

The uncommon invasive aspergillosis is very much like a malignant neoplasm which spreads to invade adjacent structures, even involving soft tissues. Proptosis of the eye may be a presenting feature and progression is slow with bone destruction often seen radiographically. Serological tests for aspergillosis antigens are usually positive. In its fulminant form aspergillosis is a rapidly progressive, destructive infection with a significant mortality usually affecting immunocompromised patients. Intracranial extension is not uncommon and may affect 20 percent of those with fulminant disease. The types of maxillary sinus aspergillosis (listed above) not confined entities but represent a progressive spectrum of the disease. It is also described as a range of disease activity, with early stage disease which may then progress to an invasive form over a period of time.

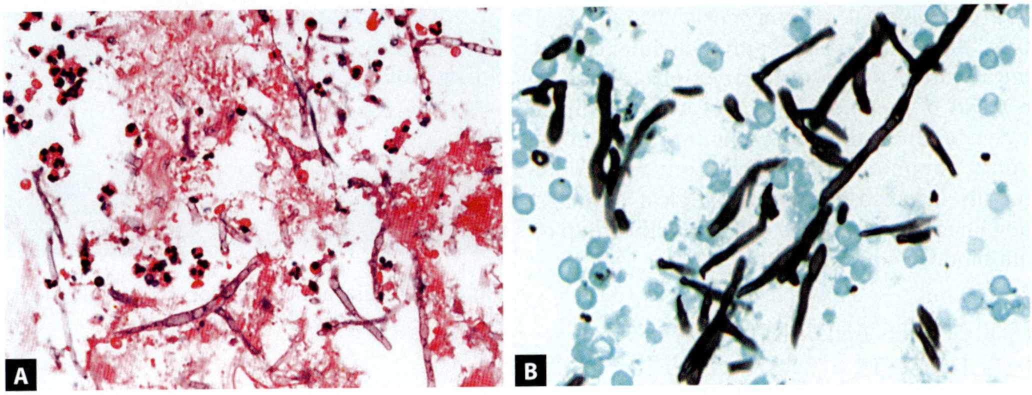

Figs 9.5A and B: Aspergillosis. (A) Branching and septate fungal hyphae in a H&E section; (B) Grocott stain showing hyphae in black color

The invasive form usually arises *de novo,* in immunocompromised patients.

Treatment

The noninvasive disease requires surgical debridement and sinus ventilation. Adjuvant antifungal agents may be needed in the semi-invasive phase. Allergic aspergillosis responds to antifungal agents and local corticosteroids if mild, but may require surgical debridement and systemic steroids in more severe cases.

Invasive and fulminant forms require more radical resective surgery with systemic antifungal agents such as amphotericin or ketoconazole (**Box 9.3**).

Box 9.3: Fungal infections of the maxillary sinuses

Key features helpful in diagnosis

- Aspergillosis represents a spectrum of disease from indolent to fulminating and invasive
- An allergic form of aspergillosis particularly affects young adults with a history of asthma
- Invasive aspergillosis invades bone and may extend into the orbit and intracranially
- There is a significant mortality in the immunocompromised
- Less commonly sinusitis may be due to blastomycosis, cryptococcosis or actinomycosis.

Blastomycosis

This is an uncommon fungal infection of the maxillary sinus caused by *Blastomyces dermatidis.* This fungus is again found endemically in soil, which produces spores that are readily inhaled. The spores can cause an intense inflammatory reaction and readily affects the nasal cavity and maxillary sinuses. However, the most affected organs are the lungs. Today the disease is almost confined to certain parts of North America particularly Ohio and Mississippi. Rarely does a disseminated blastomycosis supervene, usually in the immunocompromised, where the outcome can be fatal. The disease most often presents as a chronic maxillary sinusitis and responds to oral antifungal agents such as Amphotericin.

Cryptococcosis

This is caused by the inhalation of yeast like fungus, *Cryptococcus neoformans.* The fungus is found in bird excreta. It usually presents as pansinusitis with nasal ulceration. Treatment with antifungal agents most often results in complete resolution.

Actinomycosis

Human infection is by *Actinomyces israelii.* In the head and neck, the usual presentation is a cervicofacial actinomycosis. Trauma is a potential initiating factor although other causes are reported in the maxillary sinus, either as a result of hematogenous spread or as direct extension from the oral cavity through an oral antral communication after tooth extraction; in this instance it requires surgical drainage and an appropriate dose of a penicillin group of antibiotic or equivalent (**Box 9.3**).

MUCOCELES AND ANTRAL PSEUDOCYSTS

Mucoceles

Mucoceles and antral pseudocysts are common expansive lesions to develop in the maxillary sinus. Antral pseudocysts are mostly accidental findings presenting as dome shaped lesions in dental panoramic radiographs (**Fig. 9.6**). The reason for the causation of antral pseudocyst is accumulation of inflammatory exudates below the sinus epithelium causing elevation of the mucosa. It is not uncommon and may be found in 2 to 14 percent of the population.

Mucocele is defined as a mucosecretory respiratory epithelium surrounding mucoid secretions. Mucoceles can be an incidental finding in 10 percent of people. True sinus mucoceles occur due to obstruction of sinus ostium. They are formed when a sinus becomes obstructed and completely filled with secretions; the mucocele is often therefore larger than the obstructed sinus.

A mucous retention cyst is a mucoid filled cyst that develops when a minor gland duct becomes obstructed. It can, similarly, be an incidental finding in 10 percent of people. Radiologically therefore, the definition of a mucocele is reserved for the sinus that is airless and represents an enlarged sinus cavity filled with mucoid secretions. Progressive expansions resulting in thinning of the surrounding bone can be visualized radiographically. Occasionally an antral mucocele may elevate the orbital floor with resultant diplopia. When the same mucocele collapses enophthalmos may be the result.

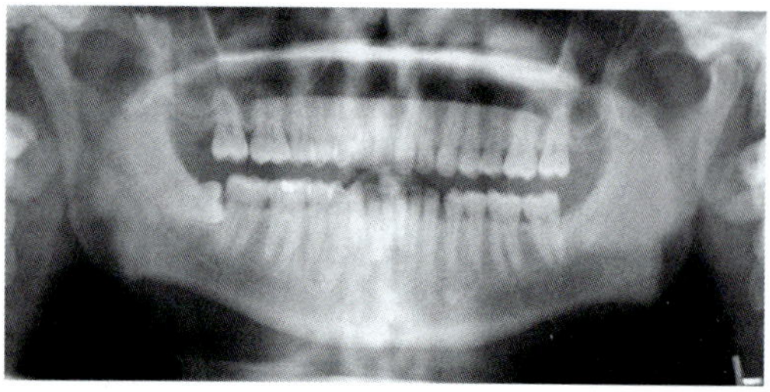

Fig. 9.6: Bilateral antral pseudocysts (antral polyps) (*Courtesy:* Dr Jimmy Makdissi)

Treatment

Radiography, occasionally with CT scan confirmation, may be all that is required to make a clinical diagnosis. Symptomatic and erosive maxillary sinus mucoceles are treated by simple enucleation. Pathological examination is usually unrewarding.

Antrochoanal Polyps

Clinical and Pathological Features

The antrochoanal polyp is a large solitary unilateral polyp usually in the posterior aspect of the maxillary sinus. It may extend through the ostium of the antrum into the middle meatus of the nose giving the appearance of a nasal polyp. Maxillary antral choanal polyps are more common in males and young patients typically up to 40 years of age. Up to 50 percent of patients with antral polyps give an allergic history. There is little difference histologically between antral and nasal polyps. Antral polyps seem to have fewer mucus glands and fewer eosinophils than ordinary nasal polyps. Atypical stromal cells representing a reactive change are sometimes visible.

Treatment

Radiographically the polyp appears as an increased soft tissue density often with an opacification of the maxillary sinus; almost 40 percent of patients have coexistent bilateral maxillary sinusitis. Antral polyps are benign in their behavior. They appear to be self-limiting in size and cause no local bony or soft tissue erosion. Complete removal results in negligible recurrence (**Box 9.4**).

Box 9.4: Antrochoanal polyps

Key features helpful in diagnosis

- Close association with a history of allergy
- Forty percent of patients have coexistent sinusitis
- Benign, self-limiting, no bone erosion

Antroliths

Clinicopathological Features

Antroliths are calcified masses that occur in the maxillary sinus. Stones arising in the antral cavities are uncommon and the development is similar to that of a sialolith. They may form around a nidus or concentrated mucus which continues to grow because of the precipitation of calcium salts in concentric layers. Antroliths are very rare. They are usually asymptomatic but may be associated with dull pain mimicking chronic sinusitis. Other features reported include facial pain, nasal obstruction, epistaxis, purulent or blood stained discharge, foul smelling postnasal drip and oral antral fistula. Occasionally patients give a history of tooth extraction. Radiographically a dense, irregular, well defined mass may be identified in the antrum (**Fig. 9.7**). Although, the nidus for calcification is usually endogenous, in some cases an exogenous source may be implicated such as tooth roots, or foreign bodies such as dental materials, glass and even paper and stone. Focal antral calcification has been seen in sinuses filled with a fungus ball of *Aspergillus*.

The differential diagnosis of antroliths include ectopic teeth root fragments, osteoma or cementoma, condensing osteitis in the periapical tissue, any form of local bony exostosis and foreign bodies. Large antroliths may even mimic neoplasia.

Treatment

A CT scan usually reveals an isolated benign, calcified, well-circumscribed lesion, and in the absence of symptoms surgical intervention is far from mandatory. Large and obstructing antroliths may require surgical enucleation (**Box 9.5**).

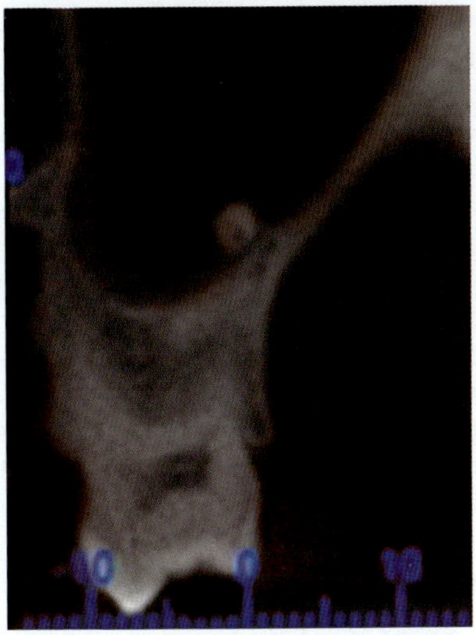

Fig. 9.7: Antrolith presenting as a well-defined radiopaque mass inside the antral cavity (*Courtesy:* Dr Jimmy Makdissi)

Box 9.5: Antroliths

Key features helpful in diagnosis

- Rare occurrence of a calcified mass forming around a nidus often of foreign material
- Usually asymptomatic, but may mimic a chronic sinusitis, or present with acute nasal symptoms or a postnasal drip
- Radio dense well-demarcated lesions may remain untreated in the absence of symptoms

TUMORS OF THE MAXILLARY ANTRUM

Benign Tumors of the Maxillary Sinuses

While the numbers of papillomas arising in the maxillary sinuses are significant, other true benign tumors are remarkably rare. Most of the benign tumors of the maxillary antrum arise from adjacent anatomical areas, such as the maxillary alveolus and nasal cavity. The majority from the former site being largely odontogenic, such as the ameloblastoma and keratocystic odontogenic tumor, while salivary tumors, fibrous lesions and even osteomas can penetrate into the sinus from an origin in the nasal cavity.

Mostly benign tumors in this situation present with facial asymmetry, facial pain or nasal discharge or bleeding. CT usually demonstrates a well-defined mass with surrounding bone remodeling or expansion reflecting the slow growth of the tumor. The notable exception to this rule is the rare juvenile angiofibroma, usually originating in the nasopharynx and invading the maxillary sinus, accompanied by significant bony destruction similar to a malignant tumor.

Schneiderian Papillomas

The schneiderian membrane is a ciliated respiratory epithelium derived from ectoderm that lines the paranasal sinuses and gives rise to three distinct papillomas (fungiform, inverted and oncocytic). Collectively Schneiderian papillomas are uncommon, accounting for around 4 percent of all sinonasal tumors (**Box 9.6**).

Fungiform (Epithelial Papilloma)

Clinicopathological Features

Fungiform papilloma comprises 20 to 50 percent of all schneiderian papillomas, occurring primarily in young and middle aged males. Primary involvement of the maxillary sinus is unusual, the papilloma tending to spread there from the lateral nasal wall. These papillomas can be multifocal but most often unilateral. Epistaxis and nasal obstruction are typical presenting features. There is evidence that the papilloma is etiologically related to the human papillomavirus (HPV) particularly types 6 and 11. Fungiform papillomas range in size from a few millimeters up to several centimeters.

The typical microscopic appearance is of papillary fronds with delicate fibrovascular cores covered by epithelium up to 20 cells thick. The epithelium varies from squamous through transitional to ciliated respiratory type. Surface keratinization is absent unless the papilloma is subjected to the trauma of nose picking. Mitoses are rare and it is generally agreed that fungiform papillomas are not associated with an increased incidence of malignant transformation.

Treatment

Complete surgical excision is the treatment of choice. Prognosis is excellent, but recurrence is possible, particularly where there is a viral association.

Inverted Papilloma

Clinicopathological Features

Inverted papillomas constitute the majority of all Schneiderian papillomas, up to 70 percent in some series. It is five times more common in men than women. Isolated lesions can occur in the paranasal sinuses without nasal involvement and indeed, inverted papillomas have been reported in unusual sites such as the posterior pharyngeal wall and hypopharynx. Ectopic migration of schneiderian membrane during embryogenesis is the proposed etiology in these instances. Nasal obstruction and epistaxis are the principle presenting features, although inverted papillomas are painful in about 10 percent of the cases. Inverted papilloma was for a long time suspected of having a viral origin. However, viral inclusions were not routinely demonstrated, both polymerase chain reaction (PCR) and hybridization techniques failed to demonstrate HPV, although involvement of Epstein Barr Virus (EBV) cannot be excluded.

Microscopically, inverted papillomas appear as hyperplastic strands of epithelium that grow endophytically into the underlying stoma. The epithelium is non-keratinized squamous and multilayered up to 30 cells thick (**Fig. 9.8**). Mitoses are not numerous and are usually confined to the parabasal and basal epithelium. In 10 to 20 percent of inverted papillomas surface keratinization can be seen, with up to 20 percent displaying varying degrees of dysplasia. Inverted papillomas are occasionally complicated by malignant transformation into squamous cell carcinoma and to a much lesser extent, verrucous, mucoepidermoid and adenocarcinoma.

The incidence of malignant change is given variously from 20 to 25 percent, although an overall figure of around 10 percent is generally accepted. The carcinoma may arise within the papilloma (carcinoma ex-inverted papilloma) and display a gradation of histological change

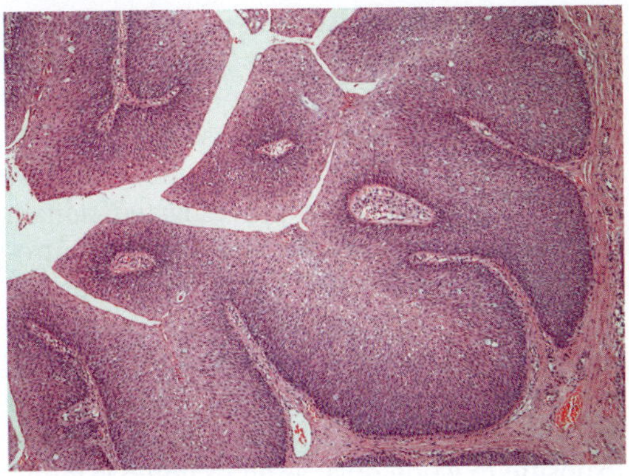

Fig. 9.8: Inverted papilloma: Nonkeratinized hyperplastic strands of epithelium extend endophytically into the underlying stoma

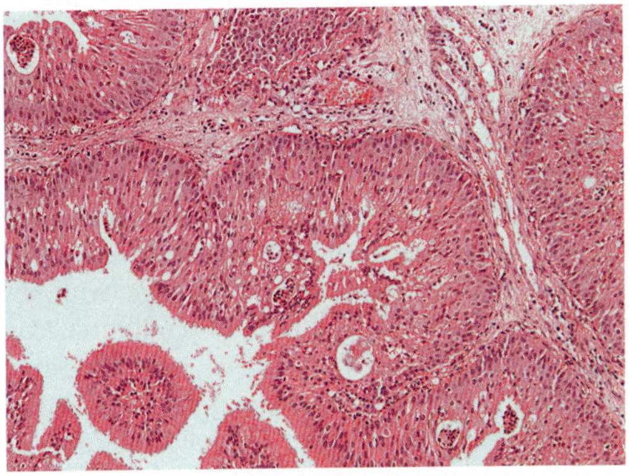

Fig. 9.9: Oncocytic papilloma (Cylindrical cell papilloma): The cells show small dark nuclei and eosinophilic cytoplasm and the cells are similar to oncocytes. Small cysts filled with neutrophils forming microabscesses within the epithelium may be present

from dysplasia to carcinoma *in situ* to invasive malignancy. However, paradoxically carcinoma may also rise in the site or where an inverted papilloma was excised many years previously.

Treatment

Treatment of choice is surgical removal and unchecked inverted papilloma has a potential to enlarge to occupy the entire maxillary sinus. Lateral rhinotomy and en bloc excision of the affected lateral nasal wall is the appropriate treatment modality. Recurrence potential is significant and even after the most thorough surgery is 16 percent.

Oncocytic Papilloma (Cylindrical Cell Papilloma)

Clinicopathological Features

Oncocytic papilloma is the least common variety constituting only about 5 percent of the total. It shares many features in common with the inverted papilloma, although has distinct microscopic features. It shows an equal sex incidence and tends to occur in patients over the age of 50. There is little, if any association of the oncocytic papilloma with human papillomavirus. Microscopically, a mixed exophytic and endophytic pattern of growth is seen. The tumor comprises a multilayered, tall columnar epithelium up to 8 cells thick. The cells show small dark nuclei and eosinophilic cytoplasm and the cells are similar to oncocytes. Small cysts filled with neutrophils, forming microabscesses within the epithelium, may be present (**Fig. 9.9**). The stroma varies from edematous to fibrous and may contain inflammatory cells. Malignant change arises in between 4 and 17 percent of all oncocytic papillomas. It is mainly squamous carcinomas but mucoepidermoid and sinonasal undifferentiated carcinoma have also been reported. As with inverted papilloma, the carcinoma may actually arise in the papilloma itself coincident with a gradation of histologic changes of dysplasia through to invasive carcinoma.

Treatment

Surgical excision is the most effective treatment, this may require lateral rhinotomy and medial maxillectomy as inadequate excision carries a recurrence rate of 25 to 30 percent.

Endoscopic sinus surgery has modified the surgical management of papillomas in general. Those confined within the maxillary sinus are considered amenable to endoscopic removal, whereas those tumors invading through the sinus walls require radical open surgery.

Box 9.6: Schneiderian papillomas

Key features helpful in diagnosis

- Comprise fungiform, inverted and oncocytic varieties
- Fungiform is the most benign
- Inverted is the most common, malignant change possible, recurrence potential significant
- Oncocytic papilloma comprises 5 percent, similar behavior to inverted type

MALIGNANT TUMORS OF THE MAXILLARY ANTRUM

The anatomical location of the maxillary sinuses makes them extremely close to vital structures such as the orbit, skull-base, infratemporal fossa, nasal and oral cavities, all within immediate proximity. The maxillary antral carcinoma can grow to a considerable size before presentation and as such aggressive therapy may be needed in an anatomically complex region. It makes these tumors highly challenging for the oncology team. Although rare, maxillary antral malignancies show few if any signs while the tumor is in its early stages. This is further complicated as the initial manifestations such as unilateral epistaxis and nasal obstruction are signs and symptoms of many common but much less serious conditions. Because the location of the maxillary sinus is adjacent to important structures such as skull-base, orbits, cranial nerves and vital vascular structures means that by the time ominous signs and symptoms occur the neoplasm is often advanced. As such, presenting features include severe headache, visual disturbance and cranial neuropathy. Similarly, attempts at curative resection may cause significant associated morbidity.

Malignancies of the maxillary sinuses are rare. They are more common in Asia and Africa than in Europe and the United States. In the western world they comprise typically just 3 percent of all head and neck cancers, though in parts of Asia the maxillary sinus carcinoma becomes the second most common head and neck cancer, after nasopharyngeal carcinoma. Men are affected five times more commonly than women. The vast majority of these tumors occur beyond the age of 45 years.

Risk factors for cancer of the maxillary sinus, although extensively investigated, remain complicated, multifactorial and perhaps controversial. It is well established that squamous cell carcinoma and adenocarcinoma of the maxillary sinus are associated with exposure to nickel and asbestos dust, mustard gas and isopropyl oil, chromium or dichlorodiethyl sulphide. Exposure to wood dust, as an example is found to increase the risk of squamous cell carcinoma and adenocarcinoma very significantly. These exposures commonly occur in the furniture making industry, the leather industry and the textile business. There is no better example of a head and neck malignancy where a careful, social and employment history should be asked. Recent studies provide mounting evidence to connect viral infection and maxillary antral carcinoma. Studies suggest that epidermal growth factor receptor and transforming growth factor alpha may be found to elevated levels, associated with carcinogenic change with an inverted papilloma. The human papillomavirus (HPV) and Epstein-Barr (EBV) infection may also be an early event between the multifactorial processes of malignant transformation in maxillary sinus cancers (**Box 9.7**).

Box 9.7: Malignant tumors of the maxillary sinus

Key features helpful in diagnosis

- The anatomical location and relations of the maxillary sinuses mean that many tumors present in their later stages and with major local complications
- Presenting features such as epistaxis and nasal obstruction occur in many less serious conditions and further delay diagnosis
- Maxillary sinus carcinoma shows marked geographical variation in its incidence, being far more common in Asia than the west
- Exposure to wood dust significantly increases the risk of both squamous cell carcinoma and adenocarcinoma
- There is evidence to connect viruses such as HPV and EBV with maxillary sinus carcinoma

Squamous Cell Carcinoma

Clinicopathological Features

Squamous cell carcinoma comprises over 80 percent of all malignancies that arise in the paranasal sinuses. The vast majority, over 70 percent occur in the maxillary sinus. Several variants of carcinoma are often considered subtypes of squamous cell carcinoma of the maxillary sinuses. These include verrucous carcinoma, basaloid squamous cell carcinoma, spindle-cell carcinoma and transitional or cylindrical cell carcinoma. The term squamous cell carcinoma indicates malignancies that have standard features widely understood to represent that entity.

Presentation is varied; they include nasal obstruction, nasal discharge, epistaxis, cranial neuropathies and pain. More advanced lesions can alter the patient's facial features in a noticeable way, causing facial asymmetry or proptosis. Visual disturbances and cranial nerve paresthesias are not uncommon in the advanced tumor invading the orbit, very occasionally the patient may present with mobility and protrusion of maxillary teeth when a mass arises from the floor of the maxilla or as a lump on the hard palate. Backward extension of the tumor sometimes leads to trismus, involving the pterygoid region. Clinical evaluation is similarly a function of the stage of the tumor, it can vary from little more than a mass or a small ulcer to advanced disease which can fungate into the oral cavity or on to the facial skin. An occipitomental view of the skull will indicate a radiopaque antrum and destruction of the antral walls. Biopsy is necessary for diagnosis and classification. Some disease conditions such as Wegener's granulomatosis may simulate the presentation of squamous carcinomas and is discussed in Chapter 20.

Treatment

The prognosis has considerably improved in those presenting early. Unlike other squamous cell carcinomas of the head and neck, lymph node involvement is rare and elective lymph node dissection is not usually advocated. Local radical surgery followed by radiotherapy forms the mainstay of curative treatment; modern neoadjuvant radiotherapy may have a role in selected cases. The overall five years survival rate is in the order of 60 percent irrespective of stage. High recurrence rates are usually encountered particularly in advanced disease.

Adenoid Cystic Carcinoma

Clinicopathological Features

Adenoid cystic carcinoma accounts for approximately 10 percent of cancers in the maxillary sinus. Therefore, it is the second most common malignancy in this site. Three histological subtypes are described; tubular, cribriform and solid based on particular growth patterns. The importance of the subtypes is centered on the fact that the solid form carries a much poorer prognosis than either cribriform or tubular and is discussed in Chapter 10.

Treatment

Cervical lymph node involvement is rare and elective neck dissection is not indicated in most cases; perineural invasion is common, it is found in approximately 50 percent of presenting cases. Late recurrence is frequent and may occur many decades after initial presentation and treatment. Surgery is the mainstay of management with radiation utilized for advanced disease, perineural invasion or surgically unfavorable margins. Overall disease free survival rates are approximately 60 percent at five years but comes down to 20 percent at fifteen years (**Box 9.8**).

Box 9.8: Maxillary sinus adenoid cystic carcinoma

Key features helpful in diagnosis

- Accounts for 10 percent of maxillary sinus cancers
- Solid form carries a poor prognosis
- Perineural invasion is found in nearly 50 percent of presenting cases
- Late recurrence is frequent

Adenocarcinoma and Variants

Clinicopathological Features

Adenocarcinoma of the maxillary sinus is historically important and is associated with specific risk factors, such as exposure to wood dust but also varnishes and other organic compounds. Both low and high grade adenocarcinomas are described and each can cause obstructive symptoms. However, pain, paresthesia and oral ulceration are more commonly found in high grade, poorly differentiated tumors. Irrespective of grade local spread to the orbits and skull-base is not an infrequent complication of the maxillary adenocarcinoma. Distant spread is unusual, when it occurs lung, liver and bone are the sites most often affected. Metastases to cervical lymph nodes are uncommon irrespective of tumor differentiation.

Treatment

Treatment is surgical resection with post-operative radiotherapy for advanced disease, unfavorable histology or positive surgical margins. Adenocarcinoma of the maxillary sinus rarely affects lymph nodes and makes elective neck dissection unnecessary. The prognostic outlook for low grade adenocarcinoma is far better than for the high grade tumors of the maxillary sinus; low grade adenocarcinoma has a 5-year survival rate of approximately 80 percent whereas only 35 percent of patients with high grade disease are alive at 3 years.

Malignant Melanoma

Clinicopathological Features

This is a rare disorder of the paranasal sinus mucosa accounting for no more than 1 percent of all malignant melanomas. However, 55 percent of the mucosal melanomas occur in the head and neck and 20 percent of these are found in the maxillary sinus. The clinical appearance of the lesion is that of a firm gray/white or pink/black ulcerated mass. Black coloration is not unusual, although predominance is an ulcerated pink mucosal color which can lead to confusion with an advanced squamous cell carcinoma. Biopsy is mandatory. However, histologically mucosal melanoma can be extraordinary variable in appearance. Immunohistochemistry plays an important role as the mucosal melanoma shows typical positivity for S-100 and HMB-45. These makers are listed in Chapter 8.

Treatment

The primary therapeutic approach is surgical resection. Retrospective data exists that demonstrates the improved local regional control with postoperative radiation, which is therefore often recommended for advanced disease. Chemotherapy is reserved for disseminated disease and palliation, even with the best therapy median survival is less than two years. Large size and extensive tumor thickness are considered as poor prognostic factors (**Box 9.9**).

Box 9.9: Maxillary sinus malignant melanoma

Key features helpful in diagnosis

- Rare tumor, accounts for only 1 percent of all melanomas
- Clinical appearance may be pigmented but predominantly ulcerated and pink mucosal color
- Surgery is the main modality of treatment
- Overall survival is poor

Verrucous Carcinoma

Clinicopathological Features

Verrucous carcinoma is a type of squamous carcinoma usually characterized by its fungating appearance and papillary nature. Verrucous carcinoma has the potential to progress to a more aggressive conventional squamous cell carcinoma. Verrucous carcinomas may cause damage by local destruction but do not metastasise unless they contain a component of squamous cell carcinoma. This component is found in approximately 20 percent of verrucous carcinoma. This may pose as a problem with treatment planning, particularly when considering an elected neck dissection. The rate of local invasion of verrucous carcinoma is also slower than usually seen with squamous cell carcinoma. Verrucous carcinomas in the head and neck are frequently associated with synchronous or metachronous tumors.

Treatment

Local resection by maxillectomy is the first line treatment. If the resection specimen contains a portion of squamous cell carcinoma further neck dissection may be considered. Overall, survival is better than many maxillary carcinomas, typically 70 percent at 5 years.

Lymphomas and Related Tumors

Primary lymphoma of the maxillary sinus is unusual. Typically the patients are aged 60 years and over. Large tumors may cause facial deformity and asymmetry. Management is similar to that generally accepted for non-Hodgkin lymphoma after staging. Chemo-therapy and radiotherapy are the main modalities of treatment, returning median survival rates close to 80 percent at five years.

A controversial type of malignant tumor is the T-cell/natural killer (NK) cell lymphoma. Throughout history it has received numerous labels including lethal midline granuloma, midline malignant reticulosis, lymphomatoid granulomatosis, angiocentric lymphoproliferative lesion and T-cell/NK cell lymphoma. According to the current knowledge this lesion is most likely a T-cell lymphoma. This tumor is an aggressive lesion presenting with obstructive symptoms, bone and soft tissue destruction and hemorrhage. It has strong viral associations and presents over a wide-age range. Modern management of T-cell lymphoma is with chemotherapy with or without radiotherapy. Survival rates up to 70 percent at five years have been reported.

Sarcomas

The maxillary sinus contains nerves, blood vessels, lymphatics, smooth and skeletal muscle, fibrous tissue and bone. However, it is surprising that the malignant tumors arising from those structures occur very rarely. Fibrosarcoma, leiomyosarcoma, rhabdomyosarcoma, liposarcoma, peripheral nerve sheath tumors amongst others have been reported. Rhabdomyosarcoma is one of the more frequent sinus malignancies in children. It has also been reported in adults. Symptoms are similar to those of other tumors and patients present in an advanced stage. Small localized lesions may be amenable to surgery. A combination of radiotherapy and chemotherapy is more often employed. Even with radical treatment overall survival is poor, below 50 percent at five years is a typical figure.

Metastatic Tumors to the Maxillary Sinus

Metastatic tumors are uncommon in the maxillary antrum. Those tumors displaying a natural tendency to metastasize to bone are usually implicated including prostate, breast, kidney, lung and thyroid. In addition, melanoma, gastrointestinal adenocarcinoma and hepatocellular carcinoma have all been reported to metastasize to the maxillary sinus. There are a small number of metastatic lesions that may cause pathological uncertainty.

SINONASAL NEUROENDOCRINE TUMORS

Sinonasal neuroendocrine tumors are a potentially confusing entity. They are a small group of four tumors:

1. Esthesioneuroblastoma (ENB)
2. Sinonasal undifferentiated carcinoma
3. Neuroendocrine carcinoma
4. Small cell carcinoma.

Studies show an overall survival of ENB of up to 93 percent at five years. Five years survival rates for undifferentiated and neuroendocrine carcinomas are typically 60 percent, whereas the highly malignant small cell carcinoma is little over 30 percent survival at five years.

Esthesioneuroblastoma

Esthesioneuroblastoma, also called olfactory neuroblastoma is an uncommon tumor that invades the maxillary sinus at an early stage. It is typically thought to originate from olfactory cells near the cribriform plate but ectopic cells do occur and they contribute tumors primarily at alternative sites. Usual presentation is with nasal obstruction and epistaxis, most patients are in the fifth decade.

Treatment of ENB has changed dramatically in recent times with the advent of craniofacial resection, which has significantly increased the five years survival. Five years survival is optimized by using craniofacial surgical resection with postoperative radiotherapy. There is some evidence that chemotherapy may add an additional benefit in the most advanced tumors. Despite a good five-year survival rate late recurrence is not uncommon, occurring in approximately one third of cases. Cervical lymph node metastases at presentation is less than 5 percent overall but cervical nodes may become involved in up to 30 percent of cases in total. Prophylactic neck dissection is recommended when the tumor is advanced at presentation.

Sinonasal Undifferentiated Carcinoma

Sinonasal undifferentiated carcinoma is an uncommon tumor of the maxillary sinus. It is an aggressive tumor frequently advanced at presentation and therefore usually treated by combined therapy unlike ENB. Tumor recurrence is common and response to further treatment is disappointing, consequently the two-year and five-year survival rates are similar. The current modality of treatment of advanced disease favors neoadjuvant chemotherapy followed by surgical resection. The tumor appears to show chemosensitivity, an unusual feature in a head and neck malignancy.

Small Cell Neuroendocrine Carcinoma

The small cell neuroendocrine carcinoma is similar to its counterpart carcinoma of the lungs. It is an unusual but reported tumor in the maxillary sinuses and occurs in a wide age range. It is an aggressive tumor, often advanced at presentation, in fact multiple paranasal sinuses may be involved. Cervical lymph node metastases and indeed pulmonary metastases are usually early. Treatment attempts using combinations of surgery, chemotherapy and radiotherapy return equally poor results. The median survival is typically less than two years.

SELF-ASSESSMENT QUESTIONS

1. Give a classification for diseases of the maxillary antrum.
2. Describe the anatomy and physiology of the maxillary antrum.
3. Discuss the clinicopathological features of acute and chronic sinusitis.
4. Outline the treatment of acute and chronic sinusitis.
5. Discuss the fungal infections which may affect the maxillary sinus.
6. Describe the clinicopathological features and management of antroliths
7. Write an account of papillomas of the maxillary sinus.
8. Describe the geographic distribution and other risk factors for the development of malignant tumors of the maxillary antrum.
9. Describe the clinicopathological features of malignant tumors of the maxillary sinus.
10. Describe the imaging modalities available to diagnose antral diseases.

SUGGESTED READING

1. Acheson ED, Hadfield EH, Macbeth RG. Carcinoma of the nasal cavity and accessory sinuses in woodworkers. Lancet. 1967:11; 311-2.
2. Batsakis JG, Rice DH, Solomon AR. The pathology of head and neck tumors: squamous and mucous-gland carcinomas of the nasal cavity, paranasal sinuses, and larynx, part 6. Head Neck Surg. 1980;2:497-508.
3. Busquets JM, Hwang PH. Endoscopic resection of sinonasal inverted papilloma: a meta-analysis. Otolaryngol Head Neck Surg. 2006;134:476-82.
4. Corey JP, Romberger CF, Shaw GY. Fungal diseases of the sinuses. Otolaryngol Head Neck Surg. 1990;103:1012-5.
5. Lanza DC, Kennedy DW. Adult rhinosinusitis defined. Otolaryngol Head Neck Surg. 1997;117:S1-7.
6. Lehmann P, Bouaziz R, Page C, et al. Sinonasal cavities: CT imaging features of anatomical variants and surgical risk. J Radiol. 2009;90:21-9.
7. Lund V. The evolution of surgery on the maxillary sinus for chronic rhinosinusitis. Laryngoscope. 2002;112:415-9.
8. Narayana Swamy KV, Chandre Gowda BV. A clinical study of benign tumors of nose and paranasal sinuses. Ind J Otolaryngol Head Neck Surg. 2004;56:265-8.

Chapter 10

Salivary Gland Disorders

John Eveson

Chapter Outline

INTRODUCTION

There are three pairs of major salivary glands—parotid, submandibular and sublingual glands. In addition there are numerous minor salivary glands dispersed throughout the oral cavity particularly in the lips and palate. Most non-neoplastic disorders of major salivary glands represent acute or chronic infections of these glands, obstruction to the salivary flow caused by calculi being responsible in most cases. Common inflammatory, autoimmune and neoplastic disorders are presented here.

NON-NEOPLASTIC SALIVARY DISORDERS

Developmental Disorders

Aplasia/agenesis: Congenital absence of one or more salivary glands is very rare, but occasionally the parotid gland is absent. Absence of all major salivary glands is even rarer. Salivary aplasia can be associated with other orofacial developmental anomalies.

Duct atresia: This is failure of a duct to canalize and it is also rare. It usually affects the submandibular duct. Absence of a patent duct lumen results in the formation of retention cysts in the submandibular and sublingual glands and progressive atrophy of the glandular parenchyma.

Heterotopia (ectopia): It is relatively common to find salivary ducts and sometimes acini in the upper cervical and intraparotid lymph nodes (**Fig. 10.1**). These inclusions are known as Neisse Nicholson rests and they may be important in the pathogenesis of Warthin tumor. Occasionally salivary tissue is seen in the middle ear and other head and neck sites. Stafne's bone cavity is a cyst-like area in the medial aspect of the angle of the mandible, below the mylohyoid line (**Fig. 10.2**). It is due to an invagination into the lingual plate which is usually filled with an extension of the submandibular gland or fibrofatty tissue. Much less commonly, an analogous defect can be seen in the anterior lingual aspect of the mandible.

Accessory ducts and lobes: These are regarded as normal anatomical variations rather than anomalies. A distinct accessory duct and lobe in

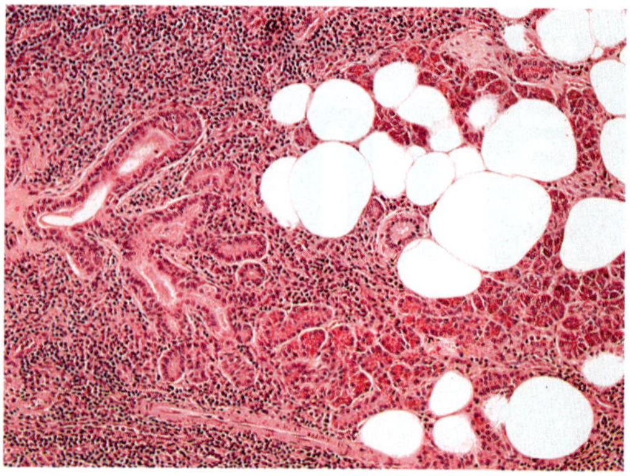

Fig. 10.1: Salivary inclusions in parotid lymph node

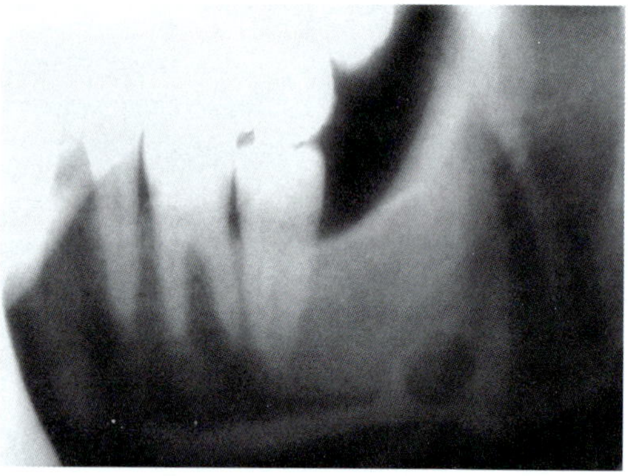

Fig. 10.2: Stafne bone cavity presenting as a cyst-like radiolucent area below the mylohyoid line

the parotid is present in as many as 50 percent of patients. Accessory ducts and lobes are, however, very rare in the submandibular gland.

INFLAMMATORY/INFECTIVE DISEASES

Acute Suppurative Sialadenitis

Ascending infection is most common in the parotid gland, possibly because it has a shorter and wider duct than the submandibular gland and lacks the sphincter-like mechanism seen in the submandibular papillae. In addition, the serous salivary secretion of the parotid gland has less bacteriostatic activity than the mucinous submandibular saliva.

Ascending parotitis was considerably more common in the past, and in preantibiotic days could be fatal. Debilitated and dehydrated post-surgical patients were particularly at risk from infection ascending from the oral cavity as a result of a combination of reduced salivary flow and oral sepsis. This type of presentation is now rare. Most cases are secondary to chronic xerostomia, usually as a consequence of Sjögren's syndrome and radiation damage, or less commonly, tricyclic medication. Occasionally, the infection is secondary to sialolithiasis or presents spontaneously.

Clinical Features

The parotid gland shows the cardinal signs of inflammation, i.e. it is red, hot, swollen and painful (**Fig. 10.3**). Pyrexia and regional lymphadenopathy are common. Pus may discharge into the oral cavity through parotid duct (**Fig. 10.4**). In severe cases, abscesses may develop and these can discharge onto the face as fistulae.

The most common causative organism are *Staphylococcus aureus* and *Viridans* streptococci. However, the infection is often mixed and a wide variety of other bacteria has been incriminated, including gram-negative bacilli, coliform organisms and anaerobes.

Histopathology

Initially there is hyperemia, edema and neutrophil accumulation. Ducts, and then acinar tissue, are progressively destroyed, leading to formation of microabscesses. In cases that are left untreated, or when the patient is immunocompromised, there can be extensive macro-abscess formation and destruction of large areas of the gland. As the infection resolves there is progressive fibrosis. This can result in distortion of the ductal architecture and permanent loss of secretory acinar tissue. This in turn can cause stagnation of saliva which predisposes the gland to further inflammatory episodes.

Treatment and Prognosis

If possible, pus should be obtained for culture and antibiotic sensitivity. In order to limit contamination from the mouth, the mucosa around the duct orifice should be wiped clean with a sterile swab, and any pus present should be milked by forward pressure on the parotid gland. It is prudent to have the microbiology swab ready before milking the gland, as it is common to lose the bead of pus if you do not. As staphylococci are frequently the causative organism, flucloxacillin is usually the first empirical choice, but is changed if the microbiological findings dictate. Metronidazole can be added because of the frequency of anaerobic infections. Sialography is contraindicated at this stage as it can force more organisms back into the gland and could result in bacteremia or septicemia. Early treatment with antibiotics, fluids to correct any dehydration and stimulation of salivary flow

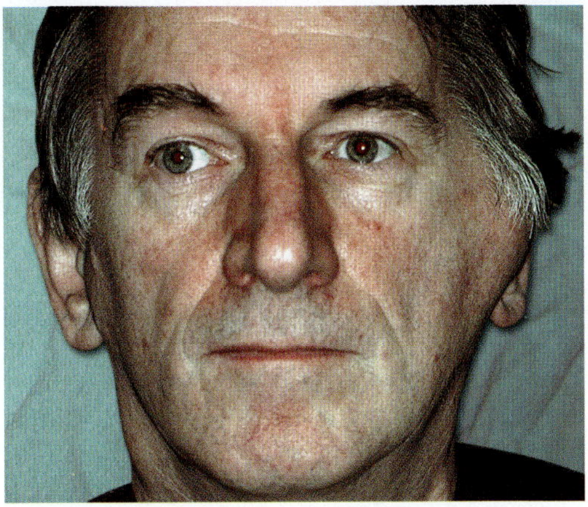

Fig. 10.3: Acute suppurative parotitis causing a large facial swelling

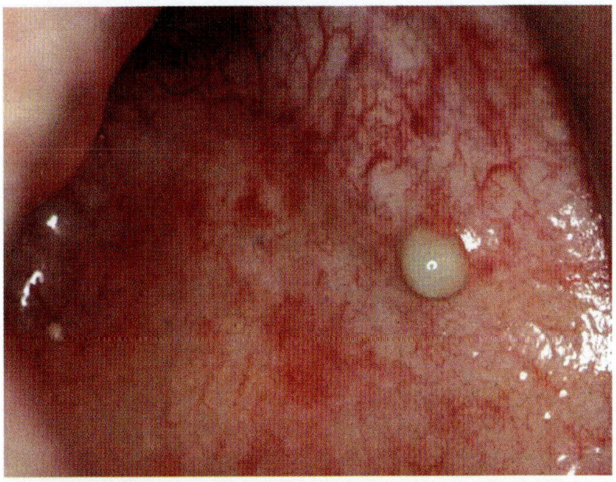

Fig. 10.4: Bead of pus milked from inflamed parotid gland

by sialagogues is usually effective. Severe cases may require emergency hospital admission for intravenous fluids and antibiotics.

Recurrent Parotitis (Juvenile Parotitis)

Clinical Features

Recurrent parotitis is a rare but well characterized condition in children, typically starting at about 6 years of age: it often resolves spontaneously around adolescence. Boys are affected twice as often as girls. Patients usually present with recurrent unilateral or bilateral parotid pain and swelling, particularly at mealtimes. Heat, redness, fluctuation and pyrexia are absent. The condition is often initially interpreted as 'recurrent mumps'. Sialography shows widespread punctuate and globular sialectasis (**Fig. 10.5A**) and ultrasound, which is increasingly the investigation of choice, shows multiple small hyopechogenic areas. The cause of recurrent parotitis is uncertain but suggestions include congenital sialectasis, viral and bacterial infections and autoimmunity. Recurrent parotitis in adults is much more common and is usually due to obstruction and/or xerostomia.

Histopathology

Microscopy shows cystic dilatation of interlobular ducts with florid periductal lymphoplasmacytic infiltration (**Fig. 10.5B**) and reactive germinal follicle formation. In addition, there can be extensive acinar atrophy and interstitial fibrosis.

Treatment and Prognosis

Despite the lack of a proven bacterial etiology, many cases respond well to antibiotics, including long-term and continuous low-dose penicillin. Progressive damage to the glands in adults can make treatment difficult and may necessitate removal of the affected gland.

Chronic Obstructive Sialadenitis and Sialolithiasis

Chronic obstructive sialadenitis is relatively common and affects the submandibular glands much more frequently than the parotid glands. This is due to the more viscid, mucinous secretion and narrower duct of the submandibular gland and its predisposition to form calculi. The very high concentration of calcium in the secretory material of the submandibular gland, which is higher than in the parotid, may also be contributory. In addition, trauma to Wharton's duct in the floor of the mouth can lead to periductal fibrosis and obstruction.

Salivary calculi consist predominantly of calcium phosphate and carbonate which crystallize around an organic matrix derived from mucus plugs, cellular debris from the duct

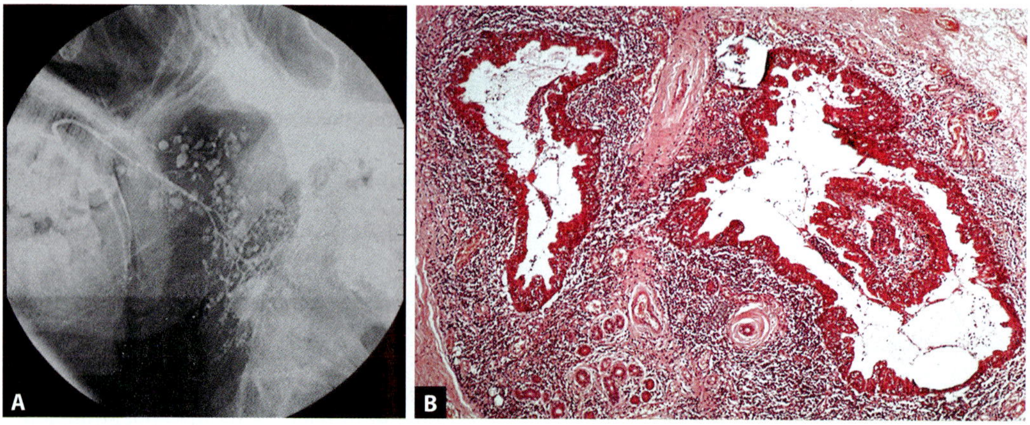

Figs 10.5A and B: (A) Sialogram of recurrent juvenile sialadenitis showing extensive punctuate sialectasis; (B) Histology showing dilated interlobular ducts and dense periductal lymphocytic infiltration

walls or bacterial colonies. An important factor is the precipitation of calcium present at high concentration in stagnant secretory material deposited on membranous debris.

Clinical Features

Most patients are 30 to 60 years old and the condition is uncommon in children. About 80 percent of cases involve the submandibular gland and ~20 percent the parotid gland. Calculi can also develop in minor salivary glands, particularly those in the upper lip. Calculi are predominantly single but multiple stones are not rare. They can develop within the gland itself or the extra glandular excretory ducts.

In the submandibular gland the most common location (~60%) is at the junction of Wharton's duct and the hilum of the gland (**Fig. 10.6**), where the duct bends around the distal aspect of the mylohyoid muscle. The next most common location is the anterior aspect of the duct in the floor of the mouth. Many cases are asymptomatic but common symptoms in the early stages include pain and swelling, particularly following eating. With progressive damage to the gland, the acute symptoms may subside and then patients often present with a hard, often painless but tender submandibular mass, or a suppurative inflammatory exacerbation.

Parotid calculi can also produce symptoms at mealtimes but are often spontaneously flushed out of the gland as a gritty discharge. Larger and more solid parotid calculi can cause more persistent diffuse swelling of the gland and discomfort on eating.

Histopathology

The main features are varying degrees of acinar atrophy, ductal dilatation and chronic inflammatory infiltration, usually predominantly lymphocytic, with widespread interstitial fibrosis in the later stages (**Fig. 10.7**). Focal foreign body type granulomas with giant cells are sometimes present (**Fig. 10.8**). Squamous metaplasia and concentrically laminated calculi may be seen in the dilated ducts. Microscopically, calculi have a lamellated or radial structure and the duct walls may undergo squamous metaplasia (**Fig. 10.9**).

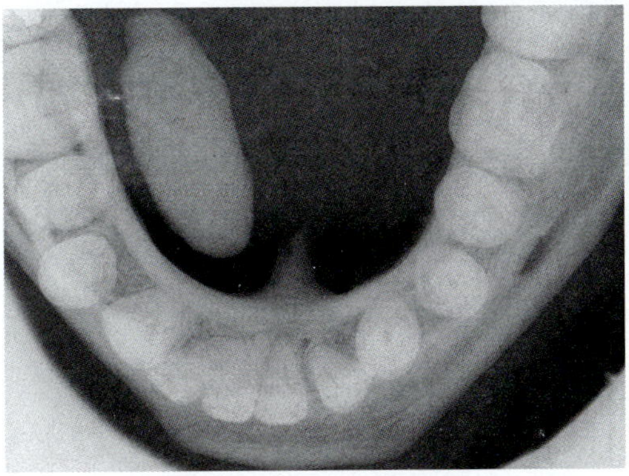

Fig. 10.6: Radiograph of a calculus in submandibular duct

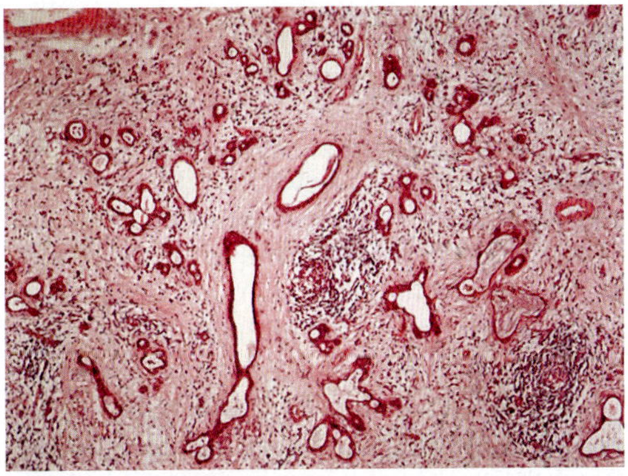

Fig. 10.7: Chronic sialadenitis showing acinar atrophy, duct dilatation, interstitial fibrosis and patchy chronic inflammatory infiltration

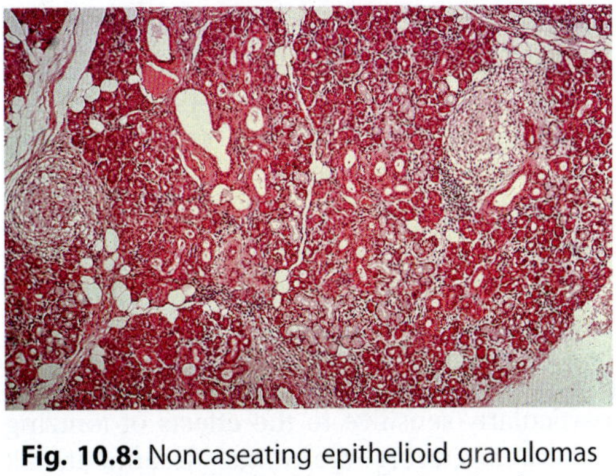

Fig. 10.8: Noncaseating epithelioid granulomas in obstructed submandibular gland

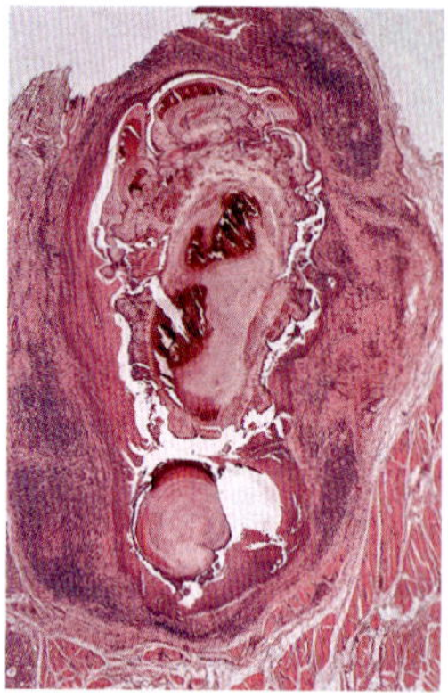

Fig. 10.9: Laminated calculus in a dilated minor salivary gland duct

Box 10.1: Salivary calculi

Key features useful in diagnosis

- Most patients 30–60 years old; slight male predominance
- Location: Submandibular gland 80 percent, parotid gland 20 percent
- Radiopaque stones: Submandibular gland 80 percent, parotid gland 20 percent
- Calculi consist of calcium phosphate and carbonate and organic nidus
- May be asymptomatic
- Pain and swelling on, or just, before eating
- Treated mainly by surgery: Basket retrieval and extracorporeal shock wave lithotripsy sometimes used.

Diagnosis and Treatment

Diagnosis is made on the basis of clinical observation, palpation and imaging. Plain radiography is very useful for submandibular calculi as 80 to 90 percent are radiopaque and thus readily visualized. However, in the parotid gland only 10 to 20 percent can be detected using this technique. Sialoliths in the accessible parts of the submandibular duct can sometimes be removed manually, sometimes using basket retrieval, or after surgical exposure. Recently, conservative surgical techniques have been used for more proximal stones but most of these cases require the removal of the entire submandibular gland. When protracted inflammation has rendered the gland virtually functionless, excision again may be the only solution. In the parotid gland distal calculi can sometimes be removed by incision into Stenson's duct but often require more extensive surgery with an extraoral approach. A non-surgical alternative treatment for both parotid and submandibular stones is extracorporeal shock wave lithotripsy, and in selected cases this can be very successful.

Postirradiation Sialadenitis

The major and minor salivary glands are particularly sensitive to the effects of ionizing radiation. During the initial treatment, all patients undergoing radiotherapy develop acute sialadenitis when the irradiated field includes the parotid or submandibular glands. The involved glands become swollen and painful within 24 hours and severe xerostomia quickly follows. The symptoms usually resolve spontaneously within a week. However, the long-term effects can be much more debilitating. There is obliterative endarteritis and progressive acinar destruction together with interstitial fibrosis. The loss of functional secretory parenchyma can lead to profound and intractable xerostomia.

VIRAL DISEASES

Mumps

The mumps virus is the most common cause of acute parotitis but many cases are subclinical. It is caused by a highly contagious paramyxovirus which is typically spread by salivary droplets. Mumps is usually a disease of childhood, but may affect nonimmune adults when it can be much more serious. The incubation period is 2 to 3 weeks and prodromal symptoms include, fever, malaise, headache and myalgia. The clinical onset usually begins with pain and swelling of one or more commonly both parotid glands and there may be associated xerostomia. The submandibular glands may also be involved. Occasionally, there are systemic complications, including encephalitis, pancreatitis, orchitis and oophoritis. Immunity following a first attack is absolute and lifelong so apparent cases of 'recurrent mumps' will invariably be due to some other cause. If there is any doubt about the diagnosis, it can be confirmed by an enzyme-linked immunoadsorbent assay for the mumps S and V antigen or by a nested polymerase chain reaction.

There are no specific remedies apart from supportive treatments and most cases resolve without complications within two weeks.

Microscopy is rarely undertaken but shows striking hyperemia, diffuse interstitial edema and a dense lymphoplasmacytic and histiocytic infiltration (**Fig. 10.10**). Despite the often severe acinar cell vacuolation and ductal dilatation, most cases show a full functional recovery.

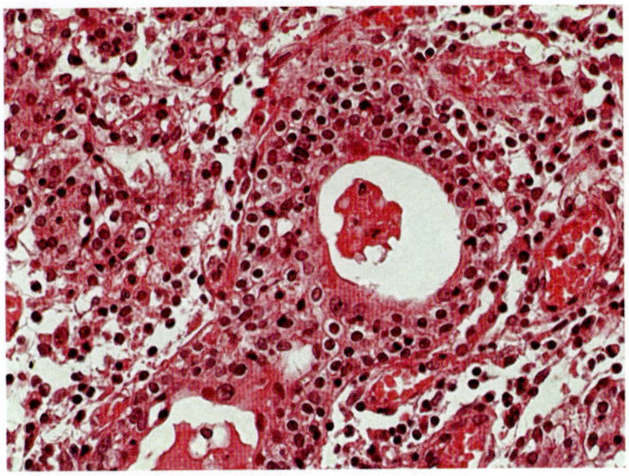

Fig. 10.10: Parotid gland mumps showing striking vascular hyperemia, acinar cell vacuolation and lymphocytic infiltration. Interstitial lymphoid infiltrate are predominantly CD8 positive

HIV-associated Salivary Gland Disease

Clinical Features

Between 1 and 10 percent of adult HIV positive patients develop salivary gland swellings due to lymphocytic infiltration, often with cyst formation (HIV-associated lymphoepithelial cysts). Cases of parotid gland Kaposi's sarcoma, however, are surprisingly rare. HIV-associated lymphoepithelial cysts are seen predominantly in children born to infected mothers and young adults. The parotid glands are mainly affected and clinically apparent disease is rare in other major and minor salivary glands. There are slow growing, painless and typically bilateral swellings of the parotid glands which can become massively enlarged. The swellings develop early in the course of the disease and are usually associated with persistent cervical lymphadenopathy. There may be other signs and symptoms of HIV infection including fever, fatigue, diarrhea and wasting. Xerostomia is an inconsistent symptom that appears to be more prevalent in children.

Unlike patients with Sjögren's syndrome, most patients with HIV-associated sialadenitis are males in a considerably younger age group. An autoantibody picture typical of Sjögren's syndrome is also not associated with the sicca syndrome of HIV infection: SS-A or SS-B antibodies are not present and rheumatoid or antinuclear factors are no more frequent than in the general population.

Histopathology

Gross examination of the affected glands shows multiple cysts of variable sizes but some may be several centimeters in diameter. The superficial lobe is usually affected more severely than the deep lobe. Microscopy shows multiple cysts in an ill-defined matrix of densely packed lymphocytes, together with large and conspicuous reactive follicles (**Figs 10.11 and 10.12**). The cysts are lined mainly by nonkeratinized stratified squamous epithelium that is permeated by lymphocytes. These include monocytoid B cells and smaller numbers of T cells. The T cells in the ducts and interstitial lymphoid infiltrate are predominantly CD8 positive.

Focally, the ductal epithelium proliferates to form solid lymphoepithelial lesions similar to those seen in Sjögren's syndrome. An important difference, however, is that in Sjögren's syndrome the infiltrate is mainly of CD4 lymphocytes, but in HIV infection there is typically dense CD8 lymphocytic infiltration. Focal periductal lymphocytic infiltration similar to that seen in Sjögren's syndrome can also be detected in labial gland biopsies. Here, once again, the lymphocytes are predominantly CD8 positive T cells.

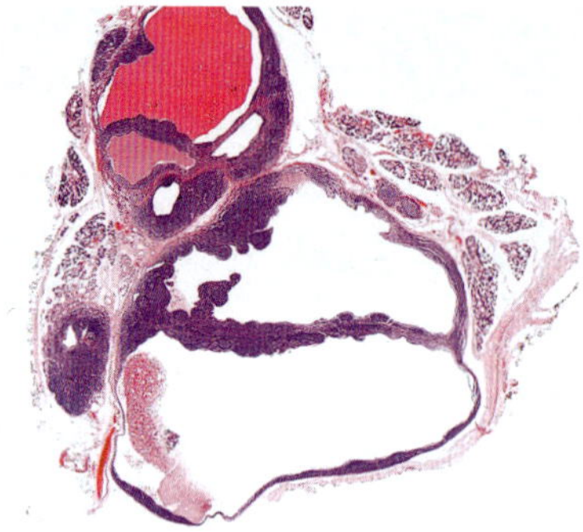

Fig. 10.11: HIV-associated sialadenitis showing multiple cysts and dense lymphocytic infiltration

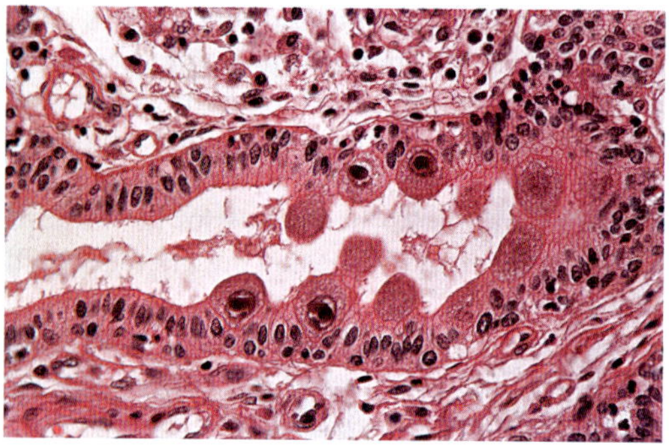

Fig. 10.13: Congenital cytomegalovirus of parotid gland showing the characteristic "owl-eye" inclusion bodies

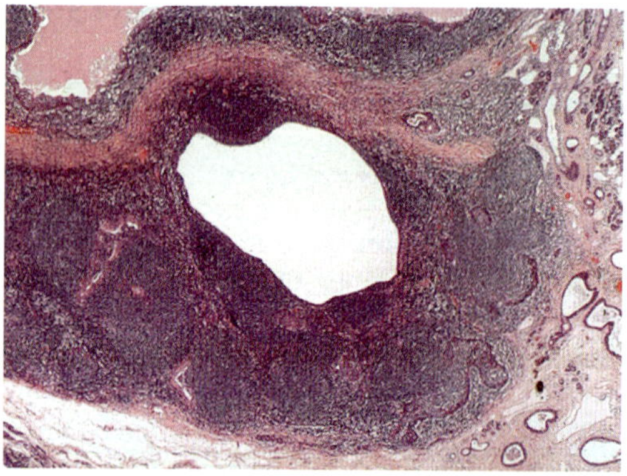

Fig. 10.12: HIV-associated sialadenitis showing epithelial-lined cysts, dense lymphocytic infiltrate and epithelial islands

Treatment and Prognosis

The parotid swellings tend to be persistent and a rapid increase in size could herald the development of a hematolymphoid tumor such as a Burkitt-type high grade B-cell lymphoma. On the other hand, the swellings can shrink dramatically following antiretroviral therapy.

Other Viral Infections of Salivary Glands

Cytomegalovirus is a member of the Herpes-virus group that infects the majority of the population. However, most cases are sub-clinical and clinically significant infections are seen predominantly in immunocompromised individuals and following transplacental transmission. Congenital cytomegalovirus infection (salivary gland inclusion disease) gives rise to a characteristic picture with double-contored 'owl-eye' intracytoplamic viral inclusion bodies in the intralobular duct cells (**Fig. 10.13**).

Acute parotitis may rarely be caused by a range of other viruses including Coxsackie, echo, Epstein-Barr or choriomeningitis viruses.

MUCOCELES

Mucoceles are the most common cystic lesions of salivary glands and are seen almost exclusively in the minor glands. There are three main types: extravasation, retention and superficial.

Extravasation Mucoceles

These account about 85 to 90 percent of mucoceles. Most are considered to be due to trauma to the excretory duct and escape of mucus into the surrounding tissues. The lower lip accounts for about half of the cases (**Fig. 10.14**). Other common sites include the buccal mucosa, floor of the mouth, ventrum of the tongue (up to and including the tip), and the soft palate. Mucoceles are uncommon in the upper lip (~5%) and the possibility of a salivary neoplasm should always be considered when dealing with cysts at this site. The peak incidence of mucoceles is in the second and third decades: occasional cases are multiple.

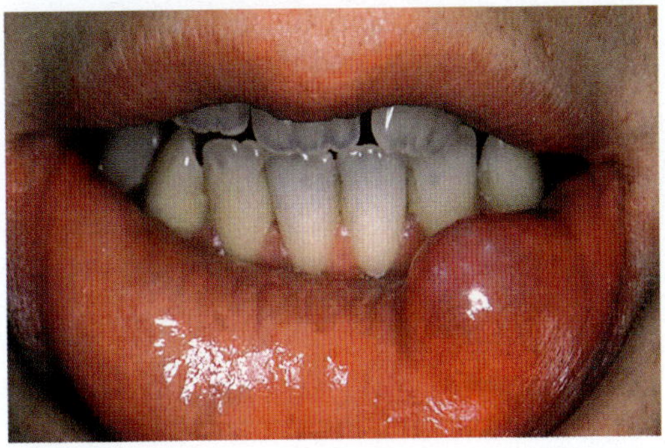

Fig. 10.14: Extravasation mucocele in the lower lip forming a domed, bluish swelling

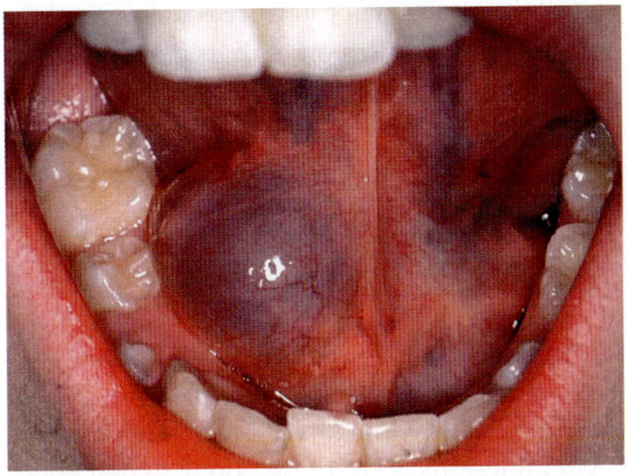

Fig. 10.15: Large ranula in the floor of the mouth

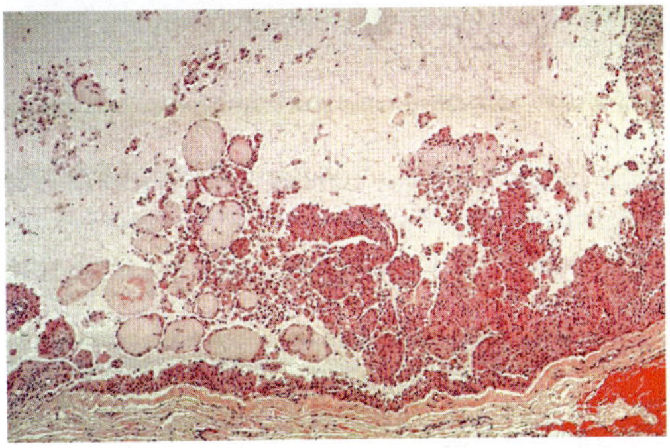

Fig. 10.16: Mucocele showing early cavitation and the cyst starting to be lined by macrophages

Mucoceles typically form bluish, domed swellings which occasionally fluctuate in size or may appear when eating. Some patients tend to nibble on them so they can eventually resemble a fibrous overgrowth. Mucoceles rarely exceed 1 cm in diameter except in the floor of the mouth where they can be several centimeters in size and are called ranulae (**Fig. 10.15**).

Microscopy of early lesions shows ill-defined pools of mucus and acute inflammatory infiltration. Eventually, a central cavity becomes more defined and the cyst is lined initially by granulation tissue (**Fig. 10.16**). This undergoes progressive fibrosis and the cyst is then lined by compressed macrophages many of which are foamy and contain mucus (mucinophages) (**Fig. 10.17**). Similar cells are present in the cyst cavity and are distinctive in fine needle aspirates.

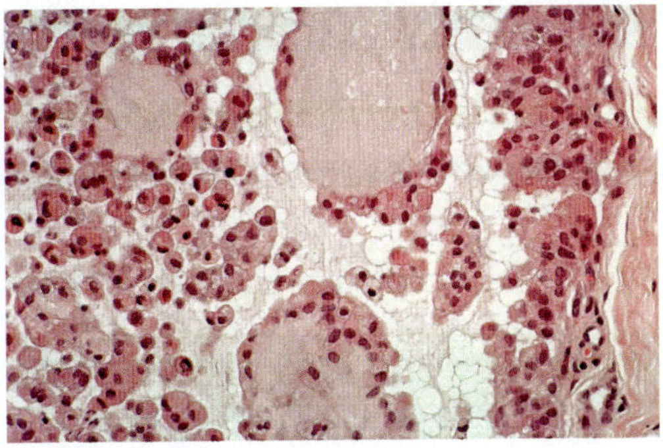

Fig. 10.17: Extravasation mucocele. High power showing numerous foamy macrophages (mucinophages)

Retention Mucoceles (Mucus Retention Cysts)

These are less common (10-15%) and are usually seen in older patients. The etiology is uncertain but it is generally believed that they are due to intermittent duct obstruction. They form unicystic cavities that are lined by modified duct epithelium. This is usually cuboidal or columnar but occasionally there is squamous, mucous or oncocytic metaplasia.

Some mucoceles are located immediately beneath the oral epithelium and raise a small subepithelial blister. These superficial mucoceles are seen most frequently in the region of the palatoglossal fold but they can present in other intraoral sites. They are frequently multiple and recurrent. For unknown reasons, they appear to be much more common in women than men. Superficial mucoceles have been reported in

Box 10.2: Mucoceles

Key features useful in diagnosis
- Most common oral soft tissue cysts.
- 85–90 percent extravasation—due to ductal damage and salivary escape—cysts lined by compressed macrophages and fibrous tissue.
- 10–15 percent retention—due to intermittent duct obstruction—cysts lined by epithelium.
- Age: extravasation 2nd and 3rd decades: retention 5th to 7th decades.
- Sites—50 percent lower lip, rest in cheek, tongue, floor of mouth. Rare in upper lip.

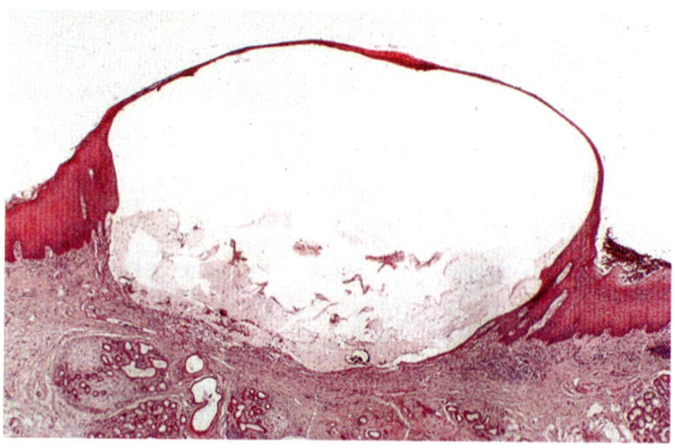

Fig. 10.18: Superficial mucocele forming a subepithelial blister covered by attenuated oral epithelium

patients with intraoral lichen planus and graft versus host disease. Superficial mucoceles are more common than is generally appreciated as they rupture readily to form shallow ulcers that rapidly heal, so there may be little to see clinically. Because they form subepithelial blisters (**Fig. 10.18**), these lesions are sometimes confused with mucocutaneous vesiculating disorders, particularly mucous membrane pemphigoid and occasionally pemphigus vulgaris, both clinically and microscopically.

Treatment and Prognosis

Mucoceles often spontaneously rupture but regeneration of the overlying epithelium can result in the secretion reaccumulating. Although surgery is often necessary, sometimes it is worthwhile delaying active treatment, as the cyst may spontaneously resolve. If removal is indicated, an incision is made through the overlying mucosa and the cyst is removed, together with the related minor salivary gland. Mucoceles in the tongue have a distinct tendency to recur, probably because the associated minor glands are mainly located deeply within the lingual musculature and are damaged further by surgery. In these circumstances, cryotherapy or diathermy may be of value.

NECROTIZING SIALOMETAPLASIA

Necrotizing sialometaplasia is a relatively rare benign and self-limiting inflammatory lesion. It is typically seen in the palate although it can also be found in other minor oropharyngeal glands and occasionally major salivary glands. The main problem with this lesion is that it can simulate malignancy, both clinically and microscopically and this can lead to an erroneous diagnosis of cancer, usually squamous cell carcinoma or mucoepidermoid carcinoma.

Clinical Features

Necrotizing sialometaplasia is of uncertain cause, though it may be associated with cigarette smoking and is sometimes seen after trauma. Bilateral lesions account for about 20 percent of cases and have been reported in the palates of patients with bulimia nervosa. For unexplained reasons, it is much more frequent in the USA than in Britain. The condition predominantly affects middle-aged males (M:F 3:1). In most cases, the patient develops a relatively painless, but often deeply ulcerated (**Fig. 10.19**), swelling on the hard palate, midway between the midline and gingival margin. The lesion, which may be several centimeters in diameter, can clinically resemble a carcinoma but resolves spontaneously within one to three months (**Fig. 10.20**).

Histopathology

Microscopically, there is coagulative necrosis of minor salivary gland tissue with ghost outlines of the acinar cells retaining a lobular distribution. There is often mucous extravasation and a mixed inflammatory infiltrate which is florid in advanced lesions. There is regenerative hyperplasia of the adjacent salivary ducts, often

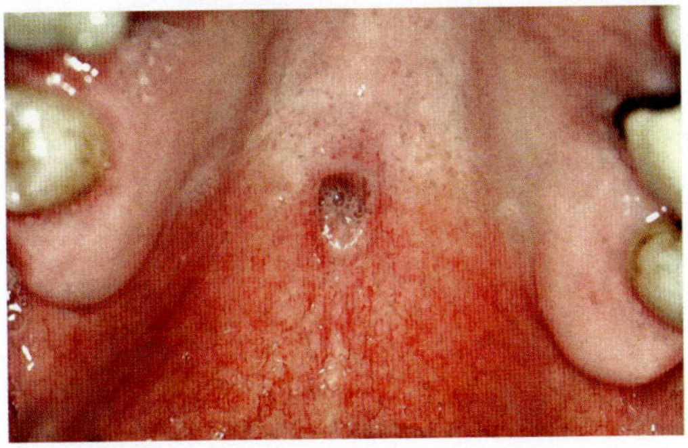

Fig. 10.19: Necrotizing sialometaplasia causing a nondescript but deep ulcer at the junction between the hard and soft palates

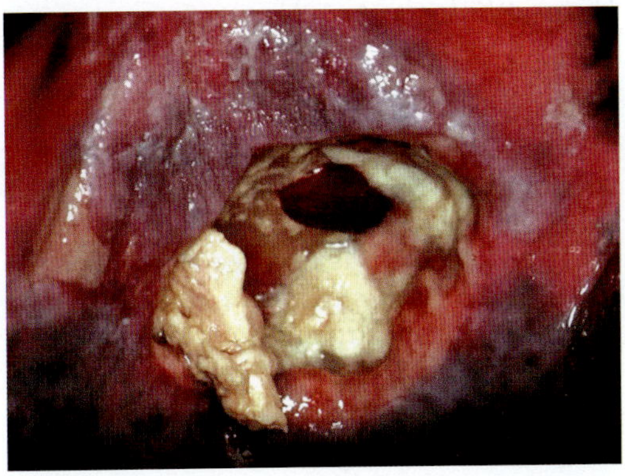

Fig. 10.20: Necrotizing sialometaplasia causing massive ulceration in the center of the palate mimicking a malignant ulcer

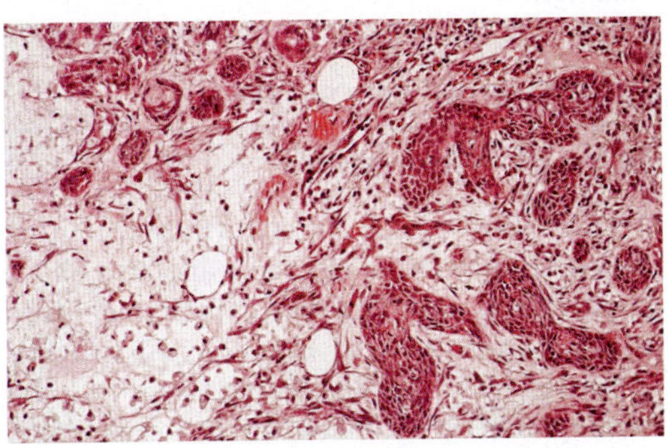

Fig. 10.21: Necrotizing sialometaplasia showing structured necrosis and ghost outlines of the infarcted mucous glands and pseudoepitheliomatous hyperplasia of the adjacent salivary ducts

with striking pseudoepitheliomatous squamous metaplasia forming islands and cords of epithelium. There is no significant cellular atypia but occasional morphologically normal mitotic figures can be seen. Mucous metaplasia may also be present. When the lesion has ulcerated there may be irregular hyperplasia of the overlying or adjacent oral epithelium which may extend into the underlying tissue as pseudoepitheliomatous down-growths (**Fig. 10.21**).

Differential Diagnosis

The lesion needs to be distinguished from squamous carcinoma and mucoepidermoid carcinoma (see mucoepidermoid carcinoma for details).

Treatment and Prognosis

Conservative treatment, including antiseptic mouthwashes and local or systemic analgesics, is all that is required and the lesion resolves spontaneously over time.

SIALOSIS (SIALADENOSIS)

Sialosis is an uncommon condition characterized by noninflammatory, non-neoplastic, persistent swellings of the salivary glands, particularly the parotid glands. It is commoner in women than men and the peak incidence is in the 30 to 60 years age range.

Clinical Features

In most cases, there are bilateral and painless parotid swellings producing a hamster-like appearance (**Fig. 10.22**). Unilateral cases have been described and in some patients aplastic or hypoplastic parotid glands are present on the contralateral side. Sialosis has been reported rarely in the submandibular gland and intraoral minor glands in the palate. Occasionally patients may experience xerostomia or sialorrhea.

The stimulated salivary flow rate and sialochemistry are usually within the standard range, apart from a raised potassium concentration. Sialography is usually normal, although some have described narrowing of the smaller ducts in sialograms.

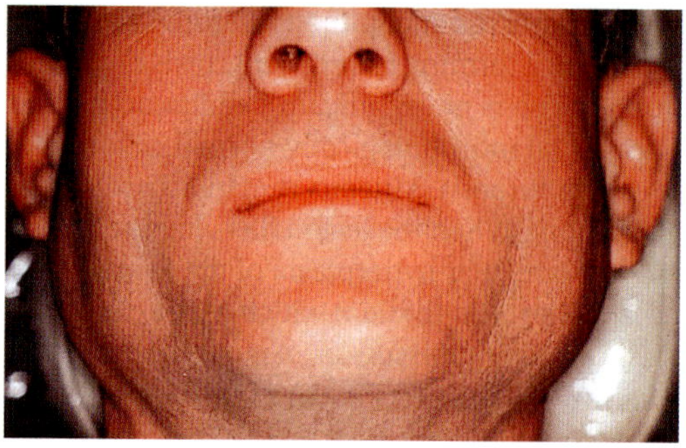

Fig. 10.22: Sialosis (sialadenosis) showing bilateral parotid swellings

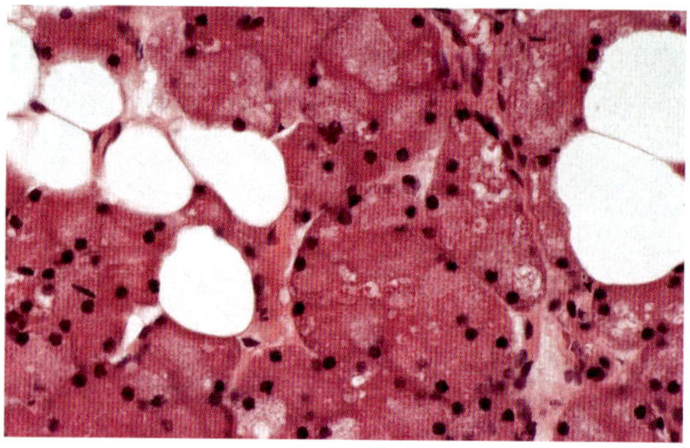

Fig. 10.23: Sialosis (Sialadenosis) of parotid gland showing hypertrophy of the serous acinar cells

The cause of sialosis is uncertain but some cases have been associated with a variety of diseases, (**Table 10.1**) particularly diabetes mellitus, liver disorders and bulimia. It has been postulated that a unifying etiopathogenesis for sialosis is related to peripheral autonomic nerve dysfunction.

Table 10.1
Conditions associated with sialosis

Hormonal
• Diabetes mellitus
• Ovarian insufficiency
• Acromegaly
• Hypothyroidism
• Uremia
Metabolic
• Cirrhosis
• Alcoholism
• Malnutrition
• Bulimia
• Chronic pancreatitis
• Chronic renal failure
Drugs
• Iodine containing drugs
• Antihypertensives
• Isoprenaline
• Lead
• Mercury
• Naproxen

Histopathology

Sialosis is rarely biopsied but microscopy shows that the acinar cells are swollen (hypertrophied) usually with densely packed zymogen granules but sometimes showing vacuolated cells with a loss of cytoplasmic granules (**Fig. 10.23**). Occasionally, there is a mixed population. In some cases, there is extensive fatty infiltration and parenchymal atrophy, but inflammation is typically absent.

Treatment and Prognosis

Nutritional and drug-related sialosis can regress if the associated factors are eliminated but in cases due to diabetes mellitus and chronic alcohol abuse, sialosis usually persists despite treatment.

AUTOIMMUNE DISORDERS

Sjögren's Syndrome

Sjögren's syndrome is one of the most common, chronic autoimmune disorders affecting about 0.5 percent of the population. It is characterized by dry mouth and dry eyes. The histological hallmark of Sjögren's syndrome is the development of lymphoepithelial sialadenitis (LESA). Affected glands show focal acinar atrophy associated with multifocal periductal lymphocytic infiltration and the development of lymphoepithelial lesions ('epimyoepithelial islands'). The damage is progressive and leads to increasing functional impairment. The etiology of Sjögren's syndrome is unknown but a variety of viral and genetic factors have been causally associated. Lesions closely resembling LESA can be seen in patients with HIV and hepatitis C infections but a direct role of viruses in the pathogenesis of Sjögren's syndrome is yet to be established.

Clinical Features

There are two main forms of the disease: primary and secondary. Primary Sjögren's syndrome (sicca syndrome) consists of dry mouth and dry eyes in the absence of any other connective tissue disease. The glandular destruction tends to be severe and is often associated with extraglandular disease. Secondary Sjögren's syndrome is the combination of dry eyes, dry mouth and a connective tissue disorder, usually rheumatoid arthritis. The sicca symptoms are frequently less severe than in the primary type.

The percentages shown in **Table 10.2** are the proportion of patients with a connective tissue disorder who also have Sjögren's syndrome. Because rheumatoid arthritis is far-and-away the most common connective tissue disorder, they form the bulk of patients likely to be seen. On the other hand, because Sjögren's syndrome is so common in patients with primary biliary cirrhosis, it is often possible through the appropriate investigations, to make a diagnosis of potentially serious hepatic disease in an otherwise symptomless patient.

There is a F:M ratio of about 9:1. Most patients are middle aged or elderly, but much younger patients can also be affected. Intermittent enlargement of the major salivary glands, particularly the parotid, affects approximately 20 percent of patients, and there is persistent enlargement in about 5 percent. Sometimes, the principle complaint is not a dry mouth itself, but one of its consequences such as disturbed taste, impaired speech, intraoral soreness or difficulty in swallowing dry food. The oral mucosa can appear dry and wrinkled but frequently seems to be unremarkable. However, there may be no obvious flow of saliva from the parotid ducts and frothy or stringy saliva, particularly in the lower vestibular sulci and floor of the mouth. In long-standing cases, the tongue becomes partially depapillated and develops a very characteristic lobulated dorsal surface (**Fig. 10.24**).

Table 10.2
Diseases most commonly associated with secondary Sjögren's syndrome

- Rheumatoid arthritis (15%)
- Systemic lupus erythematosus (30%)
- Systemic sclerosis (scleroderma)
- Dermatomyositis
- Polyarteritis nodosa
- Primary biliary cirrhosis (70%)

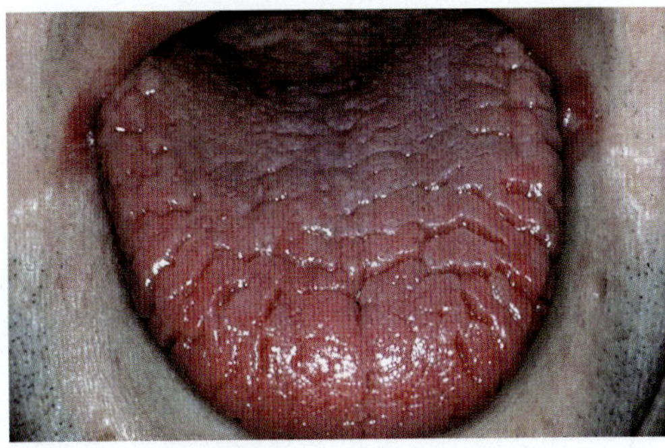

Fig. 10.24: Sjögren's syndrome showing characteristic lobulated tongue and angular stomatitis

Candidal infections are very common and these lead to redness, glazing and soreness of the oral mucosa. Obvious candidal plaques are not frequently seen but may be present in protected mucosal reflections. Angular stomatitis is also common. The xerostomia predisposes to rampant dental caries affecting the cervical collars of the teeth particularly severely. Oral dryness changes the balance of the oral flora and this, together with the compromised secretory function, predisposes patients to acute suppurative parotitis.

The dry eyes associated with Sjögren's syndrome (keratoconjunctivitis sicca) can be the most debilitating aspect of the condition. It results in burning, itching and blurring of vision. Thick secretions tend to accumulate in the conjunctival sac and the conjunctiva may become severely erythematous.

In addition, significant numbers of patients with Sjögren's syndrome, including those with the primary form, can display a wide range of extraglandular manifestations, as shown in **Table 10.3**.

Diagnosis

Patients frequently have nonspecific markers of inflammation such as a raised erythrocyte sedimentation rate and raised C-reactive protein. There is also frequently mild anemia, leukopenia and thrombocytopenia. About half of patients have polyclonal hypergammaglobulinemia. Autoantibodies, particularly rheumatoid factor and rheumatoid arthritis precipitin (RAP), are found in 90 and 75 percent, respectively, of cases of secondary Sjögren's syndrome, but in only 50 and 5 percent, respectively, in primary disease. SS-A (Ro) antibodies are more specific and found in 5 to 10 percent of cases of the primary disease, but in 50 to 80 percent of cases of secondary disease. SS-B (La) antibodies are found in about 75 percent of cases of primary disease, but in 5 percent or less of secondary disease. Gastric parietal cell, thyroid microsomal, thyroglobulin and smooth muscle autoantibodies may also be detected.

▪ Table 10.3
Extraglandular manifestations of Sjögren's syndrome

Musculoskeletal	Rheumatoid arthritis, nonerosive arthritis, myasthenia gravis
Hematolymphoid	Generalized lymphadenopathy, non-Hodgkin lymphoma (40x risk), Waldenström's macroglobulinemia
Gastrointestinal	Hepatitis (primary biliary, chronic active), pancreatitis, pernicious anemia
Cutaneous	Rashes of systemic lupus erythematosus or dermatomyositis, purpura
Respiratory	Parenchymal lung involvement (common but rarely serious)
Renal	Glomerulonephritis, renal calculi, renal tubular acidosis, interstitial nephritis
Vascular	Raynaud's syndrome, vasculitis leading to peripheral neuropathies, including benign sensory trigeminal neuropathy

Histopathology

The characteristic microscopical feature of Sjögren's syndrome is lymphoepithelial sialadenitis (LESA). The initial lesion in the salivary gland is a polyclonal B-and T-cell lymphocytic infiltration aggregating focally around small, intralobular ducts. This periductal infiltrate spreads centrifugally, destroying and replacing the surrounding salivary parenchyma (**Fig. 10.25A**). Reactive lymphoid follicles with germinal centers form in the increasingly dense lymphoid infiltrate which becomes more mixed and contains plasma cells, immunoblasts and histiocytes. Adjacent focal infiltrates eventually fuse and spread throughout the entire salivary lobule but do not cross the interlobular septa. At the same time, the intralobular ducts undergo proliferation of their luminal cells which eventually obliterates the duct lumen forming solid cords. In two dimensional sections these appear as islands. These were previously called epimyoepithelial islands (**Fig. 10.25A**) but, as the role of myoepithelial cells in their formation is questionable, they are now simply called epithelial islands. These islands frequently contain eosinophilic, hyaline droplets consisting of basement membrane material such as type IV collagen and laminin. In addition, they are infiltrated by variable numbers of monoclonal monocytoid or marginal zone B cells. Squamous metaplasia of the epithelial islands is an uncommon feature.

Focal periductal lymphocytic sialadenitis can be seen in the minor salivary glands of patients with Sjögren's syndrome. However, in minor glands the characteristic lymphoepithelial lesions with ductal proliferation are uncommon. The number and distribution of the lymphocytic foci mirror, to a degree, the extent of the disease present in major glands, and biopsies of minor glands from the lower lip have been used for diagnostic purposes (**Fig. 10.25B**). The number of defined, focal aggregates adjacent to normal appearing mucous acini and containing more than 50 lymphocytes in 4 mm^2 of tissue is

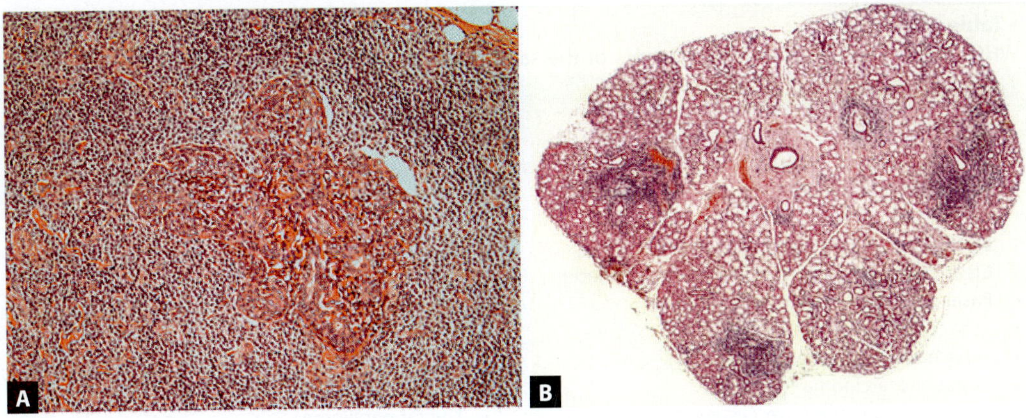

Figs 10.25A and B: (A) Sjögren's syndrome. Late stage lymphoepithelial sialadenitis showing total acinar destruction and replacement by lymphocytes and an epithelial island containing hyaline deposits; (B) Labial gland biopsy showing multifocal, periductal, lymphocytic sialadenitis

counted in at least four lobules. A focus score of 1 or more is consistent with a diagnosis of Sjögren's syndrome.

Treatment and Prognosis

This is dealt with in Chapter 11.

NEOPLASTIC SALIVARY DISORDERS

Salivary gland tumors are a diverse and complex range of neoplasms. They form only about 3 percent of tumors in the head and neck but in the current World Health Organization classification there are 13 benign and 24 malignant named epithelial tumors, and many of these have defined variants (**Table 10.4**). In addition, some benign tumors have a propensity to recur or to progress to malignancy, and some malignant tumors behave in a relatively low grade manner.

In this Chapter, only the most common and clinically signifcant tumors will be considered in detail.

BENIGN NEOPLASMS

Pleomorphic Adenoma

Pleomorphic adenoma has been defined as 'a tumor of variable capsulation characterized microscopically by architectural rather than cellular pleomorphism. Epithelial and modified myoepithelial elements intermingle most commonly with tissue of mucoid, myxoid or chondroid appearances'. Synonyms include mixed tumor and benign mixed tumor.

Clinical Features

Pleomorphic adenoma is the most common salivary gland tumor and accounts for between about half and two thirds of all tumors seen in the parotid, submandibular glands and minor glands. It is rare in the sublingual gland where, for unknown reasons, most of the tumors are malignant. The tumor has a wide age range with a peak incidence in the fourth and fifth decades. As with many other salivary neoplasms, children and adolescents can be affected. There is a female preponderance of about 2:1. About 80 percent arise in the parotid gland with most of the rest developing in the submandibular (~10%) and intraoral minor salivary glands (~10%).

In the major glands, pleomorphic adenoma usually forms a slow-growing, painless swelling (**Fig. 10.26A**). This tends to be smooth, firm and mobile. In larger tumors particularly, the surface may be knobbly or bosselated. Deep lobe tumors may present as a parapharyngeal mass. Minor gland pleomorphic adenomas usually form painless, mobile, submucosal swellings.

▪ Table 10.4
WHO histological classification of tumors of the salivary glands 2005

Malignant epithelial tumors	*Benign epithelial tumors*
• Acinic cell carcinoma • Mucoepidermoid carcinoma • Adenoid cystic carcinoma • Polymorphous low-grade adenocarcinoma • Epithelial-myoepithelial carcinoma • Clear cell carcinoma, not otherwise specified • Basal cell adenocarcinoma • Sebaceous carcinoma • Sebaceous lymphadenocarcinoma • Cystadenocarcinoma – Low-grade cribriform cystadenocarcinoma • Mucinous adenocarcinoma • Oncocytic carcinoma • Salivary duct carcinoma • Adenocarcinoma, not otherwise specified • Myoepithelial carcinoma • Carcinoma ex-pleomorphic adenoma • Carcinosarcoma • Metastasizing pleomorphic adenoma • Squamous cell carcinoma • Small cell carcinoma • Large cell carcinoma • Lymphoepithelial carcinoma • Sialoblastoma	• Pleomorphic adenoma • Myoepithelioma • Basal cell adenoma • Warthin tumor • Oncocytoma • Canalicular adenoma • Sebaceous adenoma • Lymphadenoma – Sebaceous – Nonsebaceous • Ductal papillomas – Inverted ductal papilloma – Intraductal papilloma – Sialadenoma papilliferum • Cystadenoma **Soft tissue tumors** • Hemangioma **Hematolymphoid tumors** • Hodgkin lymphoma • Diffuse large B-cell lymphoma • Extranodal marginal zone-B cell lymphoma **Secondary tumors**

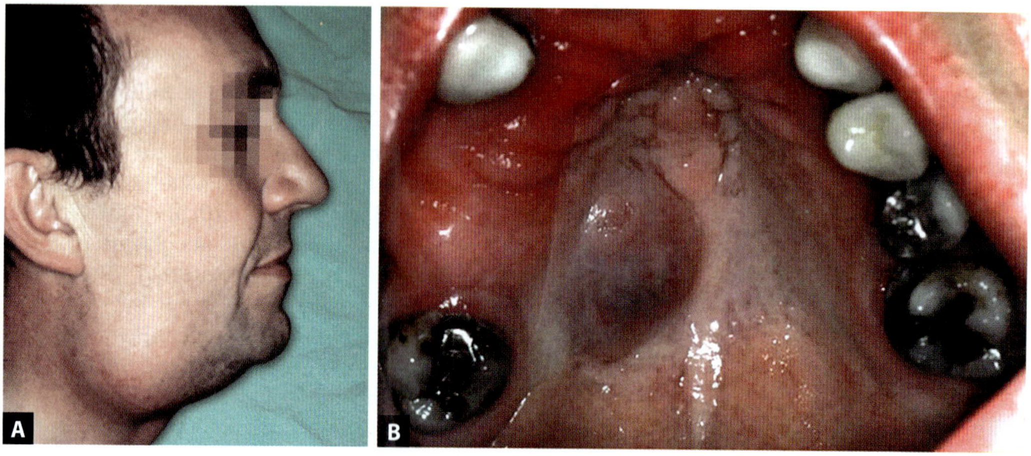

Figs 10.26A and B: (A) Large pleomorphic adenoma of the submandibular gland; (B) Pleomorphic adenoma at the junction of the hard and soft palates

In the palate, however, they typically present as unilateral swellings at the junction of the hard and soft palates (**Fig. 10.26B**). Here they tend to be fixed to the underlying mucoperiosteum. In addition, at this site particularly, they may ulcerate as a result of masticatory trauma.

Histopathology

Pleomorphic adenomas, as their name implies, can show a very wide range of morphological diversity. The principle elements are epithelial cells, modified myoepithelial cells and mesenchymal. The epithelial component shows a variety of cell types and architectural configurations. Cell types include cuboidal, basaloid and squamous epithelial cells and the myoepithelial cell component can be spindle, plasmacytoid or clear. The cellular elements can form sheets, cords or duct-like structures (**Fig. 10.27A**). The latter are frequently double layered with an inner layer of duct lining cells and an outer layer of myoepithelial cells which often have clear cytoplasm and small, hyperchromatic and angular nuclei. The duct lumina may contain eosinophilic secretions and may also dilate to form microcysts. Squamous metaplasia, with or without keratinization, is common (**Fig. 10.27B**). A very characteristic feature of some tumors is the formation of so-called hyaline or plasmacytoid cells which are modified myoepithelial cells (**Fig. 10.27C**). These tend to form sheets of loosely adherent cells.

The mesenchymal component is a product of the myoepithelial cells and can be mucoid, myxoid, cartilaginous or hyalinized (**Fig. 10.27D**). It sometimes forms the main element of the tumor. The tumor cartilage has the same structure as normal cartilage and stains for both type II collagen and the proteoglycan keratan sulfate. Occasionally bone forms either by a process resembling endochondral ossification or stromal osseous metaplasia. Mucoid areas are sparsely cellular and contain scattered myoepithelial cells whose cytoplasm tends to merge with the surrounding stroma. There is a distinct tendency for pleomorphic adenomas progressively to scar and be replaced by fibrous and elastic tissue. In old tumors there may be extensive dystrophic calcification.

Pleomorphic adenomas are often encapsulated but the capsule varies in both thickness and extent (**Fig. 10.27D**). Some tumors, particularly those that are predominantly mucoid, may show little evidence of a capsule and tumor is in direct continuity with the surrounding salivary parenchyma (**Fig. 10.27E**). In addition, tumors can show invasion of the capsule and sometimes the tumor bulges through small gaps in the capsule to produce what look like satellite tumors (**Fig. 10.27F**). There is a tendency for the tumor to split away from the capsule during surgical and pathological manipulation. This was thought by surgeons to offer a plane of cleavage but the split is intratumoral and leaves tumor adherent to the capsule.

In minor gland pleomorphic adenomas the capsule is often a poorly formed or absent.

Differential Diagnosis

When tumors show the characteristic combination of epithelial and mesenchymal components the diagnosis is relatively straight forward but in limited biopsy material there can be problems. For example, double-layered duct-like structures, as described previously, can be seen in both adenoid cystic carcinoma and epithelial myoepithelial carcinoma and it may not be possible to make the distinction in small biopsies. Areas of squamous metaplasia are common in pleomorphic adenomas but these show no cellular atypia and the presence of other components, particularly plasmacytoid cells and stromal elements, should prevent confusion with squamous carcinoma.

Treatment and Prognosis

Although pleomorphic adenoma is a benign tumor it has a tendency both to recur and undergo malignant transformation. Recurrences are mainly seen in the major glands, particularly the parotid, and they are usually multifocal. Surgery in the parotid gland is complicated by the presence of the facial nerve. In attempts to preserve this nerve, initially surgeons used to curette the tumor or remove it by dissecting around the 'capsule'. However, the relationship between the tumor and its capsule described previously militates against the success of this procedure and recurrence rates of over 50 percent have been recorded in the older literature. Most surgeons now use either superficial parotidectomy or one of its limited variants to remove these tumors. Mucoid tumors are particularly prone

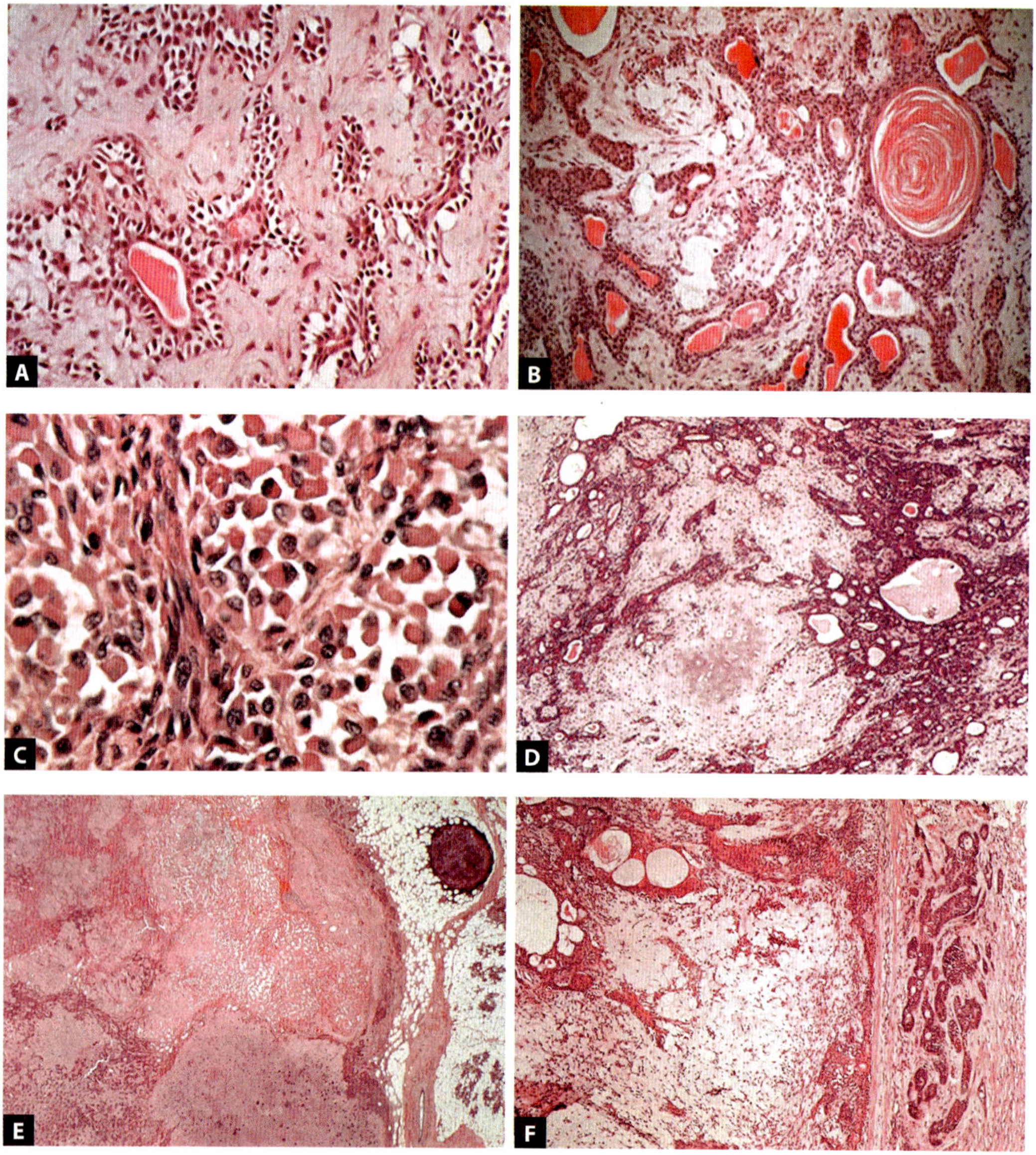

Figs 10.27A to F: (A) Low power of pleomorphic adenoma showing double-layered duct-like structures; (B) Duct-like structures containing eosinophilic secretions and a focus of squamous metaplasia; (C) Plasmacytoid (hyaline) and spindle-shaped myoepithelial cells; (D) Discrete fibrous capsule, myxochondroid areas and duct-like structures; (E) No obvious capsule and a 'satellite' nodule that is usually attached to the main tumor mass by a thin isthmus; (F) Capsular invasion

to recurrence as their diffluent nature leads to a high-risk of intraoperative rupture and it is probable that the low biological requirements of such tumors allows implanted cells to survive. In recent years the reported rate of recurrence is around about 5 percent but the longer cases are followed up, the more likely recurrences will be detected. Radiotherapy has been used to both prevent and treat recurrences but its value is debatable. The risk of malignant change is discussed in the section covering carcinoma ex-pleomorphic adenoma.

Box 10.3: Pleomorphic adenoma

Key features helpful in diagnosis

- Most common salivary neoplasm: ~60 percent of parotid, submandibular and minor gland tumors.
- F:M 2:1 Peak incidence 4th and 5th decades.
- Slow-growing, painless, mobile mass.
- Well circumscribed mass with variable encapsulation.
- Epithelial component: Duct-like structures and sheets.
- Myoepithelial component: Plasmacytoid (hyaline cell), epithelioid, spindle cell, clear.
- Mesenchymal component: Myxoid, myxochondroid, hyalinized, osseous.

Warthin's Tumor

Warthin's tumor is defined as 'a tumor composed of glandular and often cystic structures, sometimes with a papillary cystic arrangement, lined by characteristic bilayered epithelium, comprising inner columnar eosinophilic or oncocytic cells surrounded by smaller basal cells. The stroma contains a variable amount of lymphoid tissue with germinal centers'. Synonyms include adenolymphoma, cystadenolymphoma, and papillary cystadenoma lymphomatosum. Analysis of the X chromosome-linked human androgen receptor gene has shown that Warthin's tumor is nonclonal, and this makes its neoplastic status questionable.

Clinical Features

Warthin's tumor is the second most common neoplasm of the salivary glands and arises virtually exclusively in the parotid gland and para-parotid lymph nodes. It is much less frequent in dark-skinned individuals than Caucasians. Over the last 60 years, the M:F has gone from 10:1 to parity. This has been linked with the increasing frequency of women who smoke cigarettes, as it is known that the incidence of these tumors in smokers is eight times that of nonsmokers. Most patients are in the 50 to 70 years age group. Warthin's tumor usually presents as a slow-growing, soft, mobile mass in the parotid gland. It is uncommon for tumors to exceed 4 cm in size. Pain, rapid expansion and sometimes facial nerve weakness can be seen in tumors that become inflamed or infarcted. Warthin's tumor is the most common salivary neoplasm showing multifocally, both unilaterally and bilaterally, and may be seen in association with other salivary tumors.

Histopathology

Warthin's tumor is circumscribed and usually has a thin, fibrous capsule which may be incomplete. It has papillary cystic spaces of varying sizes (**Fig. 10.28A**) and these contain viscous clear or brownish fluid. Occasionally tumors are unicystic and some can be solid. The microscopical features are very characteristic. The tumor has two major components: epithelial and lymphoid (**Fig. 10.28B**). The proportion of these components is variable and either can predominate. The cysts are lined by a double layer of epithelial cells which often project into the cystic spaces as papillary infoldings. In the luminal layer, the cells are tall and columnar and contain oncocytic (i.e. pink and granular) cytoplasm (**Fig. 10.28C**). The nuclei are oval and bland and are located centrally or form a palisaded row towards the luminal end of the cell. The cell surface often shows apocrine blebbing and occasionally cilia are seen. The cytoplasm of the abluminal cells is similar, but these cells are cuboidal in shape and are less regular and abundant. Foci of squamous and mucous metaplasia are relatively common (**Fig. 10.28D**). The cystic cavities may contain variable amounts of eosinophilic material and cholesterol clefts.

The stroma consists of reactive lymphoid tissue consisting of polyclonal B and T cells, usually together with reactive follicles. Sometimes, the tumor shows a close resemblance to a normal lymph node and has a defined capsule and subcapsular sinus. Microscopic foci of inflammation, squamous metaplasia, degeneration and fibrosis are common. In some cases, however, there is virtual obliteration of the lymphoid and sometimes the epithelial component, and replacement by necrotic, inflammatory and fibrous tissue. This appearance has been called the 'infected', 'infarcted' or 'metaplastic' variant of Warthin's tumor. In some cases, there is extensive squamous metaplasia that can be confused with malignancy. In

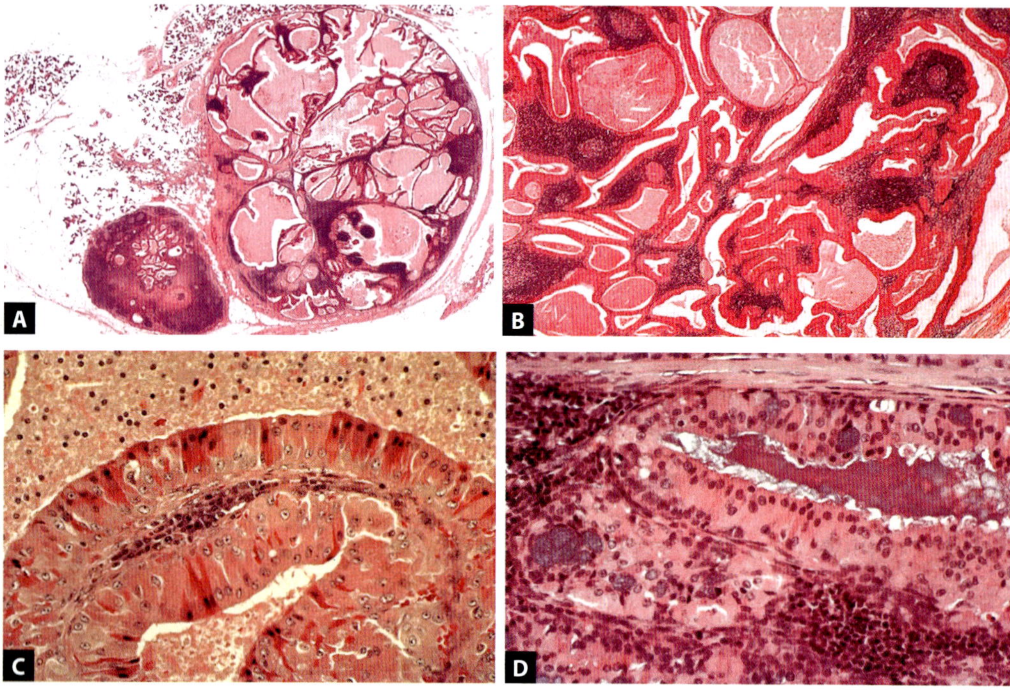

Figs 10.28A to D: (A) Low power of Warthin's tumor showing two of several nodules in the same parotid gland; (B) Papillary projections of oncocytic epithelium projecting into cystic spaces and a dense lymphocytic stroma; (C) Palisaded luminal cells and less numerous basal cells, in addition there are both 'light' and 'dark' (pyknocytes) cells; (D) Mucous metaplasia

addition, epithelioid granulomas, with or without multinucleated giant cells, can form and these have sometimes been misinterpreted as tuberculosis or sarcoidosis.

Differential Diagnosis

Typical Warthin's tumor is the easiest salivary neoplasm to diagnose microscopically. Papillary cystadenoma closely resembles Warthin's tumor but lacks a lymphoid component. As described previously, the infarcted variant is the type most likely to lead to confusion. This will probably become more frequent with the increasing use of fine needle aspiration biopsies. The presence of tumor tissue within an intra- or para-parotid lymph node, particularly if cystic, means that a metastasis may need to be considered. In such a case, the tumor is likely to show obvious cytological features of malignancy and misdiagnosis is unlikely.

Treatment and Prognosis

If the diagnosis can be confidently made on diagnostic imaging and/or fine needle

Box 10.4: Warthin's tumor

Key features helpful in diagnosis

- Second most common salivary tumor—seen almost exclusively in parotid.
- F:M ~ 1:10 Peak incidence in 6th and 7th decades.
- Slow-growing painless mass can be multifocal and bilateral.
- Circumscribed, usually cystic mass with intraluminal papillary ingrowths.
- Epithelial component—double-layered and oncocytic with columnar luminal cell and cuboidal basal cells. Mucous and squamous metaplasia.
- Mesenchymal component—dense masses of polyclonal B and T lymphocytes and germinal centers.

aspiration biopsy, active treatment may not be necessary. Conservative surgery is usually curative and the few cases of 'recurrence' are probably due to the development of new tumors. Malignant change in the epithelial and lymphoid elements of Warthin's tumor has been reported, but it is very rare.

Canalicular Adenoma

Canalicular adenoma is defined as 'a tumor composed of columnar epithelial cells arranged in thin, anastomosing cords with a beaded pattern. The stroma is characteristically paucicellular and highly vascular. Synonyms include basal cell adenoma (canalicular type), monomorphic adenoma (canalicular type) and monomorphic adenomatosis of minor salivary glands.

Clinical Features

Canalicular adenoma is uncommon and is seen almost exclusively in minor glands, particular the upper lip (80%) and adjacent buccal mucosa. It is seen predominantly in adults, with a mean age of about 65 years: there is a slight female preponderance. Occasional cases are bilateral or multifocal. Canalicular adenoma usually presents as a slow-growing, painless, mobile swelling that can appear cystic or solid. The overlying oral mucosa may appear normal or have a bluish hue. Tumors are typically 1 to 2 cm in diameter.

Histological Features

Canalicular adenomas are well circumscribed and variably encapsulated (**Fig. 10.29A**). They are usually multicystic but sometimes tumor tissue is no more than a focal area of mural thickening in a single cyst. Foci of adenomatous change can sometimes be present in adjacent minor salivary gland lobules. The tumor forms parallel rows of single columnar or, less commonly, cuboidal epithelial cells. These rows may be focally opposed, but at intervals the rows tend separate forming a characteristic 'beaded' appearance. The cells are cytologically bland and have eosinophilic cytoplasm and round nuclei with finely granular basophilic nuclei. The cellular cords are usually sharply demarcated from the loosely collagenized and sparsely cellular stroma. There is a distinct tendency for the stroma to undergo degeneration producing microcystic spaces containing a network of congested and dilated capillaries. There may be areas of inflammation, interstitial hemorrhage and hemosiderin deposition.

Differential Diagnosis

The main differential diagnoses are basal cell adenoma and adenoid cystic carcinoma. The bilayered nature of canalicular adenoma and the characteristic stromal degeneration helps to distinguish the tumor from the trabecular and tubulotrabecular variants of basal cell adenoma. Occasional tumors have components resembling both neoplasms and it may not be possible to make a meaningful distinction. Adenoid cystic carcinomas are likely to show invasion and have a different nuclear morphology. It is important to not to interpret multifocality as evidence of local infiltration.

Treatment and Prognosis

Complete, conservative surgical excision is usually curative. Recurrence is likely to be the result of multifocality.

Box 10.5: Canalicular adenoma

Key features helpful in diagnosis

- Uncommon and seen almost exclusively in minor glands, particularly upper lip (~80%).
- Slight female predominance, peak incidence in 7th decade.
- Slow-growing painless mass which can appear cystic or solid.
- Can be multifocal and bilateral.
- Well circumscribed and variably encapsulated.
- Parallel rows of single columnar cells with focal separation producing a 'beaded' appearance.
- Degenerative stroma forming micro- and macrocyts.

Basal Cell Adenoma

Basal cell adenoma is defined as 'a rare benign neoplasm characterized by the basaloid appearance of the tumor cells and absence of the myxochondroid stromal component present in pleomorphic adenoma'.

Clinical Features

Basal cell adenomas are rare and account for about 2 percent of salivary gland tumors. The large majority affect the major salivary glands, particularly the parotid (75%). The few reported cases in minor glands have mainly involved the upper lip. The tumors are usually seen in older individuals with a mean age at presentation of 58 years. In most subtypes, there is F:M of about 2:1 but in the membranous variant there is no sex predilection. The tumors usually present as a painless, mobile, solid mass that is usually less than 3 cm in diameter.

Histopathology

Basal cell adenomas are well circumscribed and encapsulated and may contain cystic spaces (**Fig. 10.29B**). Microscopy shows the tumor is composed of basaloid cells arranged in cords, sheets, nests and duct-like structures. There are two main cell types: one has scanty eosinophilic cytoplasm and round, basophilic nuclei with indistinct nucleoli and the other has a large pale nucleus and abundant cytoplasm. The cells are cytologically bland and there are few, if any, mitoses.

Basal cell adenoma can be subclassified into four subtypes: trabecular, tubular, solid and membranous, but some tumors can display more than one architectural pattern. All the variants can show cystic change. The most common subtype is solid and forms sheets of variable size and shape. The peripheral cells are cuboidal or columnar and often show palisading. These cells have the immunological characteristics of modified myoepithelial cells. There may be focal areas of cellular whorling and squamous eddies, sometimes with focal keratinzation, can be seen. Some tumors contain cribriform, pseudocystic areas. The islands are sharply demarcated from the loosely cellular fibrous stroma. In the trabecular variant the cells are arranged as interconnecting narrow cords. In some of these cases, the stroma is richly cellular and the cells have myoepithelial characteristics. The tubular variant is very uncommon and consists of duct-like structures surrounded by one or more layers of basaloid cells enclosing eosinophilic secretions. Most cases show combinations with trabecular patterns and some pathologists merge the two variants into a tubulotrabecular subtype (**Fig. 10.29C**). The membranous variant (dermal analog tumor) is rare and microscopically resembles cutaneous eccrine dermal cylindroma. The growth pattern is similar to that of the solid variant but the cell islands are surrounded by thick and distinctive hyaline membrane and coalescing globules of similar material are present in the intercellular area (**Fig. 10.29D**). This variant is often multifocal and bilateral.

Differential Diagnosis

The main differential diagnoses are basal cell adenocarcinoma, adenoid cystic carcinoma, pleomorphic adenoma and canalicular adenoma. Basal cell adenocarcinoma can show limited cellular atypia and mitotic activity and is distinguished from basal cell adenoma largely on the basis of evidence of invasion. Although cribriform areas can occasionally be seen in basal cell adenoma, the tumor is noninvasive and has different nuclear morphology from adenoid cystic carcinoma. Areas resembling basal cell adenoma can sometimes be seen in pleomorphic adenoma. However, basal cell adenomas themselves lack the other characteristic features of pleomorphic adenoma such as plasmacytoid cells, myxochondroid matrix, etc. Canalicular adenomas have characteristic double-layered trabeculae and lack evidence of myoepithelial differentiation.

Treatment and Prognosis

Basal cell adenoma is essentially benign and conservative excision is usually curative. However, the membranous variant can be multifocal and bilateral and this may lead to apparent recurrence in about a quarter of affected patients. In addition, this variant may have coexisting cutaneous tumors including multiple dermal cylindromas (turban tumors of the scalp), trichoepitheliomas, basal cell tumors and others. Exceptionally, basal cell adenomas can progress to form basal cell adenocarcinomas and, even more rarely, other forms of carcinoma.

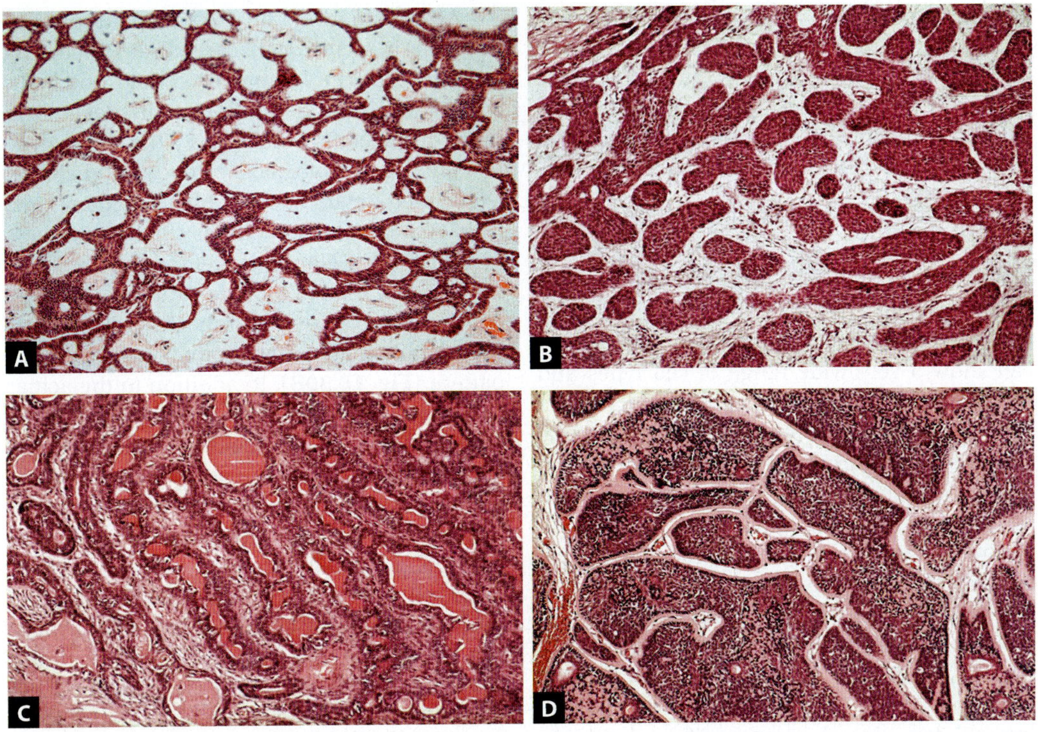

Figs 10.29A to D: (A) Canalicular adenoma showing the characteristic bilayered columnar epithelium and stromal degeneration; (B) Basal cell adenoma showing solid variant; (C) Tubulotrabecular variant; (D) Membranous variant (dermal analog tumor) containing solid islands of tumor with peri- and intratumoral hyaline material

Box 10.6: Basal cell adenoma

Key features helpful in diagnosis

- Rare: About 2 percent of salivary tumors and large majority seen in major glands.
- F:M 2:1 Peak incidence in 6th decade.
- Slow-growing painless mobile mass: Membranous variant can be multifocal and bilateral and associated with cutaneous neoplasms.
- Well circumscribed encapsulated mass.
- Basaloid epithelial and myoepithelial cells in solid, trabecular, tubular and membranous configurations.
- Some tumors have 'myoepithelial cell-rich' stroma.

MALIGNANT NEOPLASMS

Acinic Cell Carcinoma

Acinic cell carcinoma is defined as 'a malignant epithelial neoplasm of salivary glands in which at least some of the neoplastic cells demonstrate serous acinar differentiation, which is characterized by cytoplasmic zymogen secretory granules. Salivary ductal cells are also a component of this neoplasm'. Synonyms include acinic cell adenocarcinoma and acinous cell carcinoma.

Clinical Features

Acinic cell carcinoma accounts for about 3 to 6 percent of all salivary gland tumors and between 7 and 17.5 percent of malignant salivary neoplasms in major series. About 80 to 90 percent of cases arise in the parotid gland and most of the remainder involve the minor glands of the oral cavity, particularly the upper lip, buccal mucosa and palate. The tumor is relatively uncommon in the submandibular and sublingual glands. There is a slight female preponderance and the tumor affects a wide age range (3–91 years) with a mean of 44 years. Acinic cell carcinoma usually presents as a slow-growing, mobile mass, although some cases may be fixed and nodular. About half the patients complain of pain or tenderness and 5 to 10 percent show involvement of the facial nerve.

Histopathology

Macroscopically, the tumors are usually circumscribed, round or lobulated and they rarely exceed 3 cm in diameter. Microscopy can show a very wide range of cell types and morphological configurations. The archetypal cell is acinic and closely resembles normal serous cells. These cells are round or polyhedral and have abundant, pale, basophilic cytoplasm which contains dense, grayish or blue zymogen granules. These may be fine or moderately coarse and are periodic acid Schiff positive and diastase resistant. The nuclei are round, uniform, and typically located peripherally. They are usually darkly stained and basophilic or occasionally more vesicular. Other cell types include intercalated ductal, nonspecific glandular, vacuolated and clear cells. Intercalated duct cells are smaller than the acinar cells and are cuboidal in shape. They have less cytoplasm which is eosinophilic or amphophilic. The nuclei are usually centrally located. These cells surround central duct-like spaces of variable sizes. Nonspecific glandular cells are polygonal or round and are smaller than acinar cells. Their cytoplasm is amphophilic and they usually aggregate as sheets of cells with indistinct cytoplasmic borders. The nuclei are larger and more vesicular than in the other cell types and, in addition, they may show mild pleomorphism and occasional mitotic figures. Vacuolated cells are common and are sometimes a conspicuous component of the tumor. They are round or polygonal and contain clear, PAS/D negative cytoplasmic vacuoles of variable sizes and occasional zymogen granules. The nuclei have an open chromatin pattern and may also show mild pleomorphism. Cells with clear cytoplasm and distinct cell membranes may be seen singly or in small foci but they are rarely a conspicuous feature. They do not contain glycogen and, in some cases, may be a fixation or processing artefact.

A wide variety of growth patterns can be seen in acinic cell carcinoma, including solid, microcystic, papillary—cystic and follicular, and tumors may contain several of these architectural subtypes. The solid type usually consists of sheets or nodules of closely aggregated, cytologically bland acinar cells (**Fig. 10.30A**) and sometimes smaller numbers of nonspecific glandular cells or intercalated ductal cells. The microcystic pattern is the most common and consists of numerous small spaces within more solid tumor, producing a lattice-like pattern (**Fig. 10.30B**). In addition to the acinar cells, these tumors may contain intercalated ductal and vacuolated cells. The cystic spaces can enlarge and there may be intracystic papillary proliferation. In this papillary-cystic variant, luminal cells may show conspicuous hob-nailing and typical acinic cells may be inconspicuous (**Fig. 10.30C**). This variant often shows intratumoral and intracystic hemorrhage and phagocytosis of hemosiderin by tumor cells. The follicular pattern is uncommon but distinctive, and consists of multiple cystic spaces of varying sizes (**Fig. 10.30D**). These are lined predominantly by cells of the intercalated duct type and contain homogeneous, eosinophilic and proteinaceous material. The intercystic areas consist predominantly of nonspecific glandular cells. Psammoma bodies are an occasional but sometimes conspicuous feature of acinic cell carcinomas.

The stroma is usually scanty and composed of delicate fibrovascular tissue but may become more dense and hyalinized. Infiltration of the stroma by lymphocytes is common, but some tumors show very striking tumor-associated lymphoid proliferation, together with germinal center formation. These tumors tend to be of the solid or microcytic type, are well circumscribed, and have a low MIB-1 proliferation index. This variant has been termed 'well-differentiated acinic cell carcinoma with abundant lymphoid stroma' and preliminary data suggest that it has more favorable prognosis.

Differential Diagnosis

The cellular and architectural variability of acinic cell carcinoma can make precise diagnosis difficult. Solid tumors especially, can

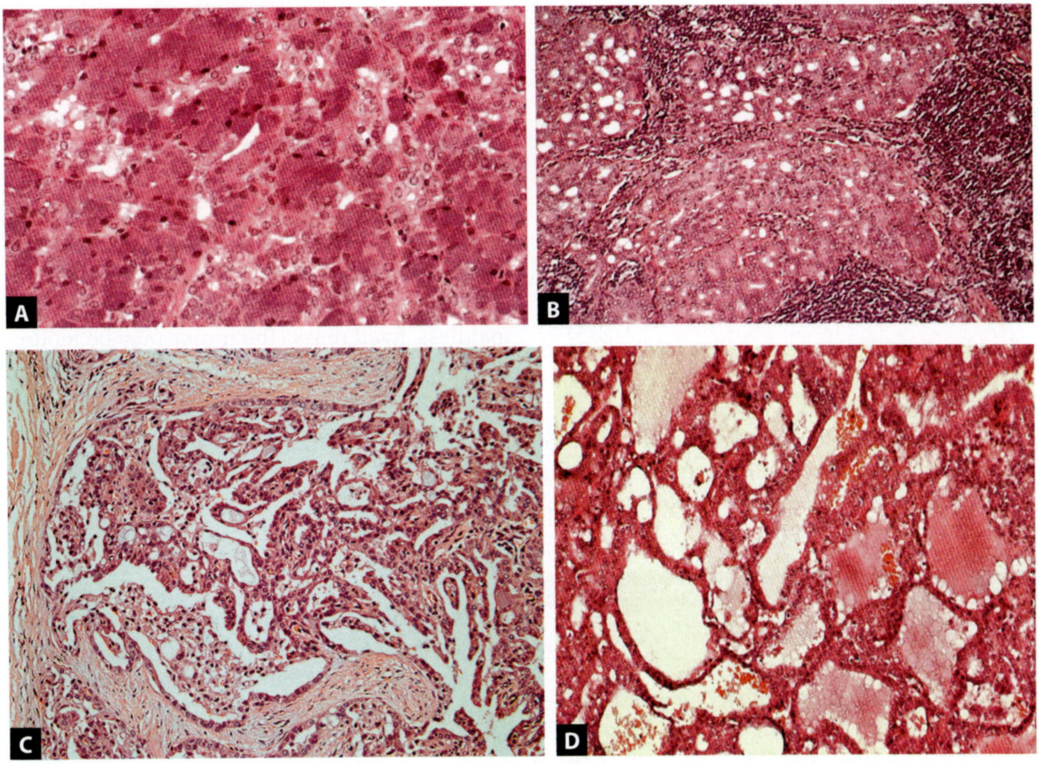

Figs 10.30A to D: (A) Acinic cell carcinoma. Solid type showing granular basophilic cells that resemble normal serous acinar cells; (B) Microcystic pattern and lymphocyte-rich stroma; (C) Papillary-cystic variant; (D) Follicular pattern

closely resemble normal salivary serous acini or sialadenitis, particularly in limited material. The lack of other structures such as intercalated or striated ducts should aid recognition. Papillary variants need to be distinguished from cystadenocarcinoma and the presence of zymogen granules and vacuolated cells may help. The microcystic spaces contain mucicarmine-positive secretions and can be misinterpreted as mucocytic differentiation in a mucoepidermoid carcinoma. These tumors, however, lack other characteristic features of mucoepidermoid carcinomas, including intermediate and epidermoid cells. The follicular variant of acinic cell carcinoma resembles follicular thyroid carcinoma but in equivocal cases staining for thyroglobulin avoids confusion.

Treatment and Prognosis

The average recurrence rate is about 35 percent and the average rate of metastasis and disease-associated death is about 16 percent but these figures mask a very wide range in the literature. In a meta analysis of over 2000 cases, the 5- and 10-year survival was 82 and 68 percent respectively. Multiple recurrences, locoregional or distant metastases, usually to lung or bone, are associated with an unfavorable outcome. Tumors in the minor glands have a better prognosis than those in major glands, and submandibular gland tumors have a particularly poor prognosis. There are no universally accepted histological grading schemes for this tumor, and no consistent relationship between the main histological subtypes and prognosis.

Histological features that may be associated with a poor prognosis, however, include high mitotic frequency, cellular pleomorphism, necrosis, perineural or vascular invasion, stromal desmoplasia and widespread invasion. Clinical staging at presentation appears to be the best predictor of clinical outcome. Large size (> 6 cm diameter) and the involvement of the deep lobe of the parotid gland are associated with a worse outcome. Multiple recurrences, multinodularity and the presence of regional or distant metastases are indicators of poor prognosis. Superficial parotidectomy is the usual treatment and neck dissection is not undertaken unless there is good evidence of regional metastasis. Failure to remove the tumor completely at the first excision is another indicator of poor outcome.

Box 10.7: Acinic cell carcinoma

Key features helpful in diagnosis

- Accounts for 3–6 percent salivary tumors: 80–90 percent parotid and minor glands next most common location.
- F:M ~ 1.5:1 Wide age range (3–91) with peak incidence in 5th decade.
- Slow-growing, mobile or fixed mass with variable pain and/or facial nerve involvement.
- Usually less than 3 cm often circumscribed but nonencapsulated.
- Characteristic serous acinar cells with other cell types including nonspecific glandular, intercalated duct, vacuolated and clear.
- Diverse architectural patterns including solid, microcystic, papillary-cystic and follicular.

Mucoepidermoid Carcinoma

Mucoepidermoid carcinoma is defined as 'a malignant glandular epithelial neoplasm characterized by the proliferation of mucous, intermediate and epidermoid cells, with columnar, clear and oncocytic features'.

Clinical Features

Mucoepidermoid carcinoma is the commonest primary malignant salivary neoplasm in most major series (12–29%). It can be seen in both adults and children and the mean age is around 45 years. About half of the cases affect the major glands, particularly the parotid gland (45% of cases). The tumor can involve a wide range of intraoral sites including the palate, buccal mucosa, lips, retromolar pad, tongue and floor of mouth. Rare, central (intraosseous) cases have been reported, mainly involving the body and angle of mandible. There is a slight female predominance of about 1.5:1. Mucoepidermoid carcinoma usually presents as a slow-growing, painless, fixed mass. The tumor may be tender, and in advanced tumors there may be neural involvement, trismus and dysphagia. Intraoral tumors may present as a bluish red, fluctuant swelling that closely resembles a mucocele or a vascular blemish.

Histopathology

Mucoepidermoid carcinoma may appear macroscopically circumscribed or partially encapsulated but they are almost invariably invasive. Mucoepidermoid carcinomas form sheets, islands and duct-like structures together with cysts of variable sizes (**Fig. 10.31A**). The cysts contain mucinous secretions and commonly rupture spreading mucus and tumor cells into the surrounding tissue and evoking a florid inflammatory reaction. The tumor consists predominantly of three cell types: epidermoid, intermediate and mucous. The proportion of each cell type can vary widely between tumors and sometimes within a single tumor mass. Less common cell types include columnar cells, clear cells and oncocytes. Intermediate cells usually predominate and range from small basal cells with scanty, basophilic cytoplasm and small, central, hyperchromatic nuclei to large, oval cells with more abundant, eosinophilic cytoplasm. Intermediate cells usually form sheets and may be the basal layer of intratumoral cysts (**Fig. 10.31B**). Epidermoid cells may be relatively uncommon and are polygonal in shape, with ovoid or elongated, vesicular nuclei and abundant eosinophilic cytoplasm. Individual cell keratinization or keratin pearl formation is usually only seen following a biopsy or fine needle aspiration. Mucocytes are large with pale, slightly blue and sometimes foamy cytoplasm that is positive for mucicarmine, Alcian blue

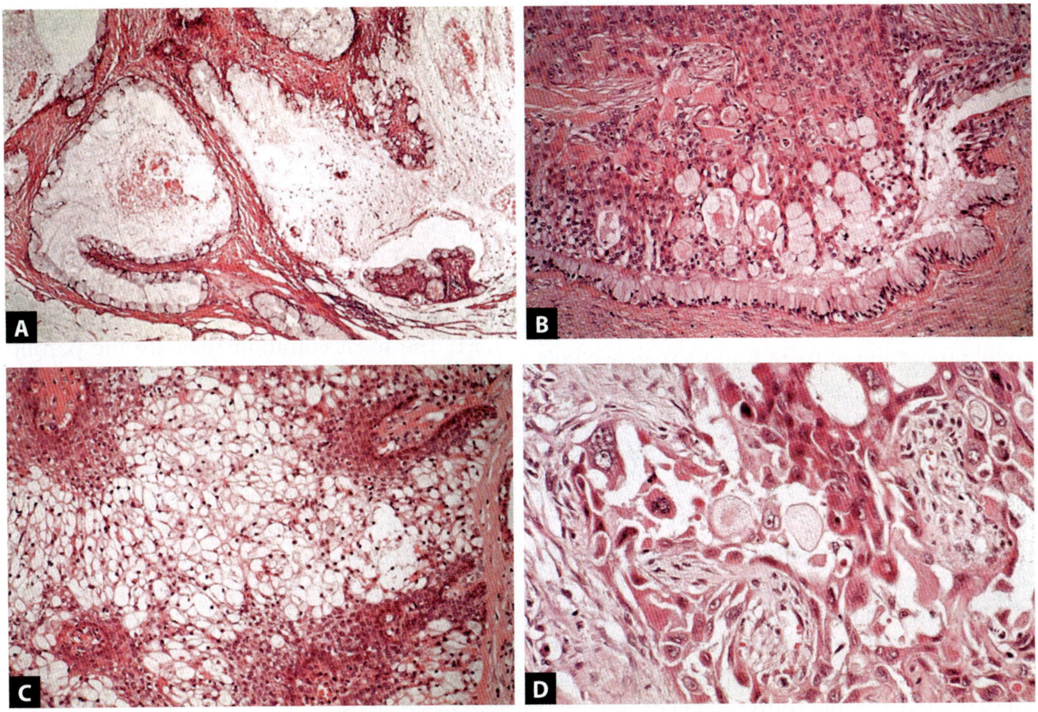

Figs 10.31A to D: (A) Mucoepidermoid carcinoma consisting predominantly of cysts lined by mucous cells and sparse numbers of intermediate cells; (B) Predominantly solid tumor consisting of intermediate cells and mucocytes, some of which are columnar; (C) Prominent intermediate and clear cells; (D) High grade mucoepidermoid carcinoma showing pleomorphic epidermoid and mucous cells

and periodic acid Schiff. They may be single or form aggregates and they frequently line cysts or duct-like structures. Sometimes broad papillary projections, often covered in mucous cells, extend into the cystic lumina. In some tumors mucocytes may be so uncommon that they may be difficult to detect without special stains. Clear cells have distinct cell boundaries, small, centrally located, hyperchromatic nuclei and water clear cytoplasm (**Fig. 10.31C**). They tend to form sheets and may be the predominant element of the tumor. Columnar cells are uncommon and are usually seen lining cyst. Oncocytes are also uncommon but rarely the entire tumor can show oncocytic metaplasia.

Mucoepidermoid carcinomas can be graded as low, intermediate and high. Low-grade tumors are cytologically bland, and the tumors are predominantly cystic with a high mucous cell content. Higher grade tumors tend to be more solid, show evidence of cytological atypia, a high mitotic frequency, neural invasion and necrosis (**Fig. 10.31D**). Some pathologists ascribe numerical values to a variety of histopathological characteristics and define the grades using a point scoring system.

Differential Diagnosis

Necrotizing sialometaplasia can be confused with mucoepidermoid carcinoma. In necrotizing sialometaplasia, however, the epithelial islands have a lobular distribution and there are usually areas showing transition from obvious ducts. In addition, there are no intermediate cells and cyst formation is not a feature. High grade tumors can resemble squamous cell carcinoma but lack evidence of keratinization, and also show foci of mucocytic differentiation. Clear cell variants need to be distinguished from epithelial myoepithelial carcinomas by the lack of an inner, duct-lining cell component and clear cell carcinoma (NOS) by the presence of more characteristic areas elsewhere in the tumor.

Treatment and Prognosis

Prognosis depends on a variety of factors including clinical stage, site, histological grading and surgical margins. The majority of tumors are low grade and the prognosis is generally good with a 5 years survival rate of over 95 percent. A small proportion of these tumors unexpectedly undergo metastasis so protracted follow-up is essential. In tumors with a high clinical stage or histological grading, and cases of incomplete surgical removal, the 5 years survival rate falls to less than 45 percent. In addition, tumors in the submandibular gland, floor of mouth and tongue have a poorer prognosis. The treatment of choice is complete surgical excision with a neck dissection if there is good evidence of locoregional metastasis. Radiotherapy has a limited impact on the course of the disease.

Box 10.8: Mucoepidermoid carcinoma

Key features helpful in diagnosis

- Most common primary malignant salivary neoplasm (12–29%).
- Over half of cases involve parotid gland and most of the remainder affect the mouth and respiratory tract.
- F:M ~ 1.5:1 Wide age range including children with peak incidence in 5th decade.
- Slow-growing, often painless, fixed mass: symptoms include pain, nerve involvement and trismus. Tumors in minor glands may ulcerate.
- May be circumscribed but usually nonencapsulated and infiltrative and variably cystic.
- Cell types include intermediate, epidermoid and mucous cells and less commonly clear, columnar and oncocytic.
- May be predominantly cystic or solid and inflammation is common.
- Tumors graded as low, intermediate or high.

Adenoid Cystic Carcinoma

Adenoid cystic carcinoma is defined as 'a basaloid tumor consisting of epithelial and myoepithelial cells in variable morphologic configurations, including tubular, cribriform and solid patterns'.

Clinical Features

Adenoid cystic carcinoma accounted for 4.4 percent of all salivary gland tumors and 11.8 percent of malignant salivary neoplasms in the largest reported series. It affects a wide age range, with a peak incidence in 50 to 70 year olds. There is a female preponderance of about 1.5:1. The most common sites are the parotid (21%), palate (17%) and submandibular gland (15%). Minor glands of the mouth and the upper aerodigestive tract account for about half of all cases. Tumors usually present as a slow growing but widely infiltrative mass of long duration and they can be mobile or fixed. They may be tender or painful, and cranial nerve lesions, particularly facial nerve palsy, can be the presenting feature. Tumors of minor glands often show ulceration of the overlying mucosa.

Histopathology

Adenoid cystic carcinoma is composed of luminal ductal cells and abluminal, modified myoepithelial cells. The latter predominate and have indistinct cell borders and frequently sparse, amphophilic or clear cytoplasm. The nuclei are uniform in size, basophilic and may be round or angular (peg-shaped). The ductal cells surround small and sometimes indistinct lumina; they are cuboidal and have more abundant, eosinophilic cytoplasm and round, uniform nuclei that may contain small nucleoli. There are three main morphological patterns: cribriform (cylindromatous), tubular and solid, in that order of frequency. A mixture of these patterns may be seen. The cribriform variant consists of islands of modified myoepithelial cells containing rounded, pseudocystic areas forming a characteristic 'Swiss cheese' appearance (**Fig. 10.32 A**). The pseudocysts are basophilic and mucoid, or consist of hyaline, eosinophilic material. They are composed of glycosaminoglycans and reduplicated basement membrane material. Foci of ductal cells are present within the myoepithelial areas but may require careful examination to detect. The tubular variant is double layered and has conspicuous ductal differentiation (**Fig. 10.32B**). There is an inner layer of eosinophilic, duct-lining cells and the abluminal myoepithelial cells may show clear cytoplasm and irregular, angular nuclei or be morphologically similar to the luminal layer. Occasionally, foci of squamous, sebaceous or oncocytic metaplasia are present. The least common, solid variant consists of islands or sheets of basaloid cells with larger and less angular nuclei (**Fig. 10.32C**). Duct-lining cells may be few and inconspicuous and comedonecrosis is common. Mitoses are sparse in the cribriform and tubular patterns but may be frequent, often together with extensive apoptosis, in the solid type. The stroma is usually fibrous and cases where hyalinization is so abundant that tumor cells are attenuated into strands have been reported as a sclerosing variant (**Fig. 10.32D**). Perineural or intraneural invasion is common and frequently conspicuous and the tumor can extend along nerves and their branches over a wide area (**Fig. 10.33**). The tumor may invade bone extensively before there is any radiological evidence of bone destruction. Lymph node involvement is uncommon (~ 5% of cases) and is usually due to contiguous spread rather than lymphatic permeation or embolization.

Differential Diagnosis

It is important to distinguish adenoid cystic carcinoma from polymorphous low-grade adenocarcinoma in tumors from minor salivary glands. Polymorphous low-grade adenocarcinoma consists of a uniform cell population with cytologically bland, round or oval and vesicular nuclei and pale eosinophilic cytoplasm, whereas cells in adenoid cystic carcinoma often have clear cytoplasm and angular, hyperchromatic nuclei and may show mitotic activity. The MIB-1 proliferative index is reported to be nearly 10x higher in adenoid cystic carcinoma than polymorphous low-grade adenocarcinoma with no overlap zone. Smooth muscle markers of myoepithelial differentiation are positive in adenoid cystic carcinoma but negative in polymorphous low-grade adenocarcinoma. In addition, this tumor shows a much wider spectrum of histomorphological differentiation. Even when cribriform areas are present in polymorphous low-grade adenocarcinoma they are typically focal and adenoid cystic carcinoma does not show papillary differentiation or the single cord arrangement of cells seen in polymorphous low-grade adenocarcinoma. Although both adenoid cystic carcinoma and polymorphous low-grade adenocarcinoma show neural invasion, in polymorphous low-grade adenocarcinoma this is often associated with a striking whorling arrangement of single file cords of cells or small ducts, and is seen predominantly within or very close to the main tumor mass. Occasional foci in pleomorphic adenoma can resemble adenoid cystic carcinoma, but the presence of typical myxochondroid matrix and plasmacytoid or spindle-shaped cells helps to avoid confusion. Basaloid squamous cell carcinoma can resemble solid variants of adenoid cystic carcinoma but typically involves the hypopharynx and glottal region, which are uncommon sites for adenoid cystic carcinoma. Both can show islands with cribriform configurations, hyaline material surrounding tumor nests and solid areas with comedonecrosis, but basaloid squamous carcinoma also has evidence of squamous differentiation and usually involves the overlying mucosa. The distinction from epithelial-myoepithelial carcinoma is covered under that entity.

Treatment and Prognosis

The average 5 and 10-year survival rates are about 60 and 40 percent respectively but the majority of patients usually die of, or with, the tumor. Local recurrence is very common, especially in the first 5 years after surgery. The main prognostic factors are site, clinical stage and histological pattern. Bone involvement and failure of primary surgery are associated with poor prognosis. Correlations between tumor morphology, grading and outcome have yielded conflicting results, particularly after 10 years follow-up due to the overall poor long-term prognosis. The tubular and cribriform variants have been reported to have a better outcome than tumors with a solid component, especially if this exceeds 30 percent of the tumor volume. Some studies suggest that tumor size and clinical stage are more reliable indicators

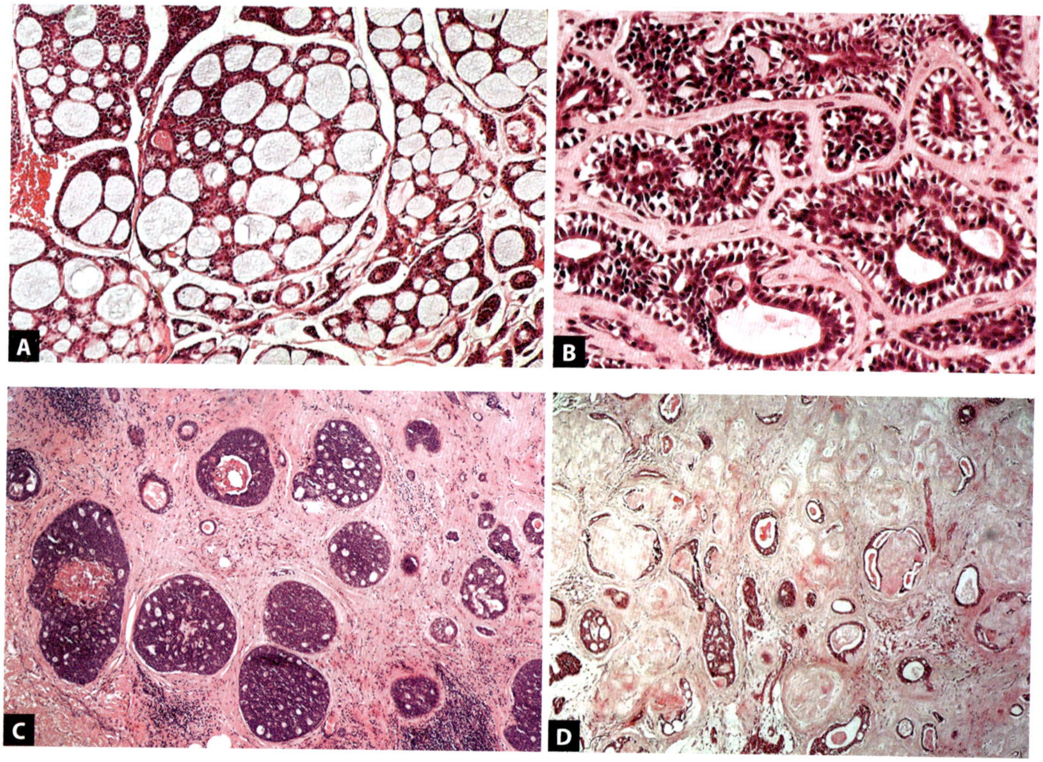

Figs 10.32A to D: (A) Adenoid cystic carcinoma showing the characteristic cribriform (cylindromatous) pattern; (B) High power of tubular variant with double-layered duct-like structures; (C) Solid variant with foci of comedonecrosis; (D) Extensive stromal hyalinization and attenuation of the tumor islands

of prognosis. Adenoid cystic carcinomas in the submandibular gland have a poorer prognosis than those in the parotid. The relationship between perineural invasion and survival is also contentious but invasion of larger nerves appears to correlate with more aggressive behavior. In a review of the literature, Barrett and Speight (2002) found 23 percent (range 2–86%) of patients had clinical evidence of neurological deficit. Histological evidence of perineural invasion was reported in 51 percent (range 8–86%) of cases. Facial nerve palsy was an indicator of poor prognosis but histological evidence of perineural invasion appeared not to be an independent factor but was associated with other adverse features such as clinically large and more aggressive tumors. In addition, large follow-up studies of patients with adenoid cystic carcinoma have found that both histological grades and perineural invasion are unreliable predictors of behavior and suggest that clinical stage is a better guide to prognosis. Lymph node involvement is relatively uncommon

Box 10.9: Adenoid cystic carcinoma

Key features helpful in diagnosis

- Accounts for about 12 percent of malignant salivary gland neoplasms.
- Parotid most common site (~20%) and half of cases involve the mouth and upper aerodigestive tract.
- F:M ~ 1.5:1 Wide age range but rare in children, peak incidence in 6th and 7th decades.
- Slow-growing, variably painful mass: neural involvement, particular facial nerve palsy, is common.
- Composed of duct-lining cells and modified myoepithelial cells.
- Main patterns are cribriform, tubular and solid
- Stroma often extensively hyalinized.
- Perineural invasion common and may be extensive.

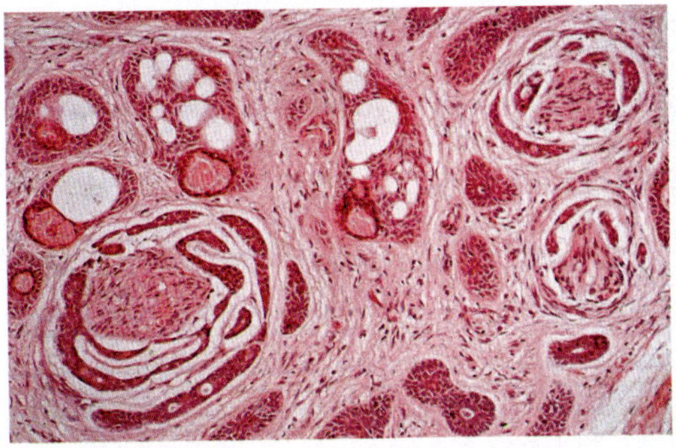

Fig. 10.33: Adenoid cystic carcinoma showing conspicuous perineural invasion

but distant metastases to lung, bone, brain and liver are seen in 40 to 60 percent of cases. Wide local excision, together with adjuvant radiotherapy, offers the best hope of local control.

Polymorphous Low-grade Adenocarcinoma

Polymorphous low-grade adenocarcinoma has been defined as 'a malignant epithelial tumor characterized by cytological uniformity, morphological diversity, an infiltrative growth pattern, and low metastatic potential'. Synonyms include terminal duct carcinoma and lobular carcinoma.

Clinical Features

Polymorphous low-grade adenocarcinoma is seen almost exclusively in the minor glands where it is one of the most common malignant tumors, accounting for about 25 percent of malignancies in these sites. The palate is the most frequent location (~60%) and other sites include the lips, particularly the upper, buccal mucosa, retromolar trigone and base of tongue. Most cases arise in the 50 to 70 years age group and there is a female predominance of 2:1. The tumor usually presents as a slow-growing painless mass which can be mobile or fixed and rarely exceeds 3 cm in diameter. Ulceration and bleeding are uncommon features.

Histopathology

Polymorphous low-grade adenocarcinoma usually appears grossly to be circumscribed but has infiltrative margins. Tumors rarely exceed 3 cm in diameter. The hallmark of the tumor is cytological uniformity and morphological diversity. The cells are isomorphic and cytologically bland. They have abundant eosinophilic cytoplasm, small- to medium-sized, round or oval nuclei containing pale and finely dispersed chromatin and relatively inconspicuous nucleoli. Mitoses are infrequent and necrosis is not a feature. The most common architectural configurations are lobular, nests or theques, cribriform areas and fascicular, duct-like structures of varying sizes (**Figs 10.34A and B**). There may be focal papillary or papillary-cystic areas. In the lobular areas, there may be palisading of the peripheral cells. The duct-like structures are usually composed of a single layer of small cuboidal cells. Both true tubular structures and pseudocystic spaces, with or without pale-staining mucoid contents, result in a cribriform appearance. The areas showing a cribriform pattern are usually localized. Columns of single tumor cells can be seen forming an "Indian-file" arrangement, especially towards the periphery of the tumor. These cells particularly, often show concentric whorling around small nerves and sometimes small vessels or duct-like structures, within or close to the edge of the tumor (**Fig. 10.34C**). Areas of oncocytic or squamous metaplasia are occasionally seen. It is common to see foci of pre-existing salivary parenchyma within the main tumor mass. Stromal fibrosis, elastosis and mucinosis are often present but chondroid or myxochondroid differentiation is not a feature (**Fig. 10.34D**). The tumor tends to abut immediately below the oral epithelium (**Fig. 10.35**) and shows invasion into the surrounding minor gland parenchyma.

Differential Diagnosis

The differential diagnosis of polymorphous low-grade adenocarcinoma includes pleomorphic adenoma, adenoid cystic carcinoma

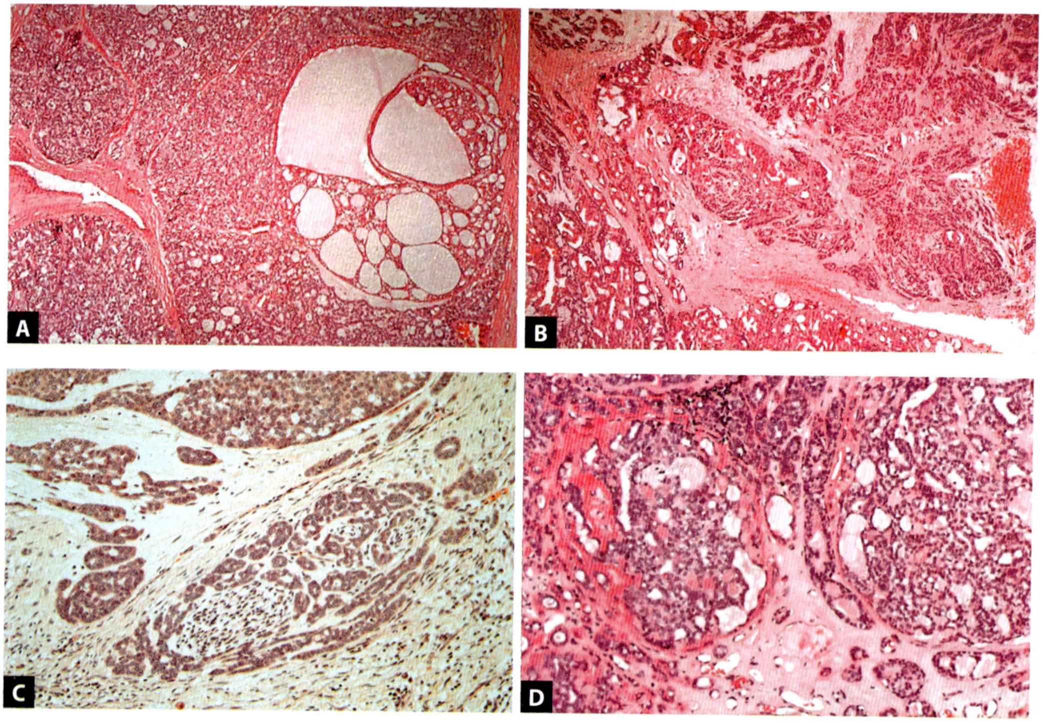

Figs 10.34A to D: (A) Polymorphous low-grade adenocarcinoma showing pale-staining cells forming sheets, islands, single-layered duct-like structures and cribriform patterns; (B) Duct-like structures of variable sizes; (C) Perineural whorling of small, single-layered duct-like structures and single-file cells; (D) Stromal hyalinization and elastosis

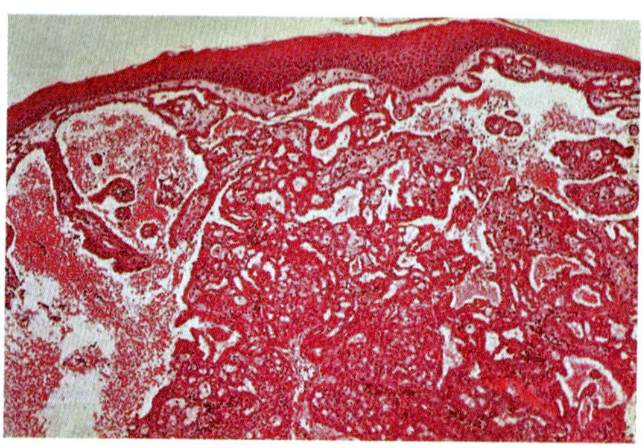

Fig. 10.35: Polymorphous low-grade adenocarcinoma abutting directly under the oral epithelium and forming papillary configurations

and papillary cystadenocarcinoma. Both pleomorphic adenoma and polymorphous low-grade adenocarcinoma consist of cytologically bland cells and show a variety of architectural configurations. However, pleomorphic adenoma is circumscribed and contains other characteristic features such as cartilaginous differentiation and plasmacytoid myoepithelial cells. In addition, the tubular structures in pleomorphic adenoma are bilayered. The distinction from adenoid cystic carcinoma is covered under that tumor. Papillary cystadenocarcinomas usually show a more uniform architecture and display more obvious cytological features of malignancy.

Treatment and Prognosis

Most polymorphous low-grade adenocarcinomas are cured by conservative and, in some cases, incomplete surgical excision. However, 9 to 17 percent of tumors recur and 9 to 15 percent involve regional lymph nodes. Despite this, the overall prognosis is excellent with more distant metastasis and death due to tumor being rare. Tumors with a significant papillary configuration appear to have a higher incidence of cervical lymph node metastasis and some consider these to be variants of papillary cystadenocarcinoma.

Box 10.10: Polymorphous low-grade adenocarcinoma

Key features helpful in diagnosis

- Seen almost exclusively in minor glands and accounts for about 25 percent of salivary malignancies in these sites.
- Palate (60%) most common site: others include lip (especially upper) buccal mucosa, retromolar pad, base of tongue.
- F:M 2:1 peak incidence in 6th to 8th decades.
- Slow-growing, painless, mobile or fixed mass. Ulceration uncommon.
- Circumscribed, usually nonencapsulated.
- Cytologically uniform and bland cells with pale staining nuclei and sparse mitotic activity.
- Morphologically diverse with multiple architectural patterns in single tumor mass.
- Characteristic concentric whorling of tumor around small nerves.

Epithelial-myoepithelial Carcinoma

Epithelial-myoepithelial carcinoma is defined as 'a malignant tumor composed of variable proportions of two cell types, which typically form duct-like structures. The biphasic morphology is represented by an inner layer of duct lining, epithelial-type cells and an outer layer of clear, myoepithelial-type cells'. It has many synonyms including clear cell adenoma, glycogen-rich adenoma, tubular carcinoma, clear cell myoepithelioma, glycogen-rich adenocarcinoma and others.

Clinical Features

Epithelial-myoepithelial carcinoma is uncommon accounting for about 1 percent of all salivary tumors. The mean age is about 60 years and the tumor is rare in children. There is a 2:1 female predominance. Most cases arise in the parotid (75%) or submandibular glands (10–12%). They usually present as a long-standing, painless mass and nerve involvement is uncommon. In the mouth, the palate and tongue are the usual sites and the tumors may ulcerate.

Histopathology

The tumor forms a circumscribed mass that is usually nonencapsulated and is often lobulated or multinodular. Most tumors range from 2 to 8 cm in diameter and cystic areas are relatively common.

Epithelial myoepithelial carcinoma is biphasic and consists of double-layered, duct- like structures (**Fig. 10.36A**). There is usually an inner layer of single cells that can be cuboidal or columnar and have a central round or oval nucleus with finely granular, densely eosinophilic cytoplasm. Cells in the outer layer are polygonal and form single or multiple layers. They have abundant, clear cytoplasm which is rich in glycogen, and vesicular, eccentrically placed nuclei. The proportion of these two cell types is widely variable, as is their distribution. The duct-like structures may be widely separated by fibrous or more hyaline connective tissue or they may aggregate forming cohesive sheets with a thequal or nested architecture. In some cases, the clear cells are the predominant feature and duct-lining cells may be infrequent and form small, solid islands that may not be immediately apparent (**Fig. 10.36B**). Sometimes, the inner and outer layers are composed of morphologically similar cells which both may have clear (**Fig. 10.36C**) or nonclear cytoplasm. About 20 percent of cases contain cystic or papillary areas. Squamous or oncocytic metaplasia, usually of the inner duct-lining cells, is an uncommon feature. Most tumors are cytologically bland with infrequent mitoses and necrosis is uncommon. Although many tumors show limited parenchymal invasion, in about 30 percent of cases there is perineural invasion and 10 percent show angiolymphatic involvement. Rare cases of de-differentiated epithelial-myoepithelial carcinoma have been reported and the tumor may be a component of carcinoma ex-pleomorphic adenoma.

Differential Diagnosis

The main differential diagnosis of epithelial myoepithelial carcinoma are other salivary gland tumors containing double layered duct-like structures and tumors composed mainly of

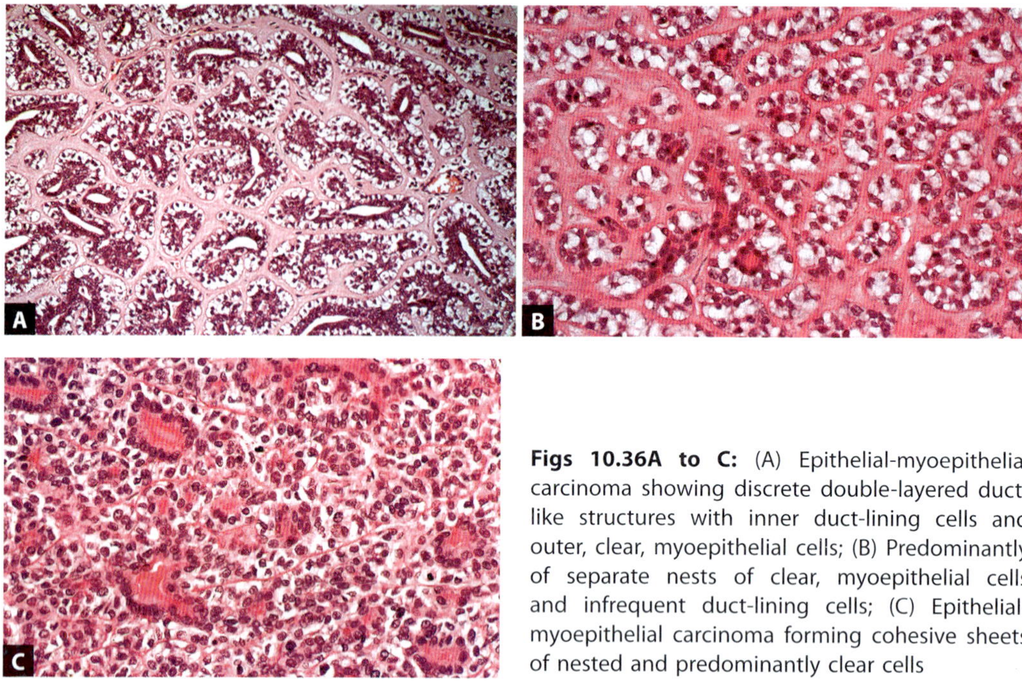

Figs 10.36A to C: (A) Epithelial-myoepithelial carcinoma showing discrete double-layered duct-like structures with inner duct-lining cells and outer, clear, myoepithelial cells; (B) Predominantly of separate nests of clear, myoepithelial cells and infrequent duct-lining cells; (C) Epithelial-myoepithelial carcinoma forming cohesive sheets of nested and predominantly clear cells

clear cells. Double-layered, duct-like structures can be seen in pleomorphic adenoma and the tubular variant of adenoid cystic carcinoma. However, the clear cells in these tumors usually have less abundant cytoplasm and their nuclei are typically more hyperchromatic and angular. In addition, these features are usually only a focal aspect of a more typical tumor. In biopsy material, the distinction may be difficult or cannot be made with confidence. Many salivary neoplasms, both benign and malignant, can show focal or extensive areas composed of clear cells. These include pleomorphic adenoma, myoepithelioma, oncocytoma, mucoepidermoid carcinoma, clear cell carcinoma and metastatic renal carcinoma. Precise differentiation of these tumors from epithelial myoepithelial carcinoma is outside the scope of this Chapter.

Treatment and Prognosis

Epithelial myoepithelial carcinoma is a low to intermediate grade tumor with a relatively high rate of recurrence (~30–40%) and metastasis to regional lymph nodes and distant sites such as lung, liver and kidney (5–25%). Notwithstanding this, the long term prognosis is generally good with a 10 year survival rate of over 80 percent. Clinical factors associated with a poor outcome include incomplete surgical excision, larger tumors, rapid growth and tumors involving minor glands. Microscopical features associated with more aggressive behavior include nuclear hyperchromasia, aneuploidy, high mitotic frequency, angiolymphatic invasion and necrosis.

The treatment of choice is surgery together with neck dissection when there is evidence of spread to the regional lymph nodes. Adjuvant radiotherapy has been used in advanced or recurrent cases, but its value is questionable.

Salivary Duct Carcinoma

Salivary duct carcinoma is defined as 'an aggressive adenocarcinoma which resembles high-grade breast ductal carcinoma'.

Clinical Features

Salivary duct carcinoma can arise *ab initio* and is also a frequent component of carcinoma ex-pleomorphic carcinoma when there may

Box 10.11: Epithelial myoepithelial carcinoma

Key features helpful in diagnosis

- Accounts for about 1 percent of all salivary tumors.
- Most common in parotid (~75%) and submandibular (~10%) glands.
- F:M ~ 2:1 Wide age range with peak incidence in 6th and 7th decades.
- Slow-growing, usually painless mass: nerve involvement uncommon.
- Circumscribed, usually nonencapsulated mass which may be lobulated or cystic.
- Double-layered duct-like structures with inner cuboidal cells and outer clear myoepithelial cells in variable proportions.
- Duct-like structures may be widely separated by stroma or aggregate into sold sheets. Papillary and cystic areas present in about 20 percent cases.
- Perineural and angiolymphatic invasion relatively uncommon.

be a history of a previous long-standing tumor. It forms about 2 percent of all salivary tumors and about 10 percent of malignant salivary neoplasms. There is a wide age range but most patients are over 50 years old and the tumor is rare in children and young adults. There is a distinct male predominance of about 4:1. Over 95 percent of cases affect the parotid gland but occasional cases have been reported in the submandibular and minor oropharyngeal glands and elsewhere. They usually present as rapidly expanding, painful masses often with necrosis, hemorrhage, ulceration and nerve involvement.

Histopathology

Salivary duct carcinoma usually shows macroscopical evidence of hemorrhage, necrosis and widespread invasion. Microscopically, the tumor closely resembles high grade ductal carcinoma of the breast. Typically, it consists of large, duct-like structures with cribriform areas, characteristic 'Roman bridging' and central (comdeo-like) necrosis (**Fig. 10.37**). Solid, papillary and squamous areas can also be present. The tumor cells are pleomorphic and show obvious cytological features of malignancy. They have pink, granular and sometimes frankly oncocytic cytoplasm. The nuclei are large and hyperchromatic and show abundant and often abnormal mitoses, together with florid apoptosis. Sometimes, these tumors are biphasic and have a spindle cell, pseudosarcomatous component. Mucin-rich and micropapillary variants have also been reported. The stroma usually shows extensive fibrosis and heavy inflammatory cell infiltration. Most tumors show evidence of perineural and angiolymphatic involvement.

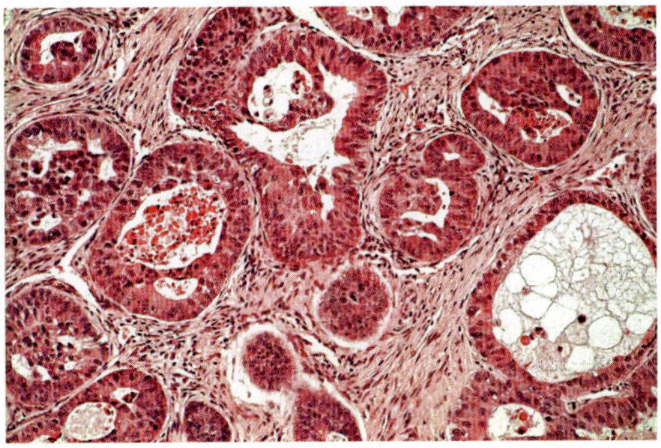

Fig. 10.37: Salivary duct carcinoma showing large pleomorphic cells forming duct-like structures with 'Roman bridging' and comedonecrosis

Differential Diagnosis

The possibility of metastatic breast carcinoma should be considered, even in men. If clinical examination is equivocal, immunophenotyping of the tumor may be helpful. Salivary duct carcinomas are androgen receptor-positive, estrogen receptor-negative, and progesterone receptor-negative. Some salivary duct carcinomas can resemble poorly differentiated squamous cell carcinoma or high grade mucoepidermoid carcinomas. Usually, however, more typical areas showing ductal or cribriform features are seen elsewhere in the tumor. Mucous cells are not a feature of salivary duct carcinoma. Predominantly papillary tumors need to be distinguished from papillary cystadenocarcinoma but these do not show the extreme cellular pleomorphism that is characteristic of salivary duct carcinoma. Some salivary duct carcinomas show extensive oncocytic elements but other characteristic features such as the cribriform architecture help to differentiate the tumor from oncocytic carcinoma.

Treatment and Prognosis

Salivary duct carcinoma is very aggressive with a local recurrence rate of about 30 percent and locoregional metastatic frequency of 60 percent. About half of the cases show distant metastases to lung, brain, bone and elsewhere. Tumors showing over-expression of HER-2/neu protein have a particularly poor outcome. Treatments include radical surgery, usually with neck dissection, and adjuvant radiotherapy. Recently, anti-androgen and transtuzumab (Herceptin) systemic therapy has been tried for patients with advanced disease and preliminary results suggest this form of treatment may offer some hope in the future.

Box 10.12: Salivary duct carcinoma

Key features helpful in diagnosis

- Accounts for ~10 percent of all malignant salivary neoplasms. Can arise ab initio or as a component of carcinoma ex-pleomorphic adenoma.
- M:F ~4:1 Peak incidence in 6th and 7th decades.
- Rapidly-growing painless mass often with necrosis, ulceration and facial nerve involvement.
- Usually solid, infiltrative mass with areas of hemorrhage and necrosis.
- Resembles high-grade ductal carcinoma of the breast, often with comedonecrosis: solid, papillary and squamous areas may be present.
- Cells cytologically pleomorphic with high mitotic frequency and florid apoptosis.
- Local, neural and angiolymphatic invasion may be extensive.

Carcinoma Ex-pleomorphic Adenoma

Carcinoma ex-pleomorphic adenoma has been defined as 'a pleomorphic adenoma from which an epithelial malignancy is derived'. Synonyms include carcinoma arising in a benign mixed tumor, carcinoma ex benign mixed tumor, carcinoma arising in pleomorphic adenoma and malignant mixed tumor.

Clinical Features

In a major review of the literature, carcinoma ex-pleomorphic adenoma accounted for about 3.6 percent of all salivary tumors and 12 percent of salivary malignancies. The true frequency may be higher as some of these carcinomas may overgrow and obliterate the original benign pleomorphic adenoma. The large majority (~70–80%) arise in the parotid gland, with smaller numbers in the submandibular, sublingual and minor glands. In the latter, the palate is the most common location. Most cases are seen in the sixth and seventh decades and there is no sex predilection. The typical presentation is that of rapid growth of a pre-existing and often long-standing swelling, but in some cases the tumor appears to arise ab initio. In addition, some cases can be seen in the site where a pleomorphic adenoma had been removed previously. As the tumor progresses pain, fixation and neural involvement become increasingly frequent. Many cases show evidence of locoregional metastasis at the time of presentation.

Histopathology

Grossly, carcinoma ex-pleomorphic adenoma is poorly circumscribed and infiltrative. The pre-existing pleomorphic adenoma may be seen as a more defined area of tumor and/or a focus of scarring.

In many tumors both the benign and malignant components are clearly visible (**Fig. 10.38A**) but in some cases there can be extensive scarring and identifying remnants of the pre-existing tumor may be difficult. Sometimes the benign elements have been totally effaced and the diagnosis can only then be inferred on the basis of the clinical history. The malignant component is most frequently a poorly differentiated adenocarcinoma (NOS) or a salivary duct carcinoma, although most other types of salivary malignancies have been reported. It is common for the tumors to have two or more defined malignant elements. Although many tumors show gross nuclear pleomorphism, frequent and often abnormal mitoses and necrosis, occasionally there is

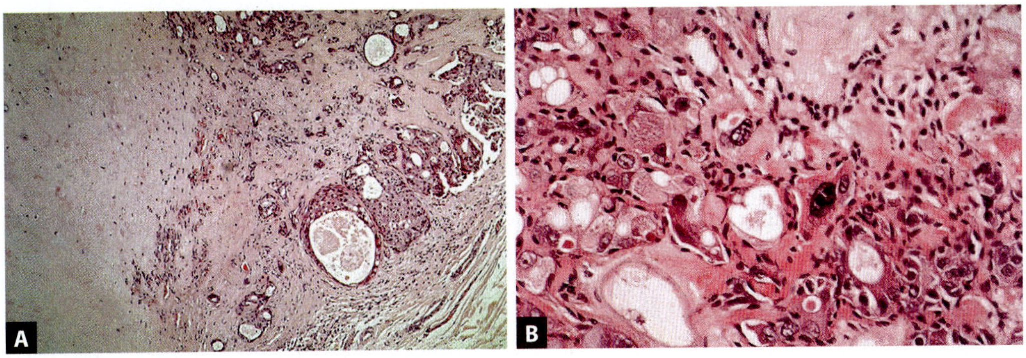

Figs 10.38A and B: (A) Carcinoma developing adjacent to a benign pleomorphic adenoma; (B) Severe dysplasia within the substance of an otherwise benign pleomorphic adenoma. This has been called intracapsular carcinoma, carcinoma *in situ* in pleomorphic adenoma and noninvasive carcinoma ex-pleomorphic adenoma

minimal cytological atypia. In many cases, there is evidence of neural and angiolymphatic invasion.

Carcinoma ex-pleomorphic can be subclassified into noninvasive, minimally invasive (<1.5 mm penetration of the malignant component into extracapsular tissue) and invasive (>1.5 mm of invasion). It is not rare to find focal or more widespread areas of dysplastic cells in pleomorphic adenomas without evidence of frank invasion, despite extensive sampling. This is termed noninvasive carcinoma ex-pleomorphic adenoma although a number of other names have been used, including *in-situ* carcinoma, intracapsular carcinoma or severely dysplastic pleomorphic adenoma (**Fig. 10.38B**).

Differential Diagnosis

Secondary changes in pleomorphic adenoma following fine needle aspiration, open biopsy or spontaneous infarction include necrosis, increased mitotic activity and squamous metaplasia, and these should not be confused with malignancy. Carcinomas often arise in old, scarred pleomorphic adenomas and these should be extensively sampled. Other tumors that can show widespread hyalinization include adenoid cystic carcinoma, salivary duct carcinoma and polymorphous low-grade adenocarcinoma. Identification of remnants of pleomorphic adenoma such as myxochondroid elements, cytologically bland ducts or plasmacytoid cells should allow appropriate classification of carcinoma ex-pleomorphic adenoma. One of the most important distinctions is between non-invasive and invasive carcinoma ex-pleomorphic adenoma, as this has significant prognostic implications.

Box 10.13: Carcinoma ex-pleomorphic adenoma

Key features helpful in diagnosis

- Accounts for ~12 percent of all salivary malignancies: large majority arise in the parotid gland with smaller frequency in submandibular and minor glands.
- M:F 1:1 peak incidence in 6th and 7th decades.
- Usually painless but rapid growth of a pre-existing and often long-standing swelling or site of previous surgery. Neural involvement common.
- Tumor poorly circumscribed and infiltrative. Remnants of benign element may be seen.
- Original pleomorphic adenoma or extensive scar together with one or more malignant elements, most commonly poorly differentiated adenocarcinoma (NOS) or salivary duct carcinoma.
- Tumors can be non-invasive, minimally invasive or frankly invasive.

Treatment and Prognosis

Carcinoma ex-pleomorphic adenoma is usually treated by wide local excision together with neck dissection. Adjuvant radiotherapy is often used for widely invasive and non-resectable tumors. If the carcinomatous component is cytologically low-grade or minimally invasive, adjuvant radiation therapy may not be deemed necessary.

Noninvasive carcinomas have a prognosis similar to that of conventional pleomorphic adenoma. Invasive carcinoma ex-pleomorphic adenoma shows a range of behavior. Minimally invasive tumors have a relatively good prognosis but tumors with a depth of invasion of more than 1.5 mm are usually high-grade and stage are associated with a poor prognosis. Local recurrence is seen in up to half of the cases and about 70 percent show regional or distant metastasis to sites including brain, lung, liver and bone (especially spine). The 5 year survival rates vary from 25 to 56 percent and the longer term prognosis is even worse.

SELF-ASSESSMENT QUESTIONS

1. Provide a classification for salivary gland disorders.
2. Describe the clinicopathological features and treatment of acute and chronic sialadenitis.
3. Describe the clinical features, investigation and treatment of obstructive salivary gland disease. What are the reasons for increased prevalence of salivary calculus in submandibular glands?
4. Describe the etiopathogenesis, presentation and management of mucoceles.
5. What is sialosis? Describe the clinicopathological presentation of sialosis and list the associated conditions.
6. Compare and contrast primary and secondary Sjogren's syndrome.
7. Compare and contrast the clinicopathological features, behavior and management of the two most common benign parotid gland tumors.
8. Give an account of mucoepidermoid carcinoma including a note on its differential diagnosis.
9. Discuss the differential diagnosis of malignant minor salivary tumors.
10. Describe the role of imaging modalities in the diagnosis and treatment of salivary gland disease. What is the role of sialography in current practice?

SUGGESTED READING

1. Auclair PL. Tumor-associated lymphoid proliferation in the parotid gland. A potential diagnostic pitfall. Oral Surg Oral Med Oral Pathol. 1994;77:19-26.
2. Barnes L, Eveson JW, Reichart P, Sidransky D (Eds). Tumors of the Salivary Glands. World Health Organization Classification of Tumors. Pathology and Genetics of Head and Neck Tumors. Lyon, IARC Press. 2005.
3. Barrett A, Speight P. Chapter 19. The controversial adenoid cystic carcinoma. The implications of histological grade and perineural invasion. In: M McGurk, Renehan A (Eds). Controversies in the management of salivary gland disease. Oxford University Press. 2002. pp.211-7.
4. Brandwein MS, Ivanov K, Wallace DI, et al. Mucoepidermoid carcinoma: A clinicopathologic study of 80 patients with special reference to histologic grading. Am J Surg Pathol. 2001;25:835-45.
5. Brannon RB, Fowler CB, Hartman KS. Necrotizing sialometaplasia. A clinicopathologic study of sixty-nine cases and review of the literature. Oral Surg Oral Med Oral Pathol. 1991;72:317-25.
6. Brook I. Acute bacterial suppurative parotitis: microbiology and management. J Craniofac Surg. 2003;14:37-40.
7. Castle JT, Thompson LD, Frommelt RA, Wenig BM, Kessler HP. Polymorphous low grade adenocarcinoma: a clinicopathologic study of 164 cases. Cancer. 1999;86:207-19.
8. Dave SP, Pernas FG, Roy S. The benign lymphoepithelial cyst and a classification system for lymphocytic parotid gland enlargement in the pediatric HIV population. Laryngoscope. 2007;117:106-13.
9. Di Palma S, Skalova A, Vanieek T. Noninvasive (intracapsular) carcinoma ex-pleomorphic adenoma: recognition of focal carcinoma by HER-2/neu and MIB1 immunohistochemistry. Histopathology. 2005;46: 144-152.
10. Ellis GL, Auclair PL. Tumors of the salivary glands. Atlas of Tumor Pathology, 4th Series, Fascicle 9. Armed Forces Institute of Pathology, Washington DC. 2008.

11. Eveson JW, Cawson RA. Salivary gland tumors: a review of 2410 cases with particular reference to histologic types, site, age, and sex distribution. J Pathol. 1985;146:51-8.
12. Gomez DR, Hoppe BS, Wolden SL, et al. Outcomes and prognostic variables in adenoid cystic carcinoma of the head and neck: A recent experience. Int J Radiat Oncol Biol Phys. 2008;70:1365-72.
13. Huvos AG. Stage means more than grade in adenoid cystic carcinoma. Am J Surg. 1992;164:623-8.
14. Lewis JE, Olsen KD, Sebo TJ. Carcinoma ex-pleomorphic adenoma: pathologic analysis of 73 cases. Hum Pathol. 2001;32:596-604.
15. Nabili V, Tan JW, Bhuta S, et al. Salivary duct carcinoma: a clinical and histologic review with implications for trastuzumab therapy. Head Neck. 2007;29:907-912.
16. Seethala RR, Barnes EL, Hunt JL. Epithelial-myoepithelial carcinoma: a review of the clinicopathologic spectrum and immunophenotypic characteristics in 61 tumors of the salivary glands and upper aerodigestive tract. Am J Surg Pathol. 2007;31:44-57.
17. Sitheeque M, Sivachandran Y, Varathan V, et al. Juvenile recurrent parotitis: clinical, sialographic and ultrasonographic features. Int J Paediatr Dent. 2007;17:98-104.
18. Teymoortash A, Tiemann M, Schrader C, et al. Characterization of lymphoid infiltrates in chronic obstructive sialadenitis associated with sialolithiasis. J Oral Pathol Med. 2004;33:300-304.
19. Teymoortash A, Werner JA. Tissue that has lost its track: Warthin's tumor. Virchows Arch. 2005;446:585-8.
20. Vitali C, Bombardieri S, Jonsson R, et al. Classification criteria for Sjögren's syndrome: a revised version of the European criteria proposed by the American-European Consensus Group. Ann Rheum Dis. 2002;61:554-8.
21. Waldron CA, El-Mofty S, Gnepp DR. Tumors of the intraoral minor salivary glands: A demographic and histologic study of 426 cases. Oral Surg Oral Med Oral Pathol. 1988;66:323-33.
22. Yoon AJ, Beller DE, Woo VL, et al. Bilateral canalicular adenomas of the upper lip. Oral Surg Oral Med Oral Pathol Oral Radiol Endod. 2006;102:341-3.

Chapter 11

Xerostomia

MAO Lewis

Chapter Outline

INTRODUCTION

The presence of adequate amounts of normal saliva within the mouth is crtical to maintaining oral health. This chapter presents an overview of the production of saliva and describes the consequences of reduced salivary secretion. The term xerostomia is widely used to describe the symptoms suffered due to altered salivary function. It should not be used as a diagnosis but rather as a clinical description that would prompt further investigation of the patient to determine the underlying cause. Xerostomia is an extremely frequent complaint amongst Western communities, having been reported in between 17 and 29 percent of some populations studied. An understanding of the investigation and management of xerostomia is an essential component of oral health care.

SALIVA

Saliva in the mouth is referred to as mixed or whole saliva since it is a combination of the secretion from all the glands. Saliva keeps the mouth wet, makes it possible to chew and swallow, helps in digestion, protects teeth from decay and prevents bacterial and fungal infections.

Physiology of Salivary Secretion

The glands which produce saliva consist of three major paired glands, the sublingual, submandibular and parotid, and more than 600 minor (accessory) glands which are distributed throughout the mouth but principally within the lips, cheeks and palate. The parotid glands account for 60 percent of the total salivary tissue, with the submandibular and sublingual providing a further 30 and 5 percent respectively.

Examination of the anatomy of salivary gland tissue reveals a complex structure of secretory units consisting of saliva producing cells (acini) and secretory ducts. The acinar cells are either serous, which produce a watery secretion or mucous which secrete a viscous form of saliva. The major glands contain different proportions of serous and mucous acinar cells and this determines the type of saliva produced by a particular gland. The parotid gland is predominantly made up of serous cells whilst the remaining glands are mainly mucous. An exeption to this generalization are the glands of von Ebner which are situated aound the circumvallate papillae on the tongue and produce a watery secretion that is believed to assist the sensation of taste. The initial fluid formed in either type of acinar celli is secreted into a ductal system, which is made up of three types of duct, namely intercalated, striated and excretory. Considerable modification of the protein and ion content of the fluid may occur within the duct before it enters the mouth. The striated ducts, which are well developed in the parotid and submandibular glands, are important sites of ion exchange, particularly sodium and chloride. The extent of exchange and level of these and other ions are influenced by flow rate which can vary considerabley between unstimulated and stimulated conditions.

Formation of saliva is under neural control, mainly through parasympathetic nerves conducting stimuli from the salivary nuclei within the brain. The parasympathetic fibers from the superior salivary nuclei travel to the submandibular and sublingual glands via the facial nerve and chorda tympani. Supply to the parotid gland is from the inferior salivary nuclei through otic ganglion and glossophayngeal nerve. Sympathetic supply to all the major glands is provided by the spinal chord via fibers from the superior cervical ganglion. Increased salivary flow is predominantly a result of parasympathetic activity that produces vasodilation in the blood vessels within the glands. A range of stimuli, including smell, taste and chewing, can lead to increased salivary secretion although the exact processes are not fully understood. In contrast, it is well recognized that anxiety can cause reduced flow. Salivary secretion under goes a diurnal variation with a peak in mid afternoon and a fall to almost zero at night. The mean unstimulated flow rate throughout the day is 0.3 mL/minute. In the past the total amount of saliva produced in a day has been reported to be in the region of 1.5 liter, although more recently it has been thought that this is an overestimate and a figure of 0.7 liter is nearer the actual amount.

Under unstimulated conditions the majority (60–65%) of saliva comes from submandibular glands with a further 20 to 30 percent from the parotid glands and 2 to 5 percent from sublingual glands. The relative contributions of the major glands changes significantly on stimulation and during eating. In these circumstances the parotid gland contributes 50 percent of stimulated saliva. It is important to remember that the "fluid" within the mouth is not just the product of the salivary glands but also conatins exudates from the gingival crevicular tissues, microorganisms, desquamated epithelial and white blood cells.

Constituents of Saliva

Saliva is 99.4 percent water with organic and inorganic solids accounting for only 0.6 percent of its content, although this does change depending on whether flow is stimulated or not. There are also differences between different glands. Although information is available for individual glands, from a clinical point of view it is probably appropriate to just look at mixed saliva (**Table 11.1**). The three most important ions in relation to the teeth are calcium and phosphate because of their direct relationship with mineralized tissues and hydrogen carbonate due to its buffering property (see blelow).

Functions

Saliva has a wide range of functions (**Table 11.2**), many of which go unrecognized until salivary production is altered or reduced. A marked reduction of saliva flow can have a devastating physical effect on the teeth due to uncontrolled dental caries, in addition to causing a distressing psychological impact on the sufferer as a result of difficulty in eating and talking. The acid buffering capacity of saliva is one of its most important functions. Ceratin bacterial species within the mouth have the ability to rapidly metabolize carbohydrates to acid end products leading to a reduction in plaque pH.

▪ Table 11.1
Inorganic and organic components of saliva

Inorganic	*Organic*
Sodium	Protein
Potassium	Serum albumin
Calcium	Gamma globulin
Magnesium	Mucoprotein
Chloride	Amylase
Hydrogen carbonate	Lysozyme
Phosphate	Proline-rich proteins
Thiocyanate	Histidine-rich proteins
Iodide	Lactoferrin
Fluoride	Fibronectin
	Statherin
	Carbohydrate
	Blood group products
	Glucose
	Lipids
	Cortisol
	Amino acids
	Urea
	Ammonia

▪ Table 11.2
Functions and properties of saliva

Function	*Property*
Acid buffer	High bicarbonate content buffers acid produced by plaque bacteria
Ion reservoir	Saliva is saturated with calcium and phosphate, which at neutral pH prevents demineralization
Pellicle formation	Salivary proteins are essential for protective diffusion barrier on tooth surfaces
Lubricant	Glycoproteins facilitates movement of soft tissues during eating and speech
Antimicrobial	Salivary proteins, immunoglobulins, lysozyme, lactoferritin, sialoperoxidase, histidine-rich proteins have a range of antibacterial and antifungal activities
Cleansing	Physically clears food from teeth and soft tissues
Taste	Substances require to be in solution for sense of taste
Digestion	Salivary amylase provides cleavage of glucose to maltose

Measurement of plaque pH over time is called a Stephan curve and can demonstrate the rate of recovery of salivary pH following ingestion of fermentable carbohydrate. Demineralization of enamel will occur at a pH less than 5.5. The ability of saliva, in relation to its bicarbonate content, to buffer bacterial acid is a major protective factor. Unstimulated saliva contains bicarbonate at a concentration of 1 mmol/l but levels up to 60 mmol/l are present in stimulated flow. Chewing of sugar-free gum can produces carbonate levels in the region of 15 mmol/l.

XEROSTOMIA

Xerostomia is a common symptom often caused by a decrease in the amount of saliva or a change in the quality of saliva.

Signs and Symptoms

A range of symptoms and signs of xerostomia have been described. The main symptoms are generalized oral discomfort, sometimes described as burning (not to be confused with burning mouth syndrome in which salivary production is normal), difficulty in talking or swallowing, altered taste, failing dental restorations, and if worn, poor retention of dentures. Usually a reduction in saliva flow of more than 50 percent is required before clinical symptoms develop. Lack of saliva will produce a generalized erythema of the oral mucosa (**Fig. 11.1**) and a lobulated/fissured appearance on the dorsum of the tongue (**Fig. 11.2**). There is also likely to be evidence of food retention between the teeth (**Fig. 11.3**), candidosis and angular cheilitis. The teeth are prone to cervical caries and existing restorations may fail due to recurrent caries (**Fig. 11.4**). Patients with xerostomia are also predisposed to recurrent episodes of suppurative sialadenitis, particularly of the parotid gland.

Etiopathogenesis

A frequent cause of reduced salivary flow is an adverse side effect of drug therapy. More than 500 different medications have been implicated in causing dry mouth. However, the

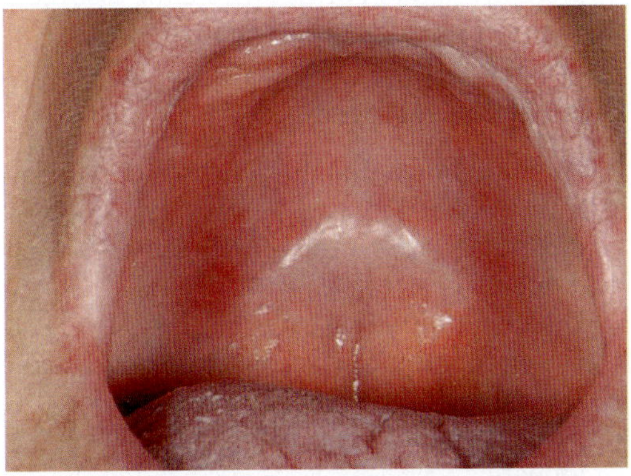

Fig. 11.1: Atrophic mucosa with areas of erythema in the palate

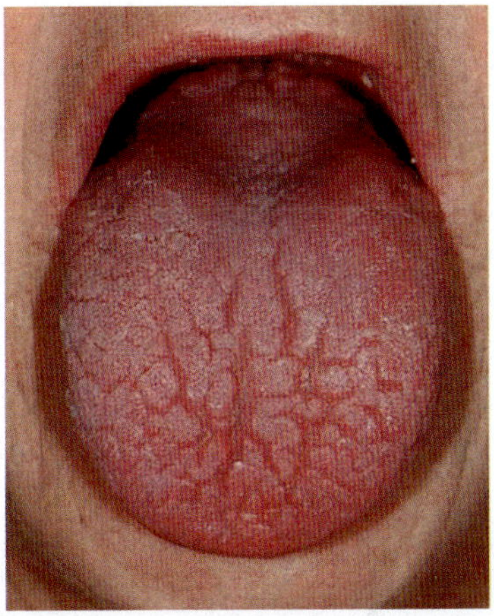

Fig. 11.2: Lobulated and fissured tongue

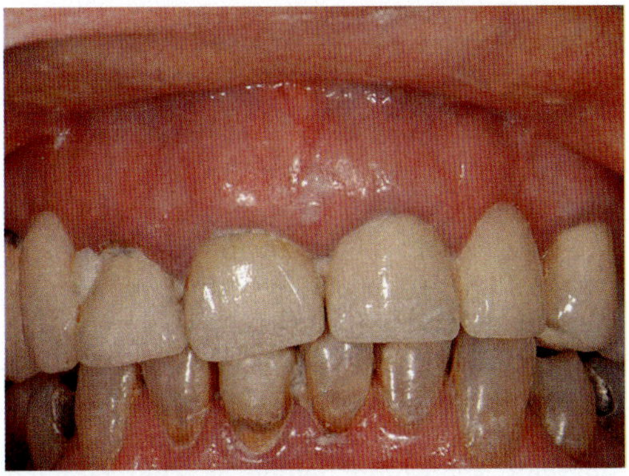

Fig. 11.3: Dry mouth with food retention between the teeth

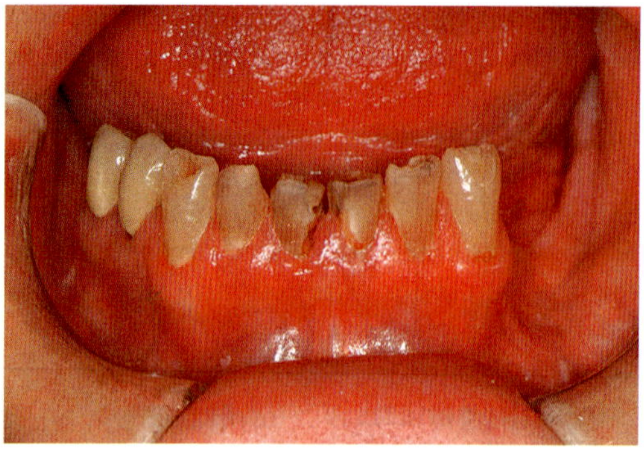

Fig. 11.4: Failing restorations and dental caries

▪ Table 11.3
Examples of drugs associated with producing reduced salivary secretion

Category of drug	*Generic name*	*Trade name*
Tricyclic antidepressants	Amitriptyline Dosulepin	(generic) Prothiaden
Selective serotonin-reuptake inhibitors	Fluoxetine Venlafaxine	Prozac Efexor
Antihistamine	Chlorphenamine	Piriton
Diuretics	Furosemide	Lasix
Anticholinergic agents	Atropine Oxybutin	(generic) Ditropan
Antipsychotic agents	Pimozide	Orap
Antiparkinsonian agents	Levadopa	(generic)
Sedative and anxiolytic agents	Diazepam	Valium

true incidence and severity of xerostomia with particular drugs has been difficult to establish. Nevertheless, certain types of medication are well recognized as producing this problem (**Table 11.3**) either by blocking stimulation from the autonomic nerve supply or inhibiting the ion exchange system.

A reduced production of saliva may also be due to the presence of the auto-immune disease Sjögren's syndrome, which is characterized by destruction of glandular acini. Sjögren's syndrome may be either primary Sjögren's syndrome, in which the patient has xerostomia and dry eyes due to lacrimal gland disease, or secondary Sjögren's syndrome, in which the sufferer has a connective tissue disorder in addition to xerostomia and/or dry eyes. Sjögren's syndrome is a relatively frequent disorder with an estimated prevalence of between 1 and 3 percent of the UK population, with a high percentage of cases occurring in middle-aged females. An increasing number of individuals receive radiotherapy to the head and neck as a part of the contemporary treatment of malignant disease. Unfortunately, salivary tissue is particularly sensitive to radiation and despite efforts to limit gland exposure by altering and refining the direction of the beam, patients frequently suffer reduced salivary production. Loss of fluid secondary to raised blood sugar levels and increase micturition associated with diabtetes also leads to reduced salivary production. Rarer causes of xerostomia included acute anxiety, cystic fibrosis, graft-versus-host disease, thyroid disorders, HIV infection, hepatic disease, renal failure, and sarcoidosis. Reduced salivary production due to the congenital absence of the salivary glands has been reported but is extremely rare.

Historically, increasing age has been implicated as a factor involved in reduced salivary production. However, it is now generally accepted that this association is unfounded. Recent research has revealed that parotid gland output is maintained throughout life. The situation is complicated by the fact that elderly individuals are more likely to being taking one or more medication or have systemic disorders that impact on salivary gland function.

Clinical Assessment

It has been shown that the presence of reduced salivary production can be correlated with a positive response to one of the five following questions:

- Does your mouth usually feel dry?
- Does your mouth feel dry while eating a meal?
- Do you have difficulties swallowing food?
- Do you sip liquids to aid in swallowing dry foods?
- Does the amount of saliva in your mouth seem too little, too much or you do not notice it?

These questions should be asked prior to examination of the patient. The medical history, especially drug history, should be obtained since this will also identify any previous exposure to radiotherapy or known presence of connective tissue disorder. An impression of the patient's general health can be gained by their appearance. Extraoral evidence of rheumatoid or other connective tissue, such as changes in the hands or facial features, can indicate the possible presence of Sjögren's syndrome. It is also worth remembering that severe deformities in the hands as a result of rheumatoid arthritis will limit the patient's manual dexterity in relation to maintaining oral hygiene if dry mouth is present. Intraoral examination in health should reveal saliva pooling in the floor of the mouth. Furthermore, external pressure applied to the major salivary glands should produce clear saliva at the duct openings. In addition, to being reduced in amount, any saliva that is present may be frothy in nature. The buccal mucosa becomes sticky and will adhere to the face of a dental examination mirror placed against it.

Investigations

Specific measurement of salivary flow rates is rarely performed outside specialist clinics. However, a crude assessment of salivary output can be achieved by collecting unstimulted saliva in a container. A level of less than 0.16 mL/minute has been proposed as being indicative of reduced function. Stimulated parotid flow rate can be measured by collection of output in Carlsson-Crittened cups placed over the parotid orifice and stimulating saliva by placement of 1 mL 10 percent citric acid on the dorsum of the tongue. Less than 5 mL/in 5 minutes can be interpreted as reduced function.

Investigation of xerostomia should include a full range of tests that will ensure that the underlying cause is identified. Routine hematological investigation must include fasting blood glucose to exclude hyperglycemia secondary to undiagnosed or poorly controlled diabetes. Blood should also be taken to determine the presence of rheumatoid factor, antinuclear antibody, SS-A and SS-B (two specific markers for Sjögren's syndrome).

Two distinct forms of imaging have been used to investigate the salivary glands. Sialography involves the infusion of a radio-opague contrast fluid up into the gland through the main excretory duct. Radiographs will reveal any structural defects within the gland. A characteristic radiographic "snow-storm effect", known as punctuate sialectasis, is seen within the parotid gland in patients with Sjögren's syndrome (**Fig. 11.5**). Scintigraphy is a technique that investgates glandular function rather than structure by measuring the active uptake of a radio-labeled marker, such as technetium-99m, after intravenous infusion. This technique is not in widespread use. More recently, ultrasound imaging is being used to investigate salivary glands since it provides a relatively simple and noninvasive assessment.

Examination of the minor salivary glands has been used as a method of determining the presence of disease in the major glands. The minor glands are easily accessible in the lower lip (**Fig. 11.6**). The procedure known as labial gland biopsy is considered one of the most helpful diagnostic tools for Sjögren's syndrome. Examination of at least five lobules of minor gland needs to performed. Histopathological feaures supportive of Sjögren's syndrome include acinar loss, duct dilation, periductal fibrosis and most importantly a focal lymphocytic infiltrate.

If the patient complains of dry eyes, and it is useful to aseses lacrimal gland function by undertaking a Schirmer's test. This involves the

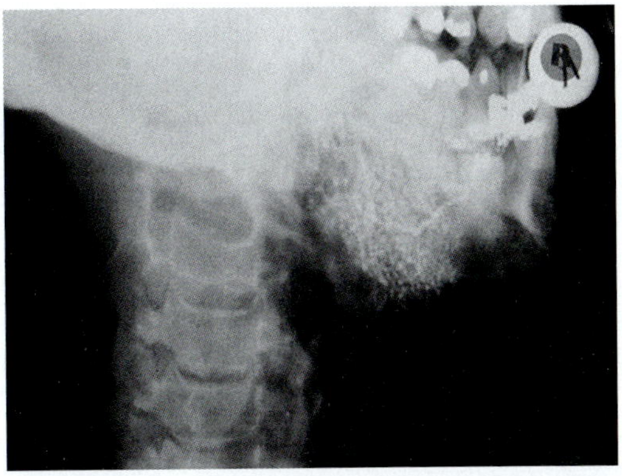

Fig. 11.5: Sialogram of the parotid gland showing sialectasis

placement of a filter paper strip under the lower eyelid for a period of five minutes. On removal the strip should show at least 5 mm of wetting.

Management

Successful management of xerostomia requires investigation of all the possible causes as described above. If the patient's drug history reveals a medication that is recognized as causing reduced salivary flow and the onset of symptoms followed the start of therapy then consideration should be given to changing the drug in question. If this situation involves a tricyclic antidepressant, such as amitriptyline, then it is worthwhile suggesting a change to an SSRI since the severity of xerostomia does appear to be less with these newer drugs. However, on many occasions it is possible to change the medication, which presents a difficult management scenario. If diabetes is discovered then establishment of glycemic control often leads to resolution of the symptoms of xerostomia.

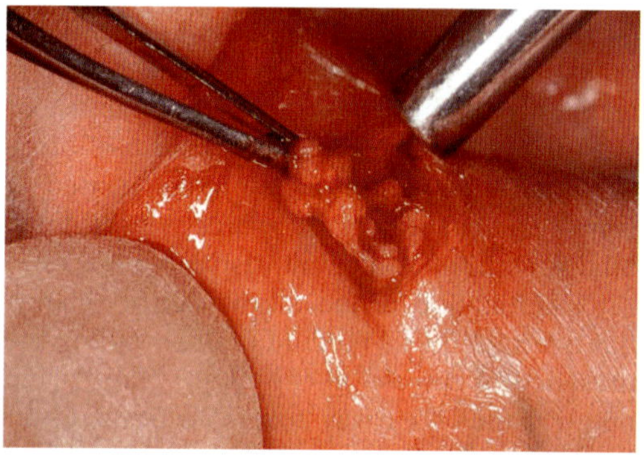

Fig. 11.6: Removal of salivary tissue during a labial gland biopsy

Management of xerostomia should focus on the relief of symptoms and prevention of the oral effects of lack of saliva. Artificial saliva substitutes, based on either carboxymethylcellulose or mucin, are commercially available and provide a form of saliva replacement. A number of preparations have been formulated in spray and gel formats (**Table 11.4**). Some preparations are based on animal gastric mucin and this must be taken into acount when advising

▪ Table 11.4

Topical saliva replacement products listed in the British National Formulary (BNF)

Product	*Content*
Saliva orthana® spray	Mucin, xylitol and sodium fluoride
Saliva orthana® lozenge	Mucin and xylitol in sorbitol basis
Glandosane® spray	Carmellose, sorbitol, potassium chloride, magnesium chloride, calcium chloride, dipotassium hydrogen phosphate
Luborant® spray	Sorbitol, carmellose, dibasic potassium phosphate, potassium chloride, monobasic potassium phosphate, calcium chloride, magnesium chloride and sodium fluoride
Biotène oral balance® gel	Lactoperoxidase, lactoferrin, lysozyme, glucose oxidase xylitol in gel basis
Bioxtra® gel	Lactoperoxidase, lactoferrin, lysozyme, whey colostrums, xylitol and other ingredients
Saliveze® spray (mint flavor)	Carmellose, calcium chloride, magnesium chloride, potassium chloride, sodium chloride and dibasic sodium phosphate
Salivix®	Sugar free, reddish amber, acacia, malic acid and other ingredients
SST tablet	Sugar free, citric acid, malic acid and other ingredients
Salinum®	Sugar-free, linseed extract (containing polysaccharides) with dipotassium phosphate

their use in vegetarians and certain religious or ethinic groups. Patients should also be advised to take frequent sips of water to moisten the mucosa. Chewing of sugar-free gum or pastilles produces salivary flow from the remaining functional tissue and is found to be helpful by many patients. Salivary stimulants (sialogues) based on glycerine and lemon preparations should only be used in edentulous patients since their low pH will encourage dental caries in dentate individuals.

The benefit of systemic pilocarpine, a drug that stimulates acetylcholine receptors within exocrine glands, has been disappointing since although salivary flow can be obtained prior to meals patients often complain of significant adverse events, in particular sweating. Cevimeline hydrochloride is another cholinergic agent that has been recommended for patients with Sjögren's syndrome but also has significant side effects that limit its use. Rigorous oral hygiene measures and preventive regimens, such as daily fluoride mouthwash or professionally applied topical fluoride therapy, should be instituted to reduce the risk of dental caries. Dietary advice should be given especially concerning the limitation of sugar intake. Opportunistic candidal infections should be treated with a systemic antifungal, such as fluconazole.

SUMMARY

Saliva is an essential fluid for oral health and its absence has a major impact on the soft and hard tissues within the mouth. Unfortunately, the signs and symptoms of xerostomia are frequently encountered in the dental surgery. Full investigation of such patients is required to determine the underlying causes of reduced salivary flow. A variety of forms of symptomatic and preventive treatment are available and these need to be provided in order to minimize the impact of this condition on sufferers.

SELF-ASSESSMENT QUESTIONS

1. Describe the production of saliva.
2. Discuss the role of saliva and hence the effects of xerostomia on the oral cavity.
3. Discuss the differential diagnosis of patient reporting a dry mouth.
4. How would you investigate xerostomia?
5. Describe a graded approach to the management of xerostomia.

SUGGESTED READING

1. Dawes C. Physiological factors affecting salivary now rate, oral sugar clearance, and the sensation of dry mouth in man. J Dent Res. 1987;66:648-53.
2. Edgar WM, O'Mullane DM. Saliva and Dental Health. London: British Dental Association; 1990.
3. Ferguson DB. Oral Bioscience. London: Churchill Livingstone; 1999.
4. Fox PC. Management of dry mouth. Dent Clin North Amer. 1997;41:863-75.
5. Ghezzi EM, Lange LA, Ship JA. Determination of variation of stimulated salivary flow rates. J Dent Res. 2000;79:1874-8.
6. Guggenheimer G, Moore PJ. Xerostomia. Etiology, recognition and treatment. JADA. 2003;134;61-9.
7. Lavelle C, Smith PM. Salivary gland function. In: Scully C (Ed). Oxford Handbook of Applied Dental Sciences. Oxford: Oxford University Press; 2002 pp. 157-63.
8. Lewis MAO, Jordan R CJ. A Colour Handbook of Oral Medicine, 2nd Edn. London: Manson; 2012.

Chapter 12

Potentially Malignant Disorders

Sol Silverman Jr, Kobkan Thongprasom, Saman Warnakulasuriya

Chapter Outline

INTRODUCTION

Squamous cell carcinoma of the oral cavity is often preceded by oral potentially malignant disorders (OPMD), the term recommended at a workshop coordinated by the WHO Collaborating Center for Oral Cancer/Precancer to entail what were earlier referred to as "precancer" or "premalignant lesions and conditions". The term OPMD is preferred as it conveys that not all lesions and conditions described under this term may transform to cancer. The full list of OPMDs encountered in clinical practice is given in **Table 12.1**. In this chapter we consider those that are common and important including oral leukoplakia, erythroplakia, lichen planus and oral submucous fibrosis (OSF) as part of the spectrum of OPMD. The global prevalence of OPMD has been reported at 1 to 5 percent. In a screening program undertaken in Sri Lanka, the prevalence of oral precancer in the 1980s was reported as 4.2 percent, but higher prevalences are described from other parts of South and SE Asia, e.g. Taiwan (12.7%), and in some Western Pacific countries, e.g. Papua New Guinea (11.7%). Such wide geographical variations are due to life-styles specific to the country or region.

▪ Table 12.1
List of potentially malignant disorders

Leukoplakia	Lichen planus
Erythroplakia	Submucous fibrosis
Erythroleukoplakia	Discoid lupus erythematosus
Palatal lesions in reverse smokers	Syphilis
	Sideropenic dysphagia
	Actinic keratosis

LEUKOPLAKIA

Leukoplakia is a term that is best described as a white plaque that can occur on any mucosal surface, that cannot be wiped off, and does not represent a specific disease entity. Several definitions have been used by various authors and working groups **(Table 12.2)** and uniformity of terminology is important to ensure that the scientific community is studying and discussing the same disorder. At the last WHO Collaborating Center's Workshop (2005) the following definition was proposed: "White plaques of questionable risk having excluded (other) known diseases or disorders that carry no increased risk for cancer". This allows exclusion of other benign conditions that appear clinically white when selecting the clinical diagnosis of leukoplakia. Leukoplakia remains a clinical diagnosis based on features noted at the initial examination.

▪ Table 12.2
Definitions of oral leukoplakia proposed in the past decades

Working group	*Definition*
WHO (1978)	A white patch or plaque that cannot be characterized clinically or pathologically as any other disease
First International Conference on oral leukoplakia. Malmo, Sweden (1984)	A white patch or plaque that cannot be characterized clinically or pathologically as any other disease and is not associated with any physical or chemical causative agent except use of tobacco
International Symposium, Uppsala, Sweden (1996)	A predominantly white lesion of the oral mucosa that cannot be characterized as any other definable disease
WHO (1997)	A predominantly white lesion of the oral mucosa that cannot be characterized as any other definable lesion
Warnakulasuriya (2007)	Leukoplakia should be used to recognize white plagues of questionable risk having excluded (other) known diseases or disorders that carry no increased risk for cancer

Demography

Leukoplakia occurs in both sexes and in all ethnic groups and is significantly more prevalent in males. The male:female ratio on average approaches 3:1, and peak age of 40 to 49 years is consistently reported in many studies. A predominance of the buccal mucosa as a typical location has been noted mainly in South Asia. A pooled estimate from 23 studies yielded a point prevalence of 2.6 percent. There are few studies that document the rate of occurrences geographically (**Table 12.3**). In a US national survey of 16,128 individuals the prevalence figure of 0.42 percent is one of the lowest reported so far. A word of caution is needed in interpreting these data as various authors have used different definitions and

▪ Table 12.3
Reported prevalence of oral potentially malignant disorders (OPMD)

Author	*Country (year)*	*Sampling method*	*Definition used*	*Age group (years)*	*Disease entity*	*Prevalence percent*
Thomas et al	PNG (2008)	Random	Axell 1984	>18	Leukoplakia	11.7
Amarasinghe et al	Sri Lanka (2008)	MSSC	WHO 1994	>30	OPMD	11.3
Chung et al	Taiwan (2005)	Random	WHO 1980	>15	OPMD Leukoplakia Erythroplakia Lichen planus OSF	12.7 7.4 1.9 2.9 1.6
Scheifele et al	USA (2003)	MSSC*	Kramer 1978 Kramer 1980	>20	Leukoplakia	0.5–0.3
Ministry of Health of Sri Lanka	Sri Lanka (2003)	MSSC*	WHO 1994	35–44 and 65–74	OPMD Leukoplakia and Erythroplakia OSF	4.1 2.6 0.4
Garcia-Pola Vallejo et al	Spain (2002)	Stratified Randomized	WHO 1978 Axell 1984	>30	Leukoplakia	1.6
Reichart et al	Germany (2000)	Stratified Randomized	Axell 1976 Zain 1995	35–44 65–74	Leukoplakia Leukoplakia	1.6 1.0
Nagao et al	Japan (2000)	All invited to a screening program	WHO 1980	Male >40 Female >20	Leukoplakia Lichen planus	0.19 0.21
Zain et al	Malaysia (1997)	Stratified Randomized	WHO 1978 Axell 1978	>25	Leukoplakia Erythroplakia OSF Lichen planus	0.96 0.01 0.06 0.38
Shepman et al	The Netherlands (1996)	Waiting room	Axell 1984	13–93	Leukoplakia	0.6
Banoczy et al	Hungary (1991)	Random	Axell 1984	All ages groups	Leukoplakia Lichen planus	1.3 0.1
Ikeda et al	Japan (1991)	Factory workers	Axell 1984	18–63	Leukoplakia	2.5
Axell et al	Sweden (1987)	Stratified, random	Axell 1976	>15	Lichen planus	1.9

Contd...

Contd...

Author	*Country (year)*	*Sampling method*	*Definition used*	*Age group (years)*	*Disease entity*	*Prevalence percent*
Axell et al	Sweden (1987)	All invited residents	Axell 1987	>15	Leukoplakia	3.6
Warnakulasuriya et al	Sri Lanka (1984)	Population screening	WHO 1978	>20	OPMD	4.2
Ariyawardena et al	Sri Lanka (2007)	Estate Workers	WHO 1978	>15	Leukoplakia Erythroplakia OSF	4.6 0.03 1.6
Warnakulasuriya et al	India (2011)	Industrial workers	WHO 1978 Axell 1984	>20	Leukoplakia	5.0

*MSSC: Multistage stratified cluster
Modified from Johnson, Jayasekara, Amarasinghe 2011. Periodontology. 2000;vol57:2011;p.27

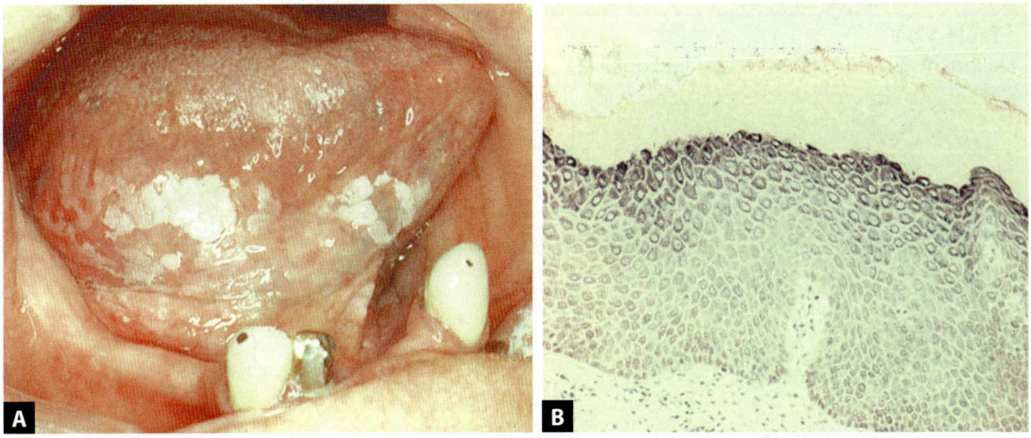

Figs 12.1A and B: Leukoplakia of the tongue and the most common histologic finding of hyperkeratosis without evidence of dysplasia. There is still a risk of transformation

criteria to detect oral leukoplakia. To further complicate prevalence rates, all leukoplakias are not the same, having different etiologies, variable clinical features, and different biologic potentials/risks. These variations require a variety of clinical approaches regarding management, which can be complex and leading to uncertain outcomes.

Epithelial Dysplasia and Malignant Transformation

The basis for the malignant potential for leukoplakia remains an enigma. The hyperkeratosis that leads to the clinical manifestation is a biochemical process, and the association between this process in oral epithelium and the potential for carcinogenesis remains unknown **(Figs 12.1 and 12.2)**. The magnitude of surface keratinization is of no importance. The malignant potential is based upon a number of studies that have reported a more than expected occurrence of carcinomas in patients with oral leukoplakia **(Table 12.4)**. A projected microscopic progression is illustrated in **Figures 12.3A to D**. Studies in cell markers may someday reveal an answer. In addition to some particular clinical features such as the site, associated erythema (redness), nodularity that an experienced clinician can recognize, there are microscopic changes that offer clues as to the degree of risk. These are the degrees of epithelial dysplasia that can be seen and to some extent quantified. Criteria used for diagnosing

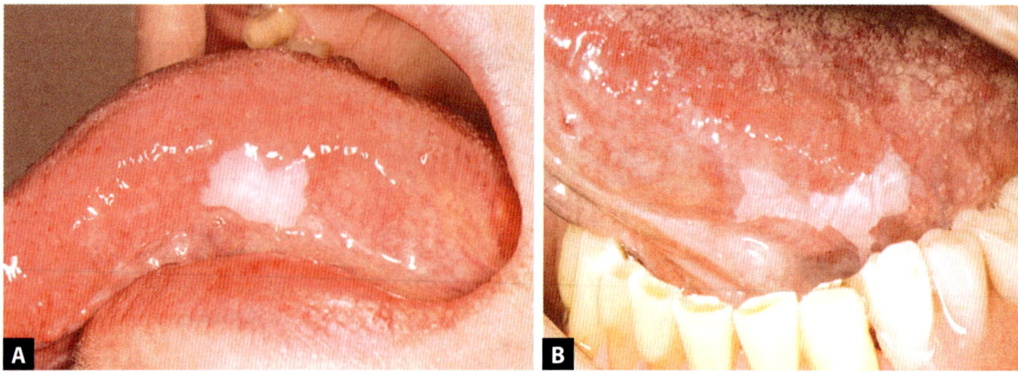

Figs 12.2A and B: Two cases of oral leukoplakia of lateral tongue with a homogeneous appearance

▪ Table 12.4
Malignant transformation in oral leukoplakia

Investigator (Country)	*Year*	*Number*	*Malignant transformation (%)*	*Years observed (mean)*
Silverman (India)	(1976)	4762	0.1	2
Gupta (India, Bhavnagar)	(1980)	360	0.3	1–10 (7)
Gupta (India, Ernakulam)	(1980)	410	2.2	1–10 (7)
Roed-Petersen (Denmark)	(1971)	331	3.6	>1
Einhorn (Sweden)	(1967)	782	4.0	1–20
Pindborg (Denmark)	(1968)	248	4.4	1–9
Kramer (England)	(1969)	187	4.8	1–16
Banoczy (Hungary)	(1977)	670	5.9	1–30 (9.8)
Silverman (USA)	(1968)	117	6.0	1–11 (3.5)
Silverman (USA)	(1984)	257	17.5*	1-39 (7.2)
Lind (Norway)	(1987)	157	8.9	6
Schepman (Netherlands)	(1998)	166	12.0	0.5–17 (2.7)
Holmstrup (Demark)	(2006)	236	12.0	7.5
Arduino (Italy)	(2009)	207	7.2	~1
Warnakulasuriya (UK)	(2011)	335	6.9	10 (4.2)

*Includes PVL

oral epithelial dysplasia are listed in **Table 12.5**. These features could be broadly categorized as changes to the architecture (strata) of the epithelium and those that manifest as cellular atypia the more prominent or numerous they are, the more severe the grade of dysplasia. There is great variability in their interpretation of the presence, degree and significance of the individual criteria. The following microscopic features have been suggested as a guidance by WHO experts to grade epithelial dysplasia to mild, moderate or severe.

Mild Dysplasia

In general architectural disturbance limited to the lower third of the epithelium, accompanied

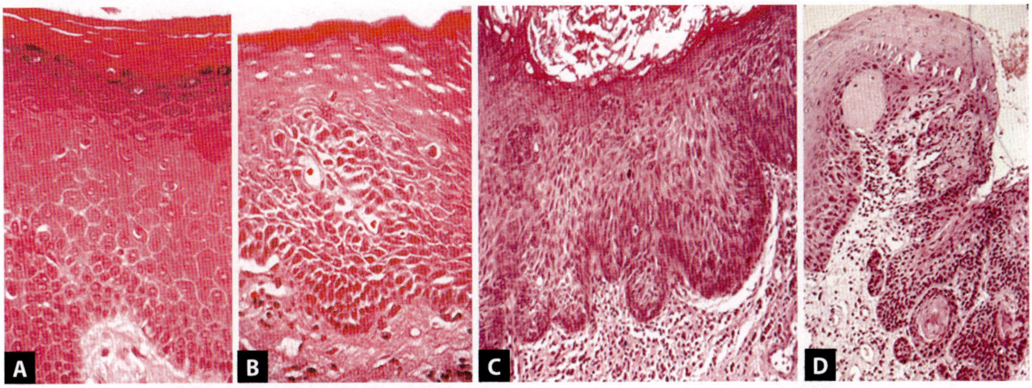

Figs 12.3A to D: Illustrations depicting increasing incidence of cellular atypia in progression of sections from leukoplakia with atypia, to squamous cell carcinoma. Note progression of cellular changes from: (A) Focal keratosis to; (B) Leukoplakia with atypia to; (C) Carcinoma *in situ* to; (D) Squamous cell carcinoma. Cellular maturation patterns are normal in focal keratosis when compared to the remaining specimens

Table 12.5
Criteria used for diagnosing dysplasia

Architecture	*Cytology*
Irregular epithelial stratification	Abnormal variation in nuclear size (anisonucleosis)
Loss of polarity of basal cells	Abnormal variation in nuclear shape (nuclear pleomorphism)
Drop-shaped rete ridges	Abnormal variation in cell size (anisocytosis)
Increased number of mitotic figures	Abnormal variation in cell shape (cellular pleomorphism)
Abnormally superficial mitoses	Increased nuclear-cytoplasmic ratio
Premature keratinization in single cells (dyskeratosis)	Increased nuclear size
Keratin pearls within rete ridges	Atypical mitotic figures
	Increased number and size of nucleoli
	Hyperchromasia

by minimal cytological atypia defines the minimum criteria of dysplasia (**Fig. 12.4**)

Moderate Dysplasia

Architectural disturbance extending into the middle third of the epithelium is the initial criterion for recognizing this category. Consideration is then given to the degree of cytological atypia. The presence of marked atypia may indicate that a lesion should be categorized as severe dysplasia despite not extending into the upper third of the epithelium. Alternatively lesions with mildly atypical features extending into the middle third of the epithelium may merit being graded as moderate dysplasia **(Fig. 12.5)**.

Severe Dysplasia

Recognition of severe dysplasia starts with greater than two-thirds of the epithelium showing architectural disturbance with associated cytologic atypia. However, as noted in the previous paragraph, architectural disturbance extending into the middle-third of the epithelium with sufficient cytologic atypia is upgraded from moderate to severe dysplasia **(Fig. 12.6)**.

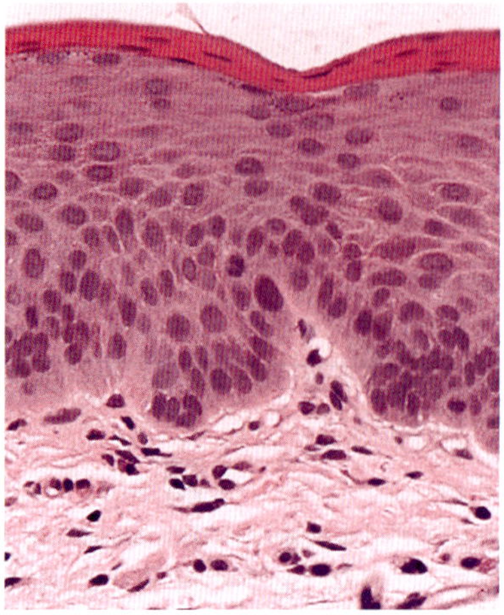

Fig. 12.4: Mild epithelial dysplasia—architectural changes are limited to the lower-third of the epithelium, cellular atypia is mild

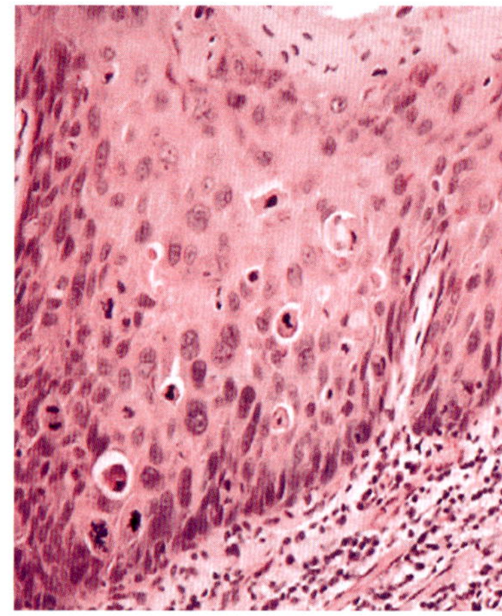

Fig. 12.6: Epithelial dysplasia graded as severe—architectural changes extend to upper-third, cellular atypia including increased mitoses

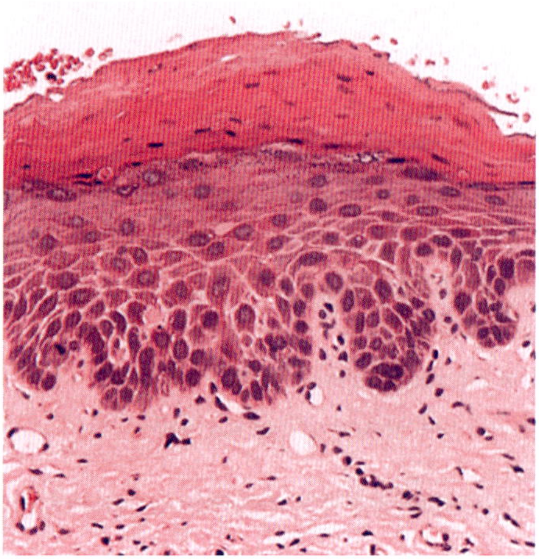

Fig. 12.5: Moderate epithelial dysplasia— architectural changes extend to middle-third of the surface epithelium, cellular atypia is moderate

Table 12.6
Interobserver agreement in the diagnosis of epithelial dysplasia

	Kappa scores	*Agreement (%)*
Brothwell et al	0.51 (0.42–0.58)	77 (75–85)
Karabulut et al	0.35 (0.27–0.45)	55 (49–69)
Abbey et al	0.46 (0.29–0.57)	82 (66–86)

Kappa values (0.35–0.51) for a diagnosis of the presence or absence of epithelial dysplasia represent only fair to moderate agreement

Dysplastic changes remain somewhat controversial as to predicting transformation to carcinoma and effective management. The varying degrees of epithelial dysplasia (mild, moderate, severe) remain our best available cell/tissue markers at this time in assessing risks for transformation but there is considerable subjectivity and only moderate agreement among observers on grading (**Table 12.6**). In a recent study, we have found that three grades of dysplasia have independent prognostic value, both for transformation and time to transformation.

Lichenoid Dysplasia

The term lichenoid dysplasia has been used when the inflammatory response associated with dysplasia is dense, concentrated subepithelially within the upper lamina propria. This terminology has been controversial and the histological appearance misjudged as of lichen planus with dysplasia (**Fig. 12.7**). The term lichenoid dysplasia implies a dysplastic lesion with a lichenoid inflammatory response.

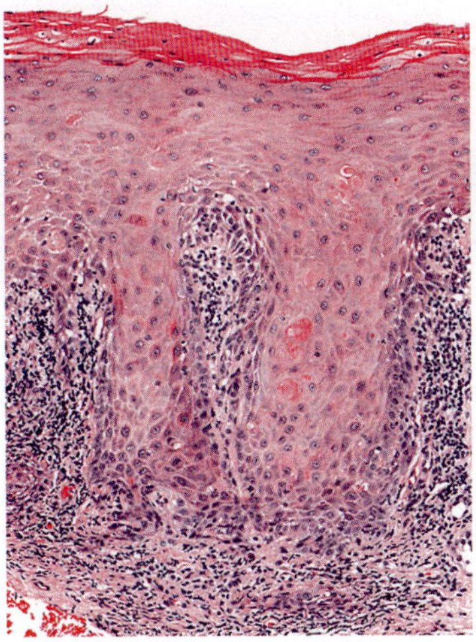

Fig. 12.7: Oral epithelial dysplasia with a lichenoid process—sometimes referred to as lichenoid dysplasia in the literature, a term that should be avoided

Cell and Molecular Markers

It is clear from a large number of reported studies that multiple genes/pathways are involved in the progression of a normal epithelium to metaplastic/dysplastic states to eventually cancer. While there are numerous papers citing work on epithelial cell markers and neoplastic risk, none have the specificity to definitively aid the clinician regarding management. The applicability of gene aberrations and altered protein expression in identifying dysplastic lesions and predicting their outcome is far from proven, especially if these findings are considered in isolation. Even a 'cocktail' of markers has not offered the specificity or practicality needed.

Some molecular alterations in genes/pathways which include cellular signaling, cell cycle, apoptosis, genomic stability, cytoskeleton and angiogenesis to predict neoplastic potential include the following examples: Loss of heterozygosity in patients with leukoplakia and/or dysplasia as evidenced by missing chromosome arms (mainly 3, 9, 17) that contain known tumor suppressor genes seem to be particularly important to predict subsequent transformation to carcinoma. The same problem of inadequate specificity exists in looking at biomarkers in dysplasia. A systematic review included seven biomarkers (p53, p73, cathepsin L, matrix metalloproteinases (MMP 1,2,9) and survivin). Growth factor receptors (EGFR), other cell cycle markers (cyclin A, B1, D), cell proliferation markers (Ki67, Mcm2) and other molecular markers that control apoptosis (e.g. pRB) have also been examined. All show wide variations in results, some with a degree of association for progression to cancer, but lack the accuracy of useful predictive positive/negative values for transformation. It is likely that morphological features seen in dysplasia are due to genetic changes in the epithelium but it is unlikely that the mutations involved are the same ones as associated with progression to cancer. Therefore, the latitude for error, as well as the lack of availability and cost, renders these approaches premature to use in the clinical management and not at the level for making definitive decisions regarding the most appropriate treatment.

Ploidy Status of Oral Leukoplakia

Chromosomal instability and DNA aneuploidy are fundamental to development of malignancy. Preneoplastic oral epithelium may show aneuploidy and it is hypothesized that DNA aneuploidy may predict malignant transformation. The prevalence of aneuploidy may also increase as lesions progress, as noted in sequential biopsies. Large scale genomic changes (DNA ploidy) can be measured using karyometry, flow cytometry and image-based analysis. Unfortunately, data from early studies are retracted and the predictive value of ploidy analysis remains untested in a routine diagnostic setting. One study has shown that epithelial dysplasia is correlated with DNA ploidy status and few have shown a predictive value for transformation.

The likely prognostic markers of value are shown in **Table 12.7**. The combined use of the dysplasia grade and ploidy status could provide the highest predictive value for transformation.

Clinical Features

All leukoplakias are not the same as well as occurring on any mucosal surface

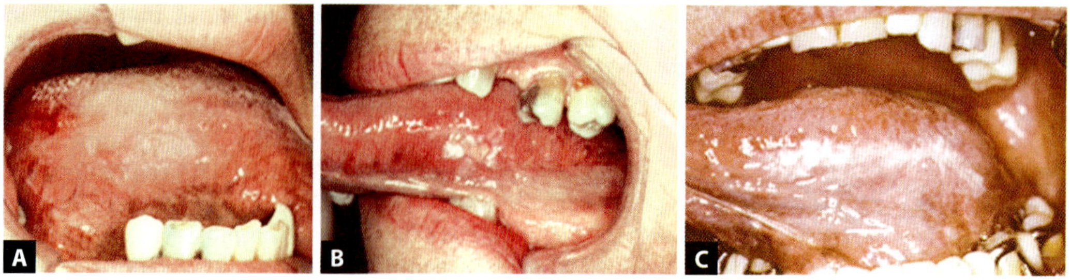

Figs 12.8A to C: Predominantly white lesions of tongue, all consistent with a diagnosis of oral leukoplakia but with varied clinical appearance

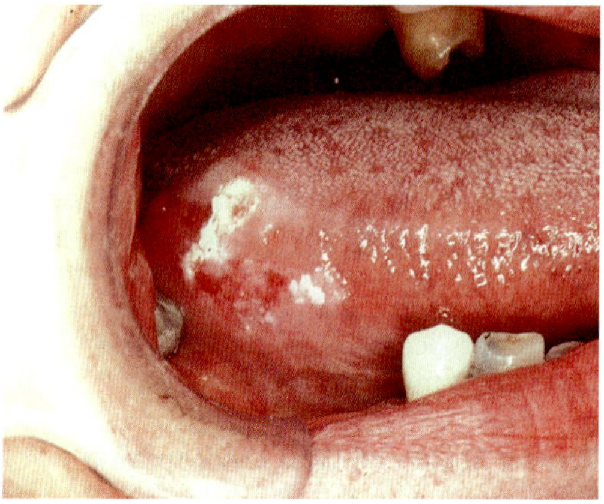

Fig. 12.9: A white patch with a red component clinically labeled erythroleukoplakia

▪ Table 12.7
Factors indicating worse prognosis

- Female gender
- Long duration (with continuation of habits)
- Idiopathic leukoplakia
- Location—Floor of mouth/Ventral tongue
- Nonhomogeneous types erythroplakia (speckled)
- Presence of *Candida*
- Severity of dysplasia
- DNA aneuploidy.

(**Figs 12.8A to C**). A range of clinical features along with patient history indicate various differences in probable causative factors, malignant potential and risk. A red component in the leukoplakia (erythroleukoplakia) indicates an increased risk for dysplasia and/or malignancy (**Fig. 12.9**). This also indicates that the diagnostic biopsy should include the red component, since this is the most likely area of dysplasia or even an early carcinoma. Some anatomical sub-sites such as floor of mouth or ventral tongue are traditionally considered as having higher risk. In the absence of a tobacco history, a leukoplakia is considered "idiopathic", though rare, are considered to have a higher risk of transformation.

The leukoplakia with the greatest potential for malignant transformation is termed proliferative verrucous leukoplakia (PVL) (**Figs 12.10A and B**). In this form, the clinical lesion increases in size over a period of time and can occur at multiple oral mucosal sites. As PVL progresses, it becomes exophytic/wart-like in appearance, and often occurs without any evident etiologic factor. Selecting representative biopsy sites can be difficult, but critical to an accurate assessment. It is found most frequently in women over 40, but can occur in younger women and in men. Margins are difficult to ascertain, so recurrences after treatment are common, accounting for an always guarded prognosis. This form can start as an unimpressive limited, flat white change, or some may have a lichenoid appearance that with time extends and becomes exophytic. PVL can show all degrees of dysplasia, transforming frequently into verrucous carcinoma or invasive carcinoma with varying degrees of cellular differentiation. The diagnosis is based upon a combined clinical-microscopic assessment.

Differential Diagnosis

There are some white patches seen on the oral mucosa that should not be confused as oral leukoplakia (**Table 12.8**). Keratotic changes (focal keratosis) from labial and cheek mucosal

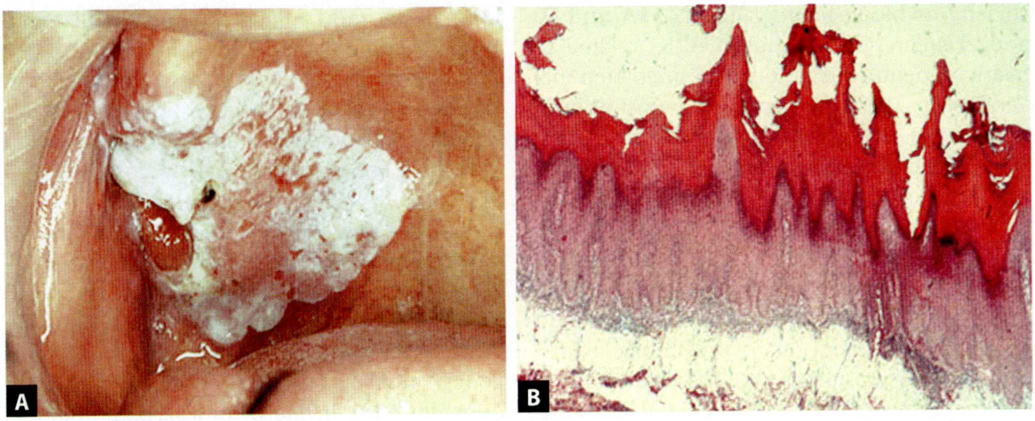

Figs 12.10A and B: Classical clinical and microscopic appearance of proliferative verrucous leukoplakia

▪ Table 12.8
White patches that should be distinguished from leukoplakia and need exclusion to diagnose leukoplakia

Disorder	*Diagnostic features*	*Biopsy*
White sponge nevus	Noted in early life, family history, large areas involved, genital mucosa may be affected	Biopsy not indicated
Frictional keratosis	History of trauma, mostly along the occlusal plane, an etiological cause apparent, mostly reversible on removing the cause	Biopsy if persistent after elimination of cause particularly in a tobacco user
Morsicatio buccarum	Habitual cheek-lip biting known, irregular whitish flakes with jagged out line	Biopsy not indicated
Chemical injury	Known history, site of lesion corresponds to chemical injury, painful, resolves rapidly	Not indicated
Acute pseudomembranous candidosis	The membrane can be scraped off leaving an erythematous raw surface	Swab for culture
Leukoedema	Bilateral on buccal mucosa, could be made to disappear on stretching (retracting), racial	Not indicated
Lichen planus (plaque type)	Other forms of lichen planus (reticular) found in association	Biopsy consistent with lichen planus
Lichenoid reaction	Drug history, or to an amalgam restoration	Biopsy consistent with lichenoid reaction
Discoid lupus erythematosus	Circumscribed lesion with central erythema, white lines radiating	Biopsy consistent with DLE supported by immunofluoresence and other investigations
Skin graft	Known history	Not indicated
Hairy leukoplakia	Bilateral tongue keratosis, other features of HIV disease	Specific histopathology with koilocytosis; EBV demonstrable on ISH
Leukokeratosis nicotina	Smoking history, grayish white palate, swollen minor salivary glands and dilated orifices	Not indicated

sucking or biting habits (**Figs 12.11A and B**) and alveolar ridge keratosis (ARK) related to overlying denture irritation are termed frictional keratoses. These forms of keratoses have little to essentially no potential for malignant transformation and are not considered under the term leukoplakia. On the buccal mucosa, when present along the occlusal plane, these changes are often termed as linea alba. Frictional keratoses in labial/buccal gingivae are rare clinical findings and also generally do not belong to the category of oral leukoplakia.

Leukoedema (**Figs 12.12A and B**) is sometimes confused with leukoplakia. But leukoedema is flat, soft, grayish in color, and a manifestation of immature keratin, epithelial hyperplasia and often some vacuolization. While in some patients this is an early stage of mucosal response to irritation, e.g. tobacco, it is often a racial disorder without any risk for neoplasia. Leukoedema tends to disappear on stretching the affected area of mucosa leaving a normal pink color of the mucosa.

White sponge nevus (WSN), a keratin defect, can be confused with leukoplakia because of the epithelial hyperplasia and some increase in surface keratin (**Figs 12.13A and B**). While WSN is a genetic defect, affecting keratin genes 4 and 13, clinical penetrance is not always apparent early in life or in a large number of family members. It is not associated with a risk for malignant transformation.

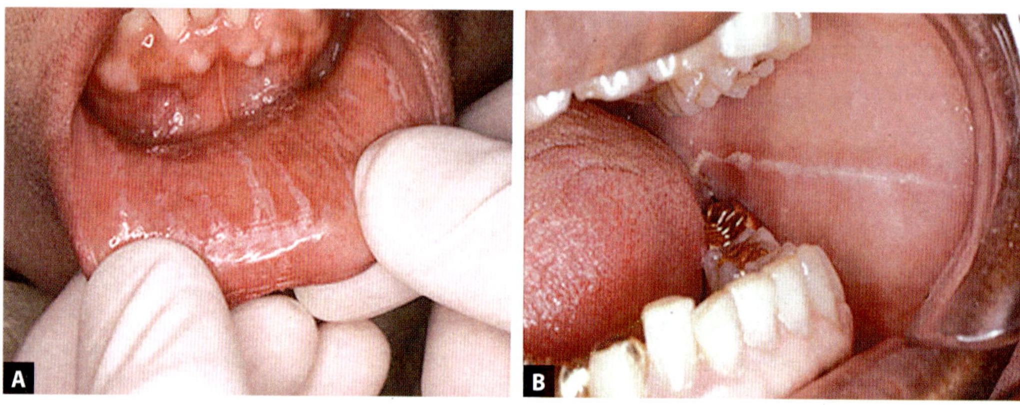

Figs 12.11A and B: (A) Frictional keratosis from lip sucking causing focal keratosis; (B) Cheek irritation causing linea alba

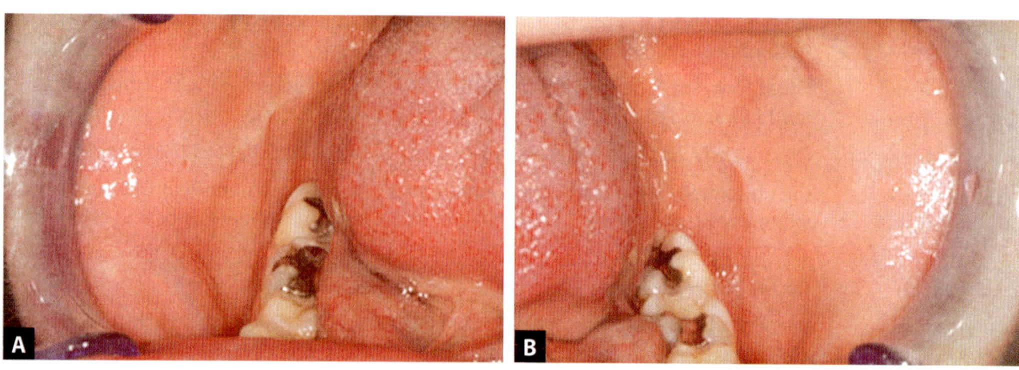

Figs 12.12A and B: Leukoedema of buccal mucosa. The white appearance will fade away on stretching the tissue leaving normal pink color

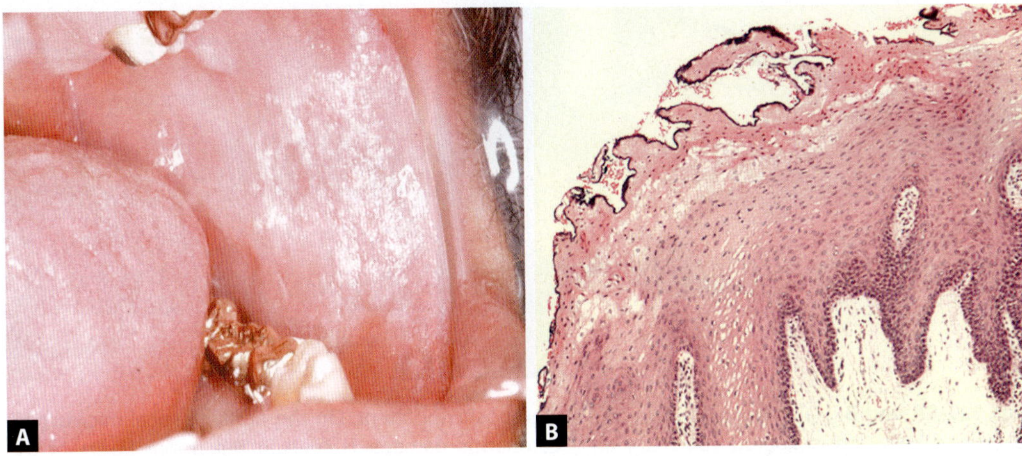

Figs 12.13A and B: Asymptomatic white sponge nevus (genetic keratin defect)

The presence of *Candida* in leukoplakia frequently confuses the clinical picture. In some instances, a trial of antifungal medicine will partially or completely modify the white plaque. Actually, candidal organisms are capable of invading the upper layers of the epithelium and stimulating keratin formation that clinically cannot be wiped off (**Fig. 12.14**). The evidence remains controversial as to whether candidal-associated leukoplakia has an increased risk for malignant transformation. Hairy leukoplakia comprising immature keratin is associated with infection with EBV in immunosuppressed or HIV seropositive subjects, and carries no documented risk for malignant transformation (**Figs 12.15A and B**). **Table 12.8** lists oral white lesions that need to be excluded while diagnosing oral leukoplakia. A schematic diagram (**Fig. 12.16**) explains the procedures to follow when investigating oral leukoplakia to achieve a correct diagnosis.

Risk Factors

The most common cause associated with leukoplakia is the use of combustible and/or smokeless tobacco and this remains the most troublesome problem during its management. The combustible forms (smoking) include the use of cigarettes, pipes, cigars and bidi. All of these forms carry an increased risk for leukoplakia and particularly among heavy users the subsequent risk for transformation to

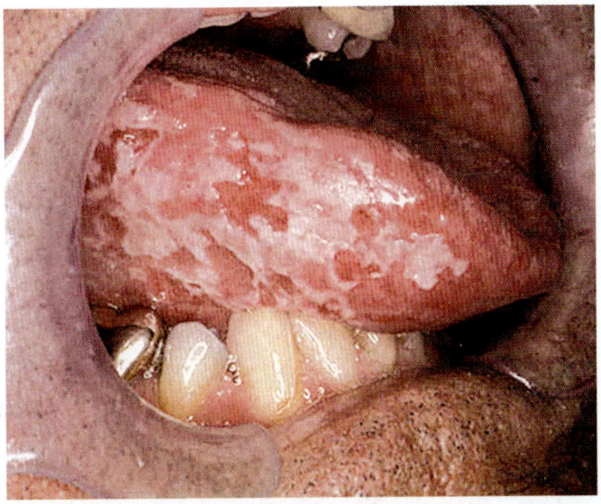

Fig. 12.14: Candidal leukoplakia on lateral tongue

malignancy. The variable clinical responses to the chemical and heat irritants depend upon the years and frequency of usage, the tobacco leaf and processing, combined with other factors such as genetic mutations, alcohol intake, and other forms of irritation such a betel quid use. Discontinuing the habit(s) is often difficult, but it is critically important in the management and control of leukoplakia. Obviously, nontobacco users can develop leukoplakia, referred to as idiopathic leukoplakia with a potential for malignant transformation, and leukoplakia can remain in ex-smokers who have discontinued the habit for a period of time. So a predictable biologic outcome remains as a variable risk. The noncombustible (smokeless) forms of

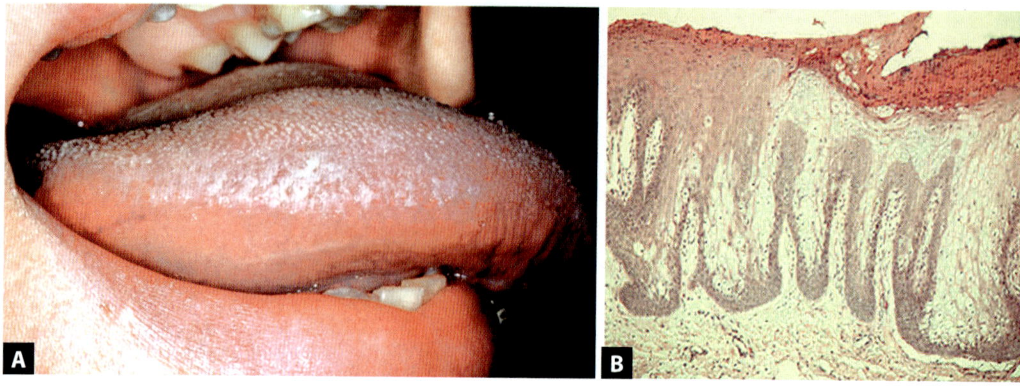

Figs 12.15A and B: Hairy leukoplakia in an HIV seropositive patient. On the right, classical microscopic feature of koilocytosis due to EBV associated cytopathic damage is seen in the upper layers of the epithelium

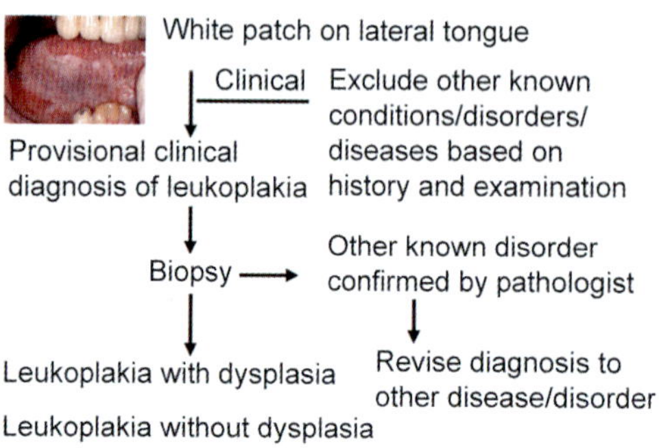

Fig. 12.16: A schematic diagram pointing out the steps to follow when investigating oral leukoplakia

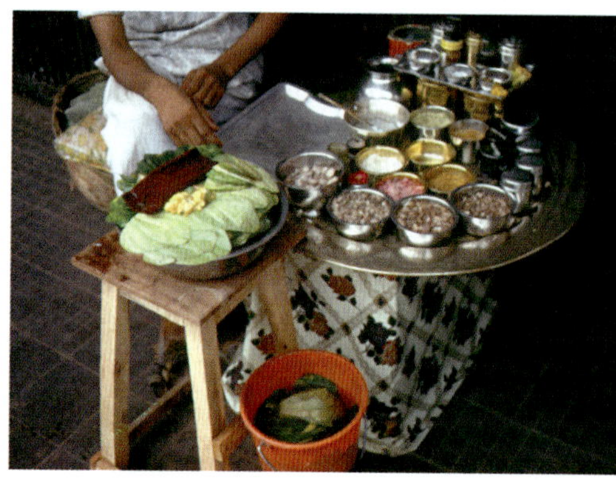

Fig. 12.17: Popular display of betel quid and ingredients

tobacco (ST) include snuff, referred to as snus in Scandinavia, chewing tobacco, gutka, and many other novel substances/forms. Nitrosamine content and availability of ST varies widely. Keratinization and transformations depend upon the product and usage. Time for development of leukoplakia and carcinoma vary widely, but usually involves many years. Prospective, well-designed epidemiologic studies are not available for definitive transformation figures.

Tobacco cessation can be by 'cold turkey' based upon will-power, by the use of counseling, incorporating nicotine replacement therapy, and using pharmacologic approaches (see Chapter 24). Smokeless tobacco (particularly snuff) associated with leukoplakia at the mucosal site of the habit is often reversible after cessation. So cessation and potential disappearance of the leukoplakia is rewarding and can be an approach to cancer prevention. Using one of these approaches is helpful to a limited degree; and combinations are the most effective. However, even with compliance and after one year follow-up, the successful cessation results are on average less than 20 percent.

Betel quid chewing is strongly associated with causation of oral leukoplakia. Betel quid entails different combinations of betel leaf with added tobacco, slaked lime, flavorings with areca nut as the main ingredient (**Fig. 12.17**). A

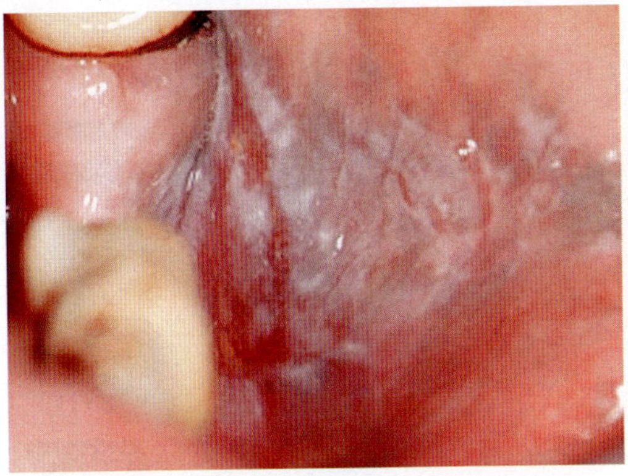

Fig. 12.18: Erythroleukoplakia arising from a betel quid-induced lichenoid lesion

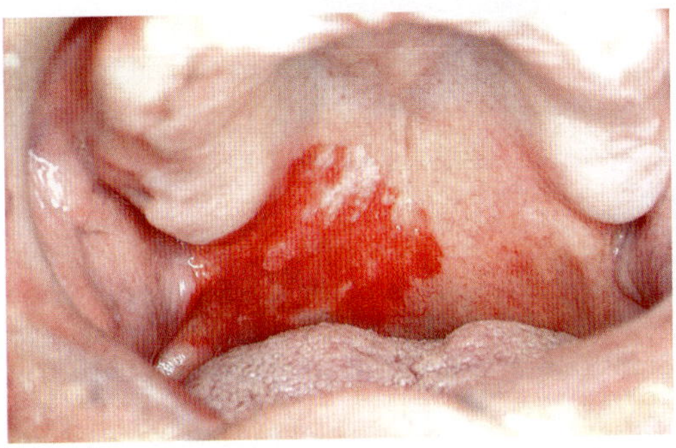

Fig. 12.19: Clinically presenting as painful erythroplakia of soft palate. On biopsy—squamous cell carcinoma

betelquid induced patch which first appeared as a lichenoid lesion and later changed to erythroleukoplakia is shown in **Figure 12.18.** In populations not adding tobacco to betel quid (e.g. Taiwan), the population attributable-risk of areca nut use was estimated at 73.2 percent.

ERYTHROPLAKIA

While quite infrequent, some dysplastic or early malignant lesions clinically will be all red with well circumscribed clinical margins. These lesions are termed erythroplakias and can represent an early carcinoma (**Fig. 12.19**). While these lesions can be mistaken for irritation or infection, if they persist a biopsy is mandated to rule out dysplasia or malignancy. In some reports from populations of drinkers and smokers, erythroplakias have been the first signs of malignancy (**Fig. 12.20**).

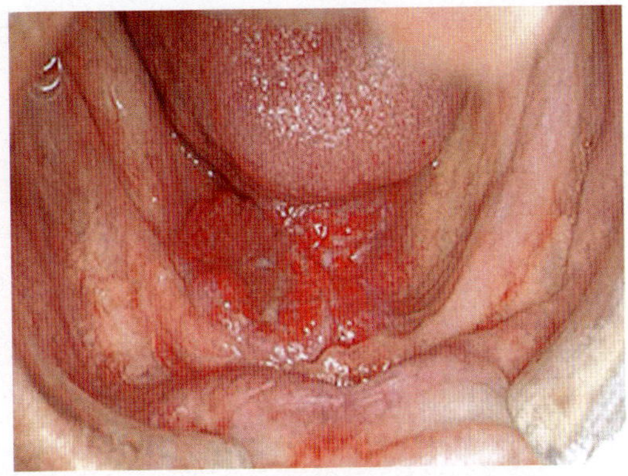

Fig. 12.20: Erythroleukoplakia in the floor of mouth in a heavy smoker and alcohol drinker that transformed into a squamous carcinoma

DIAGNOSIS AND ADJUNCTIVE TECHNIQUES

The definitive diagnosis for leukoplakia and erythroplakia is made by biopsy, usually an incisional biopsy. As indicated previously, biomarkers that have a useful predictive value are not yet available, so the presence or absence of epithelial cell dysplasia becomes helpful in lesion management and assessing malignant potential. Often, adjunctive techniques become useful for many reasons:

- Accelerating biopsy when there are otherwise reasons for delay
- Identifying the best area(s) for biopsy sampling
- To help determine margins
- For follow-up care.

Low level evidence-based data is available, indicating a benefit of several adjunctive techniques for clinicians and patients regarding early detection by accelerating biopsy in evaluating leukoplakic lesions.

At the present time, high level evidence-based data (controlled randomized prospective trials) are not yet reported to conclusively reflect the usefulness or lack of usefulness of these techniques, including cytodiagnosis (using a brush biopsy), vital staining (toluidine blue) (**Figs 12.21A to D**), and various forms of optical diagnostic techniques including

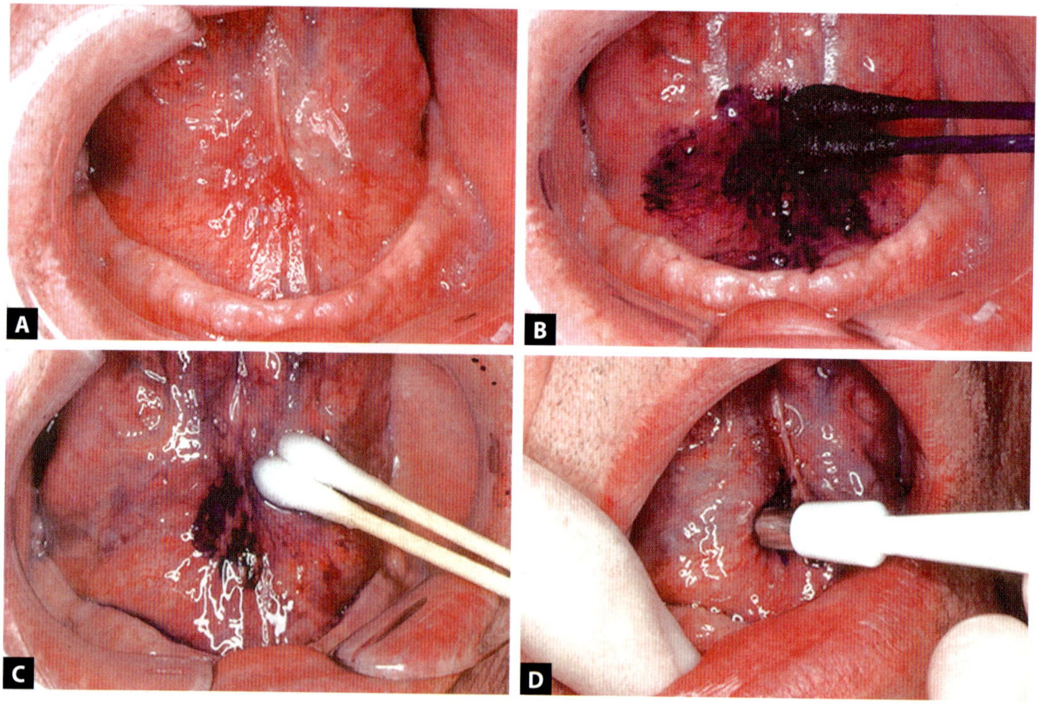

Figs 12.21A to D: Staining technique with 1 percent aqueous toluidine blue: (A and B) Application in asymptomatic erythroleukoplakia; biopsy showed severe dysplasia; (C) Toluidine blue retention after application of 1 percent acetic acid destaining; (D) Biopsy using a 5 mm dermatological punch that showed microinvasive squamous carcinoma

autofluorescence and chemiluminescence (**Figs 12.22A and B**). Their sensitivity in detecting a white or red patch is good but their specificity to detect oral dysplasia remains low. However, many reports do indicate their usefulness in accelerating appropriate tests to establish the diagnosis.

SCREENING FOR ORAL LEUKOPLAKIA AND ERYTHROPLAKIA

It must be emphasized that screening involves a thorough head and neck examination, a systematic visual examination of the oral mucosa (oral cavity) and use of adjunctive techniques (if necessary) to accelerate biopsy. Following screening any suspicious lesions found should be referred to a specialist for biopsy. The purpose is to properly assess the leukoplakia for the most appropriate management, as well as to make certain that malignant transformation has not already taken place. The differential diagnosis (**Table 12.8**) must always be considered in order to obtain the optimal, expedient, and most accurate lesion identification. As an example, frictional keratosis is the most common white lesion and would be encountered more frequently during screening. Furthermore, lichen planus, a quite common auto-immune mucocutaneous disease, would present as keratosis. Its plaque like form can mimic homogeneous leukoplakia, and erythematous forms may mimic erythroleukoplakia, or even carcinoma. Therefore, persistent lesions for which a diagnosis has not been established must be thoroughly evaluated.

Organized screening programs to detect OPMDs have been conducted in India, Sri Lanka, Malaysia, Taiwan, Japan and the UK with some benefit to these populations. The majority have used visual screening for the case-detection and a program in Taiwan in

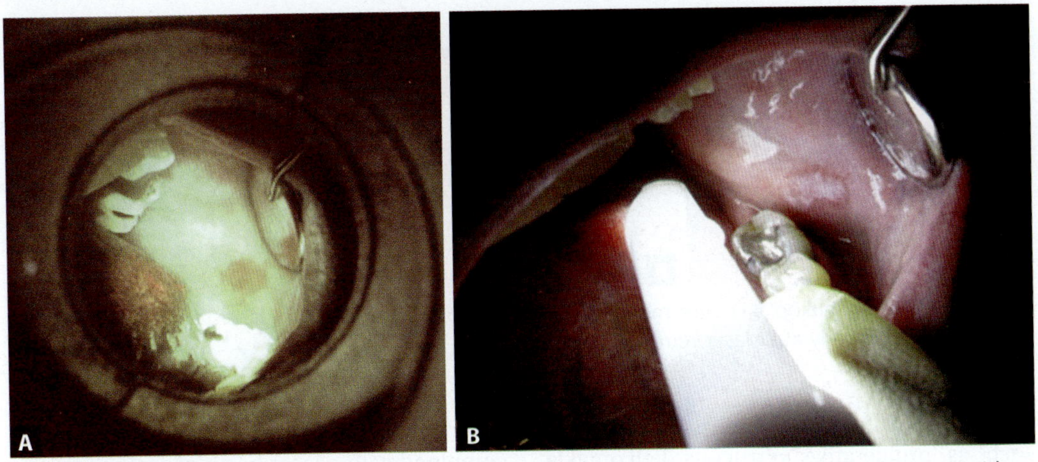

Figs 12.22A and B: (A) Newer optical techniques to detect leukoplakia. Loss of fluorescence with VelScope; (B) Enhanced whiteness under chemilumine scence using Vizilite

addition used toluidine blue. Annual screening conducted in India and Japan has established that new cases/lesions can be found by periodic screening. The role of screening as a mechanism to discover new lesions cannot be understated.

Management

If oral leukoplakia and erythroplakia can be effectively recognized, diagnosed and appropriately treated, a proportion of oral and oropharyngeal cancers could be prevented.

The natural history of oral leukoplakia- the most common OPMD lesion encountered in the oral cavity—remains unclear. Presence of oral dysplasia significantly increases the rate of transformation to cancer and this may increase with the grade. It is therefore argued that treatment of dysplastic lesions may prevent cancer development in high-risk persons with oral leukoplakia. A recent meta-analysis has provided evidence that surgical treatment of oral leukoplakia may reduce the risk of transformation but does not completely eliminate this risk. Whether we can prevent malignancy by treating precursor lesions by surgery or chemoprevention remains a complex issue. It is one of the most important problems in oral medicine and needs further research.

Management depends upon signs, symptoms, clinician experience, grading of dysplasia (± ploidy data) and patient wishes/compliance. Obviously, the most important part of management is knowing the microscopic and clinical classifications, since risk for transformation is the end point to be prevented. If removing an identified irritant will reverse a lesion, that is optimal treatment. In a persistent leukoplakia that has been already diagnosed/evaluated, management considerations include careful follow-up, incorporating adjunctive techniques, and biopsy for any changes in signs and symptoms. Discontinuing tobacco habits and other irritants (e.g. betel quid) are essential to optimal outcomes.

Definitive treatment is by surgical removal. As mentioned earlier, a recent systematic review concluded that surgical excision reduces malignant transformation but does not totally eliminate the risk. The use of laser has been effective, but any means of removal that works for the operator is in order (**Figs 12.23A to C**). The problem is one of including adequate margins to minimize chances for recurrence. The benefit of laser surgery in oral leukoplakia is that recurrences following treatment are far fewer compared with knife excision. In the leukoplakias that have a genetic basis, minimal margins with close follow-up for recurrence is a viable option. Extensive excisions are sometimes difficult in trying to attain biologically clear margins, as well as maintaining optimal comfort

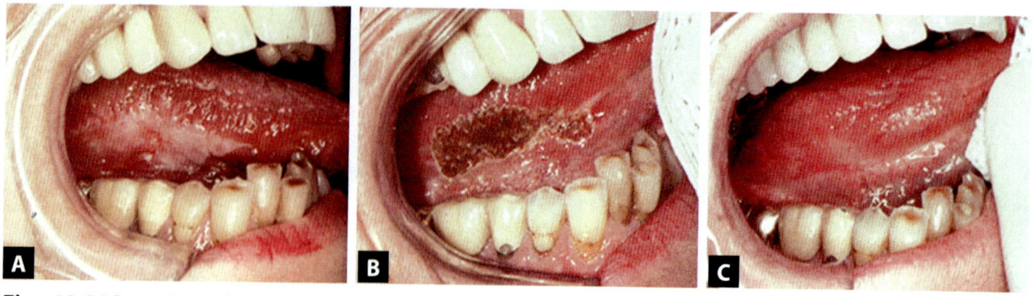

Figs 12.23A to C: Leukoplakia with moderate dysplasia controlled with CO_2 laser removal: (A) Original lesion; (B) Immediately after laser removal; (C) at 5 weeks

and function for the patient. In situations such as proliferative verrucous leukoplakia, recurrences are common. While the use of adjunctive techniques to assist identify 'safe' margins may be helpful, they are not evidence-based or reliable. Their utility is based upon the reports of experienced clinicians. If any existing habits are not discontinued, the prognosis for successful recovery is poor.

Although there have been extensive studies utilizing chemoprevention none have shown any clinical utility. The first tried were vitamin A and retinoids (retinoic acid); the results have been poor. Firstly, because all patients do not have an effective response in modifying the lesion; and secondly, high dosages must be used. In most patients, adverse side effects will occur, such as dry skin, pruritus, rash, angular cheilitis, and an increase of serum triglycerides. If there has been a response and the medicines are discontinued, unfortunately, the leukoplakia recurs (**Figs 12.24 and 12.25**). The other chemotherapeutic agent that has undergone a prospective randomized trial is lycopene. Lycopene is a carotenoid, a cyclic isomer of beta-carotene and is a natural pigment synthesized by plants, predominantly accumulated in tomatoes. A Japanese group has shown that serum levels of lycopene, among men with oral leukoplakia was significantly lower than controls. A clinical trial on 58 subjects with leukoplakia when given 8 mg or 4 mg lycopene per day for 3 months showed clinical responses of 80 and 66 percent respectively, but the study did not follow consort guidelines. More recently NSAIDs have drawn the most attention as chemoprevention agents. The ideal chemopreventive agent remains to be discovered. Radiation plays no role. Photodynamic therapy using a lesion sensitizer combined with a laser beam of a specific wave length to cause localized photo damage and cell death has not been adequately tested but may be useful in the future.

Assessing and modifying tobacco usage in young individuals is particularly important since it is at the time in life (adolescents) that adult tobacco habits are formed. While tobacco use is more prevalent in boys, usage by girls is increasing. Smoked tobacco contains numerous carcinogens (estimated to average around 60), increases the risk to those exposed individuals to develop precancerous or malignant transformations. Solutions to the problems associated with smoking depend upon passing and implementing tobacco control laws, taxes, counseling, decreased access and control of media advertising. Practical methods of tobacco cessation for patients encountered in clinical practice are given in Chapter 24.

Management also includes a thorough orientation to the patient regarding leukoplakia and periodic follow-up. Again, re-biopsy is indicated only when there are clinical changes in either signs and/or symptoms. Often, the use of an adjunctive technique might indicate the best area to sample in order to evaluate the most dangerous portion of the lesion. However, the signs and/or symptoms, including the use of markers that might yield accurate positive or negative predictive values for any specific leukoplakia are not readily available or reliable. So once again the clinical classification of the lesion, together with the histologic findings, still remain the most useful factors to support therapeutic recommendations.

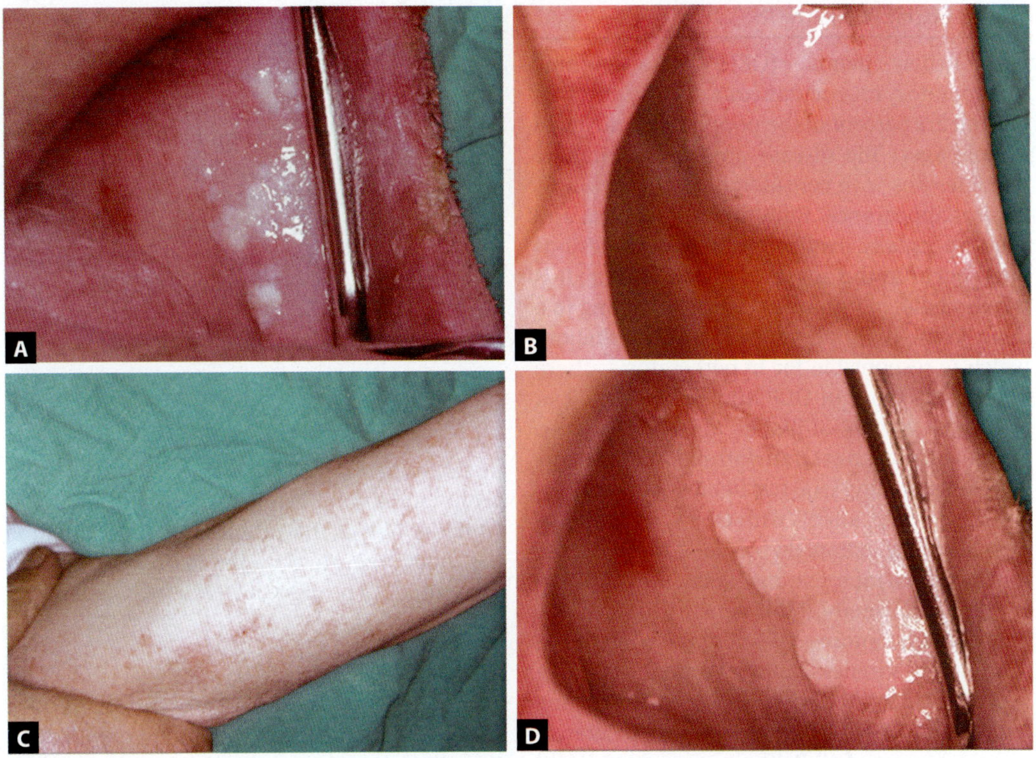

Figs 12.24A to D: Retinoid treatment of oral leukoplakia. (A) Original presentation; (B) Resolution with therapy; (C) Skin eruption during therapy; (D) The lesion has recurred on discontinuation of treatment

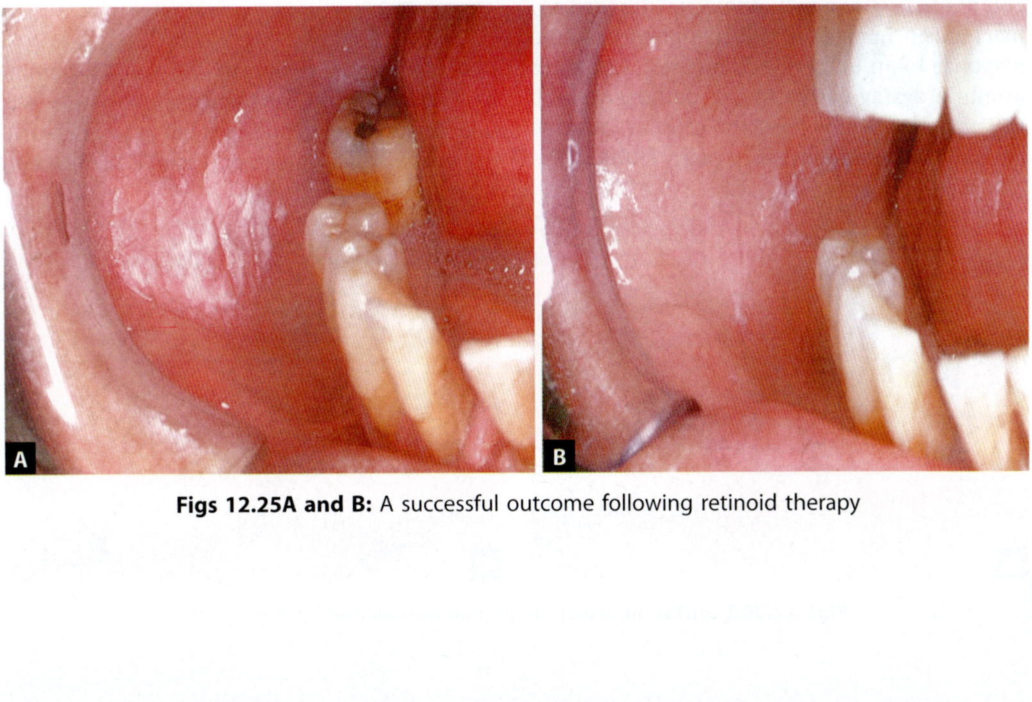

Figs 12.25A and B: A successful outcome following retinoid therapy

ORAL LICHEN PLANUS

Oral lichen planus (OLP) is a chronic inflammatory mucocutaneous disease affecting 0.5 and 2.2 percent of the population, mostly in middle ages. The disease appears as bilateral white lesions with considerable variation in its clinical appearance. Both the oral mucosa and skin are usually involved, but the oral lesions often occur in the absence of skin lesions. It is a cell-mediated immune condition leading to a delay in the maturation of mucosal epithelium which is responsible for hyperkeratosis. There are various types of OLP and some forms can affect the quality-of-life in affected patients. Moreover, malignant transformation in patients with longstanding OLP has been documented.

In general, patients with OLP are symptom-free but may complain of roughness of the mucosa. In asymptomatic subjects, the condition is often first noted by the dental practitioners. Those with symptoms often complain of burning sensation to soreness but may experience bouts of severe pain, interfering with speaking, eating and swallowing during episodes of ulcerative (erosive) forms of OLP. These symptoms could interfere with their quality-of-life.

Etiology and Immunopathogenesis

Oral lichen planus is a chronic inflammatory condition of unknown etiology. The disease mechanism involves a cell mediated immune response to an unidentified antigen. A role for immune dysregulation in the pathogenesis of OLP specifically involving the cellular immune system has been reported in many studies. The inflammatory infiltrate in OLP lesion consists primarily of T cells and macrophages. A recent study showed that activated CD8+ T lymphocytes can be found within the epithelium and adjacent to damaged basal cell keratinocytes in the OLP lesions. The basal keratinocyte degeneration observed in OLP is attributed to cytotoxic CD8+ T lymphocytes. The triggering antigen is unknown. Moreover, mast cell degranulation in OLP releases proinflammatory mediators such as tumor necrosis factor-alpha, chymase and tryptase that play an important role in the pathogenesis of OLP.

There are many factors involved in the pathogenesis of OLP such as matrix metalloproteinases, chymase, tryptase and proinflammatory cytokines. Recently, TNF-α which is one of the proinflammatory cytokine has been reported in the pathogenesis and inflammatory process of OLP.

Clinical Types of OLP

Oral lichen planus may present in various patterns and these presentations are divided into clinical types described by the criteria of the International Consensus Meeting in Chamonix, France, 2003. A variety of clinical presentations such as reticular, papular, plaque type, atrophic, and ulcerative types are described below.

Reticular Type

Reticular lichen planus is the most common type occurring on the buccal mucosa. Lesions may be localized to one area but usually involve the entire buccal mucosa (**Figs 12.26A and B**)

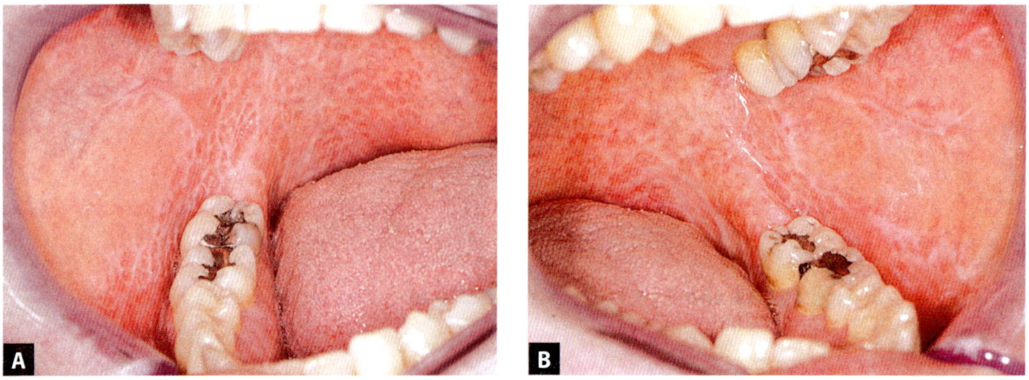

Figs 12.26A and B: Reticular lichen planus—bilateral presentation

occurring bilaterally, extending to the vestibular and retromolar area, and appear as interlacing raised lines forming a latticework. This type is also seen as keratotic white striae arranged in a reticular pattern on the lateral margins of the tongue.

Papular Type

In this type, pinhead size papules are present spaced apart but distributed close enough that the lesion has a pebble white or gray appearance. Individual small white raised papules may be obvious and these sometimes coalesce. Papular type of OLP closely resembles Fordyce's granules (**Fig. 12.27**).

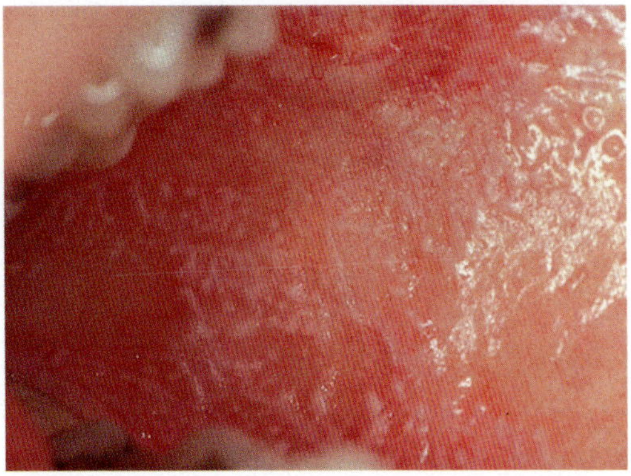

Fig. 12.27: Early papular eruption on buccal mucosa, that eventually leads to reticular form

Plaque Type

In this type of OLP, the keratotic areas are raised and appear as white plaques. Plaque type OLP closely resembles leukoplakia, but reticular elements could always be recognized in the periphery of the lesions. These white patches can be present with or without erythematous areas and the clinicians should differentiate plaque type OLP from leukoplakia or lupus erythematosus (**Fig. 12.28**).

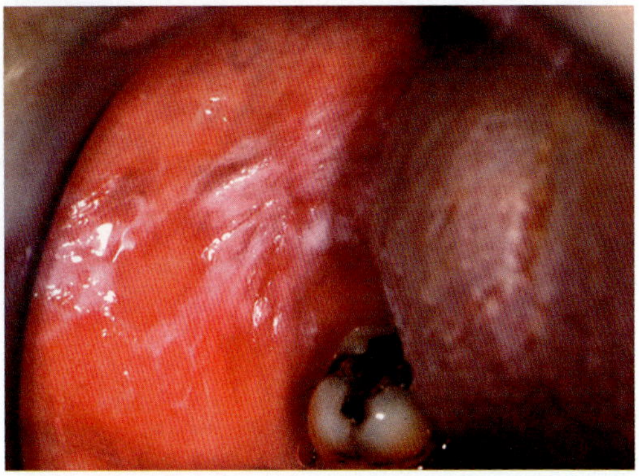

Fig. 12.28: Plaque type oral lichen planus with adjacent annular lesions

Atrophic Type

In this type, the thin epithelium overlying the basal area is weakened and this epithelium is easily lost leading to shallow erosions (**Fig. 12.29**). The OLP lesions of this type may present as erythematous areas with or without keratotic white striae. Patients usually complain of burning sensation or soreness when eating hot and spicy food. When atrophic OLP affects the gingivae, the disease may present as desquamative gingivitis.

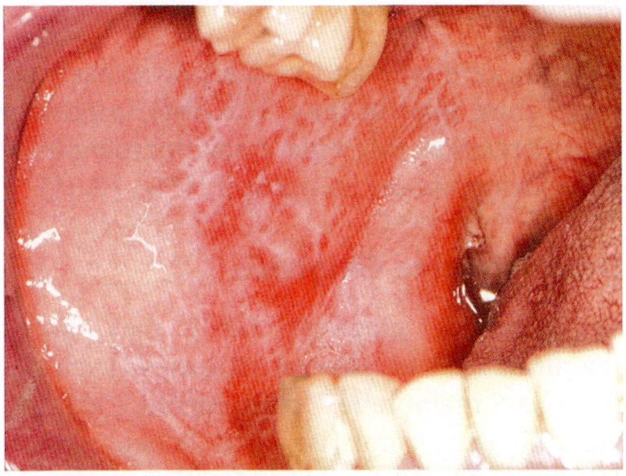

Fig. 12.29: Atrophic oral lichen planus. *Note:* There is no surface ulceration

Ulcerative (Erosive) Type

Atrophic or erosive form of OLP may rupture leaving a raw ulcerated area. Ulcerative form of OLP lesions present with serous exudates, surrounding erythema combined with white striae at the margins of the ulcer (**Fig. 12.30**). The ulcerative form of OLP may result in mucosal bleeding, soreness and fibrosis.

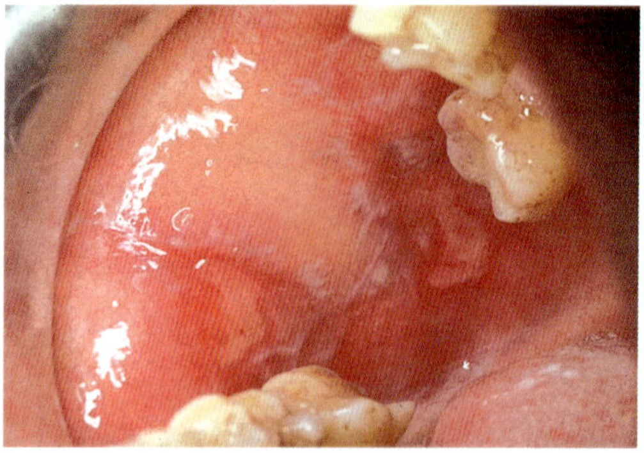

Fig. 12.30: Ulcerative oral lichen planus with associated reticular striae at margins

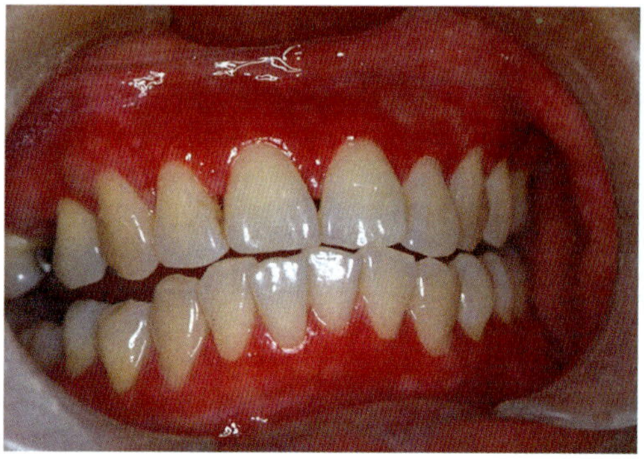

Fig. 12.32: Desquamative gingivitis often a manifestation of lichen planus

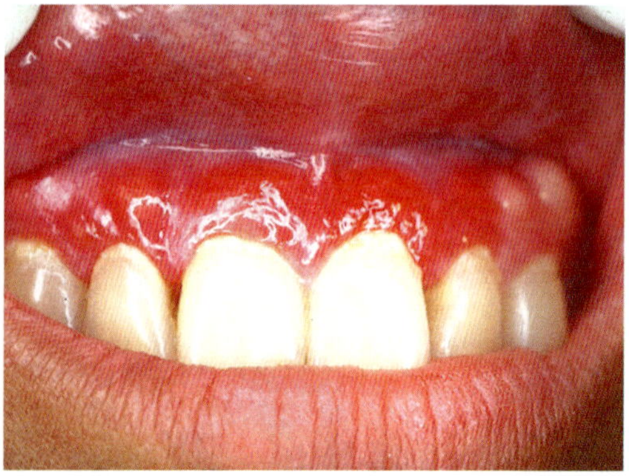

Fig. 12.31: Bullous lichen planus affective gums

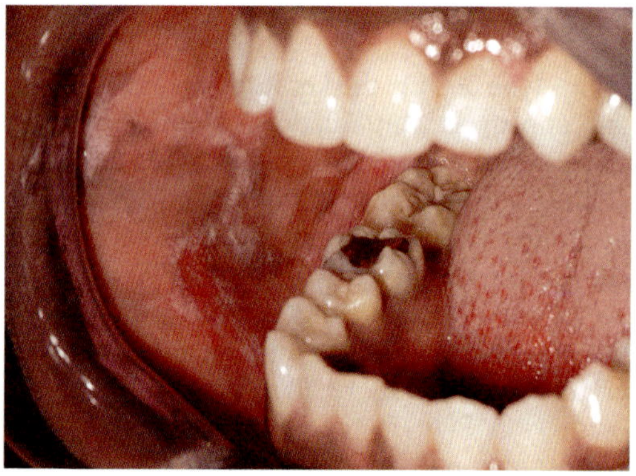

Fig. 12.33: Pigmentation in long-standing oral lichen planus

Bullous Type

This is a rare type and vesicles or bullae may occur from time to time. It is very important to differentiate this type from pemphigus or mucous membrane pemphigoid (**Fig. 12.31**).

Desquamative Gingivitis

Desquamative gingivitis (DG) may be a manifestation of several diseases such as mucous membrane pemphigoid (MMP), pemphigus vulgaris (PV) and lichen planus. However, DG is a term indicating a clinical manifestation and not a diagnosis.

Gingival presentation of DG is characterized by erythema with epithelial desquamation, atrophy, edema, and/or presence of vesiculo-bullous lesions. The gingival presentation (**Fig. 12.32**) of OLP may involve both free and attached gingiva affecting all quadrants of the mouth. Hyperkeratotic striae may be evident at the periphery. Patients may present as symptom-free or report a burning sensation. Severe pain is uncommon.

Deep brown/black pigmented areas around white striae (**Fig. 12.33**) may be found associated with active OLP or mostly with burnt out lesions of OLP and is more common in dark skinned people.

Oral Lichenoid Lesions

Oral lichenoid lesions (OLLs) and lichen planus (OLP) exhibit similar clinical and histopathological features. Several OLLs are recognized, those due to contact hypersensitivity to restorations, in association with a systemic medication (OLDR) or presenting with chronic graft verus host disease (cGVHD). It is beyond this chapter to discuss all three conditions, but it is prudent to consider oral lichenoid contact lesions (OLCL) arising due to contact with metal restorations and GVHD. During follow-up studies some authors have attributed a small risk of OLCL and cGVHD transforming to cancer.

The distinguishing feature of OLCL is the lesions direct topographic relationship to the suspected causative agent, most commonly an amalgam restoration (**Fig. 12.34**). With the removal and replacement of the putative causative material, OLCL should resolve within several months. In fact, OLCL cannot be distinguished from OLP both clinically and histopathologically.

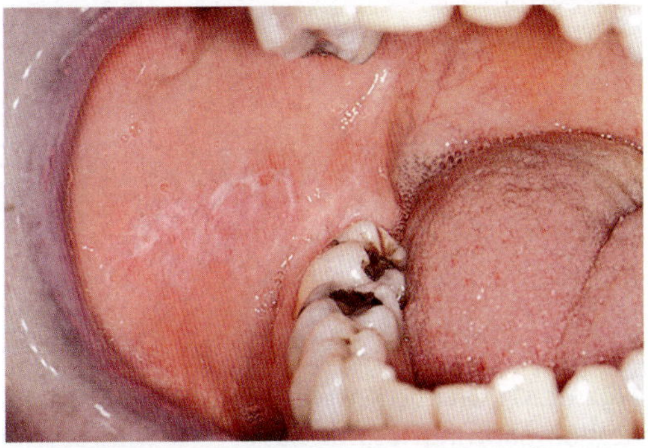

Fig. 12.34: Oral lichenoid lesion in close proximity to an amalgam restoration

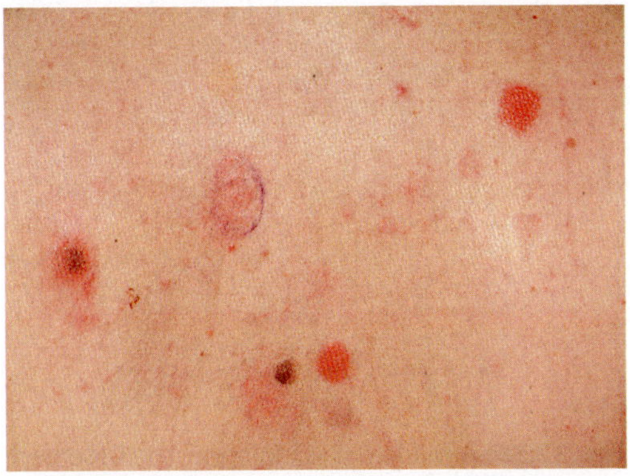

Fig. 12.35: Positive patch test result. Contact hypersensitivity to several dental materials

Skin patch testing (**Fig. 12.35**) might be helpful to the dentist in confirming a lichenoid reaction and in the determination of a suitable replacement dental material. The test substances such as mercury-containing amalgam, or salts have commonly been used. The standard tests take into account that mercury from amalgam restorations may be in the form of metal, organic substances, or organic salts. Few patients react to all three forms. There is no worldwide consensus regarding the allergens used but generally it is accepted that 5 percent amalgam and 1 percent ammoniated mercury are suitable for screening. The tests are usually carried out with additional European series and other dental materials to screen for additional allergens. These substances are applied to normal skin on the back and read after 72 hours exposure. A skin reaction with erythema (**Fig. 12.35**) and effusion with possible papulovesicles (eczema reaction) is considered a positive reaction.

Positive patch test reactions to those suspected substances have been reported with conflicting results between 8 and 78.9 percent. Some studies did not find the value of patch testing. Therefore, the value of cutaneous patch testing in OLCL remains controversial as there is a debate about the validity of extrapolating skin reactions to mucosal responses.

Oral cGVHD may also be considered a potential risk factor for the development of oral carcinoma following allogenic hemopoietic stem cell transplantation among long term survivors.

Lichenoid lesions are also encountered in betel quid users at the site of placement of the quid after prolonged use. The main distinguishing feature is from the patient's history that these OLCL arise when the quid is habitually placed and stored mostly in the buccal sulcus. The clinical appearance consists of white, linear, wavy parallel nonelevated streaks associated with a plaque like patch, the lines occasionally radiating from central erythema.

Systemic Diseases of Interest

Systemic diseases such as hypertension, diabetes mellitus, hepatitis C infection, etc. have been reported in association with OLP in many studies. As OLP occurs predominantly in middle age or older adults, many drugs used in the treatment of systemic diseases can trigger the development of OLDR. The association between OLP and systemic diseases may also be coincidental because OLP is common. Therefore, OLP apparently associated with systemic diseases is possibly to be due to drug side-effects rather than specific associations with the systemic diseases. However, there are no evidence-based studies on these aspects.

Diagnosis and Histopathology

Oral lichen planus can be clinically diagnosed by the chronicity of the history, the presence of oral and/or skin lesions, the characteristic clinical features, e.g. presence of striae and its bilateral occurrence. The oral manifestations alone may be sufficient for a correct diagnosis. Definite diagnosis of OLP is by histological examination of lesional tissue and undertaking a biopsy is important prior to commencement of treatment of this disease particularly to differentiate plaque type OLP from oral leukoplakia or erosive/ulcerative lesions from conditions such as DLE.

Oral lichen planus is characterized by a range of features seen under the microscope (**Figs 12.36 to 12.38**). Requisite histopathologic features include: liquefactive degeneration of basal cells, presence of apoptosis and a band like infiltrate of lymphocytes within the lamina propria that immediately intermingles with basal region of the surface epithelium. Additional features often present although not a prerequisite to diagnosis include: "saw-toothed" rete ridges, hyper ortho and/or parakeratosis, acanthosis or atrophy, separation of surface epithelium from underlying connective tissue, isolated individual hyaline or colloid bodies ("Civatte bodies") within the prickle cell layers. Disqualifying features include: any cellular atypia amounting to dysplasia, presence of heterogeneous round cell infiltrate, i.e. the presence of substantial numbers of plasma

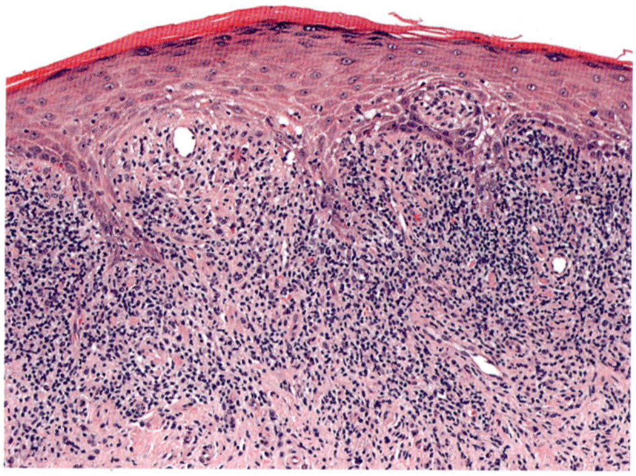

Fig. 12.36: Microscopic features of oral lichen planus. Main feature at this magnification is a dense subepithelial infiltrate of chronic inflammatory cells

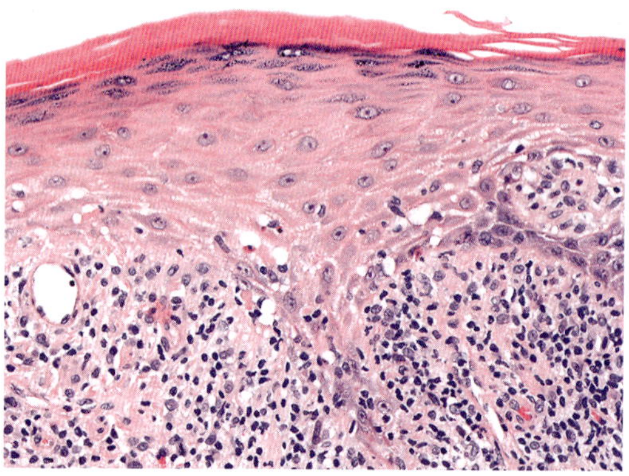

Fig. 12.37: Oral lichen planus at a higher magnification showing loss of basal cells with several apoptoses

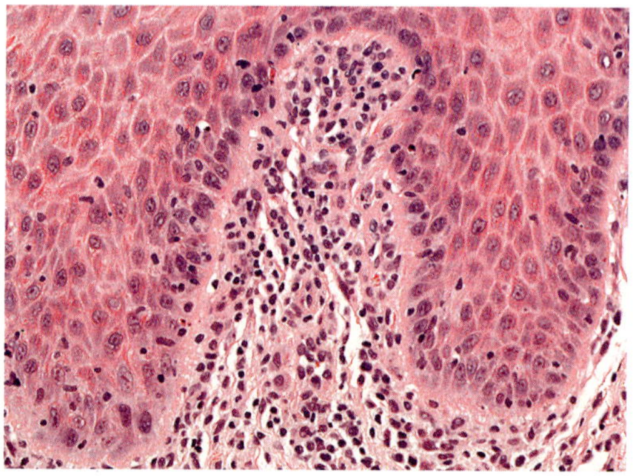

Fig. 12.38: A marked thickening of the basement membrane and migration of lymphocytes towards the epithelium

cells within the infiltrate, diffuse extension of infiltrate to involve deeper submucosal tissues or frank perivascular distribution of the infiltrate. Histopathological findings are the same irrespective of clinical type or anatomical location of the lesion.

Dysplastic changes when present termed lichenoid dysplasia remains a controversial topic and precludes a diagnosis of lichen planus. The term lichenoid dysplasia is considered above under leukoplakia and dysplasia.

Direct immunofluorescence is usually not required to make a diagnosis of OLP as there are no specific features that could be attributable to the disease. When in doubt however, this additional step is useful in the differential diagnosis of erosive and bullous types from pemphigus, mucous membrane pemphigoid or lupus erythematosus in that OLP would yield negative results by the absence of antibody binding at BMZ. Direct immunofluorescence of OLP biopsies demonstrates a shaggy band of fibrinogen in the basement membrane zone in 90 to 100 percent of cases. The presence of fibrin deposition may be used as an additional marker in the diagnosis of lichen planus. IgM-stained cytoid bodies that are present in large numbers are also considered to be suggestive of lichen planus. DIF however, has no pathognomonic features and should only be used to differentiate when OLP clinically resembles MMP or DLE.

Management

The management of OLP will vary widely both between patients, and for individual patients. Because of its recalcitrant (and chronic) nature, various factors such as patients' medical history, presenting symptoms, treatment compliance as well as possible drug interaction must be considered.

Plaque and calculus deposits are associated with an increased incidence of erythematous and erosive gingival lesions in many cases of OLP. Thus, improvement of oral hygiene is essential for eliminating dental plaque accumulation and can enhance healing of the lesions. Furthermore, there is a possibility of dental restorations inducing oral lichenoid lesions that may sometimes improve after replacement of amalgam with other restorative materials. Anxiety, depression and psychic disorders have been reported in association with OLP patients. Stress has also been found to be the most frequent cause of acute exacerbations in those patients. Reassurance is useful, and some patients may require stress management.

Various treatment regimens have been attempted to improve the refractory lesion and to reduce associated pain (**Table 12.9**), but a complete cure of OLP has not yet been accomplished because of its recalcitrant nature and lack of an apparent cause. Guidelines for

▪ Table 12.9
Empirical treatments for oral lichen planus (Adapted from Scully et al 1998)

Immunomodulators	
Immunosuppressive agents	**Anti-fungals**
Corticosteroids	Azoles
Systemic:	Griseofulvin
Prednisone	Polyenes
Methylprednisolone	
Topical:	**Surgery**
Betamethasone	Conventional
Clobetasol	Cryosurgery
Fluocinolone acetonide	Laser surgery
Fluocinonide	Grafting
Fluticasone	**UV radiation**
Hydrocortisone	UV light
Triamcinolone	PUVA
Intralesional:	
Dexamethasone	**Others**
Hydrocortisone	Eiconol
Methyl prednisolone	Enoxaparin
Triamcinolone	Glycyrrhizin
Others immunosuppressive agents	Mesalazine, etc.
Cyclosporin	
Interferon alpha	**Retinoids**
Interferon beta	Acitretin
Pimecrolimus	Etretinate
Tacrolimus	Fenretinide
Thalidomide	Iso-tretinoin
Azathioprine	Tazarotene
	Temarotene
Immunostimulants	Tretinoin
Levamisole	

the management of OLP have been published by the British Association of Oral Medicine. Topical steroids have been found to be an effective treatment of symptomatic OLP in reducing pain and inflammation. They can be used as the first line drugs in the treatment of OLP and there have been no reported serious side-effects. Topical steroids such as triamcinolone acetonide 0.1 percent paste, betamethasone sodium phosphate 500 ug (0.5 mg dissolved in 10 ml of water rinsed for 3 minutes, 4 times daily), clobetasol propionate 0.05 percent ointment (2 ml four times daily), fluocinonide 0.05 percent, fluocinolone acetonide 0.1 percent or fluticasone spray (50 ug; 2 puffs 4 times daily) are recommended as a first line therapy of oral lichen planus. Systemic corticosteroids should be reserved for acute exacerbation, multiple or widespread lesions or those unresponsive to topical steroids. Cyclosporine (1.5% or 100 mg/ml or 16 mg in bio-adhesive gel three times daily) or other immunosuppressive drugs in the family of calcineurin inhibitors such as tacrolimus (0.03%) and pimecrolimus (1% cream) when used locally have also been reported for their effectiveness. Possible mechanisms of action of tacrolimus include the suppression of the activation and differentiation of T lymphocytes, via the inhibition of nuclear gene transcription of interleukin (IL)-2 and other several proinflammatory cytokines, such as IL-4 and IL-5. In some studies adverse effects (increased burning sensation) were noted. Previous studies have documented that the use of retinoids such as tretinoin and etretinate may improve the clinical and histological state of OLP lesions.

Although a systemic form of retinoid such as etretinate has provided effective treatment for severe OLP, signs of recurrence are commonly seen after discontinuation of therapy. Because of the possible side-effects of retinoids and the fact that complete remission is rarely seen, both systemic and topical retinoids should only be used as an adjuvant therapy.

Other treatments that have been tried include aloe vera in two clinical trials and curcumin as an adjunctive treatment to prednisone. Desquamative gingival lesions of OLP have also been treated with 20 mg doxycycline twice daily or 50 mg daily for 8 weeks until symptoms resolve. The utility of doxycycline in a nonbacterial disorder suggests a potent anti-inflammatory property of the drug.

Surgical excision is recommended for isolated plaques or nonhealing erosions because it provides excellent tissue specimens for histopathologic diagnosis and may cure localized disease. CO_2 laser has been used in the treatment of plaque-like of OLP. Free soft-tissue grafts have also been used for localized areas of erosive ulcerative OLP and the symptomatic OLP completely disappeared after the treatment with free gingival graft after follow-up.

The management of OLP is often frustrating both to the patient and the practitioner. Twenty-eight randomized controlled trials included for analysis in a Cochrane review in 2011 on "Interventions for Treating Oral Lichen Planus" found only weak evidence showing the superiority of the assessed interventions over placebo for palliation of symptomatic OLP. These evaluations were based on relief of pain and reducing areas of ulceration as measures of effective treatment. There is weak evidence to suggest that aloe vera may be effective in reducing pain and clinical signs of OLP. The treatment is only for reducing pain but no cure for OLP. Cyclosporin may reduce pain and clinical signs of OLP. Toxic side-effects were commonly seen in drugs taken internally (systemic) whereas minimal side-effects were found in those applied to the oral mucosa.

Biologics

As the outcome from present treatment options remain less than satisfactory novel biologic therapies that directly and or indirectly target T cells to treat OLP may be considered in the future. Biologics may be classified by their structure and function; Structurally they include receptor fusion proteins, monoclonal antibodies and recombinant cytokines. Functionally they could be divided into T-cell or cytokine modulators (or both). Examples of biologics that have been used in other inflammatory mucosal disorders include: Alefacept, Efalizumab, TNF-α inhibitors, Basiliximab, BCG-PSN, Rituximab. Appropriateness of these agents in terms of disease control, toxicity and safety and costs to health services need to be researched.

Malignant Transformation

The risk of malignancy in oral lichen planus is small. Follow up studies mostly conducted is USA and Europe estimated a range of MT rates close to 1 percent. In one study transformation rates were high for lichenoid lesions compared with OLP. In long standing atrophic or erosive and plaque like forms particularly affecting lateral margins of the tongue there might be a higher malignant potential. At present there is no clear evidence to suggest a particular type of OLP may carry a higher risk.

The appropriate follow-up period for the early detection of any malignancy changes would depend on availability of service provision in both primary and secondary care facilities. After the first visit, OLP patients should be reviewed at frequent intervals during active treatment to assess response to treatment and to ensure that the patients apply the topical corticosteroid appropriately. Active treatment should be continued until erythema, ulceration and symptoms can be controlled. Photographic records of both initial presentation and during periodic follow-up are recommended (**Figs 12.39A and B**).

Many patients with OLP remain asymptomatic and their disease may burn out after some duration. Management will vary from individual to individual. Long-term follow-up is required for patients whose disease is recalcitrant in nature and who do not respond to medications. Patients should be educated on regarding the potential side-effects of steroid use and should be monitored to detect any such effects. Moreover, patients should understand the potentially chronic and relapsing course of OLP, as well as the need for surveillance in view of potentially malignant nature of OLP. Systemic steroid should be reserved for the treatment of recurrences with acute symptoms. If the response is satisfactory after a short burst of therapy and slow taper the patients continue to use a topical steroid until achieving symptom control. It is recommended that the lesion should be evaluated once or twice a year by their dentists. Candidal superinfection on the surface lesions of OLP during steroid use, should be treated with antifungal drugs. Those with gingival involvement need professional prophylaxis to improve their poor oral hygiene. Surveillance for possible malignant transformation in OLP is recommended, though a small group who undergo rapid development of aggressive cancers may not benefit: clear guidelines on periodical follow-up do not exist. Re-biopsy is indicated only if the lesions appear atypical or are clinically suspected of malignant change.

ORAL SUBMUCOUS FIBROSIS

Oral submucous fibrosis (OSF) is a chronic, insidious disease that affects the submucosal tissues of the oral cavity with loss of fibroelasticity. The disease manifests with

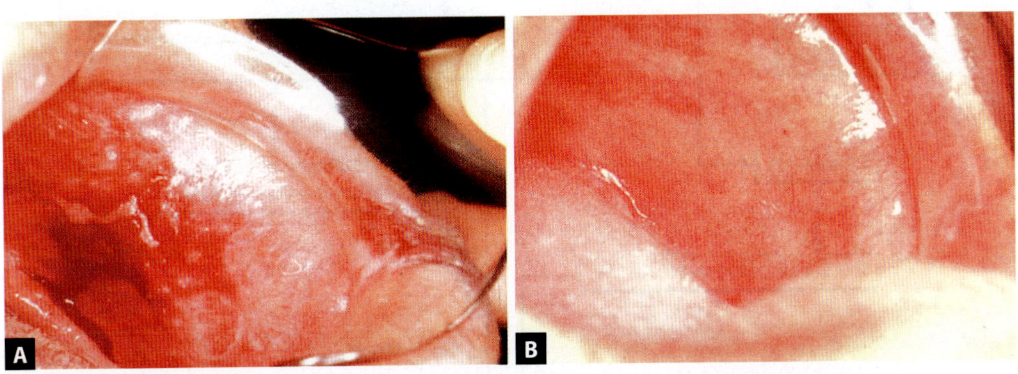

Figs 12.39A and B: An ulcerative oral lichen planus successfully treated with topical application of fluocinolone acetonide 0.1 percent in orabase

blanching and stiffening of the oral mucosa leading to limitation in opening of the mouth. The presence of fibrous bands in lips, cheeks and soft palate is a hallmark of the disease. OSF was first described by Schwartz in 1952 among five Indian females living in Kenya and he coined the term Atrophia idiopathica (trophica) mucosae oris. Several other descriptive terms have been attributed, submucosal fibrosis of palate and pillars, diffuse oral submucous fibrosis, idiopathic scleroderma of the mouth, idiopathic palatal fibrosis, and sclerosing stomatitis. The number of reported cases of OSF has rapidly risen in India from an estimated 250,000 in 1980 to 2 million cases in 1993.

Our current understanding of the pathology of OSF includes overlapping phases, an early inflammatory phase and the later fibrosis phase. In essence the disease could be described as a collagen metabolic disorder with changes observed in the extracellular matrix of the lamina propria and submucosa of the oral cavity due to both increased collagen synthesis and/or reduced collagen degradation.

Pathogenesis

There is now conclusive evidence that OSF is caused by areca nut, a masticatory substance used by Asians. Several mechanisms and biological pathways have been proposed for the pathogenesis of the disorder, a schematic diagram illustrates these factors in **Flow chart 12.1**, all based on the constituents of areca nut and genetic susceptibility to the disease. In essence the disease could be described as a collagen metabolic disorder with changes observed in the extracellular matrix of the lamina propria and submucosa of the oral cavity due to both increased collagen synthesis and/or reduced collagen degradation. Several chemicals in areca nut including arecoline, tannins and copper appear to upregulate the molecular process of deposition and/or

Flow chart 12.1: A schematic diagram to explain proposed pathogenic pathways in oral submucous fibrosis

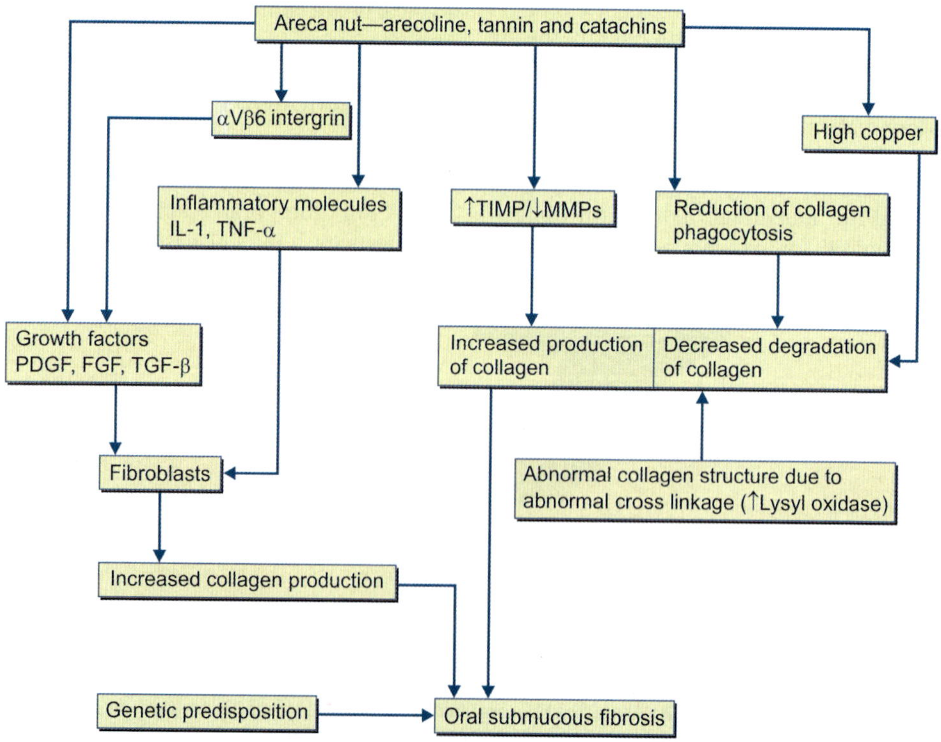

degradation and remodeling of extracellular matrix molecules contributing to collagen deposition underneath the oral epithelium. The process is influenced by increased secretion of inflammatory cytokines and growth factors. One of the key molecules found to be increased in OSF is TGF β. Extracellular matrix (ECM) remodeling phases are somewhat similar to phases of granulation tissue formation and the disease progression eventually leads to loss of ECM including elastin. Disequilibrium of ECM remodeling process is noted and has been examined in numerous studies. In areca nut chewers chronic inflammation is self-perpetuating and the process distorts the microenvironment as a result of aberrantly active transcription factors. Hypoxia has been reported to be associated with many disorders of fibrosis and Tilakaratne et al described hypoxia-inducible factor α (HIF-α) is upregulated both in protein and mRNA levels in OSF and contributes to progression of the disorder.

These authors further examined any genetic instability in OSF and described loss of heterozygocity in around 50 percent of OSF cases, predominantly in chromosome 13. These hot-spots of LOH losses harbored known onco-suppressor genes. Upregulation of αVβ6 integrin has also been described which may promote fibrosis and carcinomatous invasion.

Clinical Features

In general, chronic chewers with OSF seem to complain of three problems: inability to open their mouths a burning sensation and intolerance to spicy foods that are often the mainstay of their diet, leaving an individual handicapped both physically and psychologically.

A commonly encountered initial symptom is a burning sensation of the mouth, particularly when consuming spicy foods. Another frequently mentioned early symptom is the appearance of vesicles on the soft palate and anterior pillars of fauces though difficult to observe in clinical settings. There is gradual loss of papillae on the dorsal tongue surface. During the course of progression the labial and buccal mucosae show blanching and the mucosal texture feels tough and leathery (**Figs 12.40A and B**). Stomatitis and superficial ulceration may intervene. Gradually palpable fibrous bands appear on the lips, buccal mucosa (**Figs 12.41 to 12.43**) and soft palate (**Fig. 12.44**) contributing to a distorted, shortened or shrunken uvula (**Fig. 12.44**). The fibrosis is symmetrically bilateral but rarely unilateral in a quid chewer who prefers to carry the quid on a particular side of the oral cavity. Other OPMDs discussed earlier, namely oral leukoplakia or erythroplakia may be seen in association.

Grading of OSF

Based on the above clinical features the disease can be graded. In 1987, Warnakulasuriya introduced a grading system based on mouth opening and semiquantitative physical features. Many grading systems have subsequently evolved over the decades, some based on clinical features, others on histology and

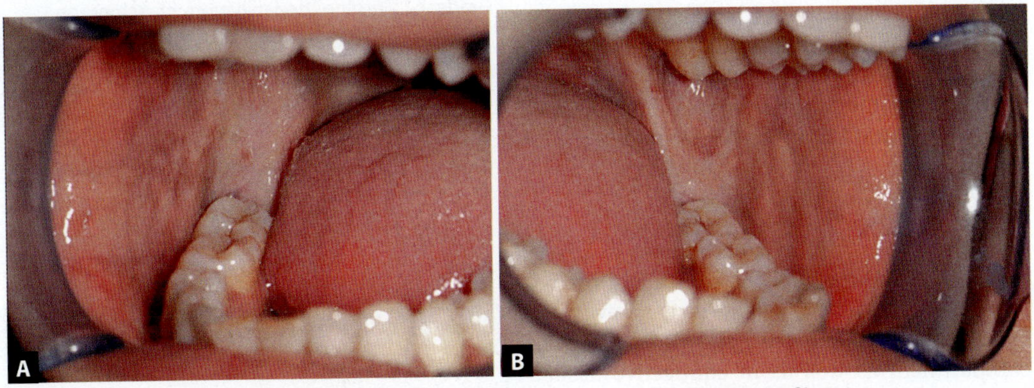

Figs 12.40A and B: Leathery appearance of oral submucous fibrosis

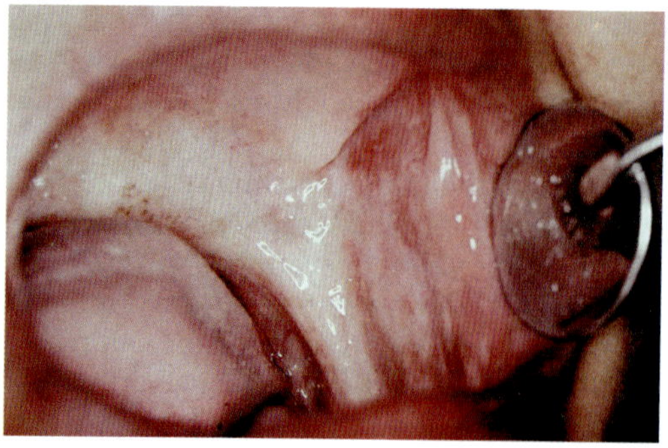

Fig. 12.41: Classical features with submucosal banding

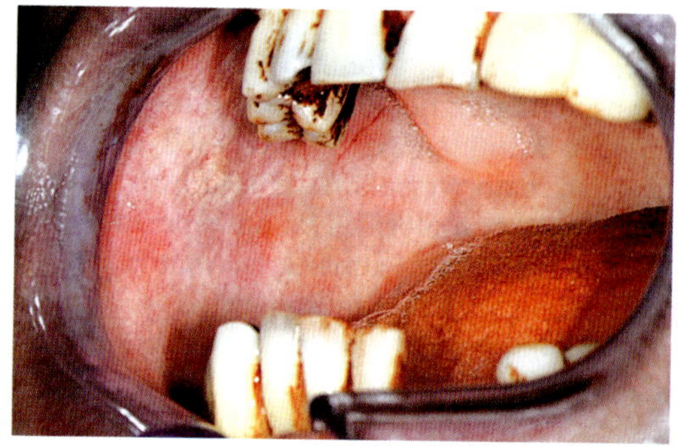

Fig. 12.43: Fibrosis of buccal mucosa and additionally oral leukoplakia (Grade 4A—see Table 12.10)

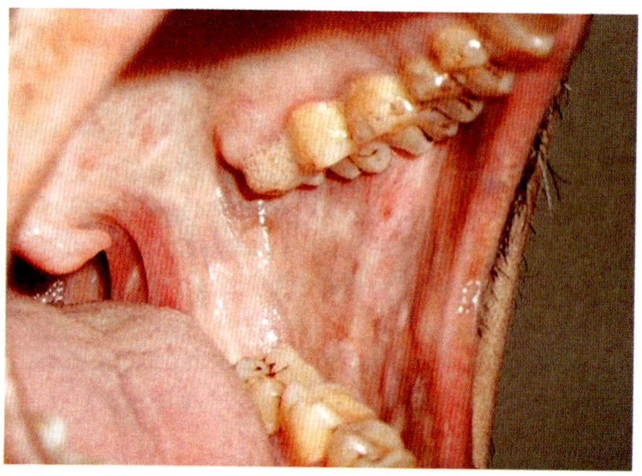

Fig. 12.42: Early oral submucous fibrosis. While mouth opening is maintained fibrous bands are just noticeable

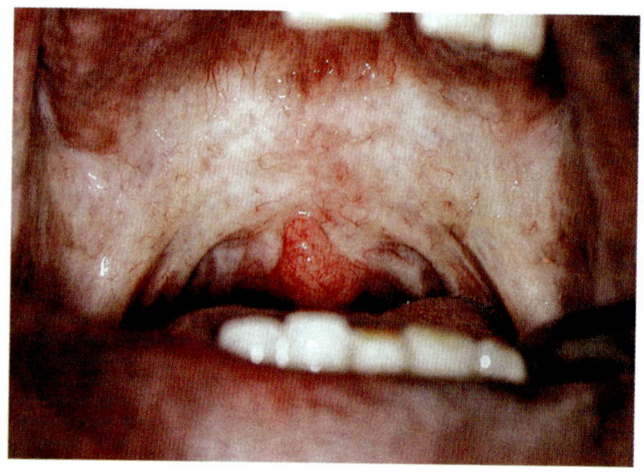

Fig. 12.44: Fibrosis affecting palatine arches and uvula

some by combination of both. Histological changes considered are based on hyalinization, thickened collagen bundles, reduced vascularity and fibrosis extending to muscle layers. Epithelial changes (dysplasia) are mostly ignored in these grading systems. The Grading System proposed by Warnakulasuriya and adopted at by the Vth World Workshop on Oral Medicine (**Table 12.10**) is a useful guide.

Table 12.10

Disease grading system for oral submucous fibrosis (OSF) (Warnakulasuriya, 2010)

Grade 1	Burning, depapillation, blanching or leathery mucosa (disease triad for OSF)–mouth opening - >35 mm
Grade 2	Moderate limitation of opening 20–35 mm
Grade 3	Severe OSF, limitation of opening < 20 mm
Grade 4A	OSF co-existing with other potentially malignant disorder, e.g. leukoplakia or erythroplakia
Grade 4B	OSF with oral epithelial dysplasia
Grade 5	OSF co-existing with squamous cell carcinoma

Histopathology

There is a spectrum of microscopic changes in the affected oral mucosa and many of the features are observed as the disease evolves. Changes are noted both in the epithelial compartment as well as in connective tissue, involving both lamina propria (**Fig. 12.45**)

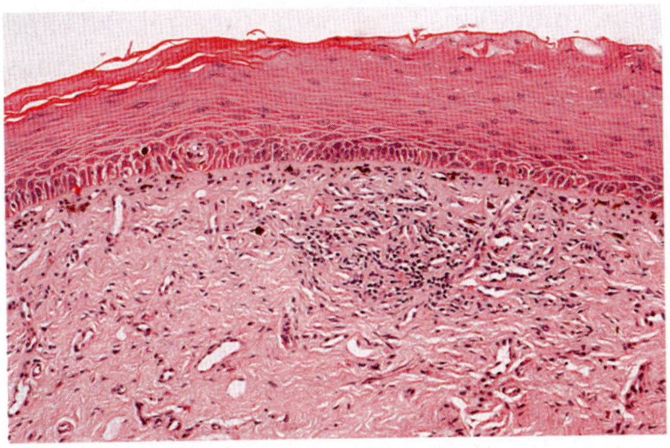

Fig. 12.45: Microscopic appearance of fibrosis affecting the lamina propria

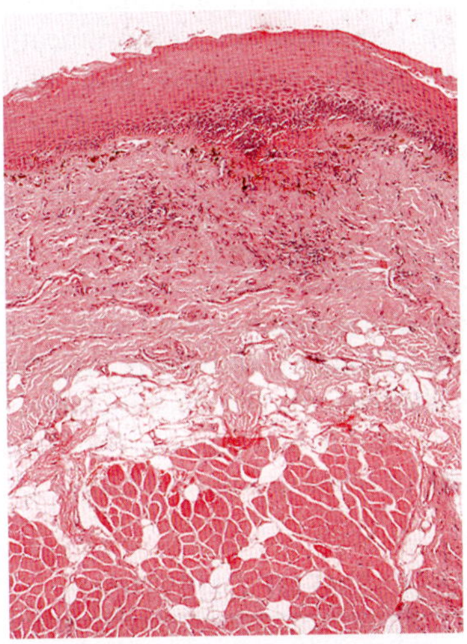

Fig. 12.46: Fibrosis extending deep to striated muscle

and submucosa. Marked atrophy of the epithelium is often noted and rete ridges may be completely lost resulting in an atrophic looking mucosa. Hyper ortho- or parakeratosis may be seen. In the early phases, the connective tissue is characterized by a finely fibrillar collagen, dispersed in edematous stroma with a strong fibroblastic response. The blood vessels could be dilated or congested. A spray of inflammatory cells mainly polymorphonuclear leukocytes are present immediately beneath the epithelium. As the disease progresses juxta-epithelial area shows early hyalinization, collagen deposition progresses and in late stages may be seen to occupy the full with of submucosa extending to muscle (**Fig. 12.46**), with obliteration of blood vessels. The inflammatory reaction is marked, occasionally eosinophils are predominant.

Malignant Transformation

Study of the natural history of OSF shows that it is an insidious disorder that progresses with time. OSF is now a well-recognized potentially malignant disorder of the oral cavity. In a long-term follow-up study in India the annual transformation rate was approximately 0.5 percent. There are no established markers to identify who may be predisposed to the disease, the presence of gene polymorphisms is the likely explanation. A possible role of *NQO1 C609T* gene polymorphism in OSF subjects and subsequent malignant transformation has been recently described. There are however, no established markers to identify the risk of malignancy in affected individuals.

Management

The treatment of patients with oral submucous fibrosis remains unsatisfactory. The primary objective is to obtain any improvement in mouth opening (interincisal distance) and tongue protrusion to enable resumption of normal eating, chewing and speech. There are other expected gains in reducing the severity of burning symptoms, reduction of discomfort or pain by repopulating the tongue papillae. One would expect to prevent cancer as a longer term objective for all patients under care.

A recent systemic review of published literature considered at the Vth World Workshop of Oral Medicine identified 4 RCTs (3 medical and one physical) conducted in India and Nepal. In clinical practice there are a number of treatments for OSF, ranging from medical interventions, surgical interventions, physical therapy, and of course habit control (i.e. cessation of areca nut use). Often a combination of strategies is used. There is a range of reported medical interventions including dietary supplementation (vitamins, antioxidants), anti-inflammatory agents (principally corticosteroids) and proteolytic agents (such as hyaluronidase and placental extracts). Based on the fact that occlusive blood vessels due to the deposition of collagen fibers could restrict nutrients and therapeutic substances from reaching the affected tissue, some groups have tried modulators that could improve vascularity. These include Pentoxifylline, Buflomedial Hydrochlorid and Nylidrin. To improve microcirculation tea pigments that are oxidized products of polyphenols derived from tea leaves have also been used in the management of OSF.

Interferon-Gamma an antifibrotic factor/cytokine was reported to be effective. This effect is attributed to the downregulation of fibroblast proliferation and a breakdown of collagen synthesis. Milk from cows immunized with human intestinal bacteria, which may suppress the inflammatory reaction and modulate the cytokine production was also reported in one study. Such agents may be administered orally, topically or via submucosal injection.

Surgical interventions are generally reserved for more severe cases of OSF. All surgical approaches begin with the surgical excision and ablation of fibrosed bands (scalpel excisions versus laser removal), and then generally followed by numerous reconstructive approaches ranging from pedicled flaps (derived from tongue flap, buccal pad, palatal island flap, nasolabial flap and temporal facia) and grafting procedures, to free flaps. Myotomy and coronoidectomy has also been attempted to release the tendons of temporalis muscle. Physical therapy may be used as a single modality intervention or combined with other interventions (principally surgical interventions).

CONCLUSION

Oral and pharyngeal mucosal lesions that have malignant potential have been well-documented. By far the most common are the leukoplakias. If these lesions can be effectively recognized, diagnosed and appropriately treated, a number of OPC could be prevented. These features are discussed and illustrated in this chapter. Control of OPMDs involves many factors. Genetic predisposition and mutations are basic to carcinogenesis. Much research is being directed at identifying and modifying implicated genes to limit/prevent these transformations. For the most part, gene mutations are both time-related and influenced by environmental influences. Thus aging is the most frequently associated factor in the development of cancer; therefore, aging itself becomes a significant risk. The paradox, of course, is that one of the goals of medicine is to lengthen life. There is solid evidence that abstaining from tobacco-use and limiting alcohol intake and abstaining from areca nut chewing will prevent many cancers from occurring in OPMDs. Screening for OPMDs and their effective management could lead to a reduction in the incidence of cancer in the screened population and thereby contribute to control of oral cancer. Community-orientated screening programs and communication also increase public awareness and knowledge of oral cancer and potentially malignant oral disorders.

ACKNOWLEDGMENTS

Professor Thongprasom would wish to acknowledge Chulalongkorn University Press for reuse of few illustrations she has included in the section on oral lichen planus. We thank Wiley Blackwell for reuse of Figures 12.4 to 12.6.

SELF-ASSESSMENT QUESTIONS

1. Compare and contrast various definitions used for oral leukoplakia and explain few difficulties if any for applying the current definition.
2. What is the natural history of oral leukoplakia and what further research may help to understand the gaps in our knowledge?
3. Explain the role of areca nut in the causation of OPMDs.
4. Compare and contrast methods of dysplasia grading. Outline additional sub features that may be applied to refine each microscopic feature used in current practice.
5. Discuss the sensitivity and specificity of adjunctive methods in the diagnosis of (1) OPMDs and (2) oral dysplasia.
6. Discuss the pathogenesis of oral lichen planus.
7. Why are current therapies failing in the management of ulcerative or symptomatic oral lichen planus?

8. "Current management of oral submucous fibrosis is unsatisfactory". Explain the reasons and what research may be needed in this area.
9. Discuss the prognostic factors for oral leukoplakia.
10. How would screening for OPMDs help in reducing the incidence and mortality from oral cancer?

SUGGESTED READING

1. Bhargava K, Smith LW, Mani NJ, Silverman S. A follow-up study of oral cancer and precancerous lesions in 57,518 workers in Gujarat, India. Indian J Cancer. 1975;12:126.
2. Epstein JB, Sciubba J, Silverman S. Utility of toluidine blue in oral premalignant lesions and squamous cell carcinoma: Continuing research and implications for clinical practice. Head Neck. 2007;29:948-58.
3. Gupta PC, Mehta FS, Daftary DK, et al. Incidence rates of oral cancer and natural history of oral precancerous lesions in a 10-year follow-up study of Indian Viallagers. Community Dent Oral Epidemiol. 1980;8:287-333.
4. Holmstrup P. Long-term treatment outcome of oral premalignant lesions. Oral Oncol. 2006;42:461.
5. Kaugars GE, Silverman S, Lovas JL, et al. A review of the use of antioxidant supplements in the treatment of human oral leukoplakia. Oral Surg Oral Med Oral Pathol. 1996;81:5-14.
6. Kerr AR, Warnakulasuriya S, Mighell AJ, et al. A systematic review of medical interventions for oral submucous fibrosis and future research opportunities. Oral Dis. 2011;17 (Sup 1):42-57.
7. Mehanna H, Ratty T, Smith J, McConkey CC. Treatment and follow-up of oral dysplasia - a systematic review and meta-analysis. Head and Neck; 2009. pp. 1600-9.
8. Napier SS, Speight PM. Natural history of potentially malignant lesions and conditions: an overview of the literature. J Oral Pathol. 2008;37:1-10.
9. Pitiyage G, Tilakararatne WM, Tavassoli M, Warnakulasuriya S. Molecular markers in oral epithelial dysplasia: a review. J Oral Pathol Med. 2009;38:737-52.
10. Ranganathan K, Mishra G. An overview of classification schemes for oral submucous fibrosis. J Oral Maxiollofac Pathol. 2006;10:55-8.
11. Silverman S, Gorsky M, Lozada F. Oral leukoplakia and malignant transformation. A follow-up study of 257 patients. Cancer. 1984;53:563.
12. Silverman S. Diagnosis and management of leukoplakia and premalignant lesions. Oral Maxillofacial Surg Clin N Amer. 1998;10: 13-23.
13. Speight PM. Update on oral epithelial dysplasia and progression to cancer. Head and Neck Pathol. 2007;1:61-6.
14. Thongprasom K, Carrozzo M, Furness S, Lodi G. Interventions for treating oral lichen planus. Cochrane Database System Rev. 2011; Issue 7. CD001168.
15. Tilakaratne WM, Iqbal Z, Teh MT, Ariyawardana A, et al. Upregulation of HIF-1 alpha in malignant transformation of oral submucous fibrosis. J Oral Pathol Med. 2008; 37:372-7.
16. Tilakaratne WM, Klinikowsky MF, Saku T, Peters TJ, Warnakulasuriya S. Oral submucous fibrosis: Review of aetiology and pathogenesis. Oral Oncology. 2006;42:561-8.
17. Warnakulasuriya S, Johnson NW, van der Waal I. Nomenclature and classification of potentially malignant disorders of the oral mucosa. J Oral Pathol Med. 2007;36:575-80.
18. Warnakulasuriya S, Kovacevic T, Madden P, Coupland VH, Sperandio M, Odell EW, Moller H. Factors predicting malignant transformation in oral potentially malignant disorders among patients accrued over a ten-year period in South East England. J Oral Pathol Med. 2011;40:677-83.
19. Warnakulasuriya S, Reibel J, Bouguot J, Dabelsteen E. Oral epithelial dysplasia classification systems: predictive value, utility, weaknesses and scope for improvement. J Oral Pathol Med. 2008;37:127-33.

Chapter 13

Oral Cancer

Saman Warnakulasuriya

Chapter Outline

INTRODUCTION

The majority of oral and oropharyngeal cancers considered in this chapter comprise a very heterogeneous group of neoplasms commonly referred to as "oral cancer". These consist of cancers arising from the lining mucosa from various anatomical sites mainly of the lip, tongue and mouth (oral cavity) [ICD-10 C00, C02-06] and that of oropharynx consisting of base of tongue (posterior third), soft palate and uvula, tonsils, tonsillar fossa and pillars and posterior walls of the pharynx that can be seen through the oral cavity [ICD-10: C01, C09-C10]. Cancers of the salivary glands [C07-08], pyriform sinus [C12] and other pharyngeal sites (naso- and hypopharynx) [C11 and 13] are excluded from this title and would not be discussed here. More than 90 percent of oral malignancies are squamous cell carcinomas. Oral cancer is a serious and growing problem in many parts of the globe. In the past few decades, there has been a significant age shift and a disproportionate number of young people are presenting with oral cancer. The large majority of oral cancers have similar risk factors, and the disease is preventable.

GLOBAL EPIDEMIOLOGY

Incidence

Oral and pharyngeal cancer, grouped together is the sixth most common cancer in the world. The annual estimated incidence is around 275,000 for oral and 130,300 for oropharyngeal cancers; two-thirds of these cases occurring in developing countries. There is a wide geographical variation (approximately 20 fold) in the incidence of this cancer.

Highest incidence rates for cancers of the lip are reported in white populations in Canada, Australia and Southern Europe (e.g. Spain). For example, more than 50 percent of oral cancers in Australians are located on the lip. Lip cancer is rare in nonwhite populations.

For intraoral cancers (excluding lip) the areas characterized by high incidence rates are found in the South and South-East Asia (e.g. Pakistan, India, Sri Lanka, Taiwan), in the Pacific regions (e.g. Papua New Guinea, Melanesia), some parts of Western (e.g. France) and Eastern Europe (e.g. Hungary, Slovakia and Slovenia) and parts of Latin America (e.g. Brazil, Puerto Alegre) (**Fig. 13.1**). Data illustrated in **Figures 13.2A to C** is based on Cancer Incidence in Five Continents (ninth volume) which has become the recognized reference source on the incidence of cancer in populations around the world and refers to latest data covering the period 1998-2002.

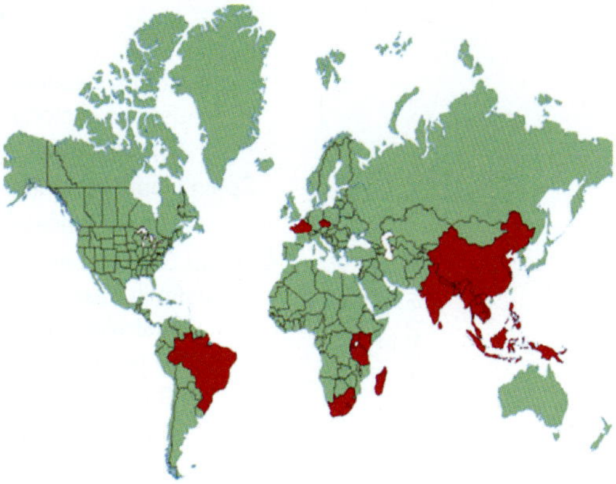

Fig. 13.1: High incidence regions for oral cancer

The relative frequency of a cancer is given as a percent of all cancers. In countries such as Sri Lanka, India and Pakistan where oral cancer is the most common cancer in men, it may contribute up to 25 percent of all new cases of cancer in a country. Where the disease is uncommon such as in the United Kingdom, USA or in Japan, oral cancer accounts for ~3 percent of all cancers.

In epidemiological terms the incidence rates (the number of new cases per 100,000 people in a given year) is a more accurate way of recording the frequency. The age-standardized incidence rates are high in several of the high incidence countries (e.g. India, Hungary, Brazil, Taiwan and PNG). The latest reported for India (2006-2008) is around 19 per 100,000 of the population.

Males have a higher incidence, and male to female ratio is currently about 2:1. The reported sex differences are attributable to heavier indulgence in risk habits (tobacco and alcohol) by men. As for other cancers of the head and neck, the age-specific incidence rates increase with

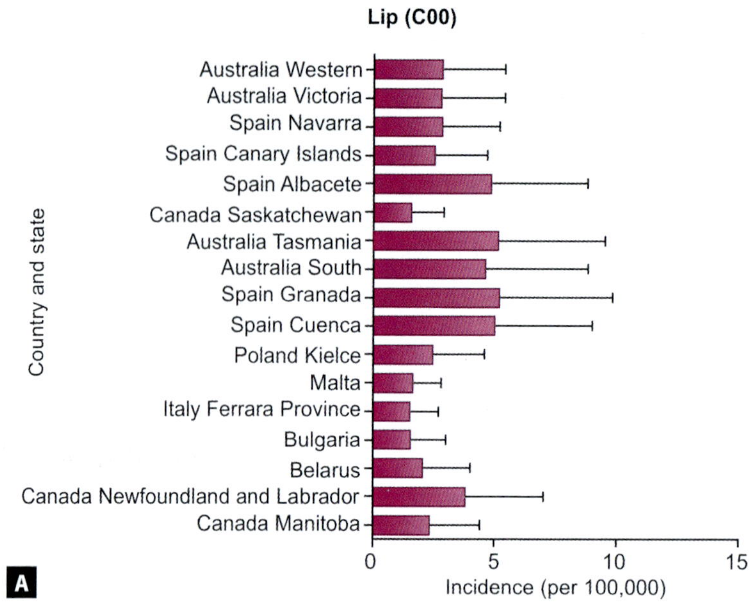

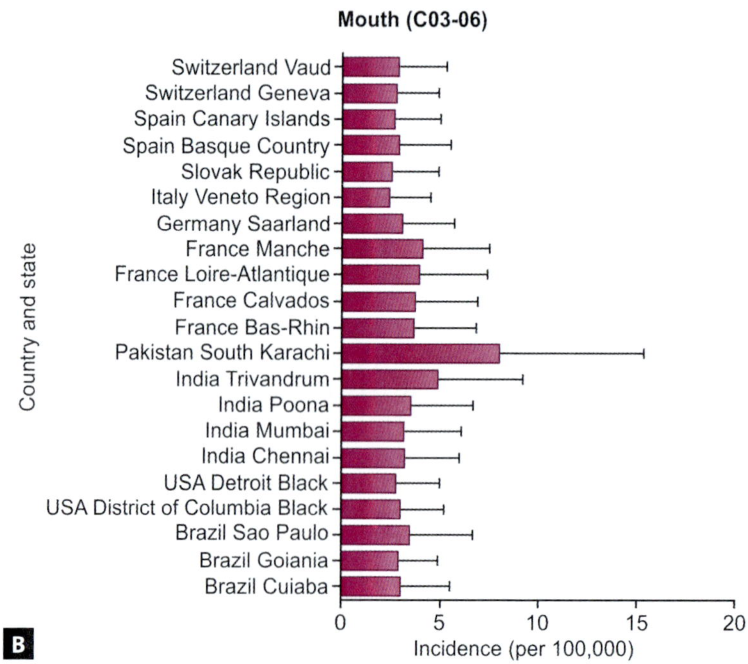

Figs 13.2A and B: Age-standardized (world) incidence (per 100,000) and standard errors for (A) Lip; (B) Mouth

age, being highest for older groups, the majority of cases occur in people aged 50 and over. The mean age range reported in many countries is around 56 to 62 years of age. **Figures 13.3A and B** illustrates age and gender profile from two countries one with a high and the other with a low incidence. Oral cancer in young people has received considerable attention in the past two decades as the incidences of the disease have increased by many folds in younger age

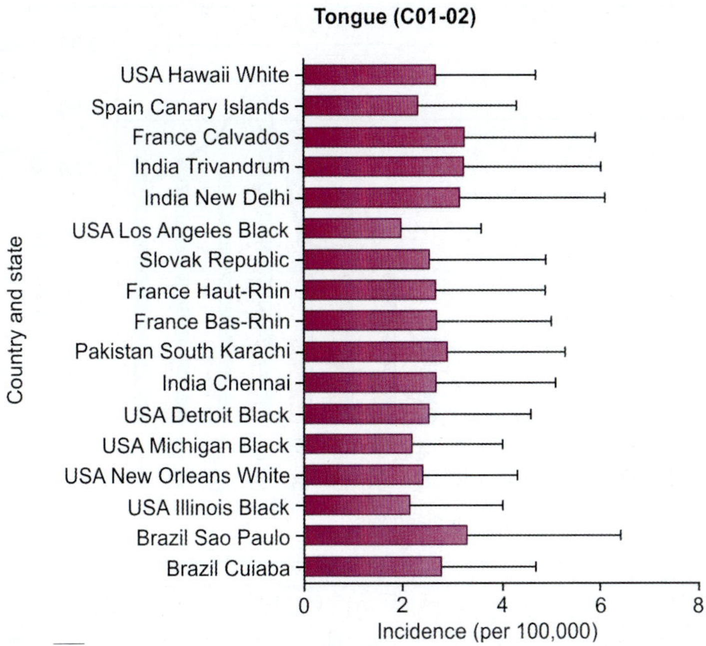

Fig. 13.2C: Tongue cancer in high incidence countries and regions (Incidence data collected by cancer registries worldwide and published in CI5 (Cancer Incidence in Five Continents) Volume IX. IARC 2007)

groups. In many cancer registry data sources about 6 percent of oral cancers occur in younger people under the age of 40 years.

Prevalence

The prevalence of a particular cancer can be defined as the number of persons in a defined population who have been diagnosed with that type of cancer, and who are still alive at a given point of time. This aspect of epidemiology is of particular relevance when discussing people living with cancer. In the world, there is close to a three quarter of a million people who previously had oral cancer and are alive 5 years after diagnosis. The proportion alive at 5 years is lower in middle and low income countries.

When discussing the epidemiology of oral cancer it is important to focus on the incidence of disease and to standardize the data to the World Population.

Mortality

For most countries age adjusted death rates from oral cancer have been estimated at 3.0-4.0 per 100,000 men and 1.5-2.0 per 100,000 for women. SEER data for USA reports mortality rates of 3.8 per 100,000 men and 1.4 per 100,000 in women based on patients who died in 2005-2009. Mortality rates for black men (5.7) are higher than for other races (white or Hispanic). Oral cancer mortality among French women has risen in the past 20 years. In 2000, rates stood at 4.7 per 100,000 an annual percentage change of +1.73 percent noted between 1980 and 2000. India ranks fourth for mortality in the world and approximately has highest rates in S. Asia.

Among young people there has been a small but steady increase in mortality rates in most Western countries. This is particularly noted for the oropharynx in the US populations. Among Scottish males deaths from oropharyngeal cancer has shown the highest increase in the recent years compared to all other cancers.

Survival

Survival following any treatment is the primary concern for cancer patients. If a person survives five years following treatment it is considered

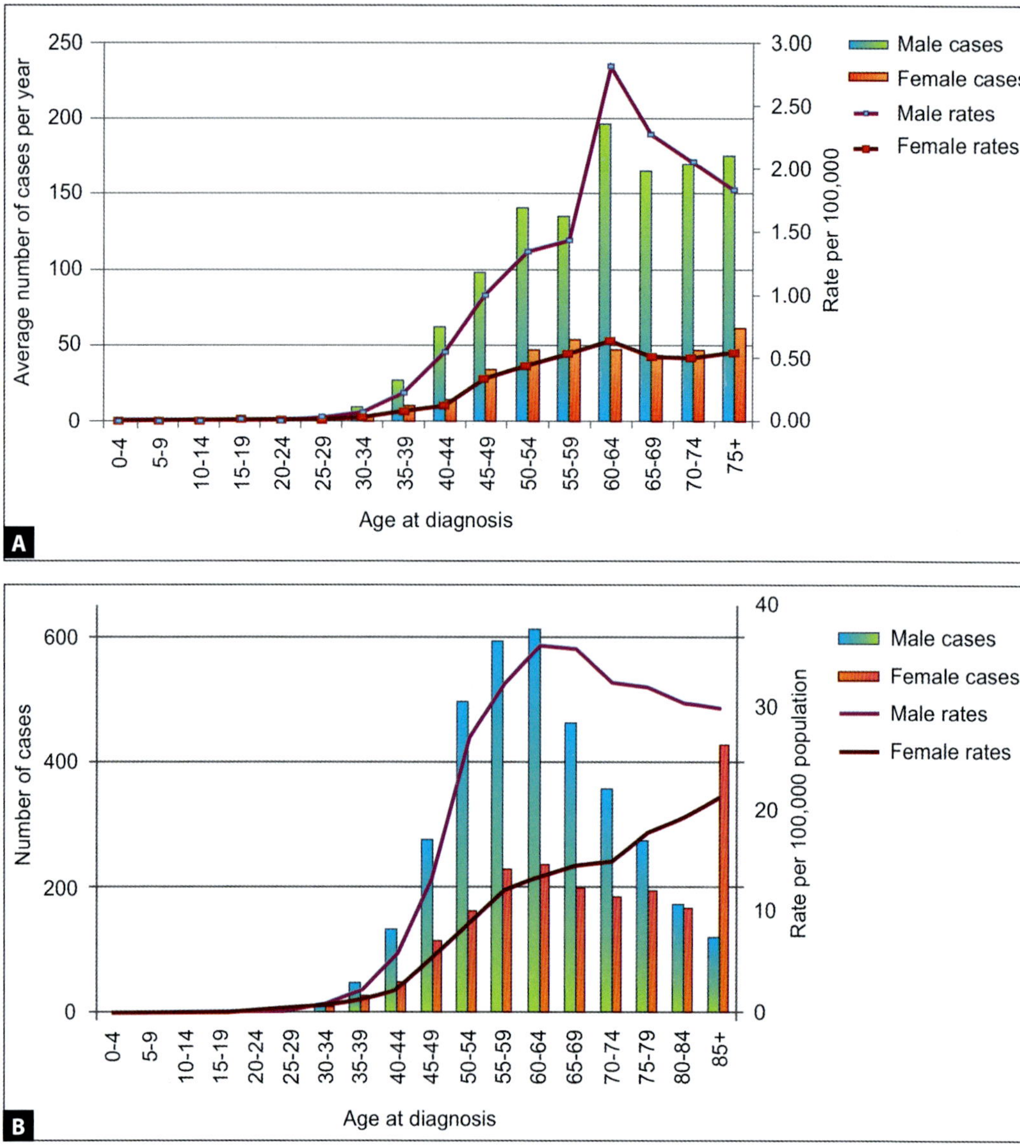

Figs 13.3A and B: Age and gender profile for oral cancer from two countries, (A) Sri Lanka; (B) UK

that the disease has been cured and therefore five years survival is a valid statistic. This is measured in two ways, as either overall survival (OS) or disease-specific survival (DSS). Most oral cancer patients are elderly and they can die of other causes and may have a life expectancy less than 5 years. For this reason OS is lower than DFS. Overall survival is relatively easy to measure where national statistics are available. The estimation of disease-free survival (DFS) requires accurate follow up data. Survival should be stratified by site and the best outcome is for cancers of the lip with over 90 percent of patients surviving five years and the worst is for pharynx. For most countries, overall 5-year survival rates for cancers of the tongue and oral cavity range from 45 percent to 72 percent, the mean is around 50 percent. In the USA overall 5-year survival has in recent years improved to 61.5 percent and within Europe varies from

Table 13.1
Survival following primary Surgery for oral cancer

Author	*Year*	*Center/Country*	*No patients*	*% DFS (5 years)*	*% OS (5 years)*
Loree	1990	US#	398	—	57
Shingaki	1995	Nigata, Japan	61*	87	80
Chen	1999	Taiwan	183	—	36
Pathak	2005	Mumbai, India**	511	57	—
Aksu	2006	Istanbul, Turkey	61	49	46
Koo	2006	Seoul, S. Korea	127	76	71
Kessler	2008	Germany	128	83	69
Rogers	2008	UK	489	74	56
Walvekar	2009	Mumbai, India**	642	53	—

DFS – Disease-free survival; OS – Overall survival
* Stages 1 & 2 only **Advanced OSCC also treated with adjunct radiotherapy when indicated
# Memorial Sloan Kettering, USA

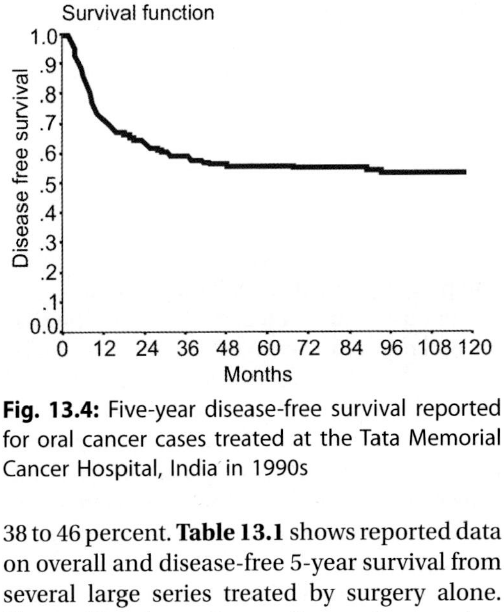

Fig. 13.4: Five-year disease-free survival reported for oral cancer cases treated at the Tata Memorial Cancer Hospital, India in 1990s

38 to 46 percent. **Table 13.1** shows reported data on overall and disease-free 5-year survival from several large series treated by surgery alone. **Figure 13.4** shows 5-year disease-free survival reported from a major cancer center in India for their cases treated in 1990s.

In general, prognosis decreases with advanced disease and increasing inaccessibility of the tumor. For both cancer of the tongue and oral cavity, women have higher survival rates than men. TNM (Tumor, Node, Metastasis) stage at presentation significantly affects 5-year survival, the presence of cervical metastasis reduces survival up to 50 percent. For mobile tongue 5-year survival for stage 1 disease is 80 percent while for stage 1V survival drops to 15 percent. As for most cancers, survival is better for affluent groups and younger compared to older patients.

Despite important advances in the approaches to treat oral cancer the survival rates for oral cancer in many countries have not shown any improvement over the past 5 decades. Poor survival is at least in part due to failure to detect small lesions and potentially malignant lesions early (Chapter 12). High throughput centers such as the Regional Maxillofacial Unit in Liverpool, UK and the Slone Memorial Hospital in US have reported improvement in survival over time in their follow-up cohorts. For surviving patients improvements in techniques of reconstruction also have helped in rehabilitation and improved quality of life.

Many patients who are successfully treated for oral cancer have to cope with the devastating consequences of their treatment. These may affect the patient's appearance and function, e.g. eating, drinking, swallowing and speaking. These residual defects may lead to other problems such as depression and nutritional deficiency. Quality of life issues are therefore especially important for this group of patients.

RISK FACTORS

Oral cancer to a large extent is a self-induced disease. In order to plan preventive measures **it is important to understand** the risk factors **associated with the disease.** The major risk **factors are well known and are** briefly described **below, there are** excellent reviews on this **subject. There are some emerging** risk factors for **oral cancer that the dentists should** be aware of, **and some controversies related** to the etiology **of this disease that needs** clarification.

Major Risk Factors – Tobacco, Alcohol and Betel (Areca Nut) Quid

Major risk factors for oral cancer are cigarette **smoking, alcohol** misuse and betel-quid **chewing. There are several key** epidemiological **studies from many countries** that confirm the **associated risk with these** three life-styles.

Tobacco use is reported as a major risk **factor both for the oral cavity** and oropharynx. **Numerous independent investigations** in the **past several decades have** confirmed a strong **association between oral** SCC and tobacco **smoking. These data come** from numerous **case-control and cohort** studies. In countries **in which epidemiological** studies have been **conducted, it is clear** that oral cancer risk **is higher among smokers.** A meta-analysis **reported 12 studies that estimated** oral cancer **risk in the USA, Uruguay, Italy, Sweden, India, China, Taiwan and Korea.** The reported pooled **cancer risk estimate was** 3.43 times higher in **smokers compared with** non-smokers (95% CI: **2.37, 4.94). The attributable** risk is close to 70 **percent in men and approximately** 25 percent **for both sexes combined.** It is evident that oral **cancer risk is related** to both intensity and **duration of tobacco smoking.** Thus, the risk of **oral cavity cancer increases** with the average **daily consumption,** duration of consumption **and lifetime cumulative** consumption of **tobacco smoked. The differential** risk between **non-smokers and heavy** smokers, and the **steady progression** of risk with increasing **amount smoked both** provide sufficient **evidence for tobacco** as a major risk factor for **oral cancer. The proportion** of smokers (~85%) **among patients with oral** SCC is nearly 3 to 4 times greater than the general population. Furthermore most studies show an inverse relation with age when starting to smoke. These risks are also increased synergistically with alcohol consumption. However, among non-drinkers, cigarette smoking was associated with an increased risk of 2.13 (95% CI: 1.52, 2.98) confirming an independent association with tobacco use.

Smokeless tobacco (ST) use and its association with oral SCC has been the subject of several studies. Most tobacco products consumed in Asia and Africa are unregulated and are often of the smokeless variety. Products such as *gutka* (tobacco, areca nut), *mishri* (powdered tobacco, i.e. rubbed on the gums), *Gudakhu* (tobacco and molasses), *Khaini* (tobacco and lime), *Naswar* (tobacco, ash and lime), *Zarda* (boiled and dried tobacco colored with dyes), *Shammah* (tobacco, ash and lime), *Chimo* (tobacco and sodium bicarbonate and ashes from *Mamon* tree-used in Venezuela), *Maras* (sun-dried powdered tobacco mixed with ash of wood) and *Toombak* (tobacco and sodium bicarbonate used in the Sudan) are strong risk factors for oral SCC. Cancers associated with these products tend to occur more often in the vestibular, gingival and buccal mucosae, as a result of placement of non-combustible carcinogenic substances in direct and prolonged contact with these areas.

In many European and US studies the risks for oral and oropharyngeal cancers are similar for cigarette and cigar smokers. Smoking *bidi* (hand-rolled and consisting of flaked tobacco rolled in temburni leaf) is a common practice in India and Sri Lanka. A meta-analysis has shown that the risk of cancer associated with *bidi* smoking is about 3 times higher compared with cigarettes.

Tobacco smoke contains between 2000 and 4000 substances, around 60 of which are identified carcinogens. Among these there are 11 human carcinogens. Some substances generated by tobacco smoke that are recognized carcinogens include polyaromatic hydrocarbons (e.g. Benzo(a)pyrene), heterocyclic hydrocarbons, tobacco-specific nitrosamines (TSNAs), aromatic amines, aldehydes, phenolic compounds, metals and metal compounds.

Tobacco smoke also contains tumor promoters (phenolics), cocarcinogens and free radicals. Most of the compounds are thought to exert their carcinogenic effects through classical genotoxic mechanisms e.g. by the formation and persistence of DNA adducts with consequent mutations. Carcinogens from smoking that are released into the saliva tend to pool in the lower anatomic areas of the mouth and could account for the frequent occurrence of oral SCC along the lateral-ventral tongue and floor of the mouth. The striking variations in oral SCC sites and incidence seen among different regional, cultural and demographic groups are largely attributable to differences in the use and mode of delivery of tobacco.

Alcohol use is the second independent major risk factor for the development of oral cancer and ethanol is classified by the International Agency for Research on Cancer as a human carcinogen. A large number of cohort and case control studies provide strong evidence that the consumption of alcohol is an independent risk factor for oral and pharyngeal cancers. The population-attributable risk of oral cavity cancer for alcohol consumption alone does not exceed 20 percent, and is lower compared to smoking. Doubling the consumption of alcohol above recommended levels increases the risk for oral and oropharyngeal cancers two to three times, compared with the risk of non-drinkers. The risk of oral cancer increases with the number of alcoholic drinks consumed per day in a dose dependent fashion. The risk is multiplicative with the combined use of alcohol and tobacco. Some population groups with inherited defects in metabolism of alcohol may have the inability to breakdown acetaldehyde (the carcinogenic metabolite of alcohol) and may be at increased risk. Oral biofilms (bacteria) assist in metabolism of alcohol to acetaldehyde and poor oral hygiene in alcoholics may potentially increase the risk of oral cancer.

There is a controversy as to what type of alcoholic drink mostly causes mouth cancer. It is not clear whether the alcohol concentration in beverages or the quantity drunk contributes to estimates of risk. There is no clear evidence that specific alcoholic drinks, i.e. spirit, wine or beer, have different effects on oral cancer. Substitution of the type of drink is not therefore advisable. The most frequently consumed alcoholic beverage in a population is likely to be associated with highest risk for that given population.

Ethanol is metabolized to acetaldehyde by alcohol dehydrogenase, releasing multiple free radicals. Although investigations that attempt to implicate alcohol alone as the main causative agent of oral SCC have yielded largely conflicting results, the correlation of alcohol with increased risk for oral SCC is indisputable. The major clinical significance of alcohol consumption seems to be its ability to potentiate the carcinogenic effect of tobacco. The effect is at least addictive and may be multiplicative in individuals with heavy alcohol consumption or at sites with the highest levels of alcohol exposure. Although the underlying mechanisms for this association are poorly understood, some proposed mechanisms include:

- Dehydration effects of alcohol render the mucosa more susceptible to the carcinogens in tobacco.
- Alcohol activates carcinogens present in tobacco by a cytochrome p450-2E1-dependent mechanism.
- Release of acetaldehyde and free radicals within the oral mucosa from local as well as hepatic metabolism of ethanol. Deposition of acetaldehyde protein adducts has recently been demonstrated in human SCC tissues among heavy alcohol users.

Joint effect of tobacco and alcohol consumption: Epidemiological studies that have examined the combined role of alcohol and tobacco specifically for oral cavity cancers indicate that the joint effect of alcohol and tobacco is multiplicative or greater than multiplicative in most studies. The population-attributable risk of oral cavity cancer related to the combined consumption of the two carcinogens is around 75 percent and those who smoke and drink could have their risk multiplied by 4.78 compared to non-users.

Betel quid is carcinogenic to humans. In parts of South and South East Asia and in Melanesia oral cancer is of high incidence and in these populations betel quid use is recognized as a risk factor for this high incidence of oral cancer. A recent evaluation by the International Agency for Research on Cancer (IARC) in 2004 concluded that areca nut, the main ingredient used in betel quid or commercially packaged as pan masala, are carcinogenic to humans. Moreover, chewing betel quid without tobacco has recently been shown to elevate the risks of various oral precancerous lesions and conditions. Cancers of the oral cavity arise in locations (mostly buccal and mandibular groves) where betel quid and areca nut are kept for long periods.

Mechanisms of action and chemicals in areca nut responsible for carcinogenicity have been ascertained in recent studies. Endogenous nitrosation has been observed in the saliva of betel quid chewers with consequent production of carcinogenic nitrosamines. Reactive oxygen species generation in buccal cells due to auto-oxidation of polyphenols in areca nut enhanced by slaked lime an ingredient in BQ has been reported. However, areca nut remains the carcinogenic agent in betel quid and pan masala products.

The estimated elevated risks from these different agents and exposures (among smokers, regular users of alcohol and betel quid; adjusted for each other) compared to non-users are reported consistently from many populations. The elevated risks are confirmed by several meta-analysis or systematic reviews providing proof of significant risks of these life-styles for oral cavity cancers. In the United Kingdom there is evidence that the rising incidence of oral cancer noted in the past two decades, especially affecting younger people, is associated with increased intake of alcohol rather than tobacco use. The synergistic effects on the carcinogenic potency of tobacco in oral cancer by alcohol consumption and/or betel quid are well documented (**Fig. 13.5**).

Emerging Risk Factors

Human papillomavirus infection

There is sufficient evidence based on recent studies (mostly conducted in US) that infection with human papillomavirus (HPA) (subtypes 16 and 18) is a risk factor particularly for the oropharynx (posterior tongue, tonsil and the (visible) part of pharynx in continuity with the oral cavity). A meta-analysis of published studies on the prevalence of HPV in SCC in Head and Neck Cancers was found to be around 25 percent; the prevalence of HPV in oropharyngeal carcinomas (35.6%) was higher than in oral cancers (23.5%). The etiological role of HPV in cervical cancer has been well established and new data confirm that a proportion of oral and particularly oropharyngeal cancers can be attributed to HPV infection and seropositive status (particularly among young subjects with no tobacco or alcohol history). Patients with HPV infected tumors tend to be younger and have an overall better survival.

Immunosuppression

Lip cancer is reported to be increased following kidney transplantation and may be associated with the use of immunosuppressive agents (azathioprine and cyclosporine). Extended use

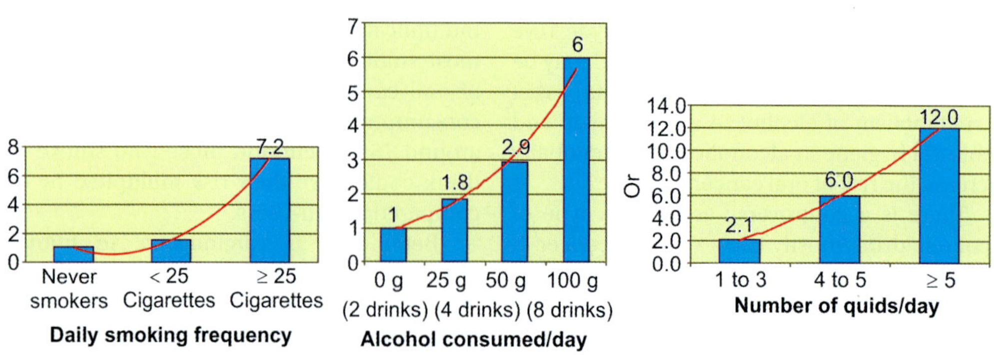

Fig. 13.5: Graphs showing the dose dependant nature of tobacco, alcohol and betel quid observed in many studies

of immunosuppressive agents (azathioprine) during the management of inflammatory bowel disorders (Crohn's disease) may also increase the risk of tongue cancer. There is no strong evidence to support that immunosuppression in HIV seropositive individuals increases the risk for oral cancer (see below).

Diet and Nutrition

There is accumulating evidence that indicates a positive correlation between low intake of fresh vegetables and fruits and an increased risk of oral cancer. An estimated 50 percent reduction in risk for oral cancer is noted among people who consume an adequate daily amount of fresh fruits and vegetables. Excess weight contributes to the increased incidence of many cancers, and may adversely affect quality of life for cancer survivors, which may worsen prognosis for several cancers. However, no data exist for oral cancer.

Mate Drinking

Mate is an infusion of the herb *Ilex paraguariensis,* cultivated throughout South America. In Argentina, Uruguay, Paraguay and southern Brazil, it is normally drunk very hot through a metal straw. The role of mate drinking in increasing the risk of cancer of the oral cavity is supported by several epidemiological studies conducted in South America that adjusted for other risks. A recent meta-analysis estimated an increased risk (OR of 2.11, 95% CI:1.39, 3.19) confirming this association. The role of mate when drunk very hot is not proven but the high temperature of this beverage could act as a cofactor by causing chronic irritation to the exposed oral mucosa.

Socioeconomic Status

Oral cancer is seen more often in people from lower socioeconomic groups and living in deprived areas. A higher prevalence of smoking, alcohol use and poor diet in these groups was thought to account for this unequal distribution. However, new research suggests that lower socioeconomic status (measured by various ways: occupation, income or education) is a significant risk factor for oral cancer independent of life style behavior.

Controversial Factors with Limited or no Evidence

Ethnicity and race

It has been speculated that susceptibility to oral cancer from tobacco and alcohol use may differ by race and ethnicity. Oral cancer incidence rates vary considerably across racial/ethnic groups in the globe. South Asians have higher rates of oral cancer than people from most other countries and black men (in US) have higher rates than whites for oropharyngeal cancer. The Mexican-American population (Hispanics) also has higher rates of oral cancer than US whites. Nutritional differences, smoking patterns (*bidi* smoking in Asians), difference in amounts smoked or alcohol drunk and the 2 way and 3 way interaction of betel quid chewing with smoking and alcohol rather than genetic factors may play a role in these observed variations in populations and high incidence in some ethnic and racial groups.

Oral Hygiene and Dentition

Although poor oral hygiene and poor dentition (faulty restorations, sharp teeth and ill-fitting dentures) have been implicated in a few epidemiological studies. It is not clear whether confounding by tobacco and alcohol have been addressed in these studies. It is likely that chronic irritation from dental factors may facilitate mucosal entry of carcinogens, so this may act as a cofactor in high-risk individuals only. Oral microbes (together with biofilms) may also be a factor in chronic alcohol users as the same microbes facilitate the metabolism of ethanol to acetaldehyde (a potent carcinogen) in the oral cavity.

Indoor Air Pollution

Studies from Germany and Brazil have reported increased risks for head and neck and upper-digestive tract cancers (including oral) from indoor air pollution due to daily exposure to fossil fuels from stove heating (with oil, coal, or wood) and from use of a wood stoves for cooking. Volatile carcinogenic compounds formed during the cooking processes have been attributed to excess mortality from oral cancer among regular cooks.

Heredity and Familial Risk

There is no evidence to suggest that oral cancer is more common among families that have an increased risk for other cancers. Oral cancers have not been reported in hereditary cancer syndromes such as Li-Fraumeni syndrome (breast cancer), Familial adenomatous polyposis (colon cancer), Familial retinoblastoma (retinoblastoma and sarcomas), Peutz-Jeghers syndrome (colorectal, breast and ovarian cancers), Gorlin syndrome (basal cell skin cancer), Multiple endocrine neoplasia (MEN2) (medullary thyroid cancer), Ataxia telangectasia (AT) (lymphoma), Bloom syndrome (solid tumors) or xeroderma pigmentosum (XP) (skin cancer) or in Fanconi anemia (acute myeloid leukemia). The only exceptions are Cowden syndrome (with few reported cases of head and neck cancer) and dyskeratosis congenita, a rare genetic disorder that may present with oral white lesions in young people that have a risk of transformation to cancer. Though oral cancer is rare in people with these disorders, if they have been diagnosed with oral keratosis they fall into a high risk group and should be under the care of a specialist for surveillance.

So far, inherited polymorphisms that may contribute to genetic predilection specifically to oral cancer have not been demonstrated. ADH polymorphism and aldehyde dehydrogenase genotypes may influence cancer susceptibility as acetaldehyde–the first metabolite of alcohol (the putant carcinogen in alcohol) may accumulate in tissues.

Despite lack of a clear hereditary trait for oral cancer, cancer cells (from oral cavity cancers) contain genetic damage due environmental exposure to carcinogens and for this reason oral cancer should be considered a genetic disease.

Marijuana (Cannabis) Smoking

Marijuana is the most commonly abused illicit drug in most countries, usually smoked as a joint or in a pipe. It is also smoked in blunts, which are *cigars* that have been (partially) emptied of tobacco and refilled with marijuana and possibly combined with tobacco ingredients. An increased risk for head and neck cancer was reported in the US but there is no consistent evidence to implicate cannabis as causing oral cancer. Any causal inference shown could be due to interaction with heavy tobacco use.

Khat (Qat) Chewing

Khat (Catha edulis Forsk) is a plant cultivated in territories of Somalia, Ethiopia, Djibouti, South and North Yemen, Madagascar, Tanzania and down to south eastern Africa. Khat leaves are extensively consumed by these populations. So far, no epidemiological studies on oral cancer and khat use have been reported and there is no evidence to link khat chewing with oral cancer. Evidence from experimental studies are also limited and there are no *in vivo* data to show any carcinogenicity of khat in animal models.

Nicotine Replacement Therapy

There is some confusion in the minds of professionals and patients whether any prolonged and chronic use of nicotine replacement therapy (NRT) could have the potential to cause cancer as these agents contain pure nicotine. There is no clear evidence that medicinal nicotine causes cancer. A recent study based on surveillance data among patients with chronic obstructive pulmonary disease in the US found no independent increased risk for any cancer among NRT users. The authors, however, noted that the surveillance time in this study was short (5 years).

HIV Infection

Though it was conceived prior to the era of highly potent antiretroviral therapy, that moderate immunosuppression in HIV disease could increase the risk for oral cancer, there is no strong epidemiological evidence based on cohort studies to confirm an association of infection of HIV or of AIDS with oral squamous cell carcinoma. Oropharyngeal cancers with a known infective cause (HPV) may be moderately

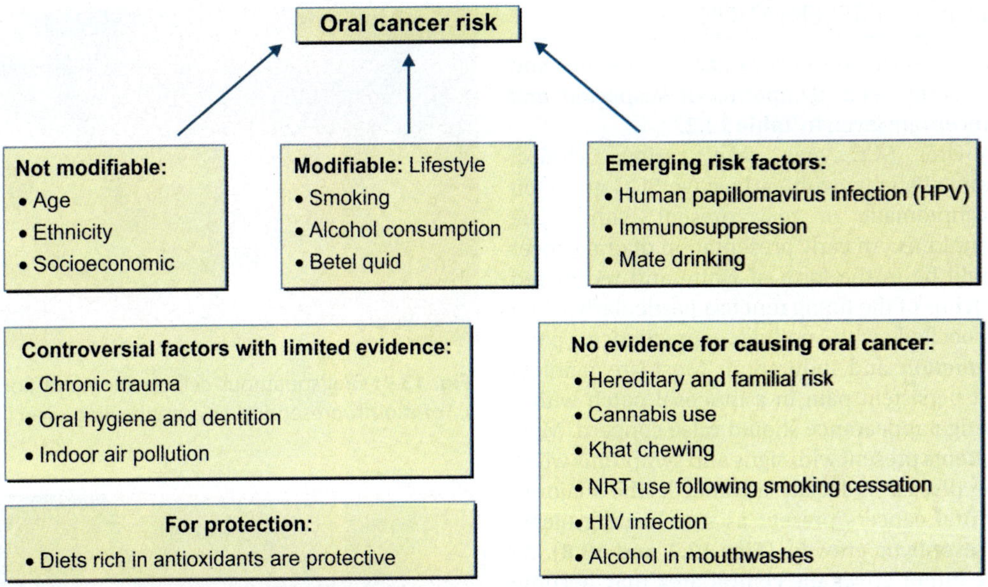

Fig. 13.6: Summary of risk factors for oral cancer

increased in people with HIV disease but the excess risk could also be attributable to tobacco use. However, it is important to note that two different neoplasms are associated with HIV disease, i.e. Kaposi's sarcoma and lymphomas, but these are normally not listed under the term oral cancer.

Alcohol in Mouthwashes

There has been some controversy about the risks of alcohol containing mouthwashes (MW) for the causation of oral cancer. While an earlier study from US distinguished non-alcohol MW from alcohol containing MWs in their study and reported an increased risk for subjects in the latter group, other studies have not considered this distinction in MW use. So far, nine epidemiological studies are available to examine any associated risks: two studies showed significant increases, two studies show nonsignificant elevated risks and four studies indicated non-significant, lower or similar oral cancer risks among mouthwash users (compared to non users). Based on these reported studies a recent meta-analysis confirmed that there is no excess risk for oral cancer from mouthwash use (with or without ethanol) (OR 1.13; 95% CI 0.89, 1.44).

It is likely that mouthwash use in people who developed oral cancer was a measure to mask their tobacco smell or was initiated after the development of symptoms in an attempt to control the disease. Two independent expert groups (FDA and IPRI) have concluded that there is no evidence for linking alcohol containing mouthwashes to oral cancer.

Figure 13.6 shows a summary of risk factors that are modifiable to reduce any risk and those with limited or no evidence which should be ignored in terms of disease causation. However, as not all persons who practice these high-risk habits will develop oral SCC, and as oral SCC in rare instances is idiopathic, there must be person-specific genetic characteristics and environmental factors which may either afford protection against the development of oral SCC, or may predispose to or even promote the development of oral SCC.

CLINICAL PRESENTATION

Most oral cancers occur in accessible sites and are easily seen. Symptoms of suspected oral cancers are given in **Table 13.2**.

Oral SCC may take various clinical forms. Patients with early stage SCC are often asymptomatic or may present with vague symptoms. An early presentation of oral cancer could be in the form of white and red or red patches of the lining mucosa particularly when associated with nodular appearance, pain, ulceration and induration. Most are painless but persistent pain in a mucosal patch with a benign appearance should raise concern. Most patients present with signs and symptoms when the disease is locally advanced. The majority of oral cancers present as non-healing ulcers or exophytic growths (**Figs 13.7 and 13.8**). As the tumor grows the central area may become necrotic largely due to poor blood supply and therefore these two features may often be seen in combination (**Fig. 13.8**). Malignant ulcers have rolled margins especially prominent in tongue and other mobile mucosa (**Figs 13.9A and B**). On palpation the base and margins of the ulcer would elicit induration and spongy areas may bleed to touch. When examined carefully there is often a leukoplakic or erythroplakic component at the margins of the tumor (**Fig. 13.10**).

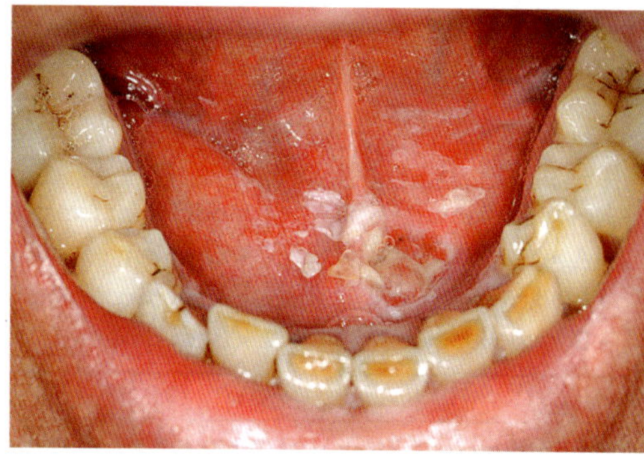

Fig. 13.7: Oral squamous cell carcinoma of floor of mouth presenting as a nonhealing ulcer

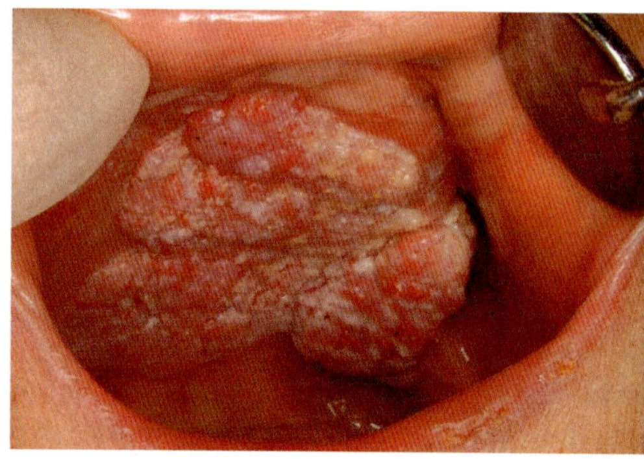

Fig. 13.8: An exophytic growth on palate, an example of a T4 tumor

▪ Table 13.2

Symptoms indicative of oral cancer (NICE Guidelines-UK)

- A non-healing ulcer
- Persistent discomfort or pain
- A persistent white and red or red patch
- A lump or thickening
- Difficulty chewing or swallowing
- Unusual bleeding or numbness in the mouth
- Loose teeth for no apparent reason
- Difficulty moving the jaw
- Speech problems
- A lump in the neck
- Sore throat and earache on same side

As a cancer spreads the mucosa may be fixed to underlying tissues, with loss of tissue mobility. The tongue may loose its mobility and cancers involving the retromolar region may lead to limitation of mouth opening and present with trismus. Tumor infiltration of the inferior alveolar nerve is associated with pain and paraesthesia found in advanced stages (**Fig. 13.11**).

Oral carcinomas appear to favor certain intraoral locations more than others. In most Western countries, the oral tongue is the most commonly reported site for oral cancer (about a third of all oral SCC), followed closely by the floor of the mouth (about a quarter). The lateral tongue and the floor of the mouth comprise more than 60~ percent of the so-called cancer-prone locations in the oral cavity. Other common

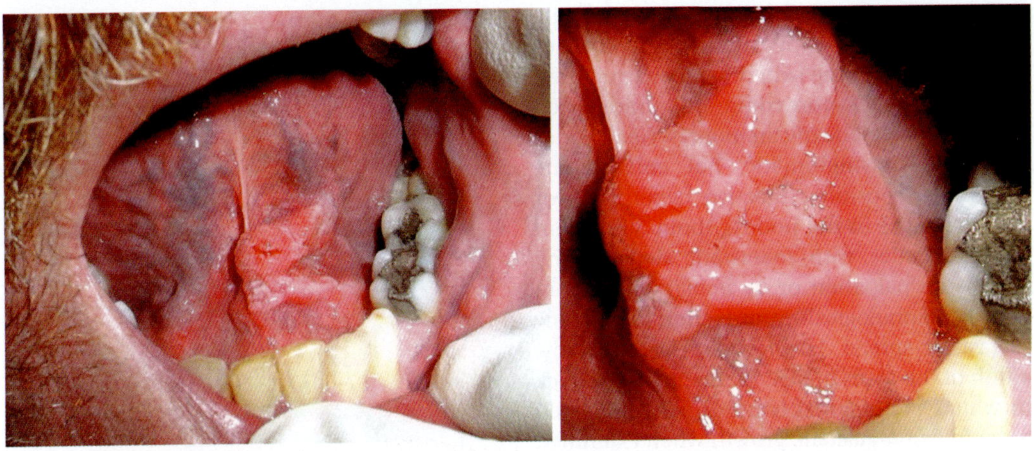

Figs 13.9A and B: A new growth on floor of mouth extending to the ventral tongue showing central necrosis and rolled margins of the ulcer

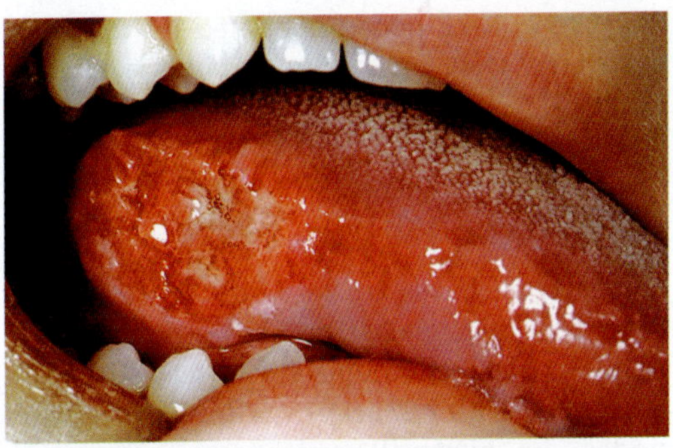

Fig. 13.10: Coexisting leukoplakia at the margin of a tongue carcinoma

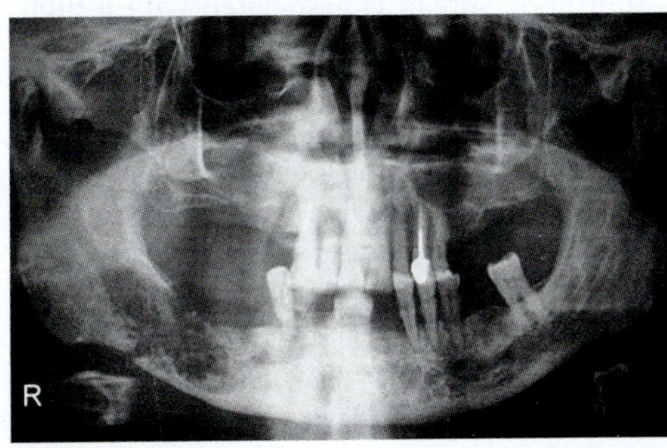

Fig. 13.11: Carcinoma of the alveolar mucosa invading adjacent mandibular bone leading to a pathological fracture

locations include the tonsillar pillars and retromolar pad areas (20%), followed by the soft palate. Gingival carcinomas are less common. In striking contrast, the buccal mucosa is the most common location for oral SCC in some other parts of the world (Central and Southeast Asia). The differences in site-specific incidence are likely attributable to cultural differences in the way tobacco and related products are used relative to their mode of delivery (smoking vs chewing). Among alcohol misusers the floor of the mouth appears to be the most affected site for oral SCC.

Oropharyngeal cancers may present with difficulty in swallowing (dysphagia), rarely with difficulty with speech, sore throat and earache.

Other clinical presentations of oral cancer include unexpected tooth mobility not associated with periodontal disease or failure of a tooth socket to heal.

METASTASIS

Spread of the tumor could occur to regional lymph nodes, underlying or adjacent bone or to distant sites.

Regional Spread

About two-thirds of oral SCC particularly those of substantial size, will have clinically detectable metastases to cervical lymph nodes at the time of diagnosis. Enlargement of one or more neck nodes with a primary in the mouth may indicate regional metastasis, especially if they feel firm or hard and fixed to the skin or deeper structures. Neck metastasis is more common with advanced stages or high grade of carcinomas. Neck nodes are mostly asymptomatic, but enlarge due to tumor deposition, reactive hyperplasia or cystic changes in the nodes. About 30 percent of neck nodes with metastatic deposits are missed on palpation or by imaging alone but on histopathological examination will show metastatic spread. Furthermore in one study, a fifth of the cases of SCC of the head and neck in which the regional lymph nodes appeared to be free of metastatic growth when examined microscopically, had on molecular analysis evidence to harbor mutations concordant to the primary site. The presence of extracapsular lymph node spread is associated with a high-rate of local and regional recurrence, distant metastasis and mortality.

The precise group of nodes likely to be affected depends on the location of the primary tumor, but submandibular, then jugulo-digastric or jugulo-omohyoid deep cervical nodes may be involved in an orderly fashion often referred to as levels 1 to 3. Neck metastases are rarely detected at levels 4 to 5, involving the posterior triangle of the neck (**Fig. 13.12**). Metastatic spread may skip one or more levels of the neck. Extensive cystic changes may be present in a neck node often leading to a misdiagnosis of a branchial cyst.

Tonsillar carcinomas may present in the neck as a metastasis without the primary being noticable. When nodal involvement of the neck is suspected the clinician should initiate investigations for an occult primary in clinically inaccessible sites of the mouth and pharynx.

Bone Invasion

It is likely that any invasion to the underlying jaws is more common with tumors centered close to the bone surface. Lesions occurring in sites of gingiva, hard palate, buccal mucosa extending to sulci, or tongue extending to floor of mouth may involve bone of the maxilla and/or the mandible (**Fig. 13.11**).

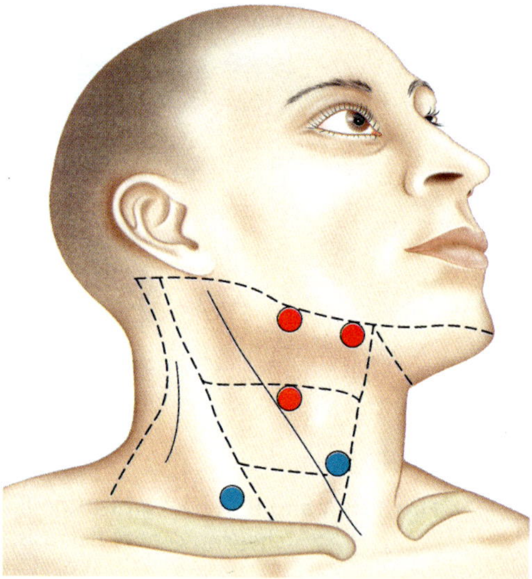

Fig. 13.12: Neck nodes associated with regional metastasis. Most oral cancers metastasize to levels 1 and 2

Distant Metastasis

Distant metastases are very rare: some authors have reported metastases in 2 to 9 percent of their patients. Metastatic disease is often associated with extracapsular spread in lymph nodes, or bilateral neck nodes. The most common distant metastases are to the lung, bones or liver.

STAGING

Oral and oropharyngeal cancers are classified according to the TNM system (**Table 13.3**). The clinical staging defines the extent of the disease in terms of anatomic spread and is vital to the development of a treatment plan. It also provides the framework that permits comparison of treatment strategies, outcomes and survival rates. The universally accepted TNM (Tumor, Node, Metastasis) staging system is used worldwide in staging malignant processes. Staging is site-specific to various anatomic organs and for oral cavity ranges from stage I (local disease) to stage IV (disseminated disease).

▪ Table 13.3
Staging of lip and oral cavity (ICD-O C00, C02-C06) cancers (TNM, 7th Edition)

	T–Primary tumor
TX	Primary tumor cannot be assessed
TO	No evidence of primary tumor
Tis	Carcinoma *in situ*
T1	Tumor 2 cm or less in greatest dimension
T2	Tumor more than 2 cm but not more than 4 cm in greatest dimension
T3	Tumor more than 4 cm in greatest dimension
T4a	(Lip) Tumor invades through cortical bone, inferior alveolar nerve, floor of mouth, or skin (chin or nose)
T4a	(Oral cavity) - Tumor invades through cortical bone, into deep/extrinsic muscle of tongue (genioglossus, hyoglossus, palatoglossus, and styloglossus), maxillary sinus, or skin of face
T4b	(Lip and oral cavity) - Tumor invades masticator space, pterygoid plates, or skull base, or encases internal carotid artery

Note: Superficial erosion alone of bone/tooth socket by gingival primary is not sufficient to classify a tumor as T4

	N-Regional lymph nodes	
NX	Regional lymph nodes cannot be assessed	
N0	No regional lymph node metastasis	
N1	Metastasis in a single ipsilateral lymph node, 3 cm or less in greatest dimension	
N2	Metastasis as described below:	
	N2a	Metastasis in a single ipsilateral lymph node, more than 3 cm but not more than 6 cm in greatest dimension
	N2b	Metastasis in multiple ipsilateral lymph nodes, none more than 6 cm in greatest dimension
	N2c	Metastasis in bilateral or contralateral lymph nodes, none more than 6 cm in greatest dimension
N3	Metastasis in a lymph node more than 6 cm in greatest dimension	

Note: Midline nodes are considered ipsilateral nodes

M-Distant metastasis	
M0	No distant metastasis
M1	Distant metastasis

Stage grouping based on TNM

Stages 1-4C

	T1	T2	T3	T4a	T4b
N0	1	2	3	4a	4b
N1	3	3	3	4a	4b
N2	4a	4a	4a	4a	4b
N3	4b	4b	4b	4b	4b

If distant metastasis is known (M1) any T any N is staged as Gp 4c

The most recent (Seventh) edition of the UICC TNM classification is identical to that published by the AJCC. Tumors are stratified into at least 32 (4 x 4 x 2) possible combinations of local tumor spread (T: 1-4b), regional lymph node involvement (N: 0-3) and presence of distant metastases (M: 0-1). For purposes of simplification the 32 possible T, N and M combinations can be reduced to clustered stages: I, II, III and IVa, b, c which are meant to reflect homogeneous survival and interstage discrimination.

The cTNM is based on clinical examination as well as ancillary techniques such as imaging. The pathological stage (pTNM), derived from the histopathological examination of the tumor specimen is generally used for decision making on adjuvant treatment and more accurate estimation of prognosis.

The present TNM system of classification lacks biological and molecular basis and overall general health and patient-based prognostic factors, such as co-morbidity. The TNM system however, is simple and therefore easy to use and adhere to and more importantly, it is universally accepted.

INVESTIGATIONS THAT AID DIAGNOSIS

Physical examination (including endoscopy particularly for tobacco users) is the primary method for diagnosis of oral and oropharyngeal cancers. A diagnostic biopsy is indicated for any mucosal lesion suspected of cancer, particularly for any ulcer or growth that persists for more than 3 weeks following the elimination of local factors. Early tissue diagnosis is the most important. Proper and timely biopsy is critical. An inadequately performed biopsy may complicate patient care and result in delay in the care pathway. Several biopsy techniques are available; the choice of biopsy is based on the size and location of the mass and the experience of the surgeon. Incisional biopsy is preferred and excisional biopsy is indicated only for small, superficial masses (<1 cm in greatest dimension), in which the probability of malignancy is low. Effective re-excision is more difficult for smaller malignant lesions that initially are unintentionally treated as benign or excised with inadequate margins when performing an incisional biopsy. During biopsy a generous wedge of tissue is removed, with minimal manipulation of tissue. Several important technical factors must be considered while performing an incisional biopsy. The incision should be oriented along the long axis, avoiding necrotic or grossly ulcerated areas and should include deeper tissue preferably including muscle. It is important that an incisional biopsy is of sufficient size and depth to include part of the advancing front of the tumor. Ideally, the deep front should be included, but if not, as in large tumors, the peripheral (lateral) front is often sufficiently representative to allow provisional assessment.

Any biopsy site should be oriented in clinic notes so that they can be resected during definitive surgery for the tumor. A biopsy enables histologic grading–an important prognostic factor in SCC and assessing infiltrative margins.

Several optical diagnostics have evolved in the past decade that include the use of chemiluminescence, spectroscopy, auto-fluorescence and optical coherence tomography. These methods of detection are discussed in more detail in Chapter 12 with reference to potentially malignant disorders.

Imaging is useful to determine the extent and depth of invasion of a primary tumor and its relation to the surrounding structures. Imaging with plain radiographs may help in identifying involvement of the underlying bone. Preoperative ultrasonography may provide a guide to the tumor thickness. This is performed with a 10 to 12 MHz intracavitary probe placed directly over the tumor and the tumor thickness measured in a vertical plane from the surface to the point of maximal depth. In cases where this measure is equal to or greater than 5 mm elective neck dissection may be considered. Imaging techniques such as computed tomography (CT) and magnetic resonance imaging (MRI) may improve staging performed by visual inspection. While CT scanning is useful in evaluating involvement of cortical bone, MRI is more informative when evaluating the extent of soft tissue and spread via neurovascular bundles. Positron emission tomography (PET) imaging with F-18-fluorodeoxyglucose (18 FDG) is a functional modality that provides additional data. Other imaging includes a chest radiograph (CXR), i.e. needed to exclude lung metastasis and followed by bronchoscopy, if the chest radiograph reveals any shadows. Liver ultrasound also may be indicated in advanced cases to exclude metastasis to the liver.

Detection of lymph node metastasis can be undertaken by CT, MRI and for clinically negative neck by ultrasound guided fine needle aspiration cytology (USgFNAC).

Sentinel node (SN) biopsy facilitates the detection of lymph nodes potentially containing malignancy. The first lymph node in a regional draining area that receives lymphatic flow from the tumor is designated the sentinel node. During the procedure the SN is identified using radioactive colloid and a blue dye. This node is excised and examined by microscopy using serial sections. Tumor negative SN precludes the presence of metastasis in regional nodes.

In preparation for surgery and anesthesia routine blood tests including FBC, urea and electrolytes, liver function and blood glucose, electrocardiography (ECG) and a cardiac echo are essential in treatment planning and identifying co-morbidities.

The pathology and imaging data are reviewed at the multidisciplinary meetings (MDM) by a panel consisting of surgeons, oncologists, pathologists, radiologists, speech therapists (SaLT), dieticians, physiotherapists and specialist nurses to draw up a treatment plan.

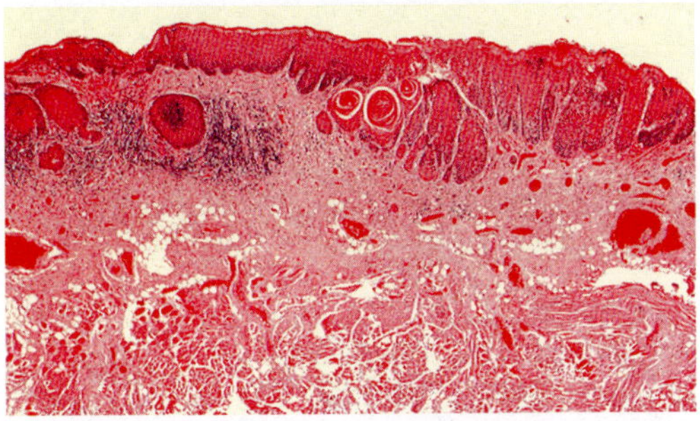

Fig. 13.13: Focal superficial invasion in a severe dysplasia

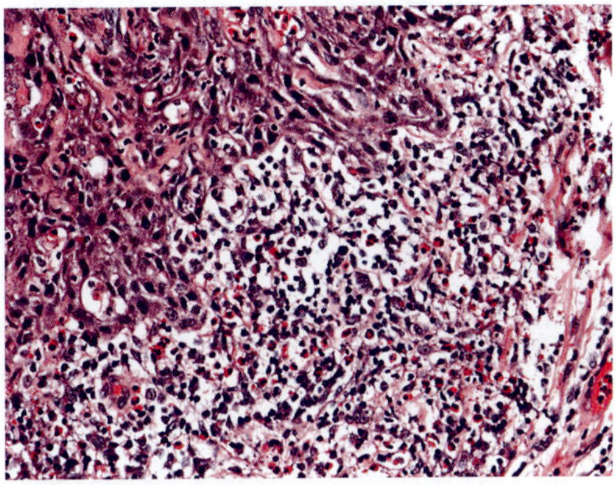

Fig. 13.14: Carcinoma that has elicited a dense host response including eosinophils and there is some killing of some carcinoma cells

PATHOLOGY

Histopathological Features of OSCC

The key histological feature that enables confirmation of a squamous cell carcinoma is invasion of deeper tissues. SCC could be superficially invasive (**Fig. 13.13**) when it involves lamina propria only and frankly invasive when invading deep submucosal tissue, muscle and fat. Tumor invasion may extend to different depths and anatomic levels. There is marked heterogeneity in the microscopic appearance of these tumors and invariably there is a host response of lymphocytes and plasma cells in the stroma, which sometimes could be dense (**Fig. 13.14**).

Pathological Grading

The histopathological grading of conventional OSCC falls into 3 categories: well (pG1), moderately (pG2) or poorly differentiated (pG3). This system is routinely used because it is simple. When the number of carcinoma islands invading are too small it is sometimes difficult to accurately grade the cancer (**Fig. 13.15**). The degree of 'differentiation' (resemblance to normal oral/oro-pharyngeal surface epithelium) is subjectively assessed in terms of keratinization, nuclear and cellular pleomorphism, mitotic activity and nuclear aberrations (**Figs 13.16 to 13.19**). In poorly differentiated tumors kerati-

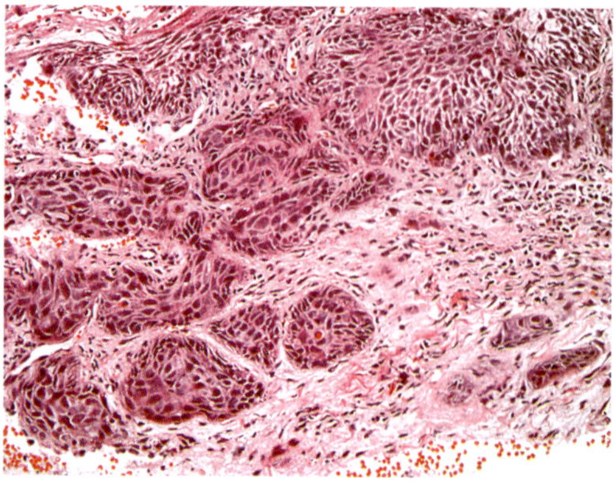

Fig. 13.15: Invasive SCC arising in oral epithelial dysplasia. Superficial carcinomas are too small for accurate grading

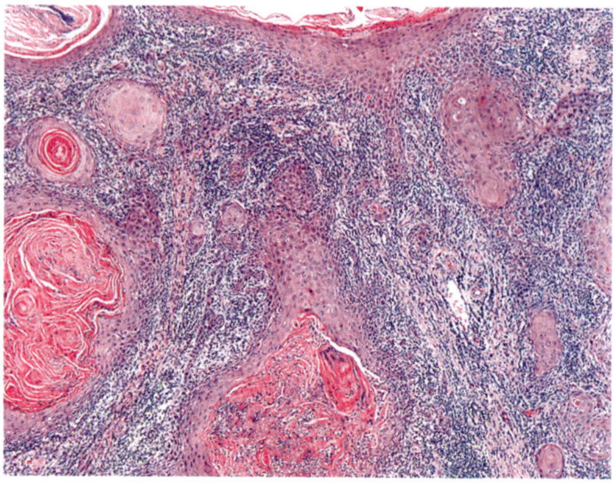

Fig. 13.16: Well differentiated carcinoma with keratinizing islands. There is a dense inflammatory infiltrate

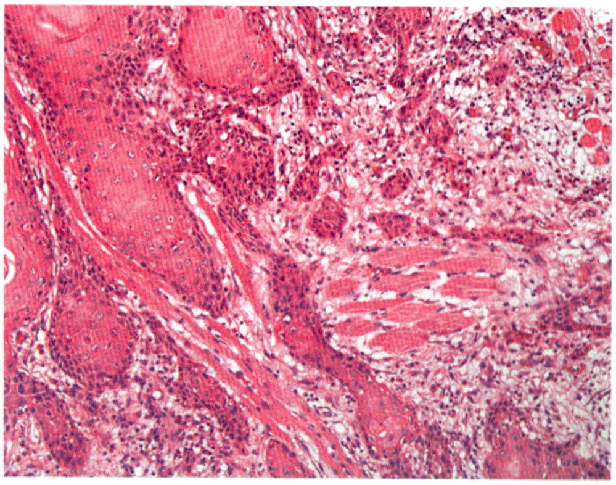

Fig. 13.17: Moderately differentiated squamous cell carcinoma invading between muscle fibers

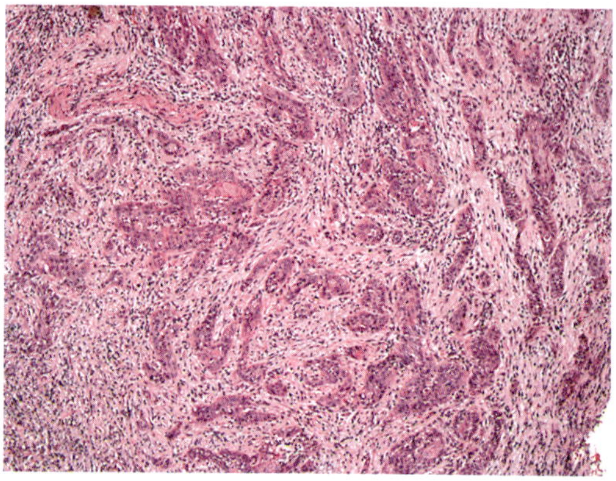

Fig. 13.18: Moderate to poorly differentiated squamous cell carcinoma with aggressive infiltratative pattern as cluster of cells

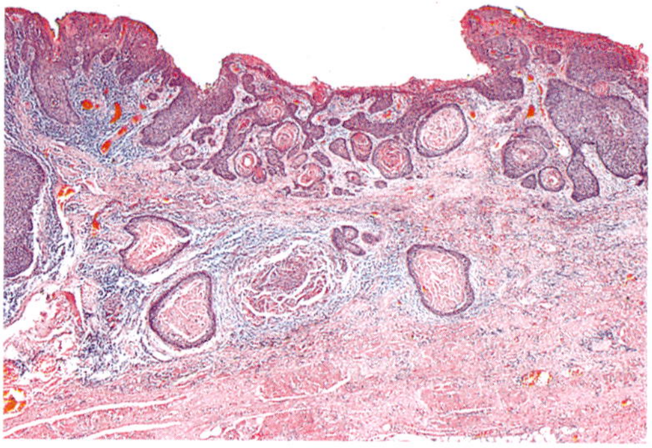

Fig. 13.19: Poorly differentiated squamous cell carcinoma. Deeper islands show necrosis

nization is inconspicuous, cellular and nuclear pleomorphism is marked with large hyperchromatic nuclei and bizarre mitotic figures (**Figs 13.20 and 13.21**). Some poorly differentiated carcinomas have a predominantly basaloid appearance (**Fig. 13.22**). Application of the grading system, which evolved from Broders' original classification, indicates that >50 percent of oral and >90 percent of oropharyngeal SCCs are moderately differentiated. Increased discrimination is, however, desirable and a panel of pathologists at the World Health Organization (WHO) has recommended that grading by differentiation is supplemented by assessment of the pattern of invasion.

Pattern of tumor invasion refers to the manner in which cancer infiltrates connective tissue at the tumor/host interphase. It is considered that neoplasia infiltrating in a widely dispersed manner is more aggressive than those growing in a bulky pushing fashion (**Figs 13.18, 13.23 to 13.26**). Four patterns of tumor invasion have been described:

- The type I pattern corresponds to tumors where the constituent cells retain cohesion and are arranged as broad, bands and columns, occasionally bulbous, which tend to penetrate at more or less the same level; this results in a rather defined, although asymmetrical 'pushing' or 'expansive' advancing front.

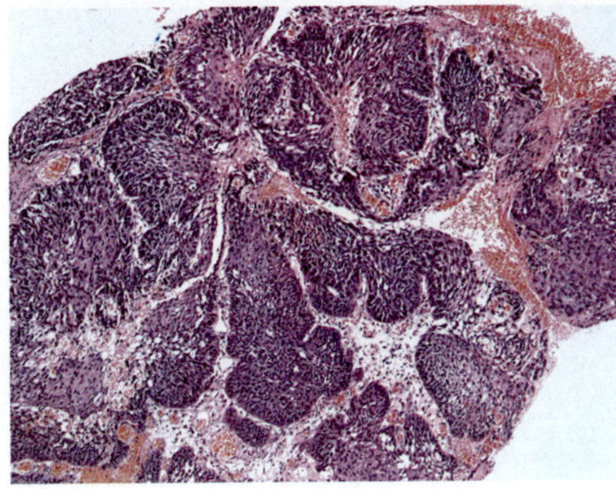

Fig. 13.22: Poorly differentiated carcinoma with a basaloid appearance

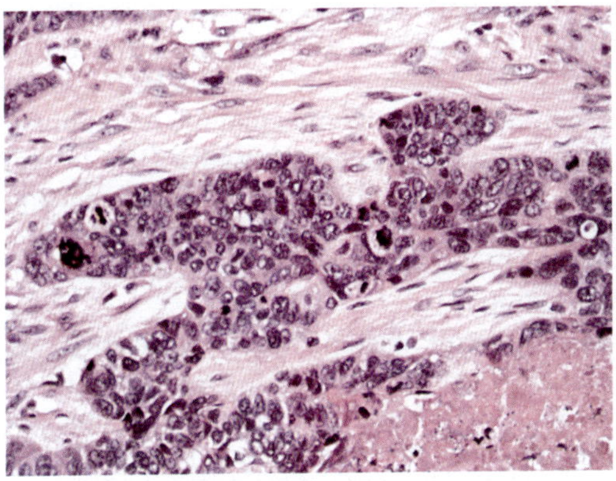

Fig. 13.20: High power view of a poorly differentiated carcinoma

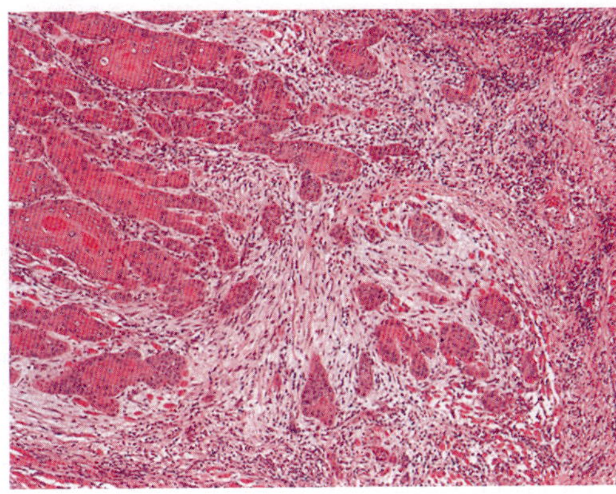

Fig. 13.23: Squamous cell carcinoma showing invasion as cluster of cells and strands

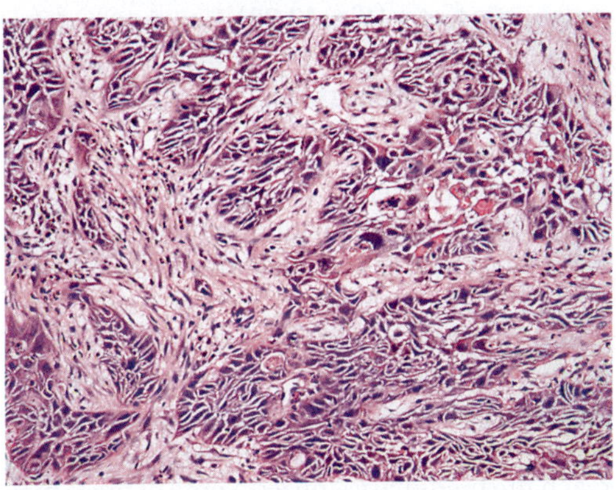

Fig. 13.21: Marked cellular pleomorphism in a poorly differentiated carcinoma with scattered markedly atypical cells and an apoptotic mitosis

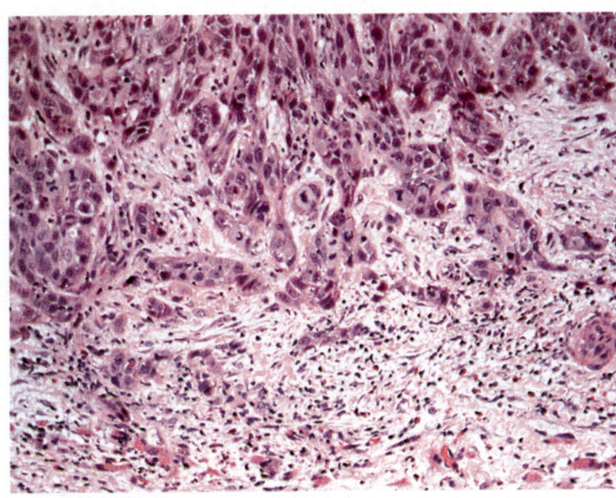

Fig. 13.24: Poorly differentiated SCC invading as clusters of cells and strands

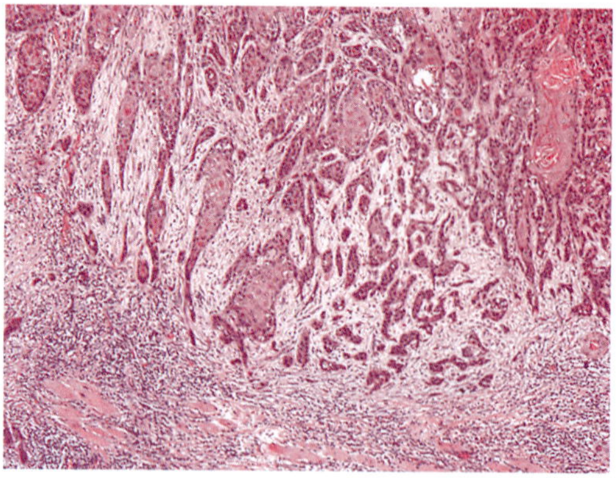

Fig. 13.25: Moderately differentiated squamous cell carcinoma with invasion as single cells and clusters in a myxoid stroma

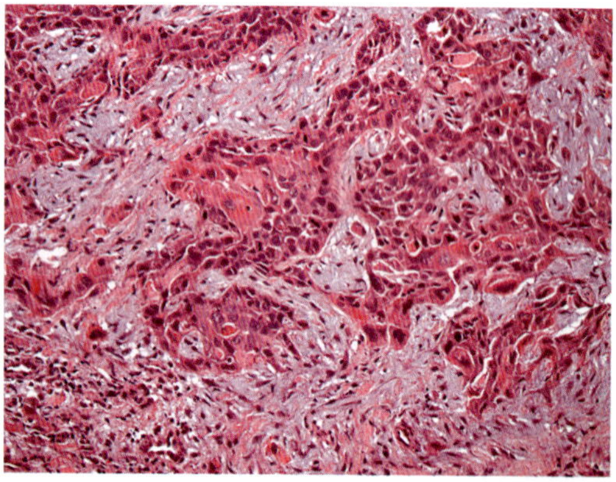

Fig. 13.26: Invasive front of a moderately differentiated SCC showing a myxoid tumor stroma and some single cell invasion

- The type II pattern is characterized by the arrangement of malignant keratinocytes as islands or sheets, rounded, irregular or spiky, which are asymmetrically distributed and penetrate at different levels; this results in an irregular tumor silhouette.
- The type III pattern resembles type II as regards the tumor silhouette, but discohesion in the form of tiny islands and cords that bud off from the larger islands and sheets, extensively affects the advancing front here.
- The type IV pattern corresponds to the archetypal non-cohesive tumors wherein the irregular advancing front shows malignant keratinocytes infiltrating as individual units because of loss of intercellular cohesion.

Tumor thickness of early oral cancers has been significantly correlated with cervical node metastases; particularly when the tumor thickness exceeds 5 mm the metastatic rate is higher. Preoperative ultrasonography may accurately measure tumor thickness.

Bryne et al select the most 'worrisome'/ unfavorable' region of the advancing front for assessment, consider features of both tumor cells and the tumor-host interface and score each feature on a scale of 1 to 4 to give a total malignancy score ranging from 4 to 24 or 28. Keratinization, nuclear aberrations and mitoses are considered in the assessment of the tumor cells whereas the tumor-host interface is assessed in terms of the pattern and level of invasion and the inflammatory cell reaction.

Some pathology laboratories now routinely screen for high-risk HPV. Without activation of p16, just the presence of high risk HPV even in the tissues is not that meaningful. A combined triple method to detect causative HPV in oral and OPCs by p16 immunohistochemistry, consensus PCR HPV-DNA and *in situ* hybridization improves the sensitivity and specificity of detection.

Important histopathological features of oral SCC are illustrated in **Figures 13.13 to 13.33**. Other features in the biopsy that are recorded include desmoplasia, spread of tumor to deep muscle (**Fig. 13.27**) lymphovascular invasion and peri- and endoneural invasion and invading minor salivary glands (**Fig. 13.31**). Lack of clearance at the margin is an important prognostic factor (**Fig. 13.28**).

Features of Metastasis

The earliest stage of pathological metastasis is lymphovascular invasion (**Figs 13.29 and 13.30**), mostly within endothelial lined lymphatic channels referred to as emboli. These emboli would normally be carried to the lymph nodes, the first echelon draining the primary tumor site **(Fig 13.12)**. These emboli would enter the node via the afferent lymphatic vessels, traverse the capsular sinuses (**Fig. 13.32**) and reach the medullary sinuses. Some of these may remain dormant or may die due to host defence systems. Some survive and form established metastasis and increase in size within the node

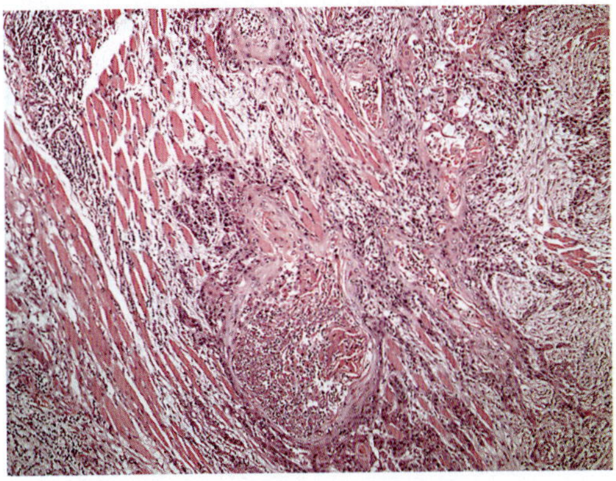

Fig. 13.27: Sarcolemmal spread of SCC

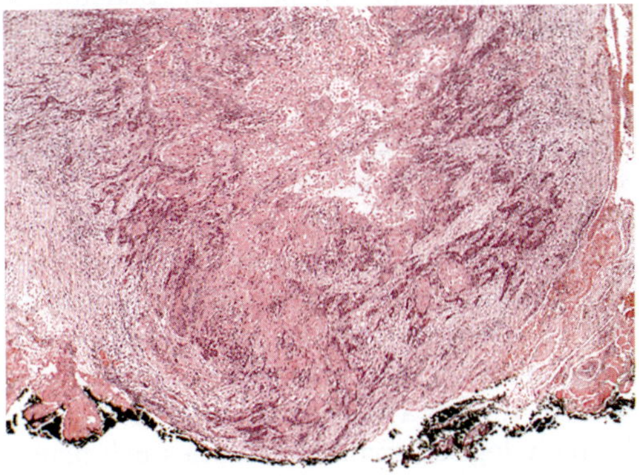

Fig. 13.28: Inflitrating single cells and small islands and strands of cells reach the surgical excision margin at the bottom of the picture

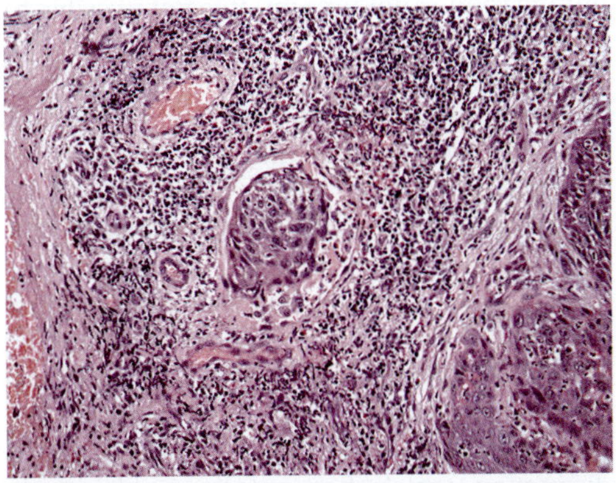

Fig. 13.29: Intravascular spread in a small mucosal lymphatic, a risk factor for developing metastasis

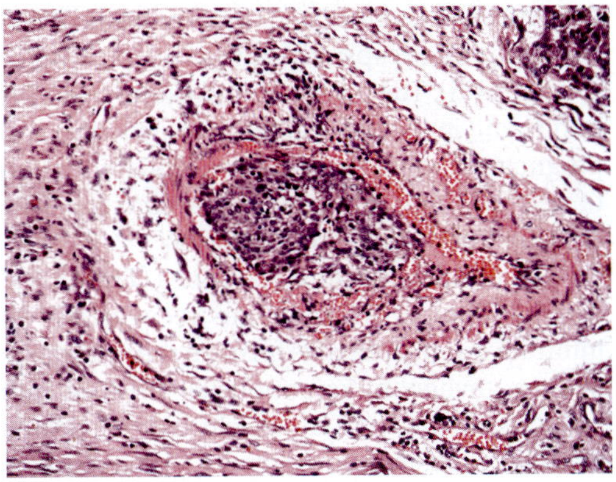

Fig. 13.30: Intravascular spread through a small vein

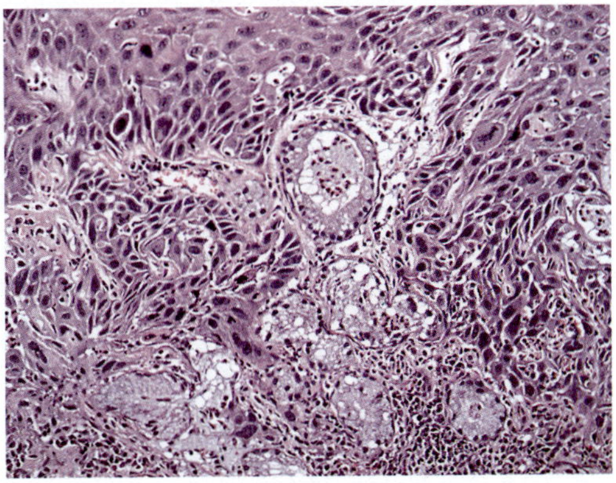

Fig. 13.31: Islands of carcinoma invading minor salivary glands, an aggressive feature

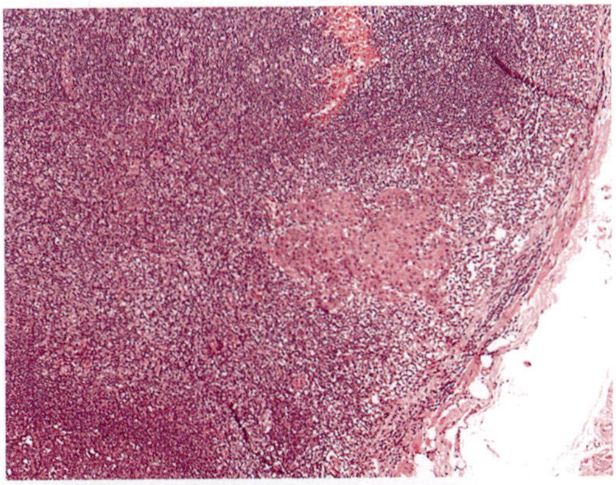

Fig. 13.32: A micrometastasis of SCC in the subcapsular sinus of a lymph node

(**Fig. 13.33**). Left untreated nodal metastasis will invade the node capsule leading to extracapsular spread (ECS). The presence and extent of ECS is important in postoperative management and prognosis prediction. Lymphovascular invasion of vessels within the mucoperiosteum covering the jaws may lead to bone invasion.

For tumors invading jaw bones (**Fig. 13.34**) two patterns of invasion are recognized; an infiltrative and an erosive form. In the infiltrative pattern, malignant keratinocytes advance into cancellous spaces in small clusters or chords with little osteoclastic activity. This requires portals of entry through the cortex, such as fenestrations on a resorbed alveolar ridge, an incompletely healed extraction socket, or perhaps a periodontal ligament. In the erosive pattern, the neoplasm advances on a broad front, with an intervening connective tissue layer and active osteoclasts separate tumor from bone. Several signal pathways initiated by products of the neoplastic keratinocytes themselves are reported to affect osteoclast function, including proteases, cytokines, and growth factors. Two major groups of proteases participate in bone invasion of OSCC: matrix metalloproteinases and cathepsins.

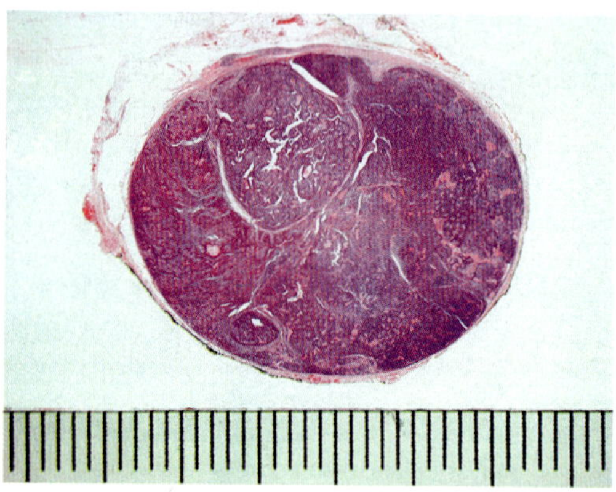

Fig. 13.33: A lymph node replaced by metastatic carcinoma but with no extra nodal spread

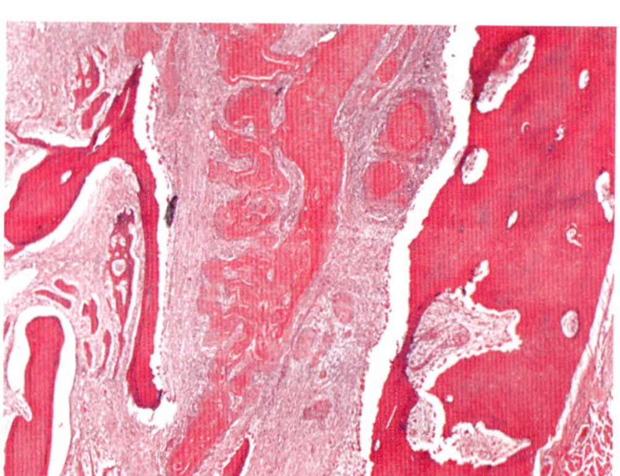

Fig. 13.34: Carcinoma islands invading bone

Perineural invasion (PNI) is a form of tumor spread exhibited by some oral SCCs that correlates with aggressive behavior. This is a form of metastatic spread similar to but distinct from vascular or lymphatic invasion. The presence of tumor cells within any of the three-layers of the nerve sheath is considered as perineural spread or even penetration of tumor cells within the nerve itself may occur - referred to as intraneural spread. The mechanism of PNI is poorly understood. The perineural space provides a suitable microenvironment for the growth of SCC cells that exhibit neurotropic behavior, probably due to cellular and growth factors that allows their growth along the nerves. Neural extension of an SCC can be demonstrated through a thorough histopathological examination and also by MRI and CT. There is a marked variation in reporting by pathologists, some laboratories use neural staining but under reporting could be frequent.

Carcinoma *In Situ*

The theoretical concept of carcinoma *in situ* is that malignant transformation has occurred, but invasion is not present. It is not possible to recognize this by visual inspection (clinically). The following is recommended for the diagnosis of carcinoma *in situ*: full thickness or almost full thickness architectural abnormalities in the viable cellular layers accompanied by pronounced cytologic atypia (**Fig. 13.35**). Atypical mitotic figures and abnormally superficial mitoses are commonly seen in carcinoma *in situ*.

The concept of, and recognition of, carcinoma *in situ* requires consideration. At the furthest end of the spectrum there is a critical distinction which has not been adequately considered and, i.e. recognition of when a lesion stops being dysplastic and is actually malignant.

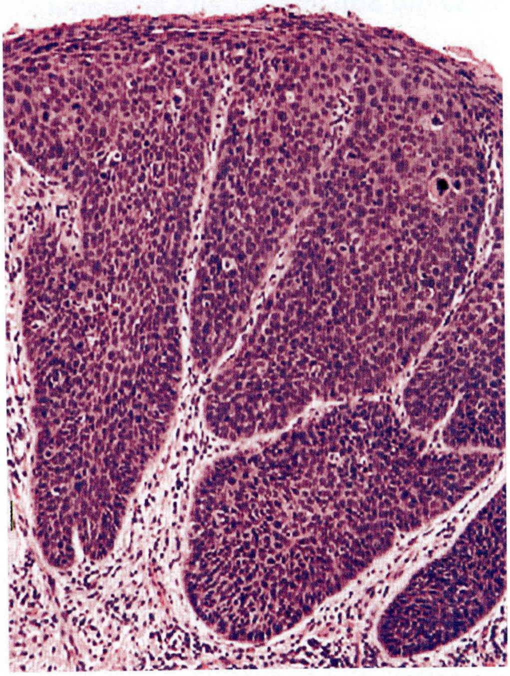

Fig. 13.35: Carcinoma *in situ*; marked cellular atypia and architectural changes extend to almost full thickness of the epithelium

Early Invasion

The histological criterion which distinguishes cancer from precursor lesions is invasion. The dictionary definition of invade includes the concepts of encroaching upon and penetrating. The earliest stage of invasion recognized by microscopy is designated microinvasive squamous cell carcinoma with a small collection of epithelial islands that penetrate subepithelial (papillary) lamina propria (**Fig. 13.36**) When unequivocal/submucosal invasion cannot be established, the question of 'early SCC' arises. The major problem here is deciding whether or not frank invasion of the lamina propria is present.

In diagnostic practice the most frequent problem is judgement about whether the earliest stages of invasion into the lamina propria are present. There is a huge literature on many aspects of invasion, but the problem the diagnostic pathologist has in identifying whether or not invasion is present has not been adequately addressed.

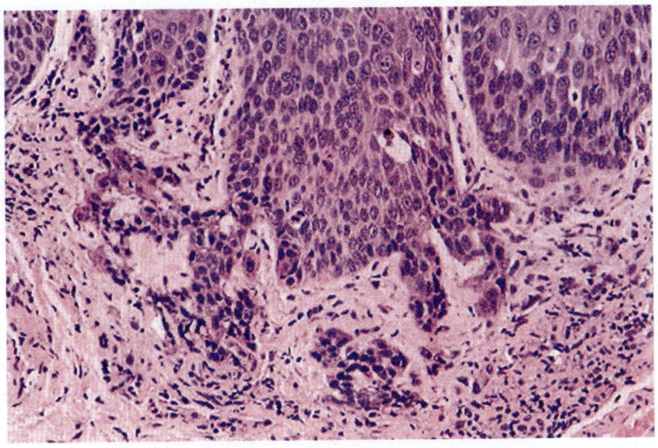

Fig. 13.36: Early invasion showing microscopic invasion

The pathologist's decision about the presence of invasion involves subjective judgement. The following features are important to recognize invasion developing from dysplastic epithelium, not necessarily in the sequence given, but in an iterative manner, often reassessing a feature in the context of another feature.

- Extent of epithelial encroachment
- Dysplasia, particularly mitotic abnormalities
- Features of the basal epithelial layer
- Interface between epithelium and lamina propria
- Eosinophilia and early keratinization

Correlation with features of dysplasia is important. Older texts emphasized loss of basement membrane, but this is not a reliable criterion. However, account should be taken of the interface between epithelium and lamina propria. A very irregular interface with pointed cytoplasmic projections of epithelium is suggestive of malignancy. Loss of a defined basal epithelial layer is important and often cells with characteristics more suggestive of stratum spinosum cells are present at the interface. Host reaction is an underexplored and possibly an important feature.

There will be occasions when the pathologist is unable to arrive at a decision as to whether or not invasion is present. If the findings in the surface epithelium justify a diagnosis of carcinoma *in situ* this should be communicated to the clinician.

PATHOLOGICAL SUBTYPES OF ORAL SQUAMOUS CELL CARCINOMA

Over 90 percent of oral carcinomas are conventional squamous type and resemble squamous epithelium except in a small proportion of anaplastic tumors. Other histological subtypes are encountered. Of these, verrucous carcinoma is particularly common in Asia. These subtypes are described below:

Verrucous Carcinoma

Favors older individuals, particularly tobacco users (chewers and cigar/*bedi* smokers). An exophytic or papillary appearance (rather than infiltrative) should raise the possibility of verrucous carcinoma. It's a slow growing tumor spreading laterally, is more indolent than that of convential SCC and lacks cellular atypia. The epithelium is highly acanthotic breaking into finger like projections with pathognomically broad bulbous rete ridges, with a pushing margin rather than an infiltrative one. Host response is dense, and tumor remains superficial without extending to muscle, but with time may transform to a more clinicopathological SCC.

Carcinoma Cuniculatum

Often involves gingival tissues and appears as a warty mass often loosening teeth. Deep keratin filled crypts are found on the superficial margins and the tumor invades on a broad pushing front and forms histologically characteristic tube-like columns.

Papillary Squamous Cell Carcinoma

Takes an exophytic and papillary form, often in elderly and speculated to be HPV positive. Papillary growth pattern is clear on histology, much basaloid, and minimal or no invasion is observed. These tumors are often p53 positive.

Adenosquamous Carcinoma

Glandular structures either duct-like or acinar structures are seen with the squamous tumor. Largely aneuploid, and known to metastasise early.

Basaloid Squamous Cell Carcinoma

Mostly arise in the posterior part of the oral cavity. Large lobules of basaloid areas are noted, packed with tumor cells with a high nuclear to cytoplasmic ratio.

Spindle Cell Carcinoma

These clinically appear as exophytic, ulcerative or polypoid lesions and is an unusual variant of SCC that frequently recur and metastasise. These neoplasms occur most frequently on the lower lip, tongue, and alveolar ridge. Mean survival time is short and often under 2 years. Histopathologic features include foci of SCC or several epithelial dysplasia, malignant dysplastic spindle cells and cellular atypia is marked. Transition between these cell compartments may be found with prominent intercellular spaces, atypical tumor giant cells, abundant mitotic figures and necrosis. These tumor cells stain positive with anti-pan cytokeratins (AE1/AE3) and are negative for the mesenchymal markers.

Giant Cell Carcinoma

This is an infrequently observed feature though laryngeal giant cell carcinomas are reported. The pathological features include numerous focal, bizarre giant cells, with multiple nuclei and prominent nuecleoli interspread within SCC. There could be associated neutrophils and cellular debris.

Immunohistochemistry with cytokeratins helps in characterization of these tumors of their epithelial origin. Clinical significance of various types is not fully established except that verrucous and papillary carcinoma may pose a better prognosis and basaloid and adenosquamous types have a poorer prognosis than conventional SCC.

MOLECULAR PATHOLOGY

The application of molecular biology techniques to assess the tumor biology of oral SCC has produced a wealth of information on disruption of normal functions and regulation, i.e. responsible for initiation and progression of cancer. It is beyond the scope of this chapter to discuss the voluminous literature on genetics of oral cancer. A short summary of some important events is given below.

Loss of heterozygosity at chromosomes 3p, 9p and 17p appear to occur in early stages of carcinogenesis and in oral epithelial dysplasias. Any alterations at 11q, 4q and of chromosome occur later in the process. Presumably if a cancer associated gene is in an area of allelic loss, this would make the host more susceptible. In the past three decades studies have identified many established and candidate genes in oral SCC. There are several putative tumor suppressor genes involved in oral SCC, but the most important so far appear to be *TP53, p16INK4A, p14ARF NOTCH1* and the retinoblastoma gene. Among these a high incidence of mutant or upregulated p53 in oral SCC has been mostly reported and correlated with prognosis. P16, retinoblastoma (*Rb*) and *TP53* are major interconnected important pathways frequently perturbed in oral SCC. Aberration of these genes causes deregulation of the cell cycle causing increased cell proliferation. The ability to proliferate continuously, without undergoing senescence is one of the hallmarks of cancer. Loss of cell cycle checkpoint control appears to promote further genetic instability. Tumor growth markers that have been studied include epidermal growth factor receptor family *(EGFR), MYC, CCND1* which encodes *cyclin D1*. These genes are mutated, deleted, amplified or over expressed in a majority of oral and oropharyngeal cancers. EGFR over-expression has been reported in many studies, and once activated, EGFR stimulates a number of downstream molecules including Ras/Raf/MAPK and STAT3. Another key pathway is PI3K/AKT/mTOR. Both contribute to malignant potential of oral SCC. Among betel quid users *ras* mutations are particularly prevalent. Alterations of *TP53* have commonly been found in oral cancer, but its prognostic value is inconclusive. A meta-analysis found there is large heterogeneity observed across published studies. Recent studies, by immunostaining found Nuclear Stat 3 and p-mTOR played a significant roles in OSCC prognosis.

Many markers examined in oral SCC appear to provide little or no definitive prognostic or predictive information that can be used in a clinical setting. Though rapid progress has been made in our understanding of molecular biology of oral SCC none of these genetic alterations are used as tumor markers at the moment. Most researchers now believe it is unlikely that any one molecular event determines tumor evolution and that the complex interaction among genes and proteins may contribute to carcinogenesis. Thus complete behavior of a tumor cannot be ascertained through the analysis of a single tumor marker and it is likely that these markers need to be combined to evolve diagnostic paradigms. The introduction of anti-EGFR and anti-m-TOR therapies for head and neck cancer are the first of the novel biological treatment modalities available for clinical use.

PROGNOSIS OF ORAL SQUAMOUS CELL CARCINOMA

Tumor size and nodal status are the most significant clinical prognostic factors for oral SCC. For early tumors, tumor thickness has been found to be a reliable prognostic marker for subclinical nodal metstasis, local recurrence and survival. Histopathologically assessed features of the surgical resection specimen and nodal pathology continue to provide information, i.e. central to determining the postoperative treatment needs and prognosis for an individual patient. Factors of significance are listed in **Table 13.4**.

TREATMENT

Surgery is the most well established mode of initial definitive treatment for a majority of oral cancers, with a longstanding history of being the accepted method of treatment for well over a century. Introduction of ionizing radiation, following the discovery of radium, became an important means of non-surgical treatment of oral cancer. However, in the majority of patients with advanced cancer radiotherapy is employed in conjunction with surgery, most often offered as postoperative treatment. Chemotherapy in the management of oral carcinoma was considered palliative in the 1950's, 60's and 70's but with the introduction of *Cis*-platinum, clinical trials of induction chemotherapy demonstrated that a good response to chemotherapy was observed

▪ Table 13.4
Factors influencing prognosis of oral SCC*

Clinical
• T stage
• Nodal status
• Tumor grade
Pathology
• Histological grade (differentiation)
• Pattern of tumor invasion
• Lymphovascular and perineural invasion
• Sialadenotrophism
• Tumor thickness; 4 mm or less vs 9 mm or more
• Bone invasion
• Margin clearance
• HPV infection
• High proliferation index (Ki 67)/rapid doubling time
• Extracapsular spread of nodal disease

*Of those listed some may not have a direct impact on the management at present but may have a significant role in determining the treatment in the future

in a significant number of patients. Unlike other sites in the head and neck area, the response to induction chemotherapy did not translate into long-term control of primary oral squamous cell carcinomas. Targeted therapies with EGFR inhibitors are an active area of investigation at this time. Immunotherapy and gene therapy are also areas of research where further work needs to be done.

The initial treatment approaches for patients with oral cancer include:

1. Primary surgery with or without postoperative radiotherapy or chemoradiation,
2. Non-surgical strategies, i.e. primary radiotherapy either by itself or combined with chemotherapy.

   Radiotherapy is typically now administered postoperatively. Chemotherapy can be given:

   a. Before surgery (induction/neoadjuvant-when treatment is administered before primary therapy, i.e it is used to shrink a tumor prior to surgery or radiation)
   b. After surgery (adjuvant-therapy, i.e. administered after the primary treatment)
   c. At the same time as radiotherapy (concomitant–also referred to as chemoradiotherapy)
   d. Alternating with radiotherapy.

Newer approaches include targeted agents directed against epidermal growth factor receptor (*EGFR*) or anti *mTOR* reported for other tumors.

In many countries, patients with stages I and II disease who have excellent outcome are most optimally treated with only one treatment modality (surgery). No randomized trial has been conducted to clarify whether surgery or radiotherapy would give a better outcome. Moreover, there have been no trials comparing different surgical modalities of the primary tumor. A substantial proportion of patients present with more locally-advanced stage (stages III and IV) disease, many patients with advanced stages are also primarily treated with curatively intended surgery and are then referred for postoperative radiotherapy or chemoradiation. The most commonly employed surgical approaches for resection of primary oral cancer are peroral, mandibulotomy, lower cheek flap approach, visor flap or Weber-Ferguson flap approach.

Involvement of bone in cases of OSCC has a major influence on functional outcome and dramatically impacts the patients' quality of life. In patients with very early invasion of alveolar bone by cancers of gum marginal mandibulectomy is sufficient. Segmental mandibulectomy is considered necessary when there is gross invasion of cancellous bone by oral cancer.

For advanced cancers the choice between primary surgical or non-surgical treatment strategies is often dependent on the site of the primary tumor and functional outcomes of treatment.

Classic radical neck dissection - removal of all cervical lymph nodes from levels 1 to 5 combined with adjacent structures with resultant postoperative morbidity is only reserved for advanced neck disease. Selective neck dissection is now preferred. For early stage tumors (T1) with clinically negative neck (N0) there is a controversy over the management of cervical lymph nodes, regarding elective neck dissection. There are no universally accepted guidelines for the treatment of clinically negative nodes in early stage SCCs and the use of elective neck dissection in such cases remains unresolved.

Along with surgery, radiotherapy plays a key role in the management of early stage and locally advanced head and neck squamous-cell carcinomas (HNSCC) either alone or more frequently combined with surgery and/or chemotherapy. Radiotherapy (RT) plays a key role in the management of these locally advanced stages. In recent years, the techniques for external-beam radiation with the intended purpose of delivering more radiation to the tumor while sparing normal tissues and adjacent vulnerable organs have evolved. Its results remain relatively poor in advanced cases. Several approaches have been developed to improve its efficacy while maintaining acceptable toxicities. In the last decades, altered fractionation has been one of the tools shown to improve the efficacy of RT. The objective of altered fractionated RT is to increase the dose intensity of RT by delivering a high total dose in an overall time as short as possible. Mainly two types of altered fractionation regimens have been tested, i.e. accelerated and/or hyperfractionationed RT. Accelerated fractionation radiotherapy (AFRT) was designed to increase the dose intensity usually by delivering 2 (or 3) fractions daily in order to decrease the overall treatment time. This acceleration aimed to reduce tumor cell repopulation between sessions to allow better local control probability. The latter was developed to overcome tumor cell repopulation during the course of therapy. Further variations exist. These include continuous hyperfractionated accelerated radiotherapy (CHART), two and three-dimensional conformal radiation therapy (2DRT and 3 DCRT), intensity modulated radiotherapy (IMRT) and image-guided radiotherapy. A Cochrane review found altered fraction radiotherapy is associated with an improvement in overall survival and local regional control. The benefit may be greater with hyperfractionated regimens rather than accelerated regimens. Proton beam therapy is less commonly used.

Hyperfractionated radiotherapy (HFRT) was designed to improve effectiveness by delivering 2 (or 3) fractions daily with a markedly reduced dose per fraction (1.1-1.2 Gy), which in turn could reduce late toxicity and allow to increase the total dose.

Chemotherapy plays an important role in the treatment of locally advanced HNSCC either as concomitant chemoradiotherapy (CT-RT) or as induction chemotherapy. A major advance in the treatment of this stage of disease has been the introduction of concomitant CT-RT.

There is some evidence that concomitant radio/chemotherapy is better than radiotherapy alone. There are over 80 trials on the use of chemotherapeutic agents but the information is limited or missing in many reports to extract meaningful outcome data. Cisplatin is the most common chemotherapy agent used, other platins used include carboplatin mostly in combination with 5-FU. The use of methotrexate, bleomycin, vincristine and cyclophosphamide is also reported. Based on a Cochrane analysis use of concomitant chemoradiotherapy is an effective treatment for oral cavity and oropharyngeal cancer and the addition of docetaxel (T) to the regimes containing cisplatin and 5-FU (PF) is associated with further reduction in mortality. There may be additional benefit in the use of induction TPF regimen prior to concomitant chemotherapy with TPF.

The epidermal growth factor receptor (*EGFR*) has been identified as an important gene target for cancer therapy. Inhibition of the *EGFR* using monoclonal antibodies (MAbs) directed against the external ligand binding domain or small molecule tyrosine kinase inhibitors has been extensively studied in the recent years. Based on promising preclinical studies on the interaction between EGFR inhibitors and ionizing radiation a number of prospective clinical investigations on molecular targeted therapies have been launched for *KRAS* wild type tumors.

Among the *EGFR* inhibitors, cetuximab (erbitux) is an immunoglobulin G1 (1gG1) monoclonal antibody (MAb) that inhibits ligand binding to the *EGFR* and can stimulate antibody-dependent cell-mediated cytoxity. Rapamycin analogs, including everolimus, temsirolimus, and ridaforolimus, are small molecules that selectively inhibit *mTOR* activity are currently used in clinical trials for other solid cancers and may be appropriate for treating oral carcinomas.

Local relapse after resection of a primary SCC is easily explained, when tumor is detected in the surgical margin and thus residual tumor is likely to remain in the patient, but the pathobiology is more complex in cases where the margins are histologically tumor-free. Molecular studies indicate that there are two different mechanisms responsible in these cases. First, small clusters of residual tumor cells that are undetectable on routine histopathological examination (known as minimal residual cancer: MRC) proliferate and this forms the basis of recurring cancer. A second cause of relapse is an undetected field of preneoplastic cells that is struck by additional genetic hits leading to invasive cancer. It is likely that within this field, that can be over 7 cm in diameter, a second primary carcinoma could emerge.

Oral and Oropharyngeal cancer is a devastating disease which has wide-ranging effects on the patient, due to the disease process and its surgical and non-surgical management (**Table 13.5**). Though acute effects of radiotherapy settle in four to six weeks after therapy some permanent late effects and toxicity remain. A patient's General Medical Practitioner and the General Dental Practitioner should be aware of the significance of these treatment effects on the poor quality of life, physical and functional changes, psychological effects and aim to provide practical advice in the management of surviving patients or those living with cancer.

Table 13.5 Complications following therapy
• Appearance
• Eating and swallowing (PEG feeding)
• Employment issues
• Fatigue
• Psychosocial distress
• Sexuality
• Shoulder dysfunction
• Speech and voice alterations
• Osteoradionecrosis (for those treated with radiotherapy)
• Dental status due to tooth loss
• Root caries
• Trismus
• Painful mucositis
• Excessive mucous production
• Taste disturbances
• Xerostomia

SCREENING AND PREVENTION

It is well established that the treatment of early stage oral cancers (**Figs 13.37 to 13.39**) achieves higher survival rates with less attendant morbidity than that at present where far too many patients present with late stage disease (**Fig. 13.40**). Therefore screening for early stage oral cancers is advocated. Several large population screening programs from SE Asia and smaller studies from England and Japan

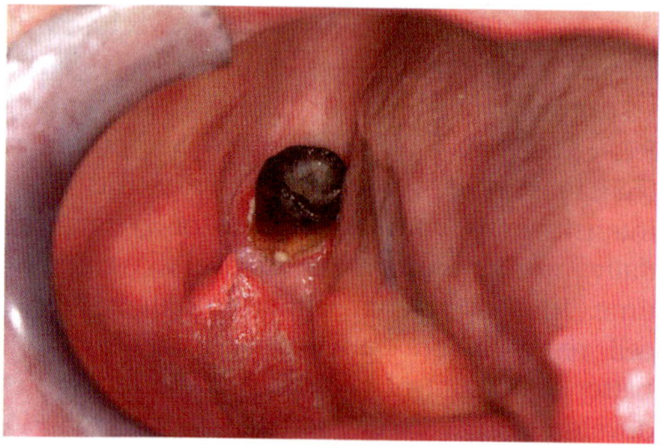

Fig. 13.37: A small T1 cancer of the gum adjacent to a mobile molar tooth. Rolled margins of this non-healing cancer indicates malignancy

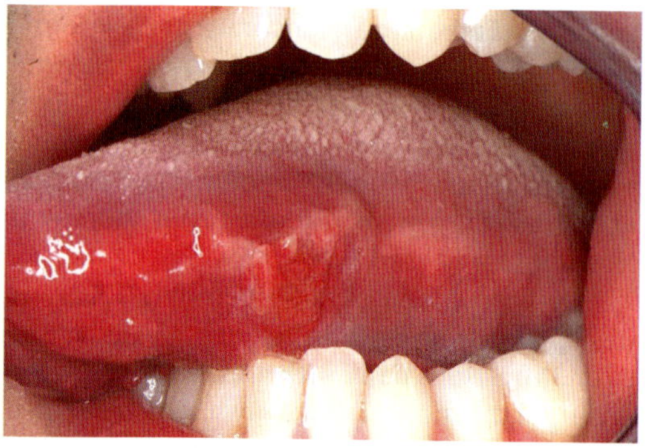

Fig. 13.38: A superficial ulcer on the lateral margin of tongue

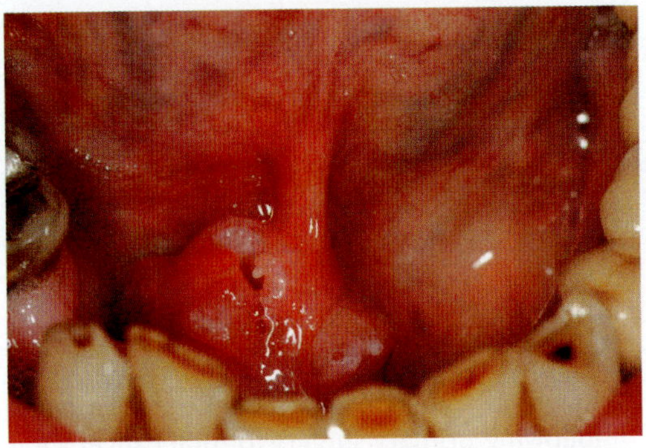

Fig. 13.39: A deeply infiltrative cancer on the floor of mouth

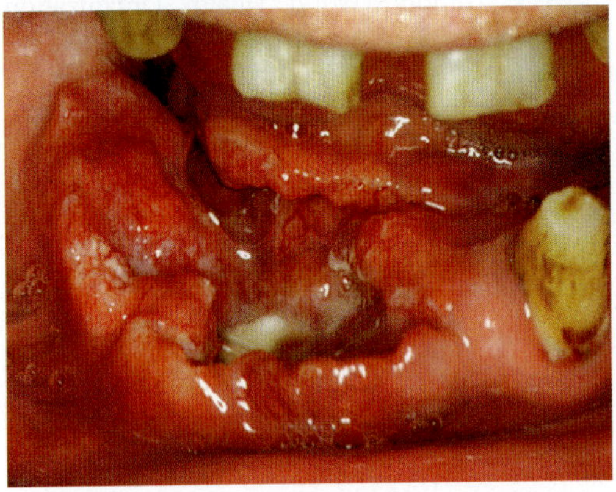

Fig. 13.40: An advanced tumor on the floor of the mouth

were reported during the period 1980 to 2000. One randomized control trial on screening for oral cancer conducted in India has demonstrated a significant mortality reduction in tobacco users. However, for low risk populations, there is insufficient evidence to support population screening. Some of the problems include the relative rarity of the disease, a lack of knowledge of the natural history of the disease, disagreement over disease management and the lack of evidence on the efficacy and cost effectiveness of different screening methods. In a high incidence country high risk groups may be targeted for screening. Opportunistic oral mucosal examinations in dental practices reduce the cost of screening and could be an effective model for countries with health care systems that support regular dental attendance. The concept underpinning screening is also based on the premise that earlier detection of the asymptomatic phases of oral precancer will allow modification of risky behaviors and to attempt other clinical interventions to prevent cancer.

To prevent cancers of the oral cavity it is important to recognize the major risk factors that are appropriate for the population. There is now clear evidence on established and modifiable risk factors (**Figure 13.5**). Any intervention should be based on good scientific evidence. It is important to take into consideration the difficulties in behavioral modification that requires multisectorial approaches.

There is good evidence to suggest that cessation of tobacco use leads to reduced risk of oral SCC though it may take up to 10 years to reach the low risk status of never users.

Most adult smokers would like to quit, and effective therapies are now available. Tobacco dependency requires targeted therapies and those with oral precursor lesions constitute a special group who need assistance for quitting tobacco use. The main role of oral health professionals is to stimulate quit attempts among their patients using brief interventions and when appropriate to refer to cessation clinics for further treatment of tobacco dependence. Methods of tobacco interventions are discussed in a later Chapter 24.

HPV vaccines (Cervarix and Gadasil) are now available. These are not therapeutic but are expected to offer protection against cervical cancer when given to young adolescent women. Results are waiting to confirm their efficacy to reduce cancer incidence in young adult women with prior exposure to HPV, or for infections in other organs other than the cervix, such as oral cavity or oropharynx.

ACKNOWLEDGMENTS

I thank Elsevier Ltd to republish Figures 13.1 and 13.2 and Wiley Blackwell for reuse of Figures 13.35 and 13.36. Figure 13.3A was kindly supplied by Dr Anura Ariyawardana of James Cook University, Queensland, Australia.

SELF-ASSESSMENT QUESTIONS

1. Explain why there is much global variation in the incidence of oral cancer.
2. What novel risk factors may be considered causative in subjects who are not exposed to the major risk factors?
3. Outline different clinical and biological characteristics of HPV-negative and HPV-positive tongue and oropharyngeal cancers.
4. Why is staging important and how would you apply TNM staging to a given tumor?
5. Explain the significance of special investigations that you would you carry-out prior to treatment planning.
6. What pathological features would you consider in assessing the prognosis of a squamous cell carcinoma?
7. What microscopic features enable the identification of variants of squamous cell carcinomas?
8. What are the features of early invasion?
9. Discuss the spread of a squamous cell carcinoma.
10. How would our understanding of the molecular alterations of oral cancer contribute to any improvement for early diagnosis and management?

SUGGESTED READING

1. Leemans CR, Braakhuis BJM, Brakehoff RH. The molecular biology of head and neck cancer. Nature Reviews Cancer. 2011;11:9-22.
2. Rogers SN, Brown, Woolgar JA, et al. Survival following primary surgery for oral cancer. Oral Oncology. 2009;45:201-11.
3. Barnes L, Eveson JW, Reichart P, Sidransky D. The Pathology and Genetics of Head and Neck Tumors (World Health Organization Classification of Tumors). IARC Press. 2005.
4. Warnakulasuriya S. Global epidemiology of oral and oropharyngeal cancer. Oral Oncology. 2009;45:309-16.
5. Warnakulasuriya S. Squamous cell carcinoma and precursor lesion: Prevention. Periodontol 2000. 2011;57(1):38-50.

Chapter 14

Recurrent Oral Ulceration

Saman Warnakulasuriya

Chapter Outline

INTRODUCTION AND CLASSIFICATION

Recurrent oral ulceration (ROU) is regarded as the most common disorder affecting the oral mucosa. Aphthous ulcers constitute the largest group of ROU, occurring in about 20 percent of the general population. A distinction should be made of the ulcers of aphthous type recurrent aphthous ulcers (RAU) from those other ROUs secondary to systemic disease or due to other causes. The diagnosis and management of different categories of ROU would be considered in this chapter. A classification is shown in **Table 14.1**.

It is also prudent to distinguish an ulcer from an erosion. An ulcer is a break in skin or mucous membrane with loss of surface tissue, and disintegration of epithelial tissue. In contrast, an erosion is the superficial destruction of the epithelial covering of the mucosa by inflammation or trauma.

▪ Table 14.1
Classification of oral ulcers related to cause

Condition/cause	*Examples*
Recurrent aphthous ulceration (stomatitis)	Minor Major Herpetiform Behçet's disease
Secondary to hematinic deficiency (Anemia)	Vitamin B_{12} Folate Iron
Secondary to other hematological cause	Neutropenia Cyclic neutropenia Pancytopenia Leukemia
Secondary to GI tract disease	Ulcerative colitis Crohn's disease Celiac disease
Secondary to a dermatological condition	Erythema multiforme Pemphigus Mucous membrane pemphigoid Erosive lichen planus Dermatitis herpetiformis Linear IgA disease
Secondary to connective tissue disease	Lupus erythematosus Reiter's syndrome
Secondary to immune deficiency	HIV disease
Secondary to drug therapy	Nonsteroidal anti-inflammatory agents Chemotherapy

RECURRENT APHTHOUS ULCERATION/RECURRENT APHTHOUS STOMATITIS

Recurrent oral ulcers of aphthous type RAU are also referred to as recurrent aphthous stomatitis (RAS). "Aphthous stomatitis" has been used interchangeably with "aphthous ulcers" and may be more accurate terminology. "Aphthous" is derived from the Greek word "aphtha" which means an ulcer. Episodic recurrences are its main characteristic feature. The frequency of recurrence varies between patients. Synonyms now mostly in disuse are:

- Mikulicz' aphthae
- Sutton's disease
- Periadenitis mucosa necrotica recurrence
- Canker sores.

Clinical Aspects

A history of RAU varies from 5 to 60 percent among adults in different populations and at a given time 20 percent may report they suffer from aphthae. RAU is more common in women. Ulceration commences usually in the second decade of life. All races are affected though reportedly it is more common in North America and less frequent in Arabia. The disease is predominant in children of higher socioeconomic status. RAU is uncommon in patients who smoke: quitting smoking seems to initiate the disease in older groups of patients.

The diagnosis of RAU is based upon a history of regular recurrence of oral ulcers and the presence of compatible clinical lesions (**Figs 14.1 and 14.2**). These ulcers, which usually occur on the nonkeratinized oral mucosa, can cause considerable pain and may interfere with eating, speaking and swallowing. For 24 to 48 hours preceding the appearance of an ulcer, most patients have a prodromal sign—pricking or burning sensation in the affected area. RAU usually occur on the nonkeratinized oral mucosa, including the lips, the buccal mucosa, the floor of the mouth, the soft palate and the ventral surface of the tongue. Regions of

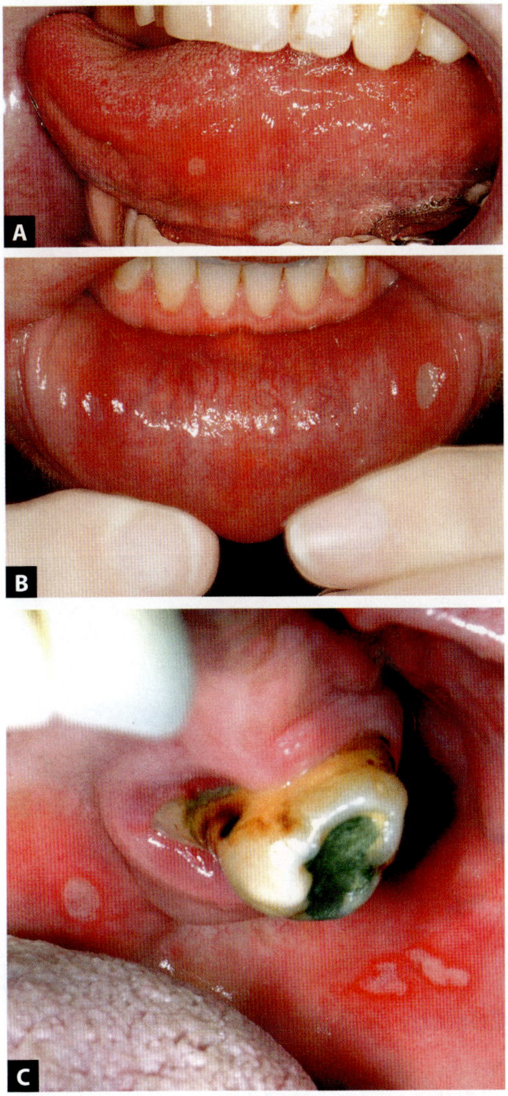

Figs 14.1A to C: Examples of minor RAU: (A and B) Minor ulcers on lower lip and tongue in the same subject; (C) A crop of minor aphthous ulcers in buccal mucosa and soft palate.
Note: Small size, pale color with surrounding erythema

keratinized oral mucosa, such as the hard palate, the gums and the dorsal surface of the tongue, are uncommon locations. Histopathological and serological findings are neither diagnostic nor exclusionary. A biopsy is therefore not undertaken except in rare circumstances when

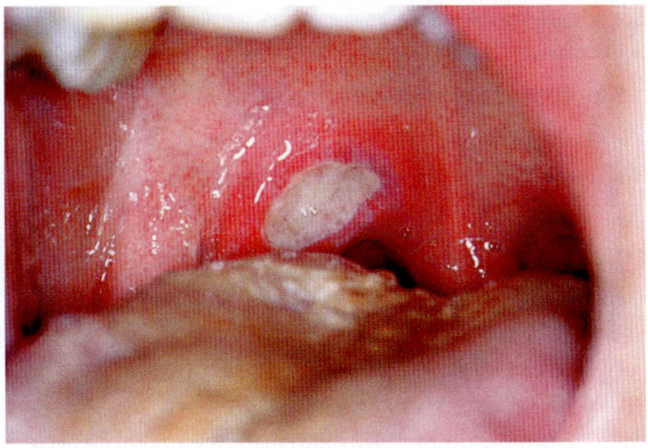

Fig. 14.2: A major aphthous ulcer in the soft palate and oropharynx.
Note: Its size is exceeding 10 mm in the longest diameter

a major aphthous ulcer (without an established history of recurrence) may mimic cancer. The patient should be evaluated thoroughly to assess the presence of micronutrient deficiencies or other associated systemic/dermatological diseases, such as Behçet's, Reiter's syndrome, erythema multiforme, celiac disease, Crohn's disease, ulcerative colitis or erosive lichen planus and classified accordingly (**Table 14.1**). Pemphigus vulgaris (*see* Chapter 15) may mimic RAU at the initial presentation but a clear note should be made that in untreated pemphigus oral ulceration is persistent. A diagnosis of RAU is made for a patient with a history of recurrent oral ulceration, in the absence of any systemic disease or hematinic deficiencies that contribute to oral ulceration.

Box 14.1: Recurrent aphthous ulcers

Key features helpful in diagnosis

- Present as crops of ulcers that recur
- No evidence of systemic disease; patient is otherwise well. Therefore, requires hematinic and immunological investigations
- Classified by their size and time taken for healing: as minor, major or herpetiform
- More common in teenagers and young adults
- In older subjects ROU are likely to be secondary to a systemic cause and should not be assumed to be RAU.

Box 14.2: Recurrent aphthous ulcers

Key features on etiopathogenesis

- Is multifactorial
- Some have genetic predisposition
- Bacterial or viral etiology is unlikely
- Immunopathogenesis involving a cell-mediated immune response mechanism is most likely
- Involves generation of T-lymphocytes, interleukins and tumor necrosis factor
- Cross reactivity with streptococcal antigens has been proposed.

Recurrent aphthae are classified into three groups:

1. Minor.
2. Major.
3. Herpetiform.

The classification is not clearly defined. It is based upon variation in the clinical presentation. The criteria used in distinguishing between the three forms of recurrent aphthae are: their size, number, localization and duration of the lesion.

- Minor type is the most common form encountered (80%). It is characterized by one or more round or oval, well-demarcated, painful ulcers of the nonkeratinized mucosa (**Fig. 14.1**). They have a depressed base covered with yellowish slough and surrounded by an erythematous margin. Normally self-limiting in nature (healing is spontaneous) they occur most frequently in the second and third decade of life.
- Major aphthae are larger in size (>10 mm in size), deep and take longer to heal (3 weeks to several months) (**Fig. 14.2**). The major form occurs less often.
- The herpetiform ulcers are the least common. These are small pin-head ulcers (**Fig. 14.3**) but may coalesce to form a large ulcer.

The characteristics of each are summarized in **Table 14.2**. Some may have mixed crops both of minor and major types or minor ulcers bordering on major type (**Fig. 14.4**). A small group with severe RAU (e.g. more than 3 episodes of ulcers per month or is rarely ulcer free) could be regarded as having atypical or complex apthosis.

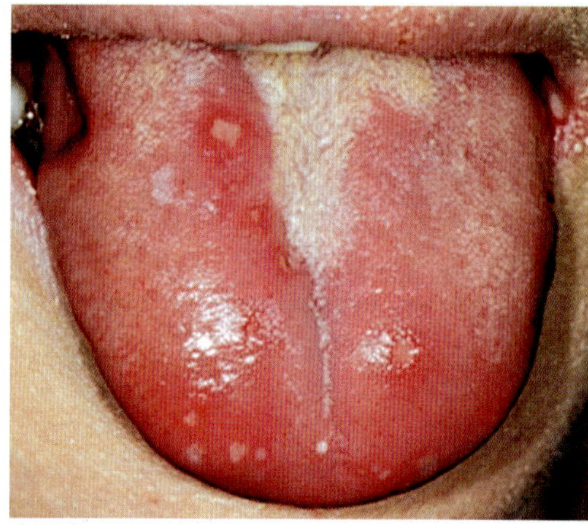

Fig. 14.3: Herpetiform recurrent oral ulceration

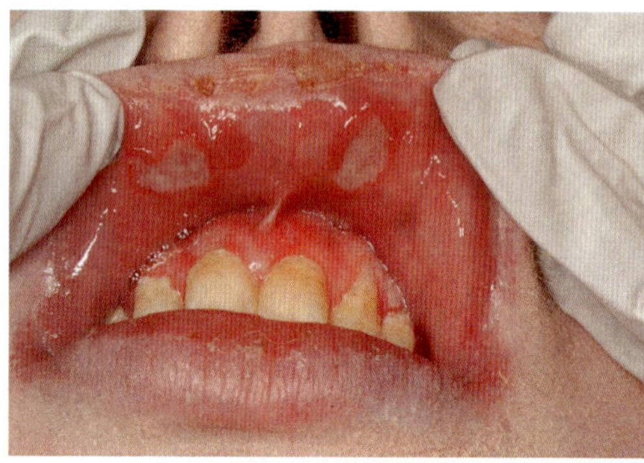

Fig. 14.4: Minor aphthous ulcers bordering on the size of major ulcers

Etiology

No single cause has been identified as causative and the etiology to date is largely unknown. RAU occur mostly in otherwise healthy people. Onset later in life suggests the possibility of an underlying cause. The most likely factors precipitating aphthous ulcers are local trauma and stress. In people susceptible to the disease trauma may often initiate RAU. Injury to the oral mucosa may result from accidental self-biting, dental procedures, toothbrush bristles and sharp-edged foods. Stress is often linked to exacerbation of oral ulcers in susceptible individuals. This association has remained controversial due to inconsistent evidence. However, emotional and environmental stress may precede the first-time an aphthous ulcer

▪ Table 14.2
Main characteristics of minor, major and herpetiform ulceration

Features	*Minor*	*Major*	*Herpetiform*
Size of ulcers	Less than 10 mm in diameter	Over 10 mm in diameter	0.5–2 mm in diameter
Shape	Oval, well demarcated	Usually oval, poorly defined margin	Round and well-defined; may coalesce to form an irregular outline
Color	Yellow/gray base with thin erythematous border	Yellow/gray base	Yellow with marked periulcer erythema
Duration	4–7 days	1–2 months	4–14 days
Site	Most, nonkeratinized oral mucosae—labial and buccal mucosae in particular	Most, nonkeratinized oral mucoase—soft palate and fauces	Nonkeratinized oral mucosa—but most often ventral surface of tongue, anterior labial sulci and soft palate
Ulcer number	1–5	2–3	10–100
Healing	No scarring	Heal with scarring	No scarring
Peak age of onset	5–20 years	10–20 years	10–30 years

manifests and is involved in a significant proportion of recurrent episodes.

Early studies by Thomas Lehner have indicated that RAU is an acquired autoimmune disorder that may manifest in a variety of clinical presentations. Recently cross-reactivity between a 65 kDa heat shock protein (HSP) of microbes and a 60 kDa human mitochondrial HSP resulting in generation of autoreactive T cell response primed to a homologous peptide has been reported. The underlying pathology of RAU is thus due to immune dysregulation, resulting in a cellular cytotoxic assault upon oral mucosal cells. An increase in T-helper cells (CD4+ cells) and a decrease in T-suppressor cells (CD8+ cells) may accompany RAU during periods of disease exacerbation and normalize during remission. The presence of activated gamma/delta T-lymphocytes in the periphery of ulcers indicates that RAU may result from an activated cell-mediated response. Interleukines and tumor necrosis factor (TNF) are involved in immunopathogenesis of the disease. New research indicates a subset of RAU patients showing a partial lack in the NK cell numbers.

Microorganisms acting as antigenic stimuli in the genesis of antibodies that cross-react with oral keratinocytes have been speculated in the causation of RAU. Several microbes *Streptococcus sanguis*, *Smitis* and *Soralis* have been suggested as causative, as well as *Helicobacter pylori* that have been detected in RAU biopsies when examined by polymerase chain reaction (PCR).

Food allergies occasionally underlie RAU.

Where a relationship to the menstrual cycle is noted, a cyclical pattern can be demonstrated. No studies so far have identified a clear hormonal cause.

Some people have a well-established fami-lial basis for RAU. However, evidence for a genetic predisposition is not strong. Patients with family history of RAU may develop the disease earlier and more severely than those with no family history. Forty to fifty percent of first-degree relatives of patients with RAU may have the condition. RAU may have a polygenic inheritance with a variable penetrance that makes it difficult to confirm familial nature of the disease.

SYSTEMIC DISEASES ASSOCIATED WITH RECURRENT ORAL ULCERATION

Behçet's Disease

ROU may be a sign of Behçet's disease (BD). In over 90 percent cases with Behçet's cases aphthous stomatitis is described. Oral ulcers may be the initial presentation and full-blown Behçet's may develop many years after onset of RAU. Behçet's is a form of vasculitis, typically arises in young adults and in about 2 percent the onset is in childhood. The signs and symptoms include genital ulceration, ocular lesions, arthritis, erythema nodosum (painful purplish nodules with a peripheral halo) and skin rashes. Other systemic manifestations (CVS—vascular thrombotic and neurological) are also described. International diagnostic criteria specify that ROU should manifest more than 3 times a year and 2 other systemic features (genital/eye/skin) to establish a diagnosis of BD. "Pathergy test"—a sterile abscess when saline is pricked into the skin (prominent 24 hours after the injection) or non-specific hyper-reactivity observed in response to minor trauma—is diagnostic of BD. In taking the initial history and during follow-up it is therefore important to question about any associated features of RAU to exclude Behçet's disease.

The cause of BD is unknown. An auto-immune reaction to some unknown stimulus is a likely explanation. This could be an infectious agent or an environmental factor. Genetical predisposition is likely as BD is observed in association with HLA haplotypes. HLA-B5 and HLA-B51 have been found in increased frequency in BD patients. The management is empirical, often unsatisfactory in controlling symptoms. Systemic steroids provide short term benefit. Steroid-sparing immunosuppressants (Colchicine, azathioprine, thalidomide) and pulse therapy with methotrexate may be helpful.

A variant of Behçet's disease where major aphthae appear with inflamed cartilage in joints is referred to as MAGIC syndrome.

Immunobullous and Systemic Diseases with ROU

There are many vesicular-bullous ulcerative conditions that may present like RAU (*see* Chapter 15). In such cases ROU is secondary in nature and many would present with dermatological disorders. In cases when the presentation is unusual of ROU and the history is vague, a biopsy may be helpful in defining the diagnosis. These cases present a diagnostic challenge. The clinical, histological and serological evaluation is often necessary to rule out many similar conditions: Primary (or recurrent) herpetic gingivostomatitis (**Fig. 14.5**), Behçet's syndrome, Sweet's syndrome, pemphigus vulgaris (**Fig. 14.6**) ulcerative lichen planus (**Fig. 14.7**), mucous membrane pemphigoid (**Fig. 14.8**), erythema multiforme (**Fig. 14.9**), and herpangina (**Fig. 14.10**). A minority patients with cyclical neutropenia

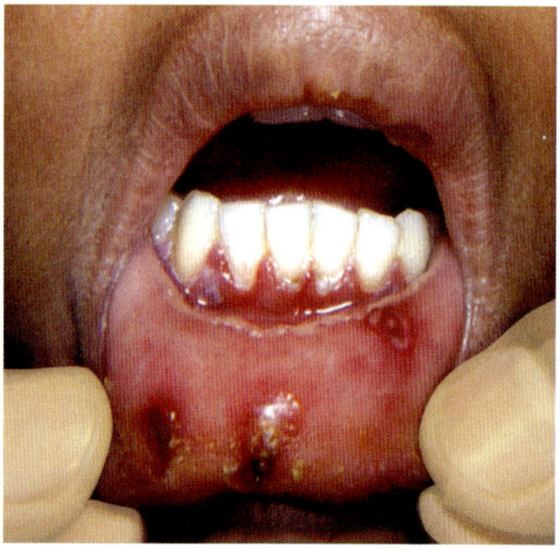

Fig. 14.5: Oral ulcers in herpes gingivostomatitis in a child

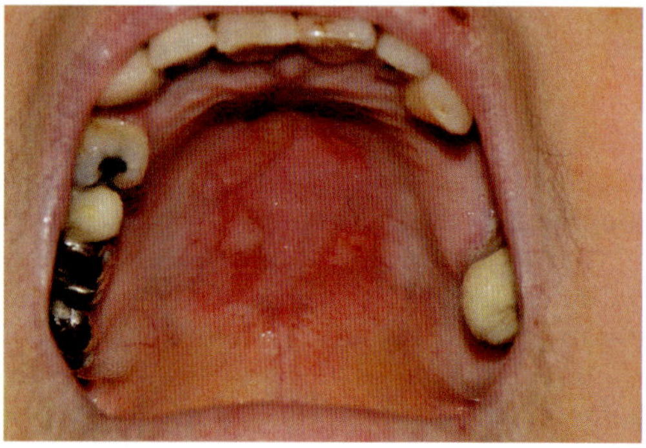

Fig. 14.6: Pemphigus vulgaris with multiple widespread oral ulceration

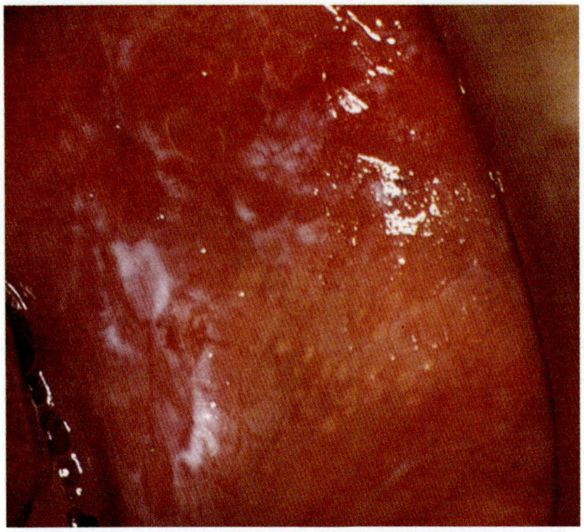

Fig. 14.7: Ulcerative lichen affecting buccal mucosa with a history of recurrent episodes. Pathognomonic feature is keratotic striae seen at the margins of the ulcer

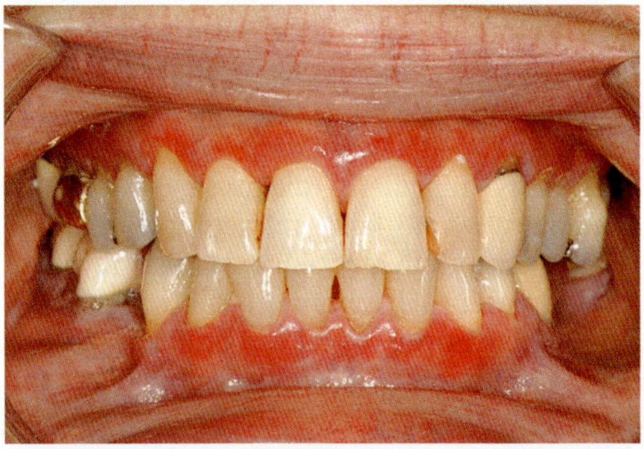

Fig. 14.8: Mucous membrane pemphigoid presenting as desquamative gingivitis. Ulcers may be found elsewhere in the oral cavity

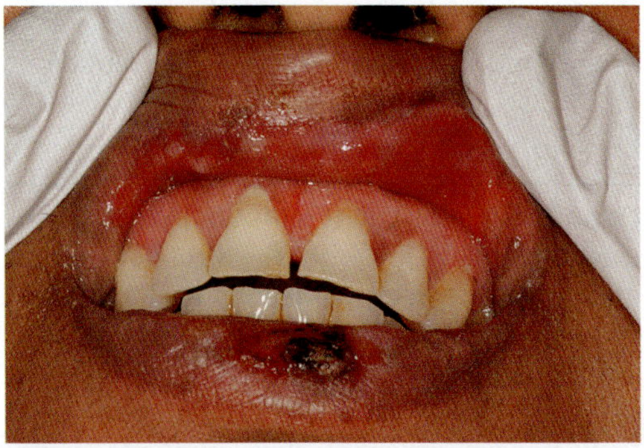

Fig. 14.9: Erythema multiforme ulceration affecting lips and labial mucosa. Crusting is a classical feature

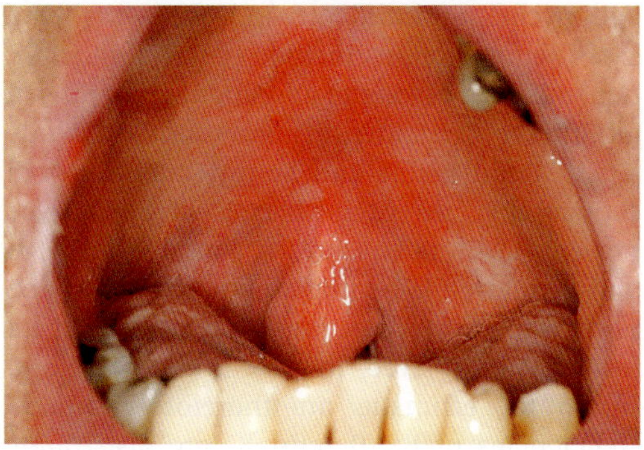

Fig. 14.10: Herpangina affecting soft palate

present with 'aphthous-type' ulceration which occurs at intervals (often monthly), reflecting their neutropenic status.

In patients who appear to present with atypical forms of RAU in later life it is advisable to assay antibodies against desmoglein 3 or to send a fresh specimen for direct immunofluorescence studies to exclude pemphigus vulgaris. These conditions should be considered prior to initiating therapies appropriate for a diagnosis of RAU.

Systemic diseases involving hematological, and nutritional deficiencies have been associated with recurrent oral ulcers. Oral ulcers have been reported in patients with cyclic neutropenia, hypogammaglobulinemia and agranulocytosis. These are discussed in detail in Chapter 20. Among hematological diseases a history of chronic anemia, myeloproliferative disorders or leukemia may be associated with oral ulceration.

Anemia and Vitamin Deficiencies

ROU may be associated with anemia commonly resulting from iron, folate, vitamin B_{12} deficiencies or due to chronic blood loss. These conditions should be excluded prior to the diagnosis of RAU or treated in primary care.

In patients with ROU (mimicking RAU) it is important to check for a history of anemia, evidence of blood loss, heavy menstrual periods, hemorrhoids or a vegetarian diet. General signs and symptoms of anemia may be present: lethargy, fatigue, shortness of breath, koilonychia, and difficulty in swallowing. Oral signs and symptoms include pallor of mucosa, depapillation of tongue and angular cheilitis in addition to ROU. Investigations should include a full blood count and serum micronutrient estimations (*see* Chapter 22). ROU may be present even before overt anemia develops and therefore the hemoglobin estimate may be normal in such cases. Measurement of serum ferritin, folate levels in serum and RBC and serum B_{12} estimates are therefore required. Deficiencies of B_1, B_2 and B_6 are also rarely reported as predisposing to ROU. Appropriate supplementation should be undertaken and hematological parameters monitored to ensure any deficiency is corrected.

GI Tract Diseases

A small cohort of patients initially presenting with RAU may on investigation be found to have these GI tract disorders. Patients with inflammatory bowel disease may develop ROU. GI tract diseases of significance are:

- Crohn's disease
- Ulcerative colitis
- Coeliac disease.

In these GI tract disorders, whether the link to ROU is related to immunologic mechanisms or nutritional deficiencies resulting from malabsorption is unknown. Patients with ulcerative colitis may present with pyostomatitis vegetans and the diagnosis needs to be confirmed by biopsy. Histology reveals a significant eosinophil response, and formation of intraepithelial miliary microabscesses.

HIV-associated ROU

ROU is common in patients with HIV disease. HIV-seropositive patients with CD4+ lymphocyte counts below 200 cells/mm^3 are more likely to have recurrent major aphthae. In HIV-infected individuals, these ulcers occur more frequently, last longer and produce more painful symptoms than in immunocompetent persons. Oral biopsy of an ulcer is required for prolonged nonhealing ulcers in order to exclude the possibility of deep fungal infections (e.g. CMV-associated disease). The management is different to RAU, for example, thalidomide

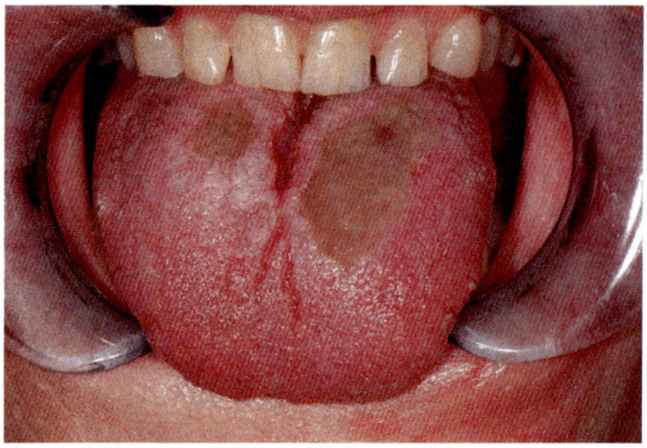

Fig. 14.11: Chronic ulcerative stomatitis affecting dorsal tongue

therapy is beneficial and is discussed later in this chapter.

CHRONIC ULCERATIVE STOMATITIS

This is an immunologically mediated often recalcitrant condition that produces chronic painful oral ulceration. Tongue (**Fig. 14.11**) and gingivae are the most common affected sites. It is difficult to diagnose clinically or histologically and fairly refractory to therapy. Direct immunofluorescence studies reveal a unique pattern of IgG immunoglobin deposition (binding) to nuclei of oral keratinocytes, mostly seen in the basal areas of the epithelium. The condition may represent a variant of Crohn's disease (regional ulcerative enteritis) as such is resistant to local therapy. High dose steroid therapy, mycophenolate mofetil may be tried. The literature indicates hydroxychloroquine (plaquenil) may be helpful. For this reason its important to distinguish CUS from other ROU as the condition is nonresponsive to steroids.

SYNDROMES ASSOCIATED WITH ROU

Other systemic conditions/syndromes associated with ROU include MAGIC (mouth and genital ulcers with inflamed cartilage) syndrome, FAPA syndrome (periodic fever, aphthous ulcers, pharyngitis and cervical adenitis) and Sweets' syndrome (fever and leukocytosis, recurrent skin eruptions, particularly localized to dorsal hands or upper neck and aphthous-like oral ulcers, arthritis and myalgia). Stevens Johnson syndrome (SJS) referred to earlier-results in wide-spread superficial oral ulceration with involvement of other mucosal sites and skin eruptions.

DRUG-INDUCED RECURRENT ORAL ULCERATION

Antineoplastic medications cause ulcerative stomatitis in a majority of patients receiving therapy for acute or chronic leukemia. The likely mechanism is accelerated detachment of oral epithelial cells. Antineoplastic drugs associated with stomatitits include methotrexate, 5-fluorouracil, doxorubicin, melphalan and hydroxyurea. Predicting which patients are most likely to manifest stomatitis is not possible. Several studies reported well circumscribed, single or multiple ovoid-shaped oral ulcers resembling either aphthous stomatitis or herpetic lesions located mostly on nonkeratinized mucosa. Also noted in patients receiving mTOR inhibitor therapy for advanced cancers.

Sometimes the effect is local such as placement of an aspirin tablet or cetiprin. Other examples of medications causing ROU include antimicrobials (sulfonamides and tetracyclins, didanosine, foscarnet), griseofulvin, non-steroidal anti-inflammatory drugs (e.g. indomethacin, salicylates, gold salts, naproxen), D-penicillamine, barbiturates, phenytoin and quinidine.

Cardiovascular medications including anti-hypertensives can cause oral ulceration—e.g. Captopril. More recently elderly patients on nicorandil (on doses above 20 mg/day) given for the treatment of unstable angina has attracted attention of specialist centres due to a flux of patients with ROU caused by this medication. A recent study has reported the visual assessment of photographs of nicorandil-associated lesions by 60 dermatologists and the outcome was that most regarded these ulcers as nonaphthous in appearance. They have some similarities with major aphthous ulcers in that they are large and have a protracted healing time, but they tend to lack the yellow base and erythematous halo that are usually associated with aphthous ulcers. These drug-induced ulcers have a punched out appearance which is not seen in aphthous

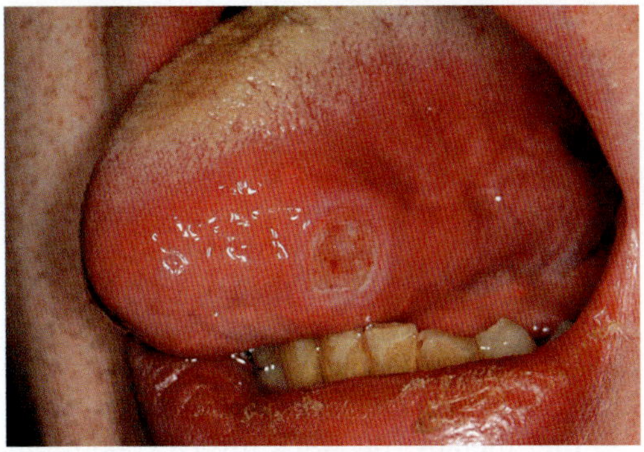

Fig. 14.12: A drug-induced ulcer (caused by nicorandil) with an aphthous like appearance. *Note:* Absence of erythema in the margins of the ulcer

ulceration. Most cases of nicorandil-induced ulceration that have had biopsies of their lesions carried out demonstrated nonspecific ulceration.

Some drug-induced ulcerative lesions may mimic erythema multiforme like lesions particularly in SJS, pemphigus/pemphigoid like reactions or present as nonspecific RAU like ulcers (**Fig. 14.12**). Drugs associated with or causing SJS include all forms of sulfonamides, trimethoprim-sulfamethoxazole, nonsteroidal anti-inflammatory agents, penicillins, anticonvulsants such as barbiturates and carbamazepine, valproic acid, allopruinol and terbinafine. The cytotoxic T-cell response in EM/SJS is presumably against keratinocytes expressing drug antigens. Thus a complete drug history at the initial assessment is essential in formulating a differential diagnosis of ROU.

MANAGEMENT

Therapy for recurrent aphthous ulcers (RAU) should concern pain relief, promotion of healing and to reduce recurrence. At the outset the roles of stress and trauma should be assessed. Before initiating medications for RAU, clinicians should determine whether well-recognized causes are contributing to the disease, in which case the presenting disorder will not be classified as RAU. Screening tests for allergies and nutritional deficiencies should be performed. Skin-patch tests for allergies to food additives, flavoring agents and essential oils may be helpful. A gluten-free diet has shown success in reducing ROU episodes both in the presence and in the absence of celiac disease. Hematologic testing (*see* Chapter 22) should be considered in patients with a history of ROU since patients with nutritional deficiencies respond well to replacement therapy.

Once these initial tests have excluded any underlying disorder the group with RAU may be managed to help their symptoms.

The therapy of RAU involves both an empirical as well as a scientific approach. The primary goals of therapy for RAU are relief of pain to reduce intensity of pain, reduction of ulcer duration, and restoration of normal oral function. Secondary goals include reduction in the frequency and severity of recurrences and maintenance of remission. There are few double-blind, placebo-controlled trial of drugs (topical or systemic) used in the treatment of RAU but only few have shown any significant benefit.

Topical Agents

For minor RAU viscous lidocaine (2%) provides symptomatic relief. Utility of both antibiotic (e.g. tetracycline) and antiseptic (e.g. chlorhexidine) mouthwashes have been studied in the management of RAU. These agents tend to help in healing thus reducing the duration of ulcers. The time required for healing of aphthous ulcers has been correlated with the ability of antimicrobial mouthwashes to reduce the population of oral mucosal flora.

Topical corticosteroids (**Table 14.3**) are usually prescribed for patients with RAU but only a few of these therapies have been tested in a randomized placebo-controlled trial. An appropriate topical corticosteroid is selected based on the size of the ulcers (minor or major) as well as the severity of symptoms that are present. Minor aphthae should be treated with low-to-mid-potency agents. Major lesions that may affect most parts of the mouth including keratinized mucosa need to be treated with mid-to-high potency agents (**Table 14.3**). Most cases benefit by regular topical use of steroids (combined with antiseptic and pain relieving mouth rinses) but few atypical cases, particularly among adults, may fail to respond to local therapy. Topical corticosteroid use in patients with RAU is intended to limit the inflammatory process associated with the formation of aphthae. Corticosteroids may act directly on T lymphocytes or alter the response of effectors cells to precipitants of immunopathogenesis. Topical corticosteroids of benefit are given in **Table 14.3** and the appropriate steroid strength should be selected as needed.

Only two double-blind, placebo-controlled trials have evaluated the efficacy of topical corticosteroids for RAU. These trials tested the application of betamethasone gel or beclomethasone aerosol spray to ulcers four times daily for four to six weeks. In both trials there were significant reductions, compared with placebo, in ulcer duration and pain severity. No-changes in the frequency of RAU were noticed.

Two nonplacebo controlled trials found no significant differences between triamcinolone ointment or betamethasone tablets and adhesive vehicles and orabase in the frequency and duration of severe RAU. A single-blind, placebo-controlled trial involving fluocinonide ointment was performed in patients with minor and

▪ Table 14.3
Topical corticosteroids for use with RAU

- Triamcinolone acetonide 0.1 percent paste applied with a dry finger to lesional sites after meals 4 times daily
- Soluble prednisolone tablets, 5 mg dissolved in 15 mL of water and used as a mouthrinse 3 times daily
- Betamethasone sodium phosphate (500 mcg dissolved in 10 of water) used as a mouthrinse up to 3 times daily
- Fluticasone propionate spray (50 mcg per puff), directed to affected areas up to 3–4 times daily
- Beclometasone spray (100 mcg per puff), sprayed 3–4 times daily on affected sites
- Clobetasol ointment (0.05%) 2 mL applied to painful areas 3–4 times daily
- Fluticasone cream (0.05%) applied to painful sites 3–4 times daily
- Fluticasone spray (50 μg; 2 puffs 4 times daily)

major RAU. Flucinonide ointment significantly reduced ulcer duration, but ulcer frequency and subjective improvement were the same as for adhesive vehicle (orabase).

It is possible to cause hypothalamic-pituitary-adrenal axis suppression with use of high potency corticosteroids. Potential absorption of the drug should be evaluated by the estimation of serum cortisol levels on a regular basis. Secondary opportunistic fungal infection may occur during therapy and all patients should be assessed for any raised candidal counts in the oral cavity and appropriately treated with antifungals. Mandatory screening procedures for patients on long term topical steroid therapies is recommended. Nonresponse to therapy should be evaluated by ascertaining patients' compliance and also that the local agent is reaching the target areas.

Nonsteroidal topical agents are also available. One such preparation is amlexanox (aphthasol) available as a 5 percent topical oral paste that has been developed for treatment of RAS. This drug has been approved by the FDA for RAS. It has anti-inflammatory properties and has been shown to accelerate healing of RAS. A recent double-blind study demonstrated its effectiveness in reducing ulcer erythema, pain, and lesional size.

Topical medications, such as antimicrobial mouthwashes and topical corticosteroids and other adhesive agents, can achieve the primary goals but have not been shown to alter recurrence or remission rates. All therapies are palliative, and none result in permanent remission. Intralesional injections of long acting corticosteroids are often effective in patients with lesions that are refractory to topical corticosteroids. When existing lesions are not controlled with topical agents, a specialist opinion needs to be sought to consider alternative systemic therapies.

Major RAU and nonhealing ROU may benefit by an intralesional corticosteroid injection and this approach should be tried prior to commencing systemic drugs.

Systemic Therapy

Systemic agents used in the past are listed in **Table 14.4**. In general these agents are only for second line of treatment when topical therapies have failed and reserved for complex or atypical RAU. Primary outcomes expected of systemic therapy include:

- Control of pain by reducing inflammation
- Reducing episode duration by promoting healing of ulcers
- Reducing episode frequency of RAU.

Systemic Corticosteroids

Systemic administration of steroids is reserved for the treatment of severe or recalcitrant disease when frequent recurrences of RAU are reported or when a patient is never ulcer-free. A low dose systemic corticosteroid, for example prednisolone 30 mg/day for a couple of weeks, then reducing by 5 mg/day to titrate to a final dose of 5 mg/day or every other day until remission have been advocated. In the author's experience longer term management on systemic steroids is rarely effective for RAU without causing serious side effects. At doses tolerated, those patients with more severe forms of atypical ulcers develop frequent crops needing to raise the dose of prednisolone too often.

Box 14.3: Therapy for RAU

Key features helpful in management

- Topical and intralesional corticosteroids are the standard therapies effective in a majority of patients
- Various systemic therapies are based on mostly open arm trials conducted on small number of cases
- The therapeutic ladder for severe aphthous ulceration ranges from topical and systemic steroid therapy through pentoxifylline, colchicine, azathioprine to oral thalidomide therapy
- When potent therapies are prescribed careful steps are needed to prevent pregnancy (e.g. thalidomide) and monitoring for neuropathy (colchicines and thalidomide) or liver toxicity (azathioprine)
- A steroid screen should be undertaken regularly for those on both topical and systemic steroids.

Table 14.4
Systemic drugs used in clinical trials

Immunomodulatory/anti-inflammatory
• Beta-glucan 1.3–1.6 (10 mg BD)
• Clofazime (100 mg OD)
• Colchicine (0.5 mg TDS)
• Levamisole (150 mg OD)
• Montelukast (leukotriene receptor antagonist) (10 mg OD)
• Pentoxifyline (400 mg TDS)
• Prednisone (25–40 mg OD-phased dose reduction)
• Sulodexide
Antimicrobials
• Subantimicrobial doxycycline (20 mg BD)
• Tetracycline (250 mg dissolved in 10 mL water; QDS)
Supplements
• Longovital (herbal + vitamin)
• Longovital (herbal alone)
• Propolis (500 mg OD)
• Vitamin B_{12}
• Multivitamin
Alternative therapy
• Camelthorn
• Homeopathy

Source: Adapted from Cochrane Database of Systematic Reviews 2005; Issue 3

Several recent reports have detailed the effectiveness of other systemic agents useful to treat oral aphthae that are nonresponsive to local steriods. These reports are all open label trials of steroid sparing agents tried on small numbers of patients.

Pentoxifylline

This is a medicine which is used in peripheral vascular disease. Results from one RCT run for 60-day suggested pentoxifylline (300 mg, 3 times/day) may have some benefit in the treatment of RAU, but the benefit is limited.

Colchicine

Prophylaxis with colchicine has been reported in several case series by authors who reported a favorable effect of this agent on patients with RAU. One RCT using colchicine (0.5 mg three times/day) compared to placebo failed to demonstrate a significant effect. Several possible mechanisms of action of the drug are discussed: it prevents recruitment of polymorphonuclear cells, interferes with their microtubular function and causes an inhibitory effect on the expression of adhesion molecules preventing the migration of white blood cells across blood vessel walls. The dose recommended is 1.5 mg/day, but it is prudent to start with a lower dose. Colchicine blood levels should be examined and toxic symptoms like myopathy and neuropathy should be regularly monitored, preferably at 3 monthly intervals. It may have potential adverse effects on male fertility when given long term to young males, and therefore sperm analysis is recommended, and the reproductive potential of treated patients carefully monitored. Most patients tolerate colchicine well, except for GI symptoms and experience a marked decrease in the frequency of oral ulceration and it is easy to use.

Azathioprine

Azathioprine, and mycophenolate mofetil have been reported to benefit patients with recalcitrant disease. Continued therapy is required to maintain the remission. Azathioprine given orally at a dose of 1 mg/kg is well tolerated but before instituting therapy selection of those who are able to metabolize the drug by performing a TPMT assay is recommended. Those with enzyme levels above 7 are usually able to tolerate this agent. Liver and hematological toxicity should be assessed with regular full blood counts and liver function tests to assess serum levels of liver transaminases. If the level of GGT or AST are more than doubled it is generally ill advised to continue therapy. The British Association of Dermatologists (BAD) has recently issued guidelines on use of azathioprine. Mycophenolate mofetil has fewer adverse side effects than azathioprine but its efficacy is less well-known. Mycophenolate mofetil is administered orally in a dose of 2 to 3 g daily. It is generally well tolerated, but gastrointestinal side-effects may limit its use in some patients. They are both slow acting and it may take at least 6 to 8 weeks to start to see the benefits.

Thalidomide

Thalidomide given per orally has recently been used for patients with major RAU or atypical ulcers in HIV seropositive subjects. NO RCTs are reported. Mechanism of action is not clear but believed to involve a decrease in inflammatory mediators, particularly tumor necrosis factor (TNF)-α and Fas-ligand. Thalidomide has been shown to selectively suppress NF-(Kappa) β activation induced by inflammatory mediators. Atypical major oral ulcers are highly angiogenic. Thalidomide may act to heal by inhibiting angiogenesis and promoting re-epithelialization. Open-label trials suggest that it is highly effective, and may result in an increase in the lymphocyte count and a decrease in the C-reactive protein level. Induction with 100 to 200 mg daily at bedtime results in improvement in 90 percent of the patients who are able to tolerate the drug. Most units however, recommend the lower dose for ROU of 50 mg a day. Toxicity commonly associated with thalidomide use includes drowsiness, headache, weight gain, amenorrhea and dizziness. Patients should be counseled on the risk of birth defects and those in childbearing ages advised to use two simultaneous forms of effective birth control starting at least 4 weeks before starting therapy and a pregnancy test performed before starting treatment. Drowsiness and dizziness may persist during the initial stages of therapy. Thalidomide neuropathy, usually sensory, and often associated with proximal weakness may limit the ability of patients to continue thalidomide on a long-term basis. Neuropathy may be reversible, but there are patients whose neuropathy has progressed despite stopping the drug. Nerve conduction (EMG) studies should be performed at the onset of therapy and periodically to screen for evidence of toxicity by checking for sensory responses. The nerve responses of superficial peroneal and sural nerves in both lower legs are evaluated by EMG for thalidomide monitoring. Antithrombotic prophylaxis for patients on thalidomide has been discussed but rarely indicated at the lower maintenance dose.

For reasons of toxicity topical thalidomide therapy has been advocated recently with some short term success.

Thalidomide is a potent teratogen and accordingly a strict program to prevent the chance of pregnancy in patients exposed to the drug should be initiated at onset and regularly monitored by the responsible physician. Unfortunately the response to thalidomide is not durable in most patients therefore long-term, low-dose maintenance therapy may be necessary.

Levamisole

Levamisole is an immunopotentiating agent that has demonstrated the ability to normalize the CD4+ cell/CD8+ cell ratio and improve symptoms in RAU patients. Correction of T-suppressor-cell deficiency may reduce the inflammatory response resulting from cellular immunity and promote resolution of aphthae. Seven placebo-controlled clinical trials assessed the efficacy and safety levamisole in patients with RAU. Four of the studies showed a reduction in the frequency and duration of aphthous ulcers during levamisole treatment with ulcer recurrences decreasing by half in up to 43 percent of patients. In six trials a complete absence of ulcers was found at the conclusion of the study in 16 of 144 patients receiving levamisole. Levamisole was well tolerated in a majority of the patients. The most frequent adverse effects were dysgeusia (21%) and nausea (16%).

Other Therapies

Other therapies that have been used in open trials include cromoglycic acid, bio-quinine, and zinc sulphate. No RCTs are published on these agents.

Longovital a herbal-based vitamin/mineral preparation has been reported to provide benefit but the evidence is limited.

Some benefit is reported by trying out toothpaste without sodium lauryl sulfate, antibacterial mouthwashes to reduce secondary infection and avoidance of foods that trigger or exacerbate the ulcers.

Further trials are needed to ascertain these claims. Future trials should assess any reduction in: the median pain score, ulcer size, number of ulcers, total number of ulcer episodes and ulcer-free periods.

SELF-ASSESSMENT QUESTIONS

1. Give a classification of recurrent oral ulceration.
2. How would you distinguish RAU from other recurrent oral ulcers?
3. Explain the features that differentiate the three types of RAU.
4. Write an appraisal of etiopathogenesis of RAU.
5. What outcomes do you expect when initiating treatment for RAU? How do you assess treatment success?
6. What systemic treatments are available for RAU that do not respond to topical steroids? Explain the mechanisms of action.
7. During an initial consultation how would you eliminate systemic disease as a cause of ROU?
8. How would you monitor a patient given corticosteroid therapy at frequent intervals to treat complex aphthosis?

SUGGESTED READING

1. Baccaglini L, et al. Urban legends: recurrent aphthous stomatitis. Oral Dis. 2011;17:755-70.
2. Eisen D, Lynch DP. Selecting topical and systemic agents for recurrent aphthous stomatitis. Cutis. 2001;68:201-6.
3. Escudier M, Began J, Scully C. Behcet's disease. Oral Dis. 2006;12:78-84.
4. Jurge S, Kuffer R, Scully C, Porter SR. Recurrent aphthous stomatitis. Oral Diseases. 2006;12:1-21.
5. Mignogna MD, Fortuna G, Leuci S. Oral pemphigus. Minerva Stomatol. 2009;58:501-18.
6. Porter SR, Hegarty A, Kaliakatsou F, Hodgson T, Scully C. Recurrent aphthous stomatitis. Clinics in Dermatology. 2000;18:569-78.

Chapter 15

Vesiculobullous Disorders

Paula Farthing

Chapter Outline

INTRODUCTION

Vesiculobullous disorders are characterized by the formation of fluid filled blisters which usually burst to leave areas of erosion or ulceration. In addition to the oral mucosa, they may affect other mucous membranes including genital, conjunctival, esophageal and laryngeal and many also affect the skin. In broad terms, there are two main causes: infective and autoimmune.

The infective causes are almost all viral and most are caused by members of the Herpes family, e.g. herpes simplex and zoster. These are outlined in detail in Chapter 16 and will not be considered further here. The others are usually the result of autoantibody production against components of the epithelium and basement membrane, so called type 2 hypersensitivity reactions.

Much work over recent years has been directed at identifying the antigens which are targeted by the autoantibodies. Broadly, they fall into two groups: those which target desmosomes, the structures which hold epithelial cells together and those which target hemidesmosomes and components of the basement membrane, which bind the epithelium to the underlying connective tissue. This research has lead not only to an increased understanding of epithelial and basement membrane structure but also has started to explain the differing clinical presentations of these diseases.

▪ Table 15.1
Vesiculobullous disorders classified by the level of separation

Intraepithelial separation	*Subepithelial separation*
Pemphigus vulgaris	Bullous pemphigoid
Pemphigus foliaceus	Mucous membrane pemphigoid
Paraneoplastic pemphigus	Cicatricial or ocular pemphigoid
IgA pemphigus	Linear IgA Disease Dermatitis herpetiformis Epidermolysis bullosa acquisita

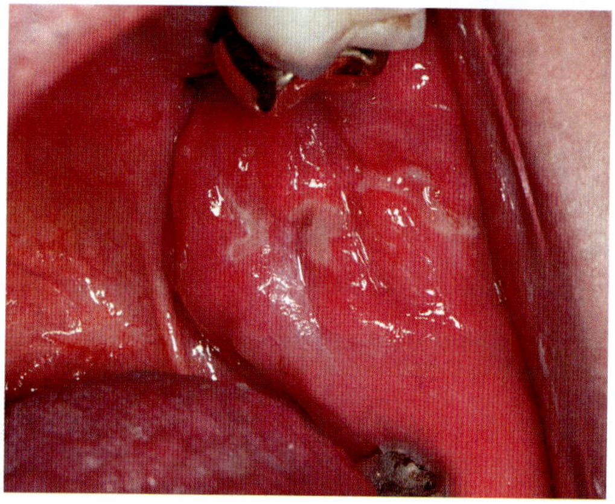

Fig. 15.1: Widespread erosions and ulceration affecting the buccal mucosa in a patient with pemphigus vulgaris

Vesiculobullous disorders may be classified according to the level of separation within the mucosa (**Table 15.1**):

a. Intraepithelial separation
b. Subepithelial separation.

This separation is the result of which structures of the oral mucosa are targeted **(Fig. 15.1)**. Intraepithelial separation occurs when autoantibodies target components of the desmosomes and subepithelial separation, when they target hemidesmosomes and basement membrane components.

DISEASES CHARACTERIZED BY INTRAEPITHELIAL SEPARATION

Pemphigus

Pemphigus is a group of autoimmune mediated disorders characterized by autoantibodies targeting the desmosomes. They are potentially life threatening and prior to the introduction of systemic glucocorticosteroids were often fatal. The most common variant affecting the oral mucosa is pemphigus vulgaris.

Pemphigus Vulgaris

Pemphigus vulgaris is a relatively rare disorder that affects between 1 to 9 per 1×10^6 of the population. Unlike most autoimmune diseases, it appears to affect men and women equally and occurs most commonly in third to fifth decades.

Higher incidences are seen in particular races such as Ashkenazi Jews (up to 32 per 1×10^6) and in individuals of Mediterranean and South east Asian origin. This genetic predisposition appears to be related to human leukocyte antigen (HLA) Class II phenotype as is common with many autoimmune diseases. In Ashkenazi Jews those with HLA-DRw4 particularly DRB1 (*0402 and *0401) alleles are susceptible and in white caucasians, Pakistani and Japanese patients, the rare HLA-DQB1 (*0503) allele confers susceptibility.

Clinical Features

Pemphigus vulgaris usually affects the oral mucosa initially (up to 70% cases) and lesions affect the posterior buccal mucosa, the gingivae and palate most commonly although any area may be affected. Initial lesions are flaccid, fragile vesicles or bullae but these easily rupture to leave ragged erosions which may ulcerate. Both the free and attached gingivae may be affected and appear fiery red and show desquamation. This condition is referred to as desquamative gingivitis but is not specific to pemphigus vulgaris and is also seen in lichen planus and mucous membrane pemphigoid. Indeed several studies have shown it is more common in the latter conditions.

Patients with pemphigus vulgaris often complain of pain and difficulty with eating as well as a history that lesions develop following trauma. Lesions of pemphigus vulgaris may be restricted to the oral mucosa but sometimes affect the larynx and pharynx and with time almost always spread to involve the skin. Skin lesions are characterized by flaccid, fragile bullae which may occur anywhere on the body. Initially they tend to affect the head and neck but then spread to the trunk and flexor areas of the limbs. They often rupture to leave painful erosions and ulcers. Without treatment the disease is fatal usually due to loss of fluids and secondary infection.

Diagnosis

Diagnosis is made on the basis of history and examination, biopsy and blood tests. Biopsy is necessary to distinguish the condition from other vesiculobullous disorders and to confirm the presence of autoantibodies in the tissues as well as the blood. It is important to biopsy peri-lesional rather than lesional tissue and either send it fresh to the laboratory or freeze it immediately. Blood should be placed in a plain tube and allowed to clot. Immunofluorescent tests detect autoantibodies in the tissues (direct immunofluorescence) and in the serum (indirect immunofluorescence) but they can only be carried out on fresh tissue as fixation destroys the antigens they detect. The basis of the test is that anti-human antibodies raised in mice against the Fc (tail) portion of human IgG, IgA, IgM and C3 (complement), are reacted with the patient's biopsy. These anti-human antibodies have been tagged with a fluorescent dye which can be identified by fluorescent microscopy. In a patient with pemphigus vulgaris a characteristic fish scale pattern of IgG and C3 is seen surrounding the cells of the prickle cell layer (**Fig. 15.2**). In indirect immunofluorescence the basis of the test is the same except that monkey esophagus or fresh normal oral mucosa is incubated with the patient's serum prior to the addition of the anti-human antibody.

Although the immunofluorescence test can localize the antibodies to either the desmosomes or subepithelial components, other tests are necessary to identify the antigens more precisely. These include immunoblotting, enzyme linked immunoabsorbant assay and

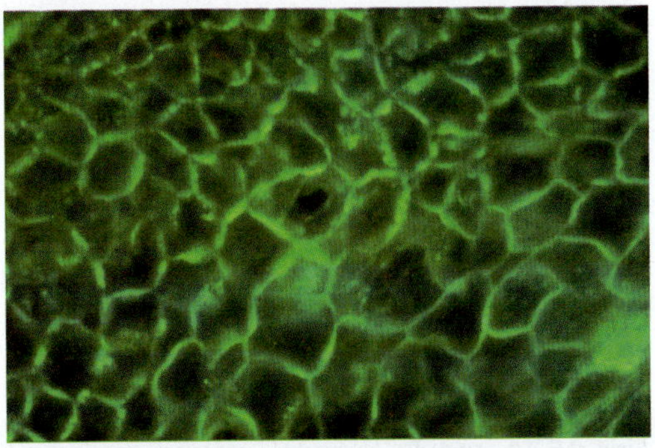

Fig. 15.2: Deposition of IgG around the periphery of cells in the prickle cell layer, so-called fish scale pattern in a patient with pemphigus vulgaris

immuno precipitation. These tests are not usually used on a routine basis to confirm diagnosis as they require specialist laboratory techniques. Their basis is that they use epithelial cell lysates or recombinant proteins which are then reacted with the patient's serum.

Histopathology

The oral mucosa shows evidence of a bullae and loss of adhesion between epithelial cells in the prickle cell layer. This occurs just above the basal cell layer and the separation is termed acantholysis. The epithelial cells appear rounded, sometimes forming groups or individual cells in the bullae. These cells are known as Tzank cells and before the advent of immunofluorescent testing were important in the diagnosis. The basal cells remain attached to the basement membrane and have been likened to a row of tombstones. There may be a mild inflammatory infiltrate in the lamina propria. (**Figs 15.3A and B**) In more advanced cases the superficial epithelium may have been lost leaving only the basal cells although often there may be total loss of the epithelium resulting ulceration. In these cases diagnosis is difficult or impossible explaining why it is important to biopsy perilesional tissue. The diagnosis is almost always confirmed by immunofluorescence tests.

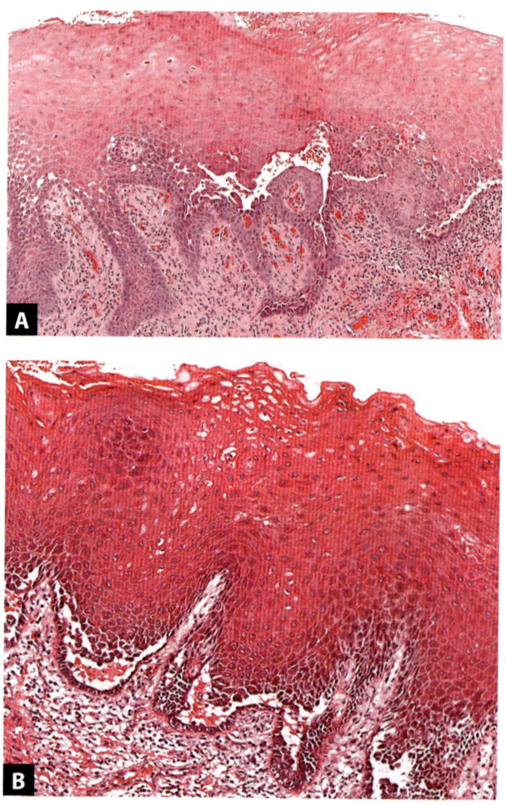

Figs 15.3A and B: H and E stained section of mucosa from a patient with pemphigus vulgaris. *Note:* The intraepithelial separation with the basal cells remaining attached to the basement membrane

Pathogenesis

Pemphigus vulgaris is the result of circulating autoantibodies produced against components of the desmosomes (**Fig. 15.4**). Desmogleins are cadherin-like proteins which cross the intercellular space between adjacent epithelial cells and almost all patients have antibodies to desmoglein 3 (Dsg3) and some in addition, against desmoglein1 (Dsg1). A small subset have antibodies to the α 9-acetylcholine receptor. The antigens targeted by the antibodies in any given patient correlate to the distribution and severity of the disease. Patients with antibodies against Dsg3 have lesions predominantly affecting the oral mucosa with few skin lesions. In contrast patients with antibodies against Dsg1 have predominantly skin lesions but in this case, the separation is towards the top of the prickle cell layer- resulting in pemphigus foliaceous. Patients with both Dsg1 and 3 antibodies have both mucosal and skin lesions. This distribution is the result of differing proportions and distribution of Dsg 1 and 3 in oral mucosa and skin.

Almost all the antibodies are IgG in class and in active disease they are IgG4. However, IgA antibodies are present in a rare variant—IgA pemphigus. There is a considerable amount of evidence to show that these antibodies are the cause of the disease. Levels of circulating autoantibodies correlate with disease severity and purified antibodies from patients with pemphigus vulgaris cause the disease when injected into mice. However the mechanisms which result in separation are not clear although

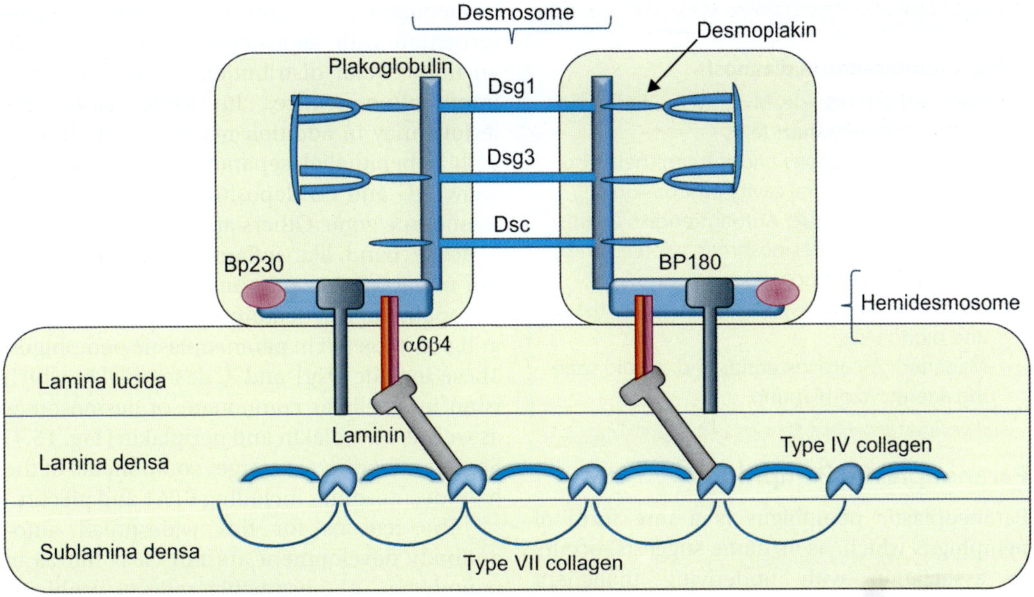

Fig. 15.4: Structure of a desmosome, hemidesmosome and basement membrane zone in stratified squamous epithelium. Dsg = desmoglein, Dsc = desmocollins

it has been postulated to involve release of proteases and proinflammatory cytokines from keratinocytes. Complement fixation occurs in almost all cases but is thought to amplify the disease rather than playing an essential role since acantholysis still occurs in complement depleted mice.

The trigger for the development of pemphigus is not known but it has long been postulated that cell-mediated immunity may be involved. The production of antibodies by B-cells is controlled by CD4 positive T-cells and T-cells autoreactive against Dsg3 have been detected in patients with pemphigus. However, these cells are also found in healthy individuals but in disease it may an imbalance between autoreactive Th2-type T cells and regulatory Th1 cells which is important since the later are only rarely detected in disease.

Management

Following diagnosis, the mainstay of treatment is immunosuppression. For localized oral lesions, topical or intralesional corticosteroids may be used but for more severe disease systemic corticosteroids are necessary and indeed this is the mainstay of treatment. Steroid sparing agents such as dapsone, azothiaprine and methotrexate are useful to reduce steroid dosage. Levels of Dsg3 and 1 antibodies correlate with disease severity and measuring the titers of each against the clinical symptoms can be useful in delivering minimum dosages to control symptoms. In some patients the initial high doses of steroids are sufficient to keep the disease under control and with time can be reduced. Indeed, some patients undergo complete remission and the proportion of these increases with time. In others, however, long-term steroids are necessary to keep the disease under control. A positive long-term response appears to be related to the initial severity and extent of the disease as well as early response to treatment.

Other forms of treatment which have been used include plasmapheresis and the use of intravenous immunoglobulins. For steroid-resistant pemphigus vulgaris the monoclonal anti-CD20 antibody, rituximab used as a single agent has been shown to be an effective therapy.

Box 15.1: Pemphigus

Key features useful in diagnosis
- Rare, 3rd-5th decade, M=F, HLA-DRw4 association and Ashkanazi Jews
- Widespread erosions and intraepithelial bullae affecting the oral cavity and/or skin
- *Autoimmune disease*: Autoantibodies against desmoglein in desmosomes, detected by immunofluorescence
- Diagnosis by biopsy of paralesional tissue and blood tests
- Managed by corticosteroids and steroid sparing agents: Azothiaprine.

Paraneoplastic Pemphigus

Paraneoplastic pemphigus is a rare form of pemphigus which, as its name suggests, occurs in association with underlying malignant disease. In a high proportion of cases this is hematological in origin and includes lymphomas and leukemia. Nonhematological causes include adenocarcinoma, squamous cell carcinoma and sarcomas. It has been suggested the disease is renamed paraneoplastic autoimmune multiorgan syndrome because of the multitude of clinical features and disease associations.

Clinical Features

In most cases, the clinical features resemble those of pemphigus vulgaris and include vesicles and bullae and widespread erosions and ulcerations. Mucosal lesions are an almost constant feature and may involve multiple sites including the naso- and oropharynx, conjunctiva and anogenital region. The skin is often also affected with blisters on the upper trunk, head and neck and extremities. Some lesions appear lichenoid and are composed small red flat topped papules particularly in children but in other cases, target lesions resembling erythema multiforme or graft versus host disease may be evident.

The disease can occur at any age and there is no gender predilection. However, because of the association with malignancy the average age is in the 7th decade.

Histopathology and Pathogenesis

The histopathological features often resemble those of pemphigus vulgaris and show intraepithelial acantholysis and bullae formation with deposition of IgG and C3 in an intercellular distribution evident on direct immunofluorescence. In some cases the lesions may in addition resemble pemphigoid with subepithelial separation and these also show IgG and C3 deposition at the basement membrane zone. Others appear lichenoid with a dense band like inflammatory infiltrate in the upper lamina propria. This variety in the histopathological features is reflected in the antigens targeted in paraneoplastic pemphigus. These include Dsg1 and 3, desmoplakin which is an intracellular component of desmosomes as well as envoplakin and periplakin (**Fig. 15.4**) Some antibodies also target components of the hemidesmosomes including BPA1 and plectin.

The reasons for this widespread autoantibody development are not clear but as in pemphigus, it presumably reflects problems with immune regulation.

Management

The disease is often fatal and may be difficult to control. Patients often die from the mucosal and skin lesions rather than the underlying malignancy. This is particularly true with low-grade malignant disease. Hig-dose corticosteroids are often used initially with the introduction of steroid sparing agents later. Immunosuppression remains the mainstay of treatment.

Box 15.2: Paraneoplastic pemphigus

Key features useful in diagnosis
- Similar clinical and histological features to pemphigus vulgaris
- Associated with underlying malignant disease
- Often fatal.

Other Variants of Pemphigus

Pemphigus Foliaceous

This rare variant usually only affects the skin and is characterized by IgG autoantibodies against Dsg1 which is expressed predominantly in the upper part of the prickle cell layer in the epidermis but at very low levels in the oral mucosa. Acantholysis and bullae formation occurs in the upper rather than the lower prickle cell layer of the epidermis and the disease is less severe than pemphigus vulgaris. Skin lesions appear scattered and scaly and may resemble psoriasis. Bullae formation is not obvious clinically and the oral cavity is rarely involved. Patients are managed by corticosteroids.

IgA Pemphigus

IgA pemphigus is characterized by deposition of IgA antibodies around the surface of keratinocytes in the prickle cells layer. Histologically, numerous intraepithelial bullae are seen filled with neutrophils. Two clinical forms of the disease are recognized SPD or subcorneal pustular dermatosis, and intraepidermal neutrophilic IgA dermatosis (IEN). Lesions are characterized by pustules forming annular patterns on the skin. Mucosal lesions may be present and show widespread ulceration. The target is desmocollins in SPD type but more heterogenous antibodies are present in IEN type.

DISEASES CHARACTERIZED BY SUBEPITHELIAL SEPARATION

There are a number of immune-mediated conditions in which autoantibodies are directed against components of the basement membrane zone. This interaction leads to separation of the entire thickness of the epithelium from the underlying connective tissue resulting in a subepithelial bullae. These conditions differ from one another in the antigens that are targeted in the basement membrane zone and this in part explains their differing clinical presentations. They are listed in **Table 15.2**.

Bullous Pemphigoid

Clinical Features

Bullous pemphigoid is the most common subepithelial, blistering disorder affecting the skin and oral lesions are uncommon (10–20% cases). Patients are often elderly and the incidence rises in patients over the age of 60 years. It is characterized by rather tense bullae which

▪ Table 15.2
Diseases characterized by subepithelial separation

Disease	*Direct immunofluorescence*	*Indirect immunofluorescence*	*Antigen targeted*
Bullous pemphigoid	Linear IgG and C3 basement membrane zone	Circulating IgG in 90% cases	BP180 and BP230
Mucous membrane pemphigoid—oral lesions only	Linear IgG and C3 basement membrane zone	Low-levels: IgG 18% patients	α6chain of α6β4 integrin
Ocular/cicatricial pemphigoid	Linear IgG and C3 at basement membrane zone Some cases IgA	Low-levels circulating IgG 7% patients	β4 chain of α6β4 integrin
Mucous membrane and skin pemphigoid	Linear IgG/IgA/C3	Circulating IgG/A in 80% cases	BP180 and BP230
Linear IgA disease	Linear IgA at basement membrane zone	Circulating IgA high proportion	BP180 and BP230 and unknown antigens
Dermatitis herpetiformis	Granular IgA basement membrane zone	None	epidermal transgluataminase 3,
Epidermolysis bullosa aquisita	Linear IgG and C3 basemment membrane zone. IgA 10%	Circulating IgG 50%	Type VII collagen and others unknown

appear to affect the lower abdomen particularly as well as the inner aspects of the thighs. Because the bullae involve the entire thickness of the epithelium they are less fragile than those of pemphigus vulgaris. Oral lesions are similarly characterized by tense bullae which may affect any area of the mucosa. They rupture to form ulcers.

Histopathology and Pathogenesis

Histologically, the lesions are characterized by separation of the entire thickness of the epidermis from the underlying dermis. Typically, accumulations of eosinophils are seen at the tips of the dermal papillae and there is variable inflammation. Direct immunofluorescence shows linear deposition of IgG and C3 at the basement membrane zone in almost all cases. Unlike pemphigus it is difficult to detect circulating autoantibodies using indirect immunofluorescence. The sensitivity of the technique can be increased by using salt-split skin. This results in separation of the epidermis from the dermis through the basement membrane thus exposing more antigens. When this is carried out circulating autoantibodies are found in almost 90 percent of cases.

Almost all patients with bullous pemphigoid have autoantibodies directed against two components of the basement membrane zone, so called BP230 and BP180. These were originally identified using immunoprecipitation but they are now recognized as components of the hemi-desmosomes which attach the epithelial cells to the basement membrane. (**Fig. 15.4**). BP230 is an intracellular component of the hemidesmosome but BP180 is a transmembrane molecule which extends into the lamina lucida where it interacts with laminin 5. BP180 is now known to be Type XVII collagen.

As with pemphigus, there is considerable evidence to show that the autoantibodies are responsible for the disease. This includes the observation that the disease can be caused when antibodies are injected into neonatal mice.

Management

Topical or systemic corticosteroids are the mainstay of treatment. Severe disease is treated with systemic corticosteroids together with steroid sparing agents such as azathioprine. Occasionally, methotrexate may be used in patients who are unresponsive to steroids. More mild cases are treated topically. Most cases resolve within 2 to 5 years.

Box 15.3: Bullous pemphigoid

Key features useful in diagnosis

- Affects skin>mucosa, elderly patients, tense subepithelial bullae and ulcers
- Autoimmune antibodies against hemidesmosomes- antigens (BP230 and BP180)
- Subepithelial blisters
- Management: corticosteroids and steroid sparing agents.

Mucous Membrane Pemphigoid

Mucous membrane pemphigoid is a condition that affects the mucous membranes. It was originally known as benign mucous membrane pemphigoid but it is a disease which may carry significant morbidity and the benign suffix has been dropped. Mucous membrane pemphigoid is heterogeneous not only in its severity and the mucous membranes affected, but also by the antibodies which target different molecules in the hemidesmosomes and basement membrane. Several clinical variants have now been recognized.

Clinical Features

Patients are usually middle-aged or elderly females in the 5th and 6th decades. The lesions present as tense fluid-filled bullae which may rupture to give widespread ulcers and erosions. In the oral cavity any area may be affected but lesions on the hard and soft palate, buccal mucosa and gingivae are common. (**Fig. 15.5**). The latter presentation is usually one of desquamative gingivitis. Lesions may

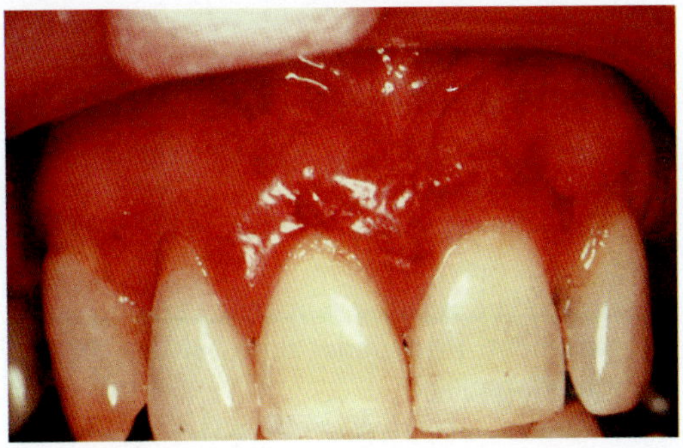

Fig. 15.5: Clinical picture of pemphigoid. *Note:* The blister formation and erosions affecting the gingivae

be induced by trauma—the so-called Nikolsky sign but this is not specific to pemphigoid and may also be seen in pemphigus. Patients often complain they have difficulty in eating and drinking and that their mucosa is 'peeling.' The lesions heal slowly and sometimes lead to scarring.

Lesions can spread to the naso-and oropharynx and may result in extreme difficulties with eating and drinking. Problems may arise with scarring and the formation of strictures in severe cases. In some patients, the mucous membranes of the genitalia and rarely the anus are affected. The conjunctiva is commonly affected and initial lesions are characterized by recurrent conjunctivitis which may last for many years. With the development of blisters, the patient may develop symblepharon (fusion of the bulbar and palprebal conjunctiva), inverted eyelashes as well as corneal scarring. This may lead to blindness and is a serious complication. Some patients develop skin lesions but this tends to be only a small proportion. The lesions resemble those of bullous pemphigoid and typically affect the trunk and head and neck.

Variants

There are a number of variants recognized depending on the sites affected and also the antibodies identified. The oral variant or oral pemphigoid as its name suggests is characterized by oral lesions only. This group have antibodies against the α6 chain of the α4β6 integrin (**Fig. 15.4**). On direct immunofluorescence, these patients show linear IgG and low levels of circulating autoantibodies.

Ocular/cicatricial pemphigoid: These patients are characterized by ocular lesions and show IgG antibodies against the β4 integrin subunit. Another group may show IgA antibodies against a 45KD antigen as yet uncharacterized.

Mucous membrane and skin pemphigoid: These patients have antibodies against BP180 and 230 antigens. Another variant is recognized which is characterized by antibodies laminin 5 (also known as epiligrin) which binds to BP180 as well as collagen VII. This variant may be associated with an increased risk of internal malignancy.

Histology

Lesions are characterized by subepithelial separation and in the early stages may be associated by very little inflammation in the underlying lamina propria (**Fig. 15.6**). Occasional accumulations of neutrophils may seen together with eosinophils but the characteristic eosinophil accumulation seen in bullous pemphigoid is not obvious. In more established lesions accumulations of chronic inflammatory cells including plasma cells may be evident. Direct immunofluorescence may show deposition of IgG, IgM, IgA or C3 at the basement membrane zone in a linear deposition (**Fig. 15.7**). Circulating autoantibodies are not often seen but as with bullous pemphigoid the sensitivity of indirect immunofluorescence tests may be increased by using salt-split skin.

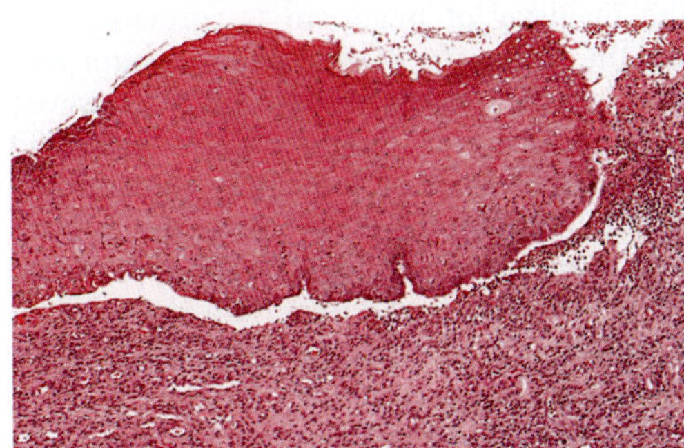

Fig. 15.6: Subepithelial separation in mucous membrane pemphigoid. The entire thickness of the epithelium has separated from the connective tissue

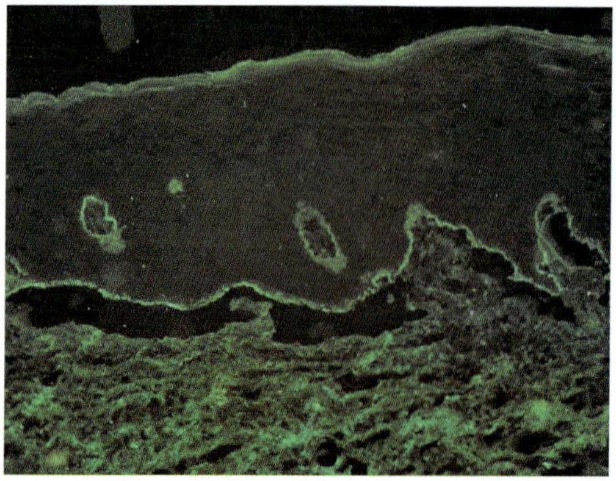

Fig. 15.7: Direct immunofluorescence in pemphigoid. Note the linear deposition of IgG at the basement membrane zone

Pathogenesis

There is considerable evidence that binding of autoantibodies to the hemidesmosomes and the basement membrane zone causes separation. The disease may be transferred passively by injection of antibodies in neonatal animals and these also cause disease in mucosa in organ culture. Blister formation appears to require complement activation and the presence of neutrophils as it does not occur in complement or neutrophil deficient mice. In addition it is thought that proteases may be important.

Management

The mainstay of treatment is corticosteroids and they bring the disease under control very quickly when taken systemically. However, patients with oral lesions may be controlled by topical steroids or sometimes intralesional steroid injections thus avoiding the serious side effects. Before deciding on the appropriate course of treatment, it is important to determine the severity of the disease. Generally, if only the oral mucous membranes are affected then topical steroids should be given. Patients with disease that affects more than one mucosal site are more high-risk and systemic steroids are advocated whilst those with any evidence of ocular lesions should be referred immediately for an ophthalmologist opinion.

Box 15.4: Mucous membrane pemphigoid

Key features useful in diagnosis

- Elderly, 6–7th decade, variable severity and manifestations
- Subepithelial bullae and erosions affecting mucous membranes
- Antibodies against hemidesmosomes and basement membrane zone: BP180, $\alpha4\beta6$ integrin, epiligrin
- *Cicatricial pemphigoid*: Affects eyes—may lead to scarring and blindness
- Low levels circulating antibodies
- Managed by topical or systemic corticosteroids.

Epidermolysis Bullosa

Epidermolysis bullosa are a group of disorders characterized by blistering of the skin and occasionally the mucous membranes. One group are inherited and are the result of genetic mutations in components of desmosomes, basement membrane or keratinocytes. They may be divided into simple, junctional and dystrophic types. The simple type is the result of mutations in keratins—intracellular components of keratinocytes. Junctional types show mutations in laminin and the dystrophic forms have mutations in Type VII collagen or in the $\beta4$ subunit of the $\alpha6\beta4$ integrin. These forms all show evidence of an inherited pattern

Epidermolysis Bullosa Aquisita

Epidermolysis bullosa aquisita is an acquired type of epidermolysis bullosa and unlike the inherited types usually although not always affects older individuals. Patients suffer from repeated and chronic subepithelial blistering which affects the skin and the oral mucous membrane in up to 50 percent of cases. It is relatively rare and accounts for about 5 percent of all cases of patients with antibodies against the basement membrane zone.

Clinical Features

It appears heterogeneous and some cases resemble the dystrophic form of inherited

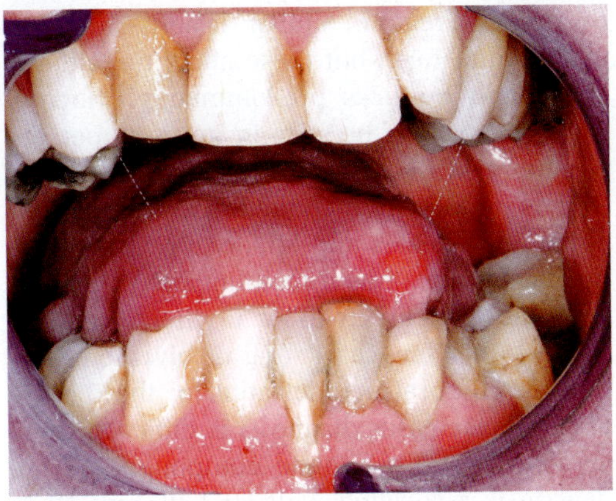

Fig. 15.8: Mucosal lesion in epidermolysis bullosa aquisita. *Note:* The ulceration and erythema on the tongue

epidermolysis aquisita. This may be because the autoantibodies target the same molecule which is mutated in the hereditary forms—Type VII collagen. Inflammatory and noninflammatory forms have been recognized. In the latter the skin is extremely fragile and trauma induces blisters and erosions. This may result in atrophy and the formation of milia. In patients with inflammatory type disease, it may be difficult to distinguish the condition from bullous pemphigoid and in these patients the flexural surfaces of the extremities are involved. The mucous membranes are also particularly affected (**Fig. 15.8**).

Histology

Histological changes include subepidermal separation which may or may not be associated with an inflammatory infiltrate in the underlying dermis. Direct immunofluorescence shows linear IgG and C3 deposition in the basement membrane zone and immunoelectron microscopy shows this is deposited in the sublamina densa region. Circulating autoantibodies are also present in the disease and are deposited on the dermal side of salt split skin. In less than 10 percent of cases, there may be deposition of IgA at the basement membrane zone.

Management

Patients are usually treated with high-dose corticosteroids but often the results are short lived and the disease may return. As a result, management can be challenging. Other adjunctive therapies include dapsone and colchicine as well as methotrexate. Patients should be advised to avoid trauma, if possible and avoid eating hard foods.

Box 15.5: Epidermolysis bullosa aquisita

Key features useful in diagnosis

- Acquired subepithelial fragile blisters, affecting skin and mucosa
- Wide age range
- Antibodies against Type VII collagen
- *Managment:* High dose corticosteroids.

Dermatitis Herpetiformis

This disease was first described by Louis Duhring in the late 19th century and it is characterized by an intensely itchy skin rash. In recent years, it has been recognized that the disease is associated with celiac disease although in many patients this may be subclinical.

Clinical Features

Patients are often young and the most common age at presentation is between 20 to 40 years although it may occur at any age. The lesions are characterized by vesicle or occasionally bullae formation which may become eroded or crusted. They may be grouped together, hence the term herpetiformis. They are intensely pruritic and in some patients are characterized by prodromal burning and stinging. The flexor surfaces are usually affected but the face, hairline and neck may also be involved. The oral cavity is rarely affected. Almost all patients have celiac disease: gluten sensitive enteropathy.

There is a genetic basis for the disease and patients have an increased incidence of HLA-A1, HLA-B8 and HLA-DR3 haplotypes.

Histopathology

Neutrophils and eosinophils accumulate at the tips of the dermal papillae immediately beneath the epidermis and this is associated with subepidermal separation and blister formation. Direct immunofluorescence shows deposits of IgA and sometimes C3 in a granular fashion at the basement membrane zone. This may also be seen in perilesional skin.

Pathogenesis

There is now evidence that the disease is the result of autoantibody to epidermal transglutaminase 3, an enzyme involved in keratinocyte differentiation. It is postulated that patients with a high gluten diet and a genetic predisposition to gluten sensitivity produce IgA antibodies against epidermal transglutaminase 3 and these are deposited at the dermal epidermal junction. Neutrophils are attracted and cause the damage possibly by the release of inflammatory mediators.

Management

Patients may be treated with dapsone or sulfapyridine and relief is usually rapid. They should also be advised to change their diet and avoid wheat products. If successful this will obviate the need for drugs but some patients find the diet difficult to tolerate.

Box 15.6: Dermatitis herpetiformis

Key features useful in diagnosis

- Affects young 20–40 years
- Associated with celiac disease: gluten sensitive enteropathy
- Itchy rash on flexor surfaces, face and neck, oral cavity rarely affected
- Autoantibodies to transglutaminase 3
- Managed by dapsone or sulfapyradine and a gluten-free diet.

LINEAR IgA DISEASE

This rare disease is characterized as its name suggests by linear deposits of IgA at the basement membrane zone in the skin and the mucous membranes. It occurs in two main forms—Linear IgA disease of childhood and Adult Linear IgA disease.

Linear IgA disease of childhood usually affects children below the age of five years and is characterized by papules or vesiculobullous eruptions which may occur around the anus or perioral region. Similar lesions are seen in the adult form but these affect the elbows, knees and buttocks predominantly. Mucosal involvement may be seen in up to 80 percent of patients with both forms of the disease. Oral lesions have been documented and these may appear as vesicles and bullae, erosions, white patches or striations resembling lichen planus. Desquamative gingivitis or erythema may be evident. In a few cases, oral involvement may be the only oral manifestation of the disease and in these cases diagnosis is difficult. There appears to be a genetic component as the disease is associated with HLA-B8 and HLA-DR3 phenotypes.

Histopathology

Subepidermal blister formation is usually seen associated with accumulations of neutrophils at the basement membrane zone particularly at the tips of the dermal papillae. Direct and indirect immunofluorescence shows linear deposition of IgA at the basement membrane zone.

Pathogenesis

The antigens targeted by the autoantibodies have not been clearly defined but using salt split skin binding occurs on the epidermal side in 80 percent of children and 30 percent of adults and in some cases bind to both the epidermal and dermal side. It is thought there are multiple antigens and some may be related to BP180 (Type XVII collagen) as well as BP230. The trigger for the disease is not known but there is evidence it may be drug related in some few cases.

Management

Diagnosis is established by biopsy and detection of autoantibodies. Most cases respond to dapsone or sulfapyridine.

Box 15.7: Linear IgA

Key features useful in diagnosis

- Two forms affecting children and adults
- Subepithelial separation and bullae with linear IgA deposition basement membrane zone
- Affects skin and mucosa in 80%
- Managed by dapsone or sulfapyridine

ANGINA BULLOSA HEMORRHAGICA

This disorder is characterized by blood filled blisters on the oral mucosa which burst to form erosions that usually heal within a week. Unlike the other disorders considered in this chapter, they are not the result of autoantibodies against components of either the desmosomes, hemidesmosomes or basement membrane zone. It will be considered here since it forms part of the differential diagnosis of vesiculobullous lesions of the oral mucosa.

Clinical Features

Patients complain of blood filled blisters which arise rapidly, burst and then heal within one to two weeks. They commonly affect the soft palate although any oral site may be affected. The patients do not have a history of blood disorders or mucosal blistering disorders. The lesions are usually solitary and may occur infrequently or with a pattern consistent for that patient. They often arise after meal times and may be associated with a burning sensation. Patients are usually middle aged or elderly.

Histopathology

This shows a subepithelial blister which is usually blood filled. There may be a mild inflammatory infiltrate in the lamina propria. If the blisters have burst the features are those of non-specific ulceration.

Management

It is important to exclude autoimmune causes of subepithelial blistering and blood dyscrasias by the appropriate tests including biopsy. Once the diagnosis is established patients should be reassured and treatment may include the use of anti-inflammatory or antibacterial mouth rinses.

Box 15.8: Angina bullosa hemorrhagica

Key features useful in diagnosis

- Blood filled blisters affecting palate, heal within a week
- Etiology unknown
- Exclude autoimmune causes and reassurance.

ERYTHEMA MULTIFORME

Erythema multiforme encompasses a range of clinical presentations which vary in severity but all are characterized by lesions which affect the mucosa and/or skin. Over the years, several attempts have been made to classify the different variants and currently, erythema multiforme minor (EM minor), erythema multiforme major (EM major), Stevens-Johnson syndrome (SJS) and toxic epidermolysis necrosis syndrome (TENS) are recognized as part of the spectrum of erythema multiforme.

Clinical Features

Erythema multiforme affects young individuals in the 20 to 40 age group and there appears to be a slight male predilection. Skin lesions are typically targeted in appearance and comprise a flat central red area surrounded by concentric edematous rings. They are usually less than 3 cm in diameter and are well defined (**Fig. 15.9**). Occasional lesions may be raised and in more severe cases, there may be evidence of bullae formation and lesions may become confluent. The extensor surfaces of the extremities are most often affected and lesions are usually symmetrical. Oral lesions are characterized by macules and blood-filled blisters which usually burst to form widespread erosions and ulceration. The lesions particularly affect the anterior parts of the mouth and the lips which become swollen and blood

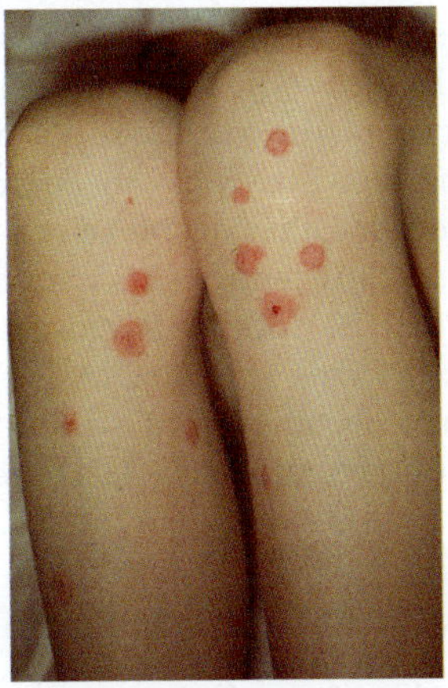

Fig. 15.9: Target lesion in erythema multiforme on the shins

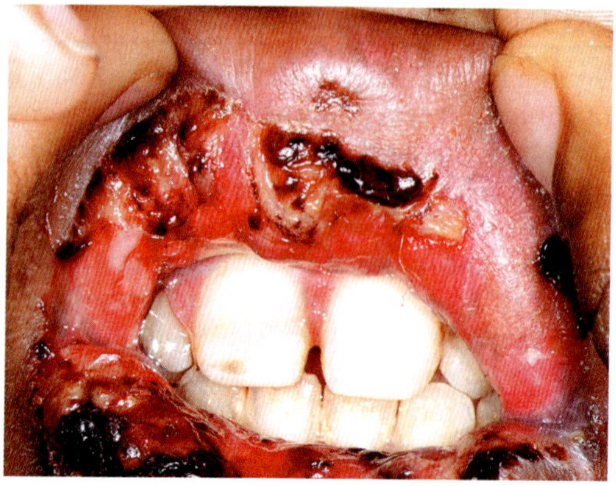

Fig. 15.10: Mucosal lesions in erythema multiforme. *Note:* The blood encrusted lips and widespread ulceration of the anterior parts of the mouth

encrusted (**Fig. 15.10**). Other mucosal surfaces may be affected and show widespread erosions and ulcers. Attacks usually last for between 10 to 20 days and the majority are single episode. However, in about 25 percent of cases the disease is recurrent with a rate of one or two per year. Most cases resolve within 10 years but the range of duration is very large and some cases are intractable.

Erythema Multiforme Minor

As its name suggests this variant is usually mild and by definition, only affects one mucous membrane—usually the oral cavity. The skin is also affected and usually typical target lesions are present on the extensor surfaces of the arms and legs. In some cases, there is evidence of fever and malaise but the disease is usually self limiting. However, it may become recurrent and very severe with widespread oral ulceration although the lips tend to be spared. There is evidence that EM minor is closely linked to EM major. In cases of recurrent EM minor the disease may become more severe with each progressive attack and may affect other mucosal sites.

Erythema Multiforme Major

This clinical variant affects not only the oral cavity but also other mucosal sites including the esophagus, larynx, genitals and eyes. There is widespread ulceration and usually typical target lesions are present on the skin. Like EM minor this form of the disease may also be recurrent.

STEVENS-JOHNSON SYNDROME

This is a very severe form of erythema multiforme and the eyes, larynx, pharynx, genitals, oral cavity and skin are all affected. Patients may complain of a flu-like illness up to 3 weeks before the onset with headache, malaise, fever, arthralgias and myalgias. Skin lesions may be atypical and flat rather than raised. Ocular lesions may resemble those of pemphigoid and patients may complain of dry eyes.

TOXIC EPIDERMOLYSIS NECROSIS SYNDROME

This is a rare variant also known as Lyells disease. Its relationship to erythema multiforme is unclear but it is almost always drug induced. TENS is characterized by widespread detachment of the epidermis from the dermis affecting almost all the skin as well as loss of oral epithelium and widespread ulceration.

Etiology

Erythema multiforme has been linked to a large number of environmental triggers including viruses, bacteria, immune reactions, drugs and foodstuffs. However there appears to be a genetic predisposition and there is an association with certain HLA phenotypes. This is particularly true of recurrent cases which are associated with HLADQ3.

Viruses are an important trigger and herpes simplex infection has been implicated in up to 70 percent of recurrent cases. Other viruses such as coxsackie, influenza and hepatitis viruses have also been reported to act as a trigger as well as a number of bacteria including streptococci, mycoplasma, ricketsia, tuberculosis and salmonella. Indeed, the number of reports showing an association with microorganisms and erythema multiforme is very large and the same is true for drugs. Sulfonamides, cephalosporins and nonsteroidal anti-inflammatory drugs have also been implicated as well as others too numerous to mention. Despite the large number of reported triggers there does appear to be an association between the nature of the trigger and the severity of the response. Viruses tend to trigger EM minor and major whereas drugs tend to trigger Stevens- Johnson syndrome and TENS. However, this association is not exclusive and a small but significant number of cases of EM minor and major are triggered by drugs and conversely, some cases of SJS are triggered by viruses.

HERPES ASSOCIATED ERYTHEMA MULTIFORME

There is increasing evidence that a preceding herpes infection may trigger a significant proportion of cases of both single episode and recurrent EM and these are known as herpes associated erythema multiforme (HAEM). The evidence for this association comes from the significant number of patients who report a preceding herpes infection 1 to 2 weeks before the episode of EM. Even in those patients who do not report such an association, the antiviral drug aciclovir is often effective. There have been several studies designed to determine whether herpes simplex virus (HSV) is present in lesions of EM. Although there is wide variability, HSV has been detected in the region of 60 percent of cases.

Histopathology

The histological appearances are very variable and diagnosis may be difficult. There is often both sub- and intraepithelial bullae formation and the epithelium is edematous and shows evidence of necrosis. This is associated with an infiltrate of T-lymphocytes and mononuclear cells in the upper dermis or lamina propria and these may extend into the epithelium and obscure the basement membrane zone. Immunofluorescence shows granular C3 deposition in basement membrane zone and around blood vessels. The extent of the inflammatory infiltrate is variable and appears to be greater in cases precipitated by herpes than those caused by drugs.

Pathogenesis

It was originally thought that EM is the result of a type 3 hypersensitivity reaction, i.e. an antibody/antigen reaction in localized blood vessels causes the destruction. However, there is increasing evidence that in some cases the disease is the result of a cell mediated immune reaction. In HAEM, it is thought the HSV-DNA fragments in epithelial cells trigger the disease. T-cells reactive to HSV DNA have been identified and these produce IFN-γ. This cytokine amplifies the immune response and recruits additional T-cells to the area which result in cell mediated tissue damage.

In drug associated lesions, it is thought that drug metabolites initiate the disease and that the destruction is not cell mediated but rather mediated by cytokines. The infiltrate which is usually sparse produces TNF-α rather than IFN-γ and this cytokine may induce apoptosis of epithelial cells directly. However, the detailed mechanisms of the damage still remain to be determined.

Box 15.9: Erythema multiforme

Key features useful in diagnosis

- Spectrum of presentations from mild to severe affecting skin and mucosa
- EM minor and major affects skin and one or more mucosal sites respectively
- Target lesions and blood encrusted lips and ulceration
- *Triggered by viruses:* Herpes, bacteria, drugs and foodstuffs
- EM minor and major associated with herpes, Stevens-Johnson syndrome with drugs
- May be recurrent, manage with aciclovir.

Management

Diagnosis can be difficult and in most cases is made on clinical features alone without the use of biopsy. In single episode disease lesions may resolve within two to three weeks and supportive care is the mainstay of treatment. In recurrent cases which are associated with herpes, aciclovir may be used either as a short course at the onset of symptoms or as a prophylaxis over a longer time period. Patients with severe symptoms may require hospitalization and supportive care. The use of steroids is controversial but may be used in patients with SJS and TENS as well as EM Minor.

SELF-ASSESSMENT QUESTIONS

1. Provide a classification for immunobullous disorders.
2. Describe the clinicopathological features of pemphigus.
3. Describe the clinicopathological features of mucous membrane pemphigoid.
4. Give an account of paraneoplastic immunobullous disease.
5. Describe the role of immunochemistry in the diagnosis of immunobullous disorders.
6. Describe the clinicopathological findings in epidermolysis bullosa.
7. Describe the clinicopathological features of erythema multiforme.
8. Describe the clinicopathological features of angina bullosa hemorrhagica.
9. Describe, using examples, the treatment of immunobullous disease.
10. Give an account of the target antigens affected in immunobullous disease.

SUGGESTED READING

1. Mignogna MD, Fortuna G, Leuci S. Oral pemphigus. Minerva Stomatol. 2009;98:501-18.
2. Schifter M, Yeoh SC, Coleman H, Georgiou A. Oral mucosal diseases: the inflammatory dermatoses. Aust Dent J. 2010;5:23-38.
3. Schmidt E, Zillikens D. Pemphigoid diseases. Lancet. 2013;381:320-32.
4. Sticherling M. Erfurt-Berge C. Autoimmune blistering diseases of the skin. Autoimmun Rev. 2012:11;226-30.

Chapter

16

Infections of the Oral Mucosa

Lakshman Samaranayake, Nipuna Parahitiyawa

Chapter Outline

INTRODUCTION

The oral mucosa, which covers a significant proportion of the oral cavity, is affected by a number of infectious diseases. The majority of these are of fungal (candidal) and viral origin and are similar to infections seen in other superficial mucosal surfaces of the body, such as the vagina although the unique oral environment laced with saliva may alter the lesion presentation and appearance.

In this section, fungal infections are discussed first with greater emphasis on candidal infection, followed by viral infections and bacterial infections. Mucosal infections other than those caused by viruses are uncommon in otherwise healthy people. However, with the increasing numbers of immunocompromised patient populations such as those with HIV, these infections are also on the rise, and therefore deserve attention of the dentist in diagnosing and managing those (**Fig. 16.1**).

FUNGAL INFECTIONS OF THE ORAL MUCOSA

Oral candidiasis (syn. Oral candidosis):

- Primary oral candidiases
- Secondary oral candidiases

Candida associated lesions:

a. *Candida*-associated denture stomatitis
b. Angular cheilitis or angular stomatitis
c. Median rhomboid glossitis
d. Linear gingival erythema.

ORAL CANDIDIASIS

Oral candidiasis or candidosis is used as an umbrella term to describe infections mainly caused by the yeasts belonging to the genus *Candida*. (**Fig. 16.2**). Although *Candida albicans* is the main etiological agent, non-albicans species do cause infection, often in the immunocompromised. All forms of oral candidiasis are considered to be opportunistic infections, and the epithet 'disease of the diseased' has been applied to these infections, which are seen mainly in the 'very young, the very old and the very sick' (**Table 16.1**). It is important to note that, particularly in the developing countries, oral candidiasis is the third most common presenting complaint of HIV infected patients.

Oral candidiases can be classified as follows:

1. *Primary oral candidiases:* Localized candidal infections present only in the oral and perioral tissues.
2. *Secondary oral candidiases:* Candidal infections that manifest in a generalized manner

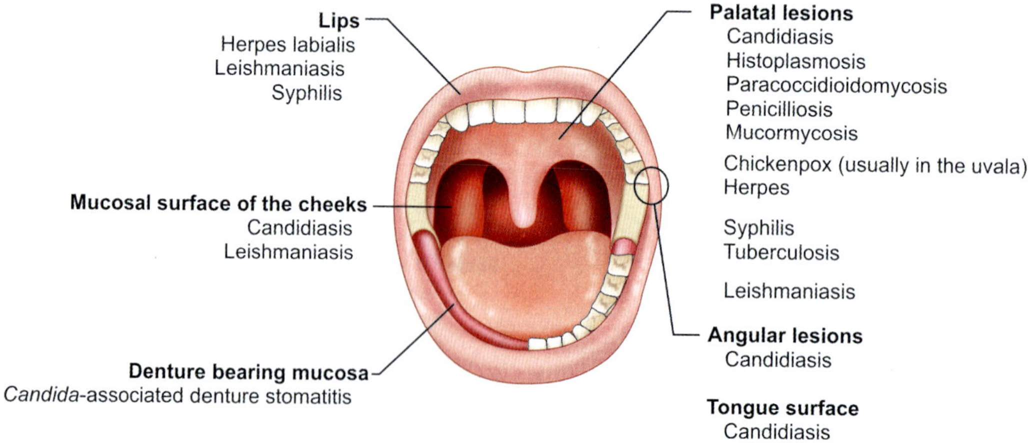

Fig. 16.1: Infections of the oral mucosa

▪ Table 16.1
Factors that predispose the host to oral candidiasis

Predisposing factor	*Mechanism or effects on host*
Physiological	Old age, infancy, or pregnancy that associate with altered host immunity, hyposalivation, etc.
Local trauma	Mucosal irritation, poor denture hygiene
Malnutrition	High-carbohydrate diet, iron, foliate and vitamin B_{12} deficiencies
Broadspectrum antibiotics	Altered oral microbiology
Corticosteroids	Steroid inhalers, systemic steroids suppressing oral immunity
Immune defects	HIV infection, AIDS, thymic aplasia
Endocrine disorders	Hypoendocrine states (e.g. hypothyroidism, Addison's disease)
Malignancies	Including blood disorders e.g. acute leukemia, agranulocytosis that impairs host's immunity
Hyposalivation	Autoimmune disease: Sjögren's syndrome; acquired: head and neck irradiation, medication including cytotoxic drug therapy

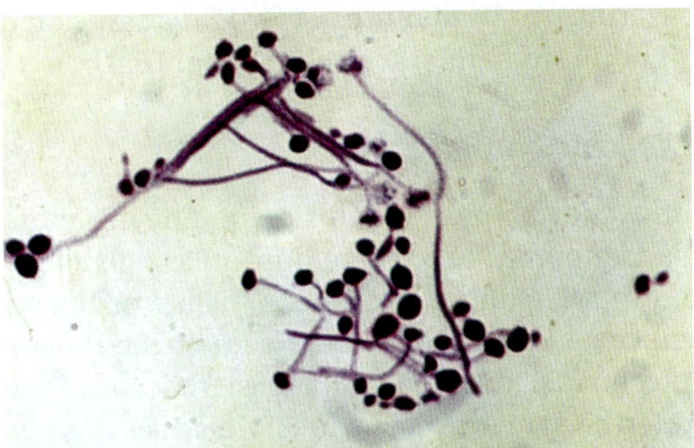

Fig. 16.2: Blastospores (yeast phase) and hyphae (filamentous phase) of *Candida albicans*

both in the oral cavity and on other mucous and cutaneous surfaces (systemic mucocutaneous candidal infections). These are due to rare disorders (except perhaps in candidiasis of human immunodeficiency virus (HIV) infection) such as thymic aplasia and chronic endocrine diseases.

The classic triad of (either primary or secondary) oral candidiases is:
- Pseudomembranous variant
- Erythematous (atrophic) variant
- Hyperplastic variant.

In addition there are a number of other *Candida*-associated lesions where the etiology is multifactorial. These are primary oral candidiases restricted to the oral cavity only. Antifungal therapy alone will not cure these diseases and underlying cofactors that perpetuate the disease need to be evaluated and eradicated for disease resolution. These variants include:
- *Candida*-associated denture stomatitis
- Angular cheilitis or angular stomatitis
- Median rhomboid glossitis
- Linear gingival erythema (the microbiologic etiology is not conclusive).

Pseudomembranous Candidiasis

Pseudomembranous candidiasis, classically termed 'thrush' (**Fig. 16.3**), is an acute infection but may persist intermittently for many months

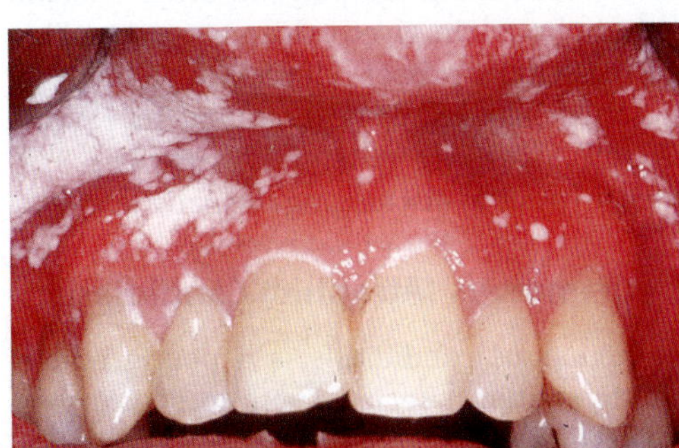

Fig. 16.3: Pseudomembranous candidiasis (thrush) in a HIV-infected young adult
(*Note:* The fungal invasion of gingival crevice)

or even years in patients using corticosteroids topically or by aerosol, in HIV-infected individuals, and in other immunocompromised patients. It may also be seen in neonates and in the terminally ill, particularly in association with serious underlying conditions such as leukemia.

Clinical Features

The lesions are characterized by white membranes on the surface of the oral mucosa, tongue and elsewhere. These develop to form confluent plaques that resemble milk curds and can be wiped off to reveal a raw, erythematous and sometimes bleeding base. Hence, some consider pseudomembranous and the erythematous variants a continuum and a single entity (i.e. two stages of the same disease).

Microbiology and Pathology

The white patches consist of necrotic material and desquamated parakeratotic epithelium, penetrated by yeast cells and hyphae which invade as far as the stratum spinosum. Oropharyngeal thrush may sometimes spread into the adjacent mucosa, particularly that of the upper respiratory tract and the esophagus. The combination of oral and esophageal candidiasis is particularly prevalent in HIV disease. Hence, it is necessary to investigate the underlying immune status of the host when this is encountered.

Management

This consists of topical antifungal preparations, mainly containing the polyene drugs nystatin and amphotericin, given as lozenges or pastilles. In recalcitrant cases fluconazole may be prescribed as second line treatment. Investigate for any underlying systemic disease (e.g. HIV disease) prior to discharging the patient.

Erythematous (Atrophic) Candidiasis

Erythematous candidiasis is a poorly understood condition associated with corticosteroids, topical or systemic broad-spectrum antibiotics, or HIV disease. It may arise as a consequence of acute pseudomembranous candidiasis when the pseudomembranes are shed, or may develop *de novo*. Erythematous candidiasis of the palate is a common *Candida*-associated lesion frequently observed in elderly people wearing full dentures (*Candida*-associated denture stomatitis; see below) (**Fig. 16.4**).

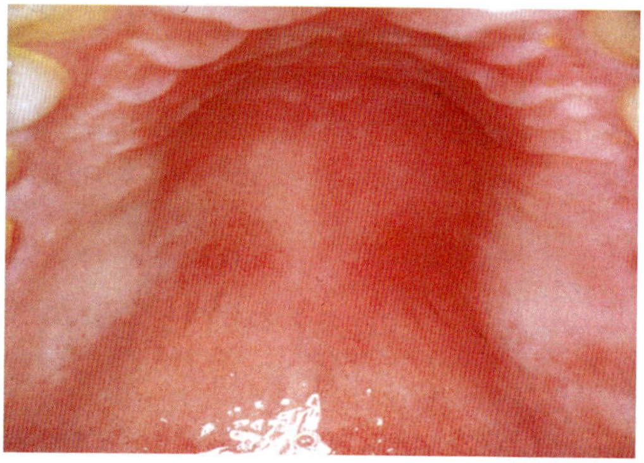

Fig. 16.4: Erythematous candidiasis of the soft palate of a HIV-infected individual

Clinical Features

The clinical presentation is of one or more asymptomatic erythematous areas, generally on the dorsum of the tongue, palate or buccal mucosa. Lesions on the dorsum of the tongue present as depapillated areas; red areas are often seen on the palate in HIV disease.

There can be associated angular stomatitis, especially in *Candida*-associated denture stomatitis.

Microbiology

Not much is known of the role of yeasts in this condition, although antifungal therapy leads to resolution of the lesions.

Management

Topical antifungal treatment, mainly nystatin and amphotericin, is given as lozenges or pastilles. Azole group agents, such as oral fluconazole tablets, are useful in HIV disease. Investigate for underlying pathology (e.g. HIV disease).

Hyperplastic Candidiasis (Candidal Leukoplakia)

The lesions in hyperplastic candidiasis present as chronic, discrete raised areas that vary from small, palpable, translucent, whitish areas to large, dense, opaque plaques hard and rough to the touch (plaque-like lesions). Homogeneous areas or speckled areas that do not rub off (nodular lesions) can also be seen. The lesions are often asymptomatic and usually occur on the inside surface of one or both cheeks (retrocommissural area) (**Fig. 16.5**). Oral cancer may supervene in 9 to 40 percent of cases of hyperplastic candidiasis, as compared with the 2 to 6 percent risk of malignant transformation cited for other oral white patches, e.g. Oral leukoplakia. Therefore, patients with recalcitrant hyperplastic candidal lesions resistant to therapy should be kept under regular surveillance (see chapter 12).

Microbiology and Histopathology

Parakeratosis and epithelial hyperplasia occur, with candidal invasion restricted to the upper layers of the epithelium. The condition has been associated in a minority with iron and folate deficiencies and with defective cell-mediated immunity. Biopsy is important as the condition is potentially malignant and shows varying degrees of dysplasia.

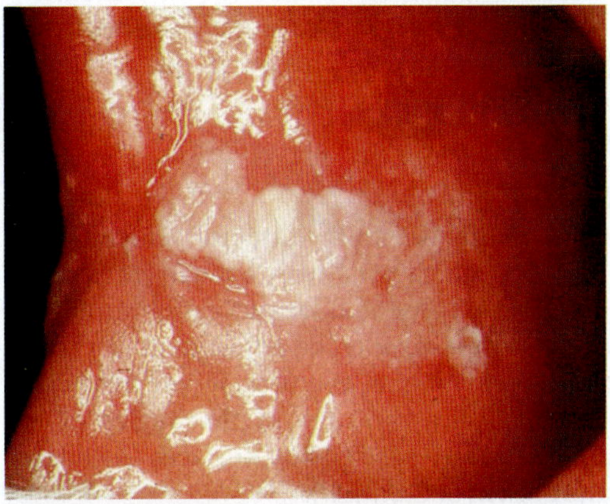

Fig. 16.5: Classic appearance of chronic hyperplastic candidiasis on the commissures of the mouth

Management

Topical antifungal treatment, mainly nystatin and amphotericin, is given as lozenges or pastilles. Azole group agents, such as oral fluconazole tablets, may help resolve chronic infections. Following successful antifungal treatment the grade of dysplasia may drop by at least one stage. Because of the possibility of malignant transformation, patients should be followed up if the condition is chronic.

CANDIDA-ASSOCIATED LESIONS

Candida-associated Denture Stomatitis

Candida-associated denture stomatitis, also called denture sore mouth or chronic atrophic candidiasis, is one of the most common ailments in wearers of full dentures; in some areas such as Scandinavia 60 percent of wearers over 60 years old were reported to suffer from the condition. It is also associated with patients wearing orthodontic appliances or obturators for cleft palate. The characteristic presenting signs are erythema and edema of the mucosa that is in contact with the fitting surface of the upper denture. The mucosa below the lower dentures is hardly ever involved.

Clinical Features

The patient may occasionally experience slight soreness but is usually free from symptoms; the only presenting complaint is sometimes an associated angular stomatitis. Depending on the severity of inflammation, the lesions may appear as:

- Pinpoint erythema of the denture-bearing mucosa (Newton's type 1)
- Diffuse and confluent erythema and edema of the denture-bearing mucosa (Newton's type 2) (**Fig. 16.6**)
- Papillary hyperplasia and inflammation, commonly involving the central part of the hard palate and the alveolar ridge (Newton's type 3).

Etiology

- *Local factors:* Poor denture hygiene, ill-fitting dentures, traumatic dentures,

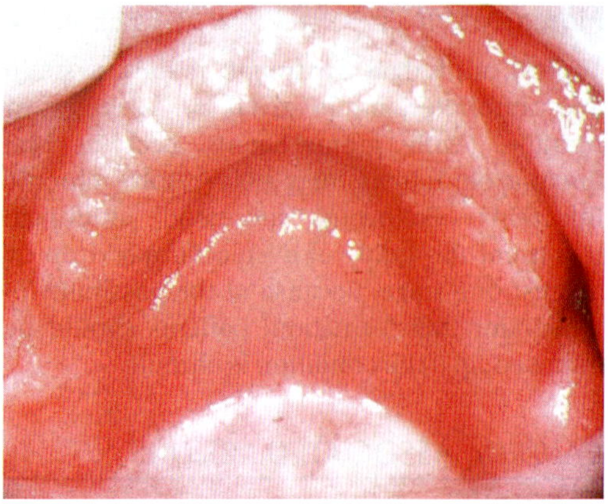

Fig. 16.6: *Candida*-associated dentures stomatitis. Classic appearance showing edematous and erythematous denture bearing mucosa of the hard palate

carbohydrate-rich diets, xerostomia (e.g. Sjögren's syn-drome).

- *Systemic factors:* Iron and folate deficiency, diabetes mellitus, immune defects.

Microbiology and Histopathology

It is generally considered to be due to accumulation of plaque biofilms with yeasts and bacteria on the fitting surface of the denture and the underlying mucosa. In the papillary hyperplastic variety, *Candida* species do not invade the epithelium. Other etiological factors, such as mechanical irritation or an allergic reaction to the denture base material (though rare) need to be excluded in persistent cases.

Management

The condition is treated by:

- Scrupulous denture hygiene and removal of dentures at night (these measures alone, without antifungals, are adequate in the majority of cases)
- Regular disinfection of dentures by steeping them in sodium hypochlorite or chlorhexidine to eradicate the reservoir of candidal hyphae adhering to the prosthesis
- Review of the denture fitness to relieve trauma, if any
- A diet with a low content of fermentable carbohydrates
- Polyene antifungals – nystatin (1;100000 units, 1 mL QDS for 10 days), amphotericin (lozenges, pastilles, etc.) 10 mg qds for 7 days
- Miconozole gel applied the fitting surface of the denture.

Angular Stomatitis (Perleche, Angular Cheilitis)

The lesions of angular stomatitis are seen in one or both angles of the mouth (**Figures 16.1 and 16.5**), especially as a complication of *Candida*-associated denture stomatitis.

Clinical Features

Characterized by soreness, erythema and fissuring, this condition is commonly associated with denture-induced stomatitis. Both yeasts and bacteria (especially *Staphylococcus aureus*) are involved as interacting predisposing factors. However, angular stomatitis is very occasionally an isolated initial sign of anemia or vitamin deficiency, such as vitamin B_{12} deficiency, and resolves when the underlying disease has been treated. The condition is also seen in HIV-associated disease.

Microbiology

Candida spp. are present with or without co-infection with *Staphylococcus aureus.* The presence of yellow crusting may indicate staphylococcal infection.

Treatment

Elimination of the intraoral reservoir of infection in patients with concurrent denture stomatitis is essential for successful resolution. Other measures include adjustment of vertical dimension of the dentures to prevent saliva drooling, and moisture at the angles of the mouth (note: moist body surfaces encourage the growth of *Candida*).

Topical antifungal therapy with nystatin, amphotericin B or miconazole (miconazole has both antifungal and anti-staphylococcal activity and is useful for mixed infections); anti-staphylococcal preparations (dictated by microbiological investigation) include fusidic acid and neomycin/chlorhexidine. Investigate also for possible underlying disease: iron or vitamin B_{12} deficiency; HIV infection.

Median Rhomboid Glossitis

Midline glossitis, or glossal central papillary atrophy, is characterized by an area of papillary atrophy which is elliptical or rhomboid in shape and symmetrically placed centrally at the midline of the tongue, anterior to the circumvallate papillae (**Fig. 16.7**). Occasionally, median rhomboid glossitis presents with a hyperplastic exophytic or even lobulated appearance. In addition to fungal infection a number of predisposing cofactors, including smoking, steroid inhalation and remnants of the tubrculum impar, have been proposed. The patients are often worried about the appearance and cancer-phobic. In this event reassurance is essential.

Linear Gingival Erythema

This condition, defined as a localized or generalized erythematous band extending along the gingival margins (between adjacent gingival papillae), was first described in HIV-infected individuals; it is however not confined to the latter group. Although *Candida* are implicated in the pathogenesis, and lesions resolve after antifungal therapy in some cases, it is likely that other cofactors such as oral hygiene play an equally important role.

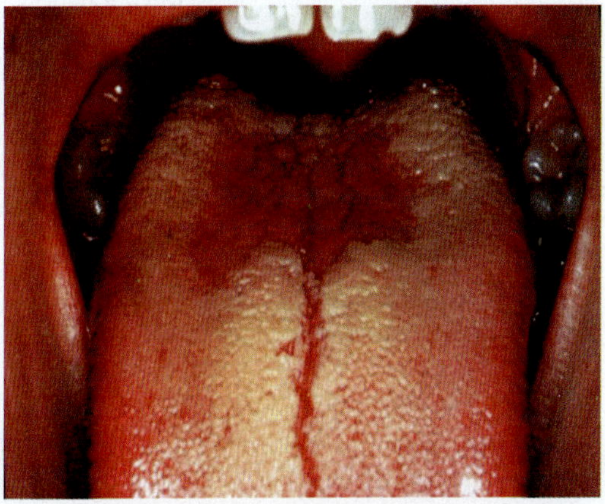

Fig. 16.7: Median rhomboid glossitis. The classic rhomboid, erythematous lesion

CANDIDIASIS AND IMMUNOCOMPROMISED HOSTS

A few patients have chronic candidiasis from an early age, sometimes with a definable immune defect, e.g. chronic mucocutaneous candidiasis. Candidal infections in these patients are seen in the oral mucosa, skin and other body parts. These secondary oral candidal infections have increased recently because of the high prevalence of attenuated immune response, consequent to diseases such as HIV infection, hematological malignancy and treatment protocols, including aggressive cytotoxic therapy.

ORAL CANDIDIASIS IN HIV DISEASE

Candidal infections, with oral thrush and esophagitis as frequent or recurrent clinical manifestations, are the most common opportunistic infections encountered in acquired immune deficiency syndrome (AIDS). It has also been shown that the occurrence of an otherwise unexpected mycoses (typically oral candidiasis) in an HIV-infected individual is a poor prognostic indicator of the subsequent development of full-blown AIDS. However, in HIV-infected populations on antiretroviral therapy, the incidence of oral candidiasis has significantly declined.

Laboratory Diagnosis

Confirmation of diagnosis requires sending a swab and/or a smear from a *Candida* suspected lesion to a microbiological laboratory. The microbiologist can give a colony count from a mouth rinse made of 10 mL of saline.

EXOTIC FUNGAL INFECTIONS OF THE ORAL MUCOSA

The infections that are dealt below are often termed as deep mycoses. These affect the tissues beyond the mucosal layers and often present as a part of systemic affection. Therefore, it is important to search for systemic signs and symptoms take a deep biopsy when oral lesions are detected (**Table 16.2**).

Aspergillosis

Aspergillosis has been reported as second only to candidiasis as the most prevalent opportunistic mycotic infection. It is also the second most frequent orofacial fungal infection in those receiving cancer chemotherapy. *Aspergillus* species are filamentous saprophytes that live in soil and decaying vegetation and the most common pathogen of the species is *Aspergillus fumigatus*. Human infections are also caused by less common, *Aspergillus flavus, Aspergillus glaucis, Aspergillus terrus* and *Aspergillus niger*. Aspergillosis may present as three clinical variants, namely: (i) saprophytic, superficial infection without invasion; (ii) allergic, as a hypersensitivity reaction; and (iii) invasive, infection into viable tissue.

Aspergillosis is generally contracted through inhalation of spores, leading to both upper and lower respiratory tract infection-bronchopulmonary aspergillosis. Infections may then spread to brain, bone or endocardium. Paranasal sinuses, larynx the eyes, ears and oral cavity may be involved in primary aspergillosis.

▪ Table 16.2
Uncommon systemic mycoses and their oral manifestations

Disease and representative agent	*Main sites affected*	*Major oral manifestations*	*Frequency of oral affection*
Aspergillosis *Aspergillus fumigatus*	Paranasal sinuses; rarely tongue, soft palate	Plaque formation and intense local pain in oral lesions	Uncommon
Blastomycosis (North American) *Blastomyces dermatitidis*	Tongue, oral mucosa, gingivae, lip, mandibular bone	Ulceration, sessile projections, indurated swellings, actinomycosis-like draining abscesses	Rare
Coccidioidomycosis *Coccidioides immitis*	Nasolabial folds, skin	Verrucous granulomas resembling carcinomas	Very rare
Cryptococcosis[a] *Cryptococcus neoformans*	Gingiva, hard and soft palate, mucosa, tonsillar pillar	Violaceous colored nodules or granulations, swellings, ulcers	Uncommon
Geotrichosis *Geotrichum candidum*	Oral mucosa	Similar to acute pseudomembranes of candidosis	Uncommon
Histoplasmosis[b] *Histoplama capsulatum* *Histoplasma duboisii*	Oral mucosa, tongue, plate, gingival, periapical area	Nodular, indurated or granular masses or tissue destruction with bone erosion	40 percent
Mucormycosis *Mucor species*	Extension from maxillary sinus through palate into the mouth	Sloughing ulcers with gray eschar and exposed bone (especially maxilla); unilateral facial pain	Common
Paracoccidioidomycosis (South American Blastomycosis) *Paracoccidioides brasiliensis*	Hard and soft palate, gingiva, tongue	Papules or vesicles leading to ulcers; extensive local destruction	Common
Sporotrichosis *Sporotrichum schenckii*	Oral mucosa	Erythematous, ulcerative lesions leading to granuloma, or papillomas	Uncommon

[a] AIDS-associated oral lesions have been described
[b] May present to the dentist with initial oral manifestations

The potential for transmission of apsergillosis from humans-to-humans is low.

Oral Considerations

Orofacial aspergillosis may affect the paranasal sinuses, nasal cavity, oral mucosa and underlying structures as well as the skin of the face. *A. fumigatus* is the usual agent of sinus aspergillosis, whereas *A. flavus* is more common in invasive lesions in immunosuppressed individuals. Orofacial aspergillosis appears to be relatively common in patients undergoing treatment for malignancies of the blood and blood-forming organs.

In general, the lesions are yellow or black in color, with a necrotic ulcerated base, typically located on the palate or posterior tongue. The hyphal elements of the fungus may invade the oral mucosa and penetrate the walls of small to medium-sized arteries and veins, producing thrombosis, infarction and necrosis finally leading to systemic spread. Aspergilloma of the maxillary antrum is not uncommon, presenting in a healthy host as a hyphal ball in chronically obstructed sinus.

Diagnosis and Management

Main differential diagnoses are from mucor and pseudomonas oral infection. Bone erosion can be more easily detected by NMR or CT imaging and the diagnosis confirmed by periodic acid schiff stained smear; immunostains may be of help. Systemic amphotericin B is the choice antimycotic, if the superficial infections do not resolve within 72 hours of other antifungals ketoconazole or clotrimazole therapy.

Blastomycosis

Although becoming more prevalent due to the HIV pandemic, blastomycosis is a relatively uncommon fungal disease. Blastomycosis is a deep mycotic infection, caused by *Blastomyces dermatitidis*, found mainly in North America particularly in rural Mississippi, Ohio and Missouri river basins as well as the Great Lakes region. In humans, blastomycosis presents as either: pulmonary, disseminated or localized cutaneous lesions. As in aspergillosis the fungal spores are found in the soil and may initiate the disease when inhaled. Transmission of blastomycosis from human-to-humans is unlikely and has not been reported.

Oral Considerations

Oral lesions may arise through disseminated blastomycosis. Oral blastomycosis is uncommon and may present as single or multiple ulcerations, sessile projections, and granulomatous or verrucous lesions. In a study of 40 patients with blastomycosis, a quarter demonstrated oral or nasal lesions and in another, seven of ten patients had nonspecific oral ulcerations in addition to systemic disease.

Diagnosis and Management

Diagnosis is based on biopsy, smear or culture. Amphotericin B, ketoconazole, miconazole and itraconazole are all effective.

Coccidioidomycosis

This condition is mainly seen in South West United States, Mexico, Central America and some parts of South America. The disease is caused by inhalation of *Coccidioides immitis* spores found in soil. Antibodies to the fungus are found in 90 percent of the population of these endemic areas. The illness is typically an acute pulmonary disease and fever, sometimes with erythema nodosum or erythema multiforme. Chronic pulmonary disease is less common. Disseminated coccidioidomycosis is seen in pregnant women, immigrant workers and immunocompromised individuals. Oral manifestations are almost always secondary to lung involvement. Transmission of coccidioidomycosis from human-to-humans is unlikely and has not been reported.

Oral Considerations

Oral lesions are rare and manifest as verrucous lesions with underlying infection of the jaw.

Diagnosis and Management

Diagnosis is by history and examination supported by histology. Coccidioidin skin test is helpful. Management is with systemic amphotericin B supplemented with azoles if necessary.

Cryptococcosis

Cryptococcosis is a chronic fungal disease involving the lungs, the central nervous system and, occasionally, the skin and mouth. The disease occurs worldwide, and the main source of the causative agent, *Cryptococcus neoformans*, is bird droppings. The disease is primarily a pulmonary infection and is usually subclinical with few if any noticeable signs or symptoms. However, in compromised individuals the disease may become rapidly systemic, involving the central nervous system, skin, mucous membranes, bone and a wide variety of other tissues. Skin lesions are not uncommon in the disseminated form of the disease, but rarely represent the site of primary infection. The face, scalp and neck are the common sites of cutaneous lesions, which present in a variety of ways, such as papules, acneiform pustules, abscesses, ulcers, superficial granulomas or sinus tracts. Cryptococcosis is unlikely to be transmitted from humans-to-humans unless in extreme situations such as in hospitals where infected patients are not adequately quarantined when other debilitated patients may acquire the disease nosocomially, through the pulmonary route.

Oral Considerations

Oral lesions occur in patients who have the disseminated form of cryptococcosis. Lesions have been described on the gingiva, the hard and soft palates, pharynx, oral mucosa, tonsillar pillar and in a tooth socket after extraction. The lesions have been variously described as violaceous nodules of granulation tissue, swellings or ulcers. The majority of reported cases of oral cryptococcosis have been reported in HIV-infected individuals.

Diagnosis and Management

Diagnosis is confirmed by microscopy. Culture and assay of serum or CSF for capsular antigen is useful. Systemic amphotericin B is the drug of choice and can be supplemented with fluconozole.

Fusariosis

Fusarium species were once considered as harmless, saprophytic, filamentous fungi living in soil. They, however, are now emerging as pathogens due to the high prevalence of compromised patients in the community. Fusariosis is the disseminated form of the disease. The disease is highly unlikely to be transmitted from human-to-humans.

Oral Considerations

Human fusarium infections may present as local, focally invasive or disseminated disease. Oral infections are rare and usually present as secondary lesions of disseminated disease where they have been described as black, necrotic ulcers occurring mainly on the palate. As these lesions are similar in appearance to those of aspergillosis and mucormycosis, definitive diagnosis should be made by histology and cultural techniques.

Diagnosis and Management

The management depends on the degree of invasion and the status of the patient. Superficial infections reportedly respond to local treatment; however, disseminated infections have a very poor prognosis. The infection can be managed by ketoconazole or voriconazole given for a prolonged period.

Geotrichosis

Geotrichum candidum is usually saprophytic but occasionally causes opportunistic infection in man. The fungus has been isolated from the skin, sputum and faeces and is carried in the alimentary tract of some individuals. Infections have been described in the bronchi, lung, mouth and intestine. Bronchial geotrichosis is the most commonly recognized form of the disease and is characterized by a persistent cough, the production of gelatinous sputum and absence of fever. Disseminated infections are seen in debilitated patients or in those receiving immunosuppressive drugs. Geotrichosis cannot be transmitted from human-to-humans.

Oral Considerations

The oral lesions of geotrichosis are indistinguishable clinically from those of acute pseudomembranous candidiasis (thrush) and the reported low incidence of the disease may be due to such misdiagnosis. Other reports indicate that the clinical appearance as edematous and erythematous gingivae and ulcerations. In one study, it was the second-most common oral yeast isolated from patients with hematologic malignancies suffering from stomatitis.

Diagnosis and Management

Diagnosis is confirmed by histology and culture. Nystatin may be effective for localized oral lesions, whilst systemic infections respond well to itraconazole therapy.

Histoplasmosis

Histoplasma capsulatum, a dimorphic fungus is endemic in Mississippi and Ohio river valleys and found in Latin America, India the Far East and in Australia. The organisms are found, especially in bird and bat feces. Infection ensues when microconidiae or hyphae are inhaled into the lung and develop into yeast or when old foci of infection are reactivated. AIDS patients are particularly at risk due to impairment of cellular immunity.

Clinical presentations include acute and chronic pulmonary cutaneous histoplasmosis, with or without disseminated disease. The latter is particularly common in immunocompromised persons. Histoplasmosis is unlikely to be transmitted from human-to-humans.

Oral Considerations

Oral lesions are mostly chronic with nodular, indurated or granular masses and ulceration; tissue destruction with bone erosion. Up to 40 to 50 percent case with systemic histoplasmosis presents with oral lesions. The major oral sites affected are the mucosa, tongue, palate, gingivae and the periapical region of teeth. The severity of the disease in AIDS patients is greater when CD4 count is below 200 cells/cm^2.

Diagnosis and Management

Diagnosis is confirmed by microscopy, culture and serology. Amphotericin B is the first choice drug, whilst fluconazole and itraconazole are alternatives. Relapse rates may be high as 80 percent for patients not placed on maintenance regimens following initial treatment with amphotericin B.

Mucormycosis (Zygomycosis; Phycomycosis)

The term mucormycosis refers to a distinctive group of diseases caused by ubiquitous, saprophytic fungi of the order Mucorales. The organisms are common inhabitants of soil and may be found in the nasal cavities of healthy individuals. Infection arises by inhalation of spores that are deposited in pulmonary alveoli. Other modes of infection include contamination of traumatized tissues and direct inoculation. The infection may present in different anatomic sites; especially the paranasal, rhino-orbital, rhinocerebral, cerebral pulmonary and gastrointestinal areas. It can also appear in the soft tissues of the extremities or as disseminated disease. The fungus preferentially erodes arteries, resulting in thrombosis with subsequent necrosis of the surrounding tissues. The host response is suppurative rather than granulomatous although chronic forms of mucormycosis occasionally occur. The infection is often associated with acidosis due to diabetes, diarrhea, or uraemia. Diabetic acidosis was considered to be the predisposing condition in 50 to 70 percent of the reported patients with mucormycosis prior to the HIV pandemic. More recently it is commonly seen associated with HIV infection and AIDS. Other predisposing conditions are blood dyscrasis, malignant disease, hepatitis, burns, malnutrition, irradiation, tuberculosis, and the administration of corticosteroids and immunosuppressive drugs. Mucormycosis is highly unlikely to be transmitted from human-to-humans.

Oral Considerations

Symptoms involving the oral, cranial and facial structures account for about 60 percent of all cases. Oral ulcerations and sinusitis and/or facial cellulitis have been described in mucormycosis. The mortality from mucormycosis is high, 50 to 100 percent, and there is little doubt that the fulminating nature of the infection, late diagnosis, and lack of rational therapy account for the poor prognosis. Other important symptoms include blood-tinged nasal discharge, unilateral facial pain or numbness. Occasionally, the most significant presenting symptom is necrotic ulceration or sloughing of the maxillary or palatal mucosa.

Diagnosis and Management

Diagnosis is confirmed by smear and histological demonstration of tissue invasion by hyphae. MRI may show thickening of the mucosa with patchy destruction of the antral walls in sinus infection. Management of mucormycosis comprises of, (i) detection of acidosis or other predisposing factors (ii) antifungal therapy using amphotericin B, and (iii) surgical debridement.

Paracoccidioidomycosis (South American Blastomycosis)

South American blastomycosis caused by *Paracoccidioides brasiliensis* is a chronic granulomatous disease which primarily infects the lungs and then disseminates to form ulcerative granulomas of the oral and nasal mucosa or other organ systems. This infection cannot be transmitted from human-to-humans.

Lymph nodes are commonly involved in mucormycosis and local extension to skin or systemic involvement of multiple organs may occur. The disease is restricted to South and Central America, especially Brazil. The source of the infection is thought to be soil and vegetative material and is acquired by direct inhalation or by direct contact. Infection is present 10 times more commonly in males that females, especially in the 20 to 40 year-old age group. Clinical cases of South American blastomycosis can be classified in one of three categories: pulmonary, mucocutaneous, lymphangitis or disseminated.

Oral Considerations

The oral manifestations of this fungal infection are common and may present in all three forms of the disease. Primary infection of the mouth or gastrointestinal tract is thought to be rare and hence oral lesions are mainly secondary. In the mucocutaneous form of the disease the oral lesions may be the most apparent presenting symptom. The lesions appear initially as small papules or vesicles, which then ulcerate and appear as shallow ulcers with a rolled edge and a white exudative base studded with small hemorrhagic dots. The lesions have a granulomatous appearance and spread slowly, causing extensive local destruction. Pain is not usually a feature of early lesions but may become severe as the disease progresses, leading to cachexia as a result of acute pain on eating. In severe cases, infection may extend into bone, leading to perforation of the hard palate. Gross fibrosis and scarring may occur as a result of attempted healing. Lesions have been described in almost all parts of the mouth and pharynx including the hard and soft palates, gingiva, tongue and tonsils. Infections in the gingival and periodontal tissues may lead to loosening and loss of teeth. Infiltration of the oral tissues, especially the lips and cheeks, may severely reduce facial mobility and radically inhibit movement of the mandible. The face may become grossly swollen, and the mouth held open with a constant escape of saliva at the angles. Regional lymph nodes draining the areas involved enlarge and often suppurate with the formation of sinus tracts. The fluid which drains from the sinuses contains numerous fungal cells.

Diagnosis and Management

Diagnosis is confirmed by histology and culture. Sulphonamide or amphotericin B, alone or in combination, is the treatment of choice. The doses used and length of administration are matters for expert clinical judgment in individual cases. Ketoconazole has been successfully used in the management of paracoccidioidomycosis.

Penicilliosis

Penicillium marneffei is a yeast-like fungus and cause disease—penicilliosis, in the normal host, as well as in immunosuppressed patients, but significantly, it has now become a major opportunistic pathogen in HIV-infected patients in Indochina, particularly Northern Thailand. Imported cases of *P. marneffei* infections have been reported from Australia, France, Italy, Netherlands, UK and United States. Human-to-human transmission of penicilliosis is highly unlikely.

P. marneffei infection may either be disseminated or focal in patients who are otherwise healthy, but in HIV disease disseminated infection is the norm. The clinical and histological appearances of focal infection strongly resemble tuberculosis. Fungaemia may be present in systemic disease together with skin affections, reticuloendothelial system, lung and gut. Patients usually present with non-specific symptoms of fever, anemia and weight loss.

Oral Considerations

Skin lesions are usually located on the face, trunk and extremities. The most common skin lesions are papules often with a central necrotic umbilication with or without subcutaneous abscesses that may ulcerate. Intraorally the lesions may be seen as papules, as erosions or shallow ulcers of varying size covered with yellow necrotic slough. The palate, gingiva, labial mucosa, tongue and oropharynx are the most common sites involved.

Diagnosis and Management

Diagnosis is confirmed by histology and culture. Although itraconazole is extremely effective against *P. marneffei* infection, initial treatment is usually amphotericin B followed by oral itraconazole up to 10 weeks. As relapse is common, long-term maintenance therapy with itraconazole is recommended.

Sporotrichosis

Sporotrichosis is a chronic nodular subcutaneous mycotic disease with a worldwide distribution, but is most frequently found in Central America, Brazil and Mexico. The causative agent is *Sporotrichum schenckii*, a fungus found in moss, soil and rotting wood, with the result that such persons as agricultural workers, florists and miners have a higher incidence of the infection than the general population. Sporotrichosis is highly unlikely to be transmitted from human-to-humans.

Sporotrichum schenckii gains access to the subcutaneous tissues via traumatic lesions, and proliferation of the fungus leads to the appearance of a nodule or small ulcer as soon as five days or as long as six months after inoculation. The nodule becomes a bubo, which may change color from pink to purple then ulcerate. The common site of the primary lesions is the finger, although the face can also be involved. After several weeks or months the initial lesion tends to heal with scarring, as new buboes develop in other areas. The regional lymph nodes become infected and the spread of the fungus can be recognized by the inflammation of the lymph vessels draining the initial lesion. The infection usually becomes chronic and locally destructive or may disseminate to the skin, oral mucosa, bone and other organs.

Oral Considerations

The oral manifestations of *sporotrichosis* may be primary, which is rare, or secondary as a result of dissemination from the skin or lung. The lesions are initially erythematous, ulcerative and suppurative and eventually become granulomatous, vegetative or papillomatous. The oral lesions are usually painful and the regional lymph nodes are hard and enlarged. The mucosal lesions usually heal without residual scarring. Oral sporotrichosis may resemble aphthous ulcers, lichen planus, secondary cutaneous leishmaniasis. On rare occasions the nose and sinuses may be involved with extension of infection to the orbit.

Diagnosis and Management

Diagnosis is confirmed by histology and culture. Amphotericin B is the most effective drug for treating relapsed lymphocutaneous sporotrichosis or the pulmonary and disseminated forms of the disease. Itraconazole is an alternative.

Box 16.1: Oral fungal infections

Key features useful in diagnosis

- Most common oral mucosal infection is candidiasis
- Candidiasis is usually seen in 'the very young, the very old and the very sick'
- Candidiasis could be primary (restricted only to the oral mucosa) or secondary (as a part of widespread systemic affection)
- Most oral fungal infections (80–90 %) are caused by *Candida albicans*
- Primary candidiasis is often due to an underlying predisposing factor such as a poorly fitting denture
- The classic triad of oral candidiasis are pseudomembranous (most common), erythematous and hyperplastic (least common) variants
- Pseudomembranous candidiasis is characterized by easily wiped off, creamy white, curd-like patches on protected sites of oral mucosa, such as in sulcal areas with low salivary flow and tongue movement
- A Gram stain of the pseudomembrane shows necrotic epithelial tissue held together by matted filamentous elements of *Candida*, with or without polymorphonuclear leukocytes
- Erythematous lesions are usually seen as red patches over palatal (mostly posterior) mucosa, and as depapillated areas of the tongue
- Hyperplastic lesions are discrete raised plaques often seen in retrocommissural area, that cannot be wiped off (compare pseudomembranous variant)
- Candidiasis in immunocompromised patients may take a more widespread form with contiguous lesions of erythematous and pseudomembranous variants (multifocal candidiasis) on the mucosa, and represents a more widespread affection
- Oral lesions of deep mycotic lesions are rare and often present as nodules or necrotic ulcerations and they are almost exclusively found in patients with compromised immune systems
- Differential diagnosis of a chronic oral ulcer in compromised patients should include rare mycoses such as histoplasmosis and cryptococcosis.

ORAL VIRAL INFECTIONS

The vast majority of virus infections of the oral mucosa are due to the herpes group of viruses. Of some 80 known herpesviruses eight are human pathogens of which herpes simplex virus causes a contagious infection with a large reservoir in the general population. Occasionally other viruses, such as coxsackieviruses, papillomaviruses and paramyxoviruses (which cause measles and mumps), may manifest with oral symptoms.

Primary Herpes Simplex Infection: Herpetic Stomatitis (HHV-1, HHV-2)

Herpetic stomatitis is the most common viral infection to affect the mouth; it is caused by human herpesviruses 1 and 2 (HHV-1, HHV-2). The incubation period is about 5 days and the virus is transmitted by contact with skin lesions or infected saliva. Children may carry the virus asymptomatically, or as convalescent carriers, in saliva for several months, but the virus is rarely isolated from adults once the primary lesion heals. The early-childhood infection is usually subclinical, frequently dismissed as 'teething', but if the infection occurs in adults the symptoms are obvious and severe. In countries with high standards of hygiene, there is an increasing frequency of adults presenting with primary herpes.

Clinical Features

In the initial stages there is mild to severe fever and enlarged lymph nodes, with pain in the mouth and throat; then a variable number of vesicles develop haphazardly on the oral mucosa, the tongue and gingivae. These vesicles rupture quickly to form small round or irregular superficial ulcers with erythematous haloes and grayish-yellow bases. The gingivae are inflamed and the infection may be confused with acute necrotizing ulcerative gingivitis (ANUG) of bacterial origin. In some, ANUG may develop secondary to primary herpetic stomatitis. The mouth is sore and eating and swallowing may be difficult. The lesions resolve without scarring within 5 to 10 days. Intraoral viral shedding may persist for several weeks after clinical resolution.

Secondary Herpes Simplex Infection: Herpes Labialis (HHV-1, HHV-2)

About one-third of the patients who have had primary infection develop herpes labialis (cold sore) in later life as a result of reactivation of the latent virus, which usually resides in the trigeminal ganglion. The stimulus for reactivation could be:

- Stress
- Trauma
- Exposure to sunlight
- Menstruation
- Debilitating disease.

The lesion develops at the mucocutaneous junction of the lip or on the skin adjacent to the nostrils. Characteristically the lesions are preceded, some 24 hours before, by a premonitory sign of itching, prickling or a burning sensation. Blisters then develop, enlarge, coalesce, rupture, become encrusted and heal within 10 to 14 days.

Intraoral recurrent herpetic infections are infrequent; they involve the hard palate, alveolar ridges and gingiva. These lesions develop in a similar manner to those of the lips, and appear as a cluster of small, shallow ulcers with red, irregular margins. Pain is not a common feature and the intraoral lesions may or may not recur intermittently for years.

Herpetic Dermatitis and Herpetic Whitlow (HHV-1 and HHV-2)

Primary herpetic dermatitis is localized and characterized by pruritus, burning and pain. Multiple vesicles appear, persist for 4 to 5 days and burst, with resultant crusting scabs which heal within 2 to 3 weeks. Dentists who escaped exposure in childhood may contract herpetic dermatitis from patients who have either primary or secondary herpes. Infection may take the form of a herpetic whitlow on the finger, resulting in an intensely painful lesion. Herpetic whitlow may recur, but less frequently than the perioral infection.

Laboratory Diagnosis of Herpetic Infection

It is useful to establish definitive diagnosis of the lesion through laboratory tests. These include viral isolation in tissue culture, cytological examination, direct fluorescent antibody tests, serological assays and DNA detection by PCR based methodology.

Direct Examination and PCR Technology

Smears of lesions stained with monoclonal fluorescent antisera to herpes simplex virus type 1 or 2 (HHV-1 or -2) provide specific and rapid diagnosis. Although PCR based techniques have superseded antibody based cytology, the former is more expensive and not readily available as yet.

Culture

Herpes simplex virus is readily isolated from samples of oral lesions in a variety of tissue culture systems. Appropriate transport media should however, be used when sending samples for virology tests.

Serology

In primary infection a fourfold or greater increase in antibody titer between the acute and convalescent sera is indicative of recent infection with herpes simplex virus. The demonstration of immunoglobulin M (IgM) antibodies by immunofluorescence techniques in a single sample can also be used in diagnosis.

Management

Moderate to severe primary herpetic stomatitis is treated with oral and topical aciclovir, together with symptomatic measures. However, the use of aciclovir in recurrent herpetic infections should be limited to immunocompromised patients and those who have a past history of severe, extensive or frequently recurring lesions. The patients should apply the drug before vesicles form to obtain the best results. For those not responding to topical applications a low prophylactic dose of acyclovir may assist to prevent recurrent infections.

Varicella and Zoster (HHV-3)

Primary infection with the *varicella-zoster* virus causes chickenpox. Zoster or shingles is the secondary (synonym: post-primary, reactivation) infection due to the reactivation of the virus hiding in the latent form in sensory ganglia.

Chickenpox

Chickenpox is a common infectious disease and is usually contracted in childhood.

Oral Manifestations

Before the typical skin rash develops, lesions may be found in the mouth, especially on the hard palate, pillars of the fauces and uvula, although any area of the oral mucosa may be involved. The characteristic skin rash, which is centripetal, and progresses from macular to papular, vesicular and pustular forms before scabbing, helps to differentiate chickenpox from other causes of oral ulceration. The oral lesions consist of small ulcers surrounded by an area of erythema. The vesicles are quickly ruptured in the mouth and therefore rarely noticed. The lesions may be painful in adults, but children rarely complain of discomfort.

Shingles (Zoster)

Shingles is a localized eruption due to the reactivation of the herpes zoster virus. It involves an area of skin supplied by one or more sensory ganglia in which the virus is residing. In some 10 percent of cases zoster reflects an underlying immune-deficiency state, possibly a neoplasm such as lymphoma or HIV disease.

Oral Manifestations

The trigeminal nerve is affected in about 15 percent of cases, with the ophthalmic, maxillary and mandibular divisions involved in that order of precedence. The lesions of shingles may be found on the skin, on the oral mucosa, or both. Severe localized oral pain often precedes the rash and mimics the pain of toothache. The most common intraoral sites affected are the anterior half of the tongue, the soft palate and the cheek. The vesicles break down intraorally within a few hours to give very painful ulcerated areas with a yellowish-gray surface and erythematous borders. The oral lesions heal more quickly than the skin lesions and rarely scar.

Laboratory diagnosis of chickenpox and shingles.

The clinical presentation is characteristic, but in unusual circumstances the disease can be confirmed in the laboratory by submitting:

- Vesicle fluid for electron microscopy and virus isolation
- Smears from an ulcer for immunofluorescence
- Acute or convalescent sera to test for the presence of specific IgM antibodies by immunofluorescence.
- PCR based assays.

Management

Chickenpox is self-limiting; but an effective vaccine is available to prevent infection. For zoster, high-dose aciclovir (800 mg five times daily) should be prescribed as soon as possible, especially in immunocompromised patients.

Epstein–Barr Virus (Human Herpesvirus 4)

Epstein-barr virus (EBV) is widespread in humans, and most adults have antibody to the virus. The virus persists in latent form within lymphocytes after primary infection (lymphotrophic, unlike HSV and varicella-zoster virus, which are neurotrophic). The genome resides in a latent form in B cells; latent EBV infection is common in the population. It is the etiological agent of a number of diseases:

- Infectious mononucleosis (glandular fever)
- Burkitt's lymphoma and other B-cell lymphomas
- Nasopharyngeal carcinoma (especially in southern Chinese populations)

- Oral hairy leukoplakia
- Post-transplant lymphoproliferative diseases.

Infectious Mononucleosis

An acute infection affecting lymphoid tissue throughout the body, infectious mononucleosis is commonly seen in teenagers, with a peak incidence at 15 to 20 years of age. The organism responsible—EBV, is present in saliva and is postulated to be transmitted during kissing—hence it is called the 'kissing disease'.

Incubation Period

Incubation is 4 to 7 weeks; possibly shorter (10–40 days) in young children.

Signs and Symptoms

These include low-grade fever with generalized lymphadenopathy and abnormal lymphocytes in the blood (note that a similar illness, glandular fever-like syndrome, develops during the first fortnight after infection with human immunodeficiency virus (HIV)). Fever, tonsillitis and fatigue are common, and many patients have splenomegaly. Lymphocytosis is a characteristic feature, hence the term 'mononucleosis'; some 10 percent of the lymphocytes are atypical, with enlarged misshapen nuclei and increased cytoplasm.

Chronic, Persistent or Reactivated EBV Infection

This may take many clinical forms and is less common than acute mononucleosis, described above. The syndrome is characterized by persistent fatigue, with or without physical or laboratory findings.

Epidemiology

The virus is ubiquitous and humans are its only known host. Spread of EBV is via respiratory secretions, primarily through oral contact. Those from lower socioeconomic classes are exposed to EBV at an early age and typically develop asymptomatic infections, while in higher socioeconomic classes, particularly in developed countries, primary infection is usually delayed to adolescence or young adulthood.

Diagnosis

As EBV cannot be easily propagated in culture, serological diagnosis is common:
- *Indirect immunofluorescence is used to detect EBV-specific immunoglobulin M* (IgM): The antibody is directed against both the capsid antigen and a non-capsid early antigen
- *Hematology:* A blood film is useful for demonstrating atypical lymphocytosis in infectious mononucleosis
- *Heterophile antibody* (non-specific): Infectious mononucleosis is characterized by the appearance of heterophile (hetero: other, phile: liking) antibodies in the patient's serum, which agglutinate sheep or horse red blood cells. This property is made use of in the Paul-Bunnell diagnostic test.

Treatment

Infectious mononucleosis is generally mild and self-limiting, hence therapy is usually symptomatic.

Burkitt's Lymphoma

Burkitt's lymphoma is a highly malignant tumor which spreads rapidly, with widespread metastases; it is particularly common in African children. The disease is especially common in areas of Africa with endemic malaria. Hence, it is thought that the effect of the malarial parasite on the reticuloendothelial system could cause an abnormal response to infection with EBV. Under these conditions the EBV may become frankly oncogenic, producing a malignant transformation in lymphoid tissue (lymphoma) instead of the benign proliferation seen in infectious mononucleosis.

Nasopharyngeal Carcinoma

A tumor with a remarkable geographic and probably racial distribution, it is particularly common among the southern Chinese. EBV DNA is regularly present in the malignant epithelial cells of the tumor.

Hairy Leukoplakia

The term 'hairy leukoplakia' is given to raised, white areas of thickening, particularly on the lateral border of the tongue. Although this new clinical entity was first described in HIV-infected patients, other immunosuppressed patients may develop the lesion, which is very closely associated with EBV. The DNA of EBV is present in the epithelial cells of hairy leukoplakia. The lesion is non-malignant but about a third of HIV-infected individuals who develop hairy leukoplakia may develop acquired immune-deficiency syndrome (AIDS) in 3 to 5 years. Demonstration of EBV in biopsy tissue of hairy leukoplakia is essential for a definitive diagnosis.

Cytomegalovirus (Human Herpesvirus 5; HHV-5)

Cytomegalovirus (CMV) rarely causes disease unless other precipitating factors, such as immunocompromising states, are present. However, it can infect the fetus during pregnancy.

Clinical Disease

Symptomless infection: The majority of infants show no signs of infection and diagnosis is made by serology. Although a large proportion of the infants are unharmed, a significant number of neonates with congenital infection show neurological sequelae, such as deafness and mental retardation, later in life. A minority develop a severe, often fatal illness associated with infection of the salivary glands, brain, kidneys, liver and lungs.

Postnatal infection: Later in life the virus may be activated by pregnancy, multiple blood trans-fusions or immunosuppression. Infection in immunocompromised patients can be severe and involve many organs, such as the lungs, liver, gastrointestinal tract and eyes.

Epidemiology

Infection appears to increase during the perinatal period and during early adulthood; patients with neoplastic disease or AIDS and transplant recipients often have local and disseminated CMV disease. The route of CMV transmission is not clear.

Diagnosis and Treatment

Diagnosis is by viral isolation in human embryonic fibroblast tissue cultures; it is confirmed using immunofluorescence and DNA hybridization.

There are no proven regimens for therapy and prevention of CMV infections.

Oral Manifestations of Other Herpesviruses (HHV-6 to HHV-8)

Other herpesvirus infections are generally of minor consequence, except for Kaposi's sarcoma caused by HHV-8.

Coxsackie Virus Infections

Two diseases caused by group A coxsackie viruses produce oral signs and symptoms:

- Hand, foot and mouth disease, caused mainly by coxsackie virus A16 and, less commonly, by types A4, A5, A9 or A10
- Herpangina, caused by coxsackie viruses A2, A4, A5, A6 and A8.

Oral Manifestations of Herpangina

This febrile disease is characterized by sore throat, dysphagia, anorexia and occasionally a stiff neck. Accompanying oral signs and symptoms are small, papulovesicular lesions about 1 to 2 mm in diameter, with a grayish-white surface surrounded by red areolae, especially in the palate. The disease lasts for about 3 to 4 days, the fever abates and the oral lesions heal promptly.

Paramyxovirus Infections

Measles, mumps, parainfluenza and respiratory syncytial viruses are categorized as paramyxoviruses. Of these, measles and mumps are of concern in dentistry as they commonly manifest with oral signs or symptoms. Measles is discussed in Chapter 10; mumps is described later under salivary gland infections.

Human Papillomavirus Infections

Papillomavirus is a DNA virus and there are more than 80 serogroups. Some are associated with mucosal and skin malignancies than others. It has been found that nearly 40 percent of the adult population carry the virus in the oral mucosal surfaces, suggesting that mouth is a reservoir of the virus. Serotypes 16 and 18, which are the etiological agents of cervical cancer in women, are also linked to oral cancers.

Box 16.2: Oral viral infections

Key features useful in diagnosis

- Herpes simplex lesions present as painful shallow ulcers over the oral mucosa often associated with fever
- In secondary herpes simplex infections (reactivation) there is often a preceding history of exposure to trigger factors such as exposure to sun, stress, and menstruation
- Itching sensation of a focal area is usually a prodromal symptom of herpetic labialis
- Intraoral lesions precede the generalized rash in chickenpox, but the maculopapular lesions may not be easily noticed due to bursting of the papule
- EBV and CMV manifest as pharyngitis with associated lymphadenopathy and fever with generalized malaise.

BACTERIAL INFECTIONS OF THE ORAL MUCOSA

- Tuberculosis
- Syphilis
- Gonorrhea
- Streptococcal infections
- Actinomycosis.

Tuberculosis of the Oral Mucosa

Mycobacterium tuberculosis and, rarely other mycobacterial species can cause chronic granulomatous lesions of the oral mucosa. It has been noted primarily in patients affected by HIV infection. Lesions could be primary or secondary (secondary to active pulmonary tuberculosis). Chronic, deep, irregular and painful ulcers on the lateral surfaces of the tongue are a common feature of primary tuberculosis, while secondary lesions are indurated painful ulcers.

Diagnosis

Tuberculosis lesions are best diagnosed through histological examination of an oral biopsy.

Syphilis

Syphilis has regained prominence as a sexually transmitted disease as a result of increasing high-risk sexual behavior across populations in the world. Oral syphilis may therefore be the presenting feature of a wide spectrum of sexually transmitted diseases including HIV. The disease is caused by a bacteria *Treponema pallidum*. Because the presentation of different stages of syphilis is highly varied, it is often called the 'great imitator' of diseases.

Primary Syphilis

The chancre is the defining lesion of primary syphilis. It is not as common as genital lesions occurring in some 10 percent of the cases. Transmission is primarily due to orogenital or oroanal contact and rarely through kissing. Lips and the tongues are the common sites affected. The ulcers are usually deep, with a red, purple, or brown base and an irregular raised border. The lesions usually heal within about five weeks. Regional lymph node enlargement is a common feature during the early phase of the infection. Due to its painless nature the chancres may go unnoticed or mistaken for other solitary ulcerations on the oral mucosa. The lesions contain live organisms and are considered highly infectious.

Diagnosis

The detailed analysis of the sexual/social lifestyle including the details about sexual partners is necessary to arrive at a presumptive diagnosis. The early laboratory diagnosis may be difficult because the first line of non specific tests (Rapid Plasma Reagin, RPR and Venereal Disease Reference Laboratory, VDRL) take time to become positive. The specific tests for IgG antibodies to *T. pallidum* become positive before VDRL and RRP tests, and thus should be carried out when a diagnosis of primary disease is likely.

Although the lesions are full of live treponemes, which can be demonstrated through dark field microscopy, it is generally not recommended to do so for the risk of nosocomial transmission and the confusion with the treponemes of the normal oral flora (*T. denticola, T. pectinovorum* and *T. vincentii*).

Secondary Syphilis

Oral lesions in secondary syphilis is the result of blood-borne spread of *Treponema pallidum*. Unlike primary syphilis, the oral manifestations are more varied and can be extensive. Nearly one-third of the patients with secondary syphilis may have oral lesions. Mucosal patches are the most common lesion found on the oral mucosa. These are usually distributed over the tonsils, soft palate, tongue and cheek (**Fig. 16.8**). Regional lymph node enlargement is a common feature and they tend to have a rubbery consistency.

The grayish surface of the lesions are easily removable and contains numerous spirocheates. Therefore, the lesions themselves are infectious. Coalescence of these lesions lead to serpiginous lesions termed as 'snail tract ulcers'. Sometimes snail tract ulcers occur *de novo* as well. These lesions heal spontaneously within 2 to 6 weeks and recurrences are seen in about 25 percent of the patients. However, unrelated antimicrobial treatment can expedite the healing of these lesions.

In addition to the maculopapular and mucosal patches, nodular necrotic lesions can be seen on the oral mucosa (lues maligna). These necrotic lesions are associated with systemic symptoms like fever, headache and myalgia and are common among patients who are also infected with HIV. The nodular lesions are commonly seen on the oral mucosa and may mimic malignant lesions.

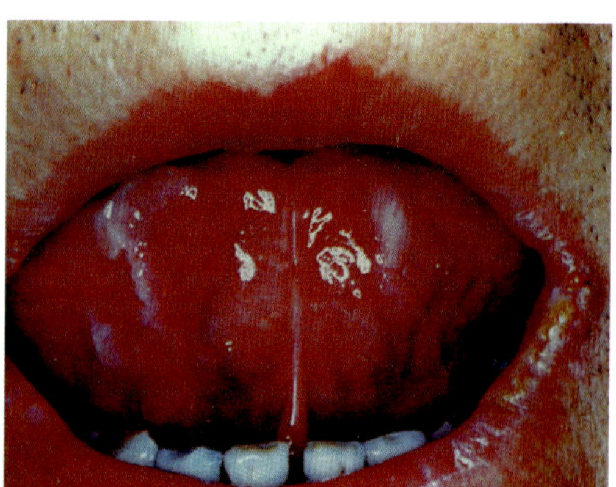

Fig. 16.8: Mucosal patches of secondary syphilis

Diagnosis

Although *T. pallidum* can usually be detected on the surface of erosions or ulcers by darkfield microscopy, it is best avoided for the reasons mentioned above. The histopathological features of secondary syphilis vary. However, perivascular infiltrates with a preponderance of plasma cells are a major feature.

Tertiary Syphilis

Approximately one-third of patients with untreated secondary syphilis progress into a much more systemic form of the disease called tertiary syphilis. The characteristic lesion of this stage of the disease is the formation of gumma. Inside the oral cavity gummata are commonly seen on the hard palate .The lesions start as small, midline, pale, raised and painless area. Ulcerations follow and rapid progression to large necrotic zone with exposure of bone is a common feature. The palate may get perforated into the nasal cavity. Unlike in the primary and secondary disease no treponemes could be found in gummata.

More rarely, interstitial glossitis which manifest as atrophy of filiform and fungiform papillae develops. These lesions lead syphilitic leukoplakia and are thought increase the development of oral squamous carcinoma.

Diagnosis

Histological examination of the gummata characteristically show endarteritis obliterans, necrosis with epithelioid and giant cells and a plasma cell infiltrates. At this stage, the nonspecific tests (VDRL and RPR) may not be positive; the most reliable serological test is FTA which might remain positive long after the treatment is finished.

Gonorrhea

Oral gonococcal infections principally affect the tonsillar surfaces and the oropharynx, but gingivostomatitis is also common. The causative organism is *Neisseria gonorrhoeae*, a Gram-negative diplococcus. The clinical presentation varies from mild erythema to deep ulcers covered by a pseudomembrane. The disease is often transmitted sexually through orogenital contact and thus is common among the sexual active persons and can affect the male and female alike. It often coincides with the genital infections and isolated oral infections are rare. Moreover, transmission of pharyngeal infection to other sites is also uncommon. Disseminated gonococcal infection occurs particularly in patients with complement deficiency, particularly the membrane attack complex (C5b, C6, C7, C8, and C9).

Box 16.3: Oral bacterial infections

Key features useful in diagnosis

- The typical lesion in primary syphilis is a chancre; a deep reddish purple painless ulcer with raised edges (differential diagnosis includes carcinoma and tuberculous ulcer)
- Oral chancres are uncommon and demands a high degree of suspicion
- Chancres are full of live treponemes but interpretation of direct smears may be difficult as commensal treponemes can affect the interpretation of the findings
- Secondary syphilis lesions present as mucosal patches over the oral mucosa with associated lymphadenopathy
- Coalescence of these lesions lead to serpiginous lesions termed as `snail tract ulcers`
- Lues maligna is a type of nodular lesion found over the palatal surfaces in secondary syphilis
- Tertiary syphilis is a more systemic form of disease and characterized by the formation of gummata
- Gummata are common over the palatal surface and have a nodular appearance
- Left unattended these lesions can become necrotic leading to widespread palatal perforations.

Diagnosis

Diagnosis is made through microbiological examination of the purulent material collected from the lesions. A Gram stained smear will show Gram-negative diplococci. Definitive diagnosis and antimicrobial susceptibility of the isolates are determined by culturing in Thayer-Martin medium.

Uncomplicated infections respond well to a single dose of intramuscular ceftriaxone. Oral cefixime, ofloxacin or ciprofloxacin has also been shown to be of equal efficacy. It is important to note that in the presence of one sexually transmitted disease there can be other concomitant infections. For example, chlamydial infections are seen in approximately 50 percent of gonorrhea patients.

Other Bacterial Infections

Streptococcal infections take the form of very erythematous painful and inflamed lesions over many parts of the oral mucosa. *Klebsiella rhinoscleromatis* causes a chronic granulomatous infection as a part of respiratory scleroma, which can manifest as oral granulomas. Although the site of entry of different *Actinomycosis spp.* is the oral mucosa, oral actinomycosis seldom present as mucosal ulcers and is caused by *Actinomyces israelii, A. viscosus, A. naeslundii* and *A. odontolyticus.*

PARASITIC INFECTIONS OF THE ORAL MUCOSA

Mucocutaneous Leishmaniasis

As opposed to viral and fungal infection of the oral mucosa, parasitic infections are a rarity. Out of them by far the most common is leishmaniasis, which is caused by the protozoan parasites of the genus *Leishmania.* Of the three clinical types of leishmaniasis (cutaneous, mucocutaneous and visceral) the mucocutaneous variant (Espundia) affects the oral mucosa. The disease is generally confined to certain geographical areas and 90 percent of all cases seen in Bolivia, Peru and Brazil. However, increased human movement has resulted in cases reported sporadically in more than 90 countries of the world. There are more than 20 species of the parasite that affects humans. Four species known as the Viannia subgroup (*L. braziliensis, L. amazonensis, L. panamensis,* and *L. guyanensis*) cause the mucocutaneous lesions. The disease is transmitted through the bite of sand flies, *Phlebotomus* and *Lutzomyia*.

The most common presentation of mucocutaneous leishmaniasis is persistent nasal congestion and erosive erythematous ulcers can be seen around the nares and lips in advanced cases. In more severe cases palatal ulceration, gingival edema, and periodontitis develops. Eventually, progressive destruction mucosa, and cartilaginous facial and upper airway structures, resulting in secondary infection, disfiguration and airway obstruction.

Diagnosis

Biopsy and demonstration of intracellular amastigotes are required for diagnosis. Histological examination of the biopsy material or touch smears from lesions may only show few parasites. However, specimens commonly reveal granulomatous reaction.

Myiasis

Oral myiasis often associated with severe underlying immunocompromised status such as neutropenia and malignancies. Malignant ulcers can be infested with fly eggs and they are hatched into larval forms which may be visible at the time of examination.

Treatment

Therapy with ivermectin and manual removal of the larvae is the standard mode of treatment but the lesions are very difficult to eradicate unless the underlying condition is treated.

Box 16.4: Oral parasitic infections

Key features useful in diagnosis

- Mucocutaneous leishmaniasis may present as lip nodules, often represent a part of a more widespread disease.
- In more advanced cases there can be erosive erythematous ulcers seen around the nares.

SELF-ASSESSMENT QUESTIONS

1. Provide a classification for candidal lesions of the oral cavity.
2. Discuss the importance in '*in toto*' assessment of a dental patient in relation to the diagnosis of candidal and other fungal infections.
3. List the predisposing factors for the development of oral candidiasis together with examples of the situation in which they may occur.
4. Describe the orofacial presentation of human herpes virus infection.
5. List the common bacterial infections of the oral cavity and describe their clinical presentation.
6. Discuss the interpretation of laboratory tests in the diagnosis of the different stages of syphilis.
7. Discuss the relevance of a direct smear in the diagnosis of viral infections of the oral mucosa.
8. Give an account of parasitic infections of the oral mucosa.
9. List the oral manifestations associated with systemic viral infections.
10. List the (i) common and (ii) uncommon infectious diseases that may cause oral ulceration.

SUGGESTED READING

1. Samaranayake LP. Essential Microbiology for Dentistry, 3rd edn. Edinburgh: Churchill Livingstone Elsevier; 2006.
2. Scully C, de Almeida OP. Orofacial manifestations of the systemic mycoses. J Oral Pathol Med. 1992;21:289-94.

Chapter 17

Connective Tissue Diseases

Richard J Cook

Chapter Outline

INTRODUCTION

Autoimmune and connective tissue disorders represent a group of conditions in which the humoral and cell based immune defense system has malfunctioned and recognized host tissue and cell structures as hostile. Accordingly, the patterns of disease can be specific but more often are a mixture of common and less common symptoms and signs requiring interpretation and judgment to establish a diagnosis. Connective tissue disorders are characterized by a series of signs and symptoms linked (to variable extents) by a common etiology of multiple autoantibody production, immune complex deposition and vasculitis, causing joint, soft tissue and muscle pain with inflammation.

The most classical hard tissue condition a rheumatologist would manage is rheumatoid arthritis. In terms of the soft tissue conditions, the three classic conditions a rheumatologist might consider in this group are:

1. Systemic lupus erythematosus (SLE) (and the discoid/DLE variant).
2. The poly and dermatomyositis groups of conditions.
3. The systemic sclerosis group.

Such conditions are regarded as nonorgan specific. In contrast, organ specific conditions feature an autoantibody targeted at a specific tissue or cell function, e.g. pemphigus, pemphigoid, myasthenia gravis, pernicious anemia and Grave's type hyperthyroidism. These conditions will not be considered further here (See Chapter 15).

A patient with an autoimmune disease is most likely to be female, the more prevalent tissue types in the group being HLA B8, B51 (Behçet's) DR3 and DR4 (rheumatoid). Autoantibodies may well be detectable in the serum, which can be indicative of the condition, but rarely diagnostic, without additional clinical evidence. Circulating autoantibodies may be detectable in clinically uninvolved relatives too, but a family history is common in these conditions. In general terms, the disease group is managed by immunomodulatory drugs.

While it is convenient to consider these diseases as separate entities in descriptive terms, they have many symptoms, signs and investigation results in common, leading to the concept of "overlap syndrome" or "mixed connective tissue disease"—which includes common elements of two or more of these conditions (**Fig. 17.1**). Of additional interest to oral care practitioners are the hard tissue rheumatological disorders, classically rheumatoid arthritis and its variants, sharing the same fundamental etiopathological mechanism but typically manifesting in joint damage. These conditions all have a common link as potential primary causes of secondary oro-ocular and genital dryness, i.e. Sjögren's syndrome—discussed in Chapter 11. The terminology designating primary/secondary is currently under revision.

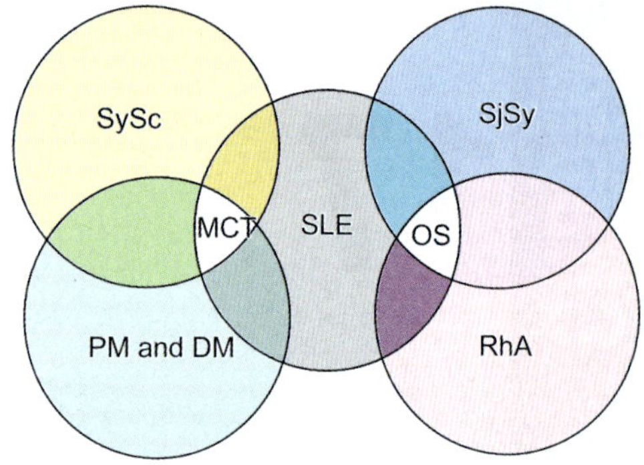

Fig. 17.1: Complex mixes of autoimmune conditions—overlaps and mixed patterns are common and some of the more common overlaps are shown here. SySc: Systemic sp sclerosis; PM and DM: Poly and dermatomyositis; SLE: Systemic lupus erythematosus; SjSy: Sjögren's syndrome; RhA: Rheumatoid arthritis; MCT: Mixed connective tissue disease; OS: Overlap syndrome. Readers should note these are illustrative: Many more overlaps occur—particularly between right and left side—as if the diagram was a continuum arranged around a cylinder

SOFT TISSUE CONDITIONS

Systemic Lupus Erythematosus

Systemic lupus erythematosus can present with a host of symptoms, being a multisystem disorder, and consequently is the most common

▪ Table 17.1
Etiological factors in development of lupus

Genetic	Increased incidence in HLA-B8 and DR3 Also 25% concordance for SLE between identical twins suggesting a heritable predisposition
Infection	Viral agents are thought most likely agents to be able to trigger such an immunologic condition
Drugs	Procainamide and hydralazine use can cause mild lupus like symptoms which resolve on drug withdrawal
Immunological	Unknown antigen promotes polyclonal B cell activation yielding elevated serum ANAs—possibly permitted by T cell and complement control dysfunctions. Most tissue damage reflects inflammation provoked by local anti-DNA/DNA complex deposition
Gender	Female gender predominance

Source: Ballinger A, Patchett S. Essentials of Clinical Medicine. 3rd edn. Saunders.

connective tissue disorder, characterized by elevated serum autoantibodies against elements of the cell nucleus—the ANAs, in particular the double-stranded DNA autoantibody (**Table 17.1**). Lupus can be subdivided into the systemic, drug related and benign discoid forms. The title "lupus" refers to tissue damage as resembling "wolf bites" and erythematosus describes the red lesions—particularly butterfly rash over the nasal and malar regions, induced by bright artificial and sunlight UV sensitivity.

Epidemiology

With a peak incidence in women in their third and fourth decades, approximately 0.1 percent of the western population are said to be affected, with a predilection for those with African heritage.

Etiology

Unsurprisingly in a multifactorial condition this remains obscure, but a series of factors have been identified as likely agents (risks or risk factors) for developing lupus (**Table 17.1**).

Signs and Symptoms

The majority of SLE symptoms are driven by the immune complex deposition associated vasculitis and the condition can vary in severity, from minor symptoms to life-threatening organ involvement (particularly renal). In small vessels, immune complexes lodge and fix, whereas in larger vessels, more active complexes bind to vessel wall ligands (and can precipitate in large vessel wall microcirculations too) to exert their proinflammatory effects and establish patterns of inflammation, capable of irritating and subsequently obstructing vessels as endothelium and flow both degenerate.

A flitting asymmetrical polyarthralgia (painful joints) is one of the most common symptoms. Unlike rheumatoid arthritis, joint swelling and damage is very rare in pure lupus.

The definitive butterfly rash, fanning out onto the cheeks from across the nasal bridge, reflects a solar sensitive cutaneous vasculitis—but is not always present **(Figs 17.2A and B)**. Nonspecific features such as recurrent fevers, low mood, and a general sense of ill health may dominate the clinical presentation although many features may present (**Table 17.2**).

The benign variant: Discoid lupus may only involve orocutaneous epithelial tissue. Typically a solar sensitive, patchy, crusting lupine rash arises in exposed skin, which can develop to include scarring, depapillation in hairy skin, and later pigmentation, along with a lichen like, reticular hyperkeratotic lesion in the oral mucosa, which can also erode and settle leaving postinflammatory pigmentation **(Fig. 17.2)**—often the buccal epithelium. Joint pains are often the only other complaint. A diagnostic biopsy may show a perivascular rather than purely subepithelial inflammatory infiltrate—helping to discriminating it from lichen planus. Serological investigations are usually negative but elevated serum ANAs are noted in the majority and other immune markers may be weakly positive only. It is considered unlikely for DLE to herald SLE development in most cases, and is best controlled with topical steroid preparations.

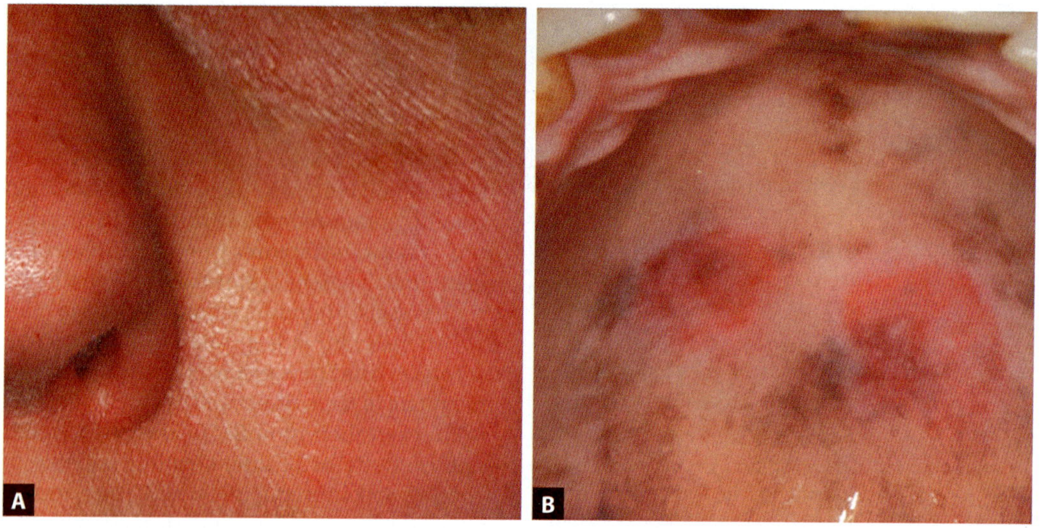

Figs 17.2A and B: Lupus features. (A) Typical photosensitive lupus rash across nasal bridge and into cheeks; (B) Intraoral lesions forming discoid erosions and pigment deposition at sites of former inflammatory processes

Diagnostic Investigations

In lupus, a chronic disease (normochromic, normocytic) anemia pattern is often seen on blood film. Consumption of inflammatory mediators during active flares produces a low complement level, leukopenia and thrombocytopenia, typically with a raised ESR but unaltered CRP. The classic autoantibody detectable is the antidouble-stranded DNA (dsDNA) which may be regarded as diagnostic for SLE—but is only positive in approximately 50 percent of cases. Rheumatoid factor is positive in approximately 25 percent of cases and anticardiolipin antibodies are detectable in 30 to 40 percent of patients too.

A biopsy of involved tissue may (inconsistently) show a vasculitis pattern—of importance in an oral biopsy of suspected Lichen planus—which can alter the diagnosis to discoid lupus instead. Basement membrane thickening, acanthosis and epithelial thinning with inconsistent grainy immunofluorescence against immunoglobulins, and complement at the basement membrane and perivascularly, are present both in normal and lesion/peri-lesional immunofluorescence biopsies.

Immunological findings in lupus:

- ANA+ve ~90 percent cases
- Anti-DNA—especially dsDNA—positive
- Rheumatoid factor positive ~30 percent cases
- Anti-RNA antibody +ve
- Anti-Smith antibody positive (highly specific but not sensitive for SLE)
- Positive LE cell preparation (neutrophil/macrophage containing phagocytosed nuclear material (Hematoxylin body) indicating cell damage.
- Elevated ESR and γ globulins
- False positive syphilis serology (VDRL test) (useful to discriminate from rheumatoid)

The American College of Rheumatology defines a diagnosis of lupus as having at least four of the main criteria found both in **Table 17.2**, and the immunological features listed.

Therapies

Lupus management is usually proportionate to the signs, symptoms and degree of disease activity at the time which can characteristically flare and remit over years. Nonsteroidal

Table 17.2
The features of lupus disease

Common > 75% cases	*Frequent 50–75% cases*	*Less common <50% cases*
Skin **Photosensitive butterfly rash** **Discoid rash** Purpura, Urticaria	Pyrexias	Raynaud's phenomenon
Joint pains Asymmetric multijoint **Arthralgias and arthritis** (crossover with rheumatoid)	*Psychological* Low mood and affect Mood swings	*Coronary* **Endo and pericardial Inflammation** (Libman-Sacks endocarditis) Aortic valve damage
Hematological changes Chronic disease **anemia** (normochromic, normocytic) occasionally hemolytic **Leukopenia and lymphopenia** **Thrombocytopenia** and purpurae	*Respiratory* Pleuritic pain and/effusions pneumonitis *Neurological* **Fitting, psychoses** Polyneuropathy including cranial nerves Ataxia and plegias	*Renal disease* **Glomerulonephritides—proteinuria and hematuria** *Myopathy* Ophthalmic Conjunctivitis Retinal damage *Gastrointestinal* Hepatomegaly, pancreatitis Red/white mucosal patches **Oral ulceration** Sjögren's syndrome

The American College of Rheumatology requires at least four of the highlighted features (bold) for a lupus diagnosis supported by the immunological findings given in the text

analgesia can be useful to control arthralgias and mild symptoms. Hydroxychloroquine (with an ophthalmology review—the chloroquine drug group are ototoxic) can assist with more intense symptoms (especially articular and cutaneous symptoms) and cutaneous involvement. As severity of disease increases, systemic steroid courses, tailing off after a short period of maintenance at high levels, may be employed alone, or in conjunction with steroid sparing immunosuppressive agents such as azathioprine.

The benign discoid lupus variant is conventionally managed with topical steroid therapies to both cutaneous and oral mucosal disease sites.

Drug Induced Lupus

The condition is typically associated with use of methyldopa, procainamide, hydralazine, isoniazid and chlorpromazine—can be predominated by rash, fever, arthritis, pleuritic and pericardial involvement, with appropriate serological changes (**Table 17.3**). The effects resolve slowly on drug withdrawal.

Outlook

Improvement in the control of inflammatory damage have limited the mortality of the condition (approximately 90% 10 years survival) particularly by controlling renal failure.

Oral Care Importance

Oral lesions—erosions, erythematous and white patches are usually late manifestations of lupus and are considered less common signs. The white lesions can resemble lichen planus, as can the lichenoid reaction occasionally generated in response to antimalarial (hydroxychloroquine) use.

▪ Table 17.3
Serological changes in connective tissue disorders

Antibody group	*Antibody target*	*Diagnostic value*
Rheumatoid factor (against Fc IgG)	Agglutination tests Direct (IgM only) > 1:16 Sheep red cells >1:32 Latex beads >1:20	Rheumatoid arthritis Occasionally SLE (30% cases) and Sjögren's syndrome
Antinuclear antibodies ANAs		
General DNA	Double-stranded (dsDNA)	Positive in 95% SLE cases titer can correlate to severity in acute disease. Can be +ve in rheumatic and chronic inflammatory disease
	Single-stranded (ssDNA)	Positive in >50% of drug induced lupus and in 85% active and 40% of inactive lupus cases.
Indirect immunofluorescence patterns		
Diffuse (homogeneous) pattern	Deoxyribonucleoprotein	High titer- SLE; low titer; other rheumatol disease
Speckled pattern	Deoxyribonucleoprotein	Mixed connective tissue disease
Rim pattern	dsDNA	Highest specificity for SLE—most likely associated with photosensitivity, serositis and nephritis
Centromere pattern	Centromeres	Limited pattern scleroderma only (CREST)
Nucleolar	Nucleolus specific RNA	Scleroderma
Extractable nuclear antibodies (ENAs)	*Nuclear components soluble in saline*	
	Smith (Sm) antigen	Specific for SLE but not sensitive test
	U1 RNP	Mixed connective tissue disease, SLE, scleroderma (muscle involvement U3 also), Raynaud's
	Scl 70 (antitopoisomerase)	Scleroderma (lung involvement likely)
	JO1	Polydermatomyositis
	Ro (SSA—Sol substance A/Robair)	Sjögren's, SLE (photosensitivity)
	La (SSB—Sol substance B/ Lattimer))	Sjögren, SLE (photosensitivity)
	Histones	Drug induced lupus
Cytoplasmic antibodies		
Antineutrophil cytoplasmic antibodies (ANCA)	Cytoplasmic proteinase 3 PR-3	Wegener's granulomatosis
	Perinuclear myeloperoxidase	Polyarteritis nodosa
Serological proteins		
Lupus anticoagulant, anticardiolipin and β2 glycoprotein antibodies	Serum phospholipids β2 glycoprotein	Antiphospholipid/Hughes syndrome—coagulopathies, miscarriages, thrombocytopenia and CNS involvement

Box 17.1: Lupus

Key features helpful in diagnosis

- Female predominance typically in their 30-40s in majority of Western cases (>90%)
- Photosensitive facial butterfly rash or discoid rash/erythema
- Multisystem involvement especially arthritis/arthralgias and renal

Diagnosis

ANA positive—especially dsDNA
ENA positive—antismith
LE preparation

Management

Analgesics—especially NSAIDs
Steroids and steroid sparing immunosuppressant regimes

Any trauma or surgical intervention can aggravate lupus and is best deferred until the disease is quiescent or well-controlled. Any surgery—particularly under sedation or general anesthesia should be planned being mindful of the likely chronic disease pattern (normochromic, normocytic) anemia, and possible thrombocytopenic bleeding risks. Occasionally antibiotics such as penicillins can aggravate lupus and tetracyclines can exacerbate UV sensitivity. Renal disease can demand modified or alterative drug therapies, from all practitioners involved in such a case.

Antiphospholipid (Hughes) Syndrome

Initially considered a part of SLE, this condition—prevalent in young women—is now considered distinct from lupus. Plasma borne proteins bound to anionic phospholipids and phospholipids themselves are thought to be the antigenic targets in this condition, characterized by detection of one or more of the pathognomonic antibodies—lupus anticoagulant, anticardiolipin and β2 glycoprotein I antibodies (**Table 17.3**). Antibody binding is believed to trigger thrombosis via interactions with platelet and endothelial cell membranes along with procoagulants such as prothrombin, protein C and protein S.

The clinical picture is predominated by thrombotic events such as TIAs, CVAs and MI in an unusually young and female patient population. DVTs are common, as are Raynaud's phenomenon and migrainous neuralgias. Rarely, hepatic vein obstruction (Budd-Chiari syndrome) may develop, while placental interruptions cause frequent and multiple consecutive spontaneous miscarriages. The condition can develop in isolation or in association with other connective tissue diseases—in particular SLE and Sjögren's syndrome. Patients are managed with NSAID anticoagulation and coumarin drugs if necessary. Healthcare providers should be watchful for associated respiratory and systemic circulation hypertension in such cases.

Box 17.2: Hughes syndrome

Key features helpful in diagnosis

- Typically young—mid age female
- History of multiple thrombotic/coagulative events including multiple miscarriages
- Positive definitive autoantibody:
- Antiphospholipid or lupus anticoagulant or Beta2 GP1
- Commonly associated with lupus

Systemic Sclerosis or Scleroderma (Greek—Hard Skin)

This chronic multisystem disorder has an 8:1 predominance in women, typically presenting before the sixth decade. Cutaneous damage is frequently accompanied by Raynaud's phenomenon.

Etiology

While many humoral and cellular immunity disturbances have been suggested, there remains no definitive etiopathological mechanism for the condition. Systemic sclerosis is characterized by loss of cutaneous elastin and excess collagen deposition in the subcutaneous tissues, leading to the characteristically tight, restrictive and scarred appearance of the skin. Positive autoantibody titers to centromere and topoisomerase molecules (**Table 17.3**) allude to a mechanism of antibody driven type 1 collagen production by fibroblasts. Triggers for the condition may include exposure to trichlorethylene (dry cleaning solvent), vinyl chloride, adhesives and polymer coating materials as well as viral infections.

Signs and Symptoms

The majority (~60%) of cases are limited to cutaneous involvement, while the remaining cases may show more diffuse cutaneous involvement but can demonstrate accelerated progression and involvement of additional viscera. Scarring of the subcutaneous tissue (excess collagen 1) and loss of elastin tightens the skin producing the characteristic scar type tight skin lesions, most noticeable over the hands and face.

Cutaneous limited disease usually develops from or with a background of Raynaud's phenomenon.

Localized scleroderma is confined to the skin and subjacent structures only—never becoming systemic. In the mildest disease form, known as morphea, red patches develop on the torso, which thicken and turn pale as scar tissue bulk establishes. This usually fades within 5 years. A linear form, typically confined to arms or legs—resembling a healing laceration or Coup de Sabre is also recognized.

Systemic sclerosis involves deeper tissues and organs and develops in either limited or diffuse patterns. Limited scleroderma develops slowly, typically involving skin of the hands, feet and face. Stiffening of the fingers, polished skin and an appearance of the digits tapering to the nails (sclerodactyly), with limited movement of the small joints, are often seen later in the disease process. Similar changes occur in the legs and feet. The inflexible skin can occasionally split and pain is aggravated by continued Raynaud's phenomenon in cold weather **(Figs 17.3A to D)**.

Facial tissue involvement can lead to a poverty of facial expression, beaked nose, microstomia with skin creases perpendicular to the vermillion border and limited jaw movements. In addition, telangiectasiae (dilated superficial small vessels in the skin) and calcinosis (deposits of calcium salts) can develop in the skin.

The combination of calcinosis, with Raynaud's phenomenon, esophageal stricture (reflux disease and dysphagia due to impaired peristaltic function), sclerodactyly and telangiectases has been used to summarize the CREST condition. Cutaneous, vascular (Raynaud's) and esophageal involvement occurs in over 80 percent of cases.

A significant minority of cases will have a diffuse cutaneous involvement, with more rapid progress to sclerosis after onset of Raynaud's phenomenon. More significantly, accelerated involvement of the hands, face, proximal limbs and torso are accompanied by major organ system involvement in 20 to 40 percent of cases. Organ system involvement may progressively include—lung (pulmonary fibrosis and pulmonary hypertension), cardiac (fibrosis and deranged rhythms), renal (kidney failure and hypertension) and musculoskeletal (myopathies, inflammation and joint damage). Approximately 10 to 15 percent of cases have oro-ocular dryness symptoms and signs, consistent with secondary Sjögren's syndrome diagnosis. Early onset pulmonary and renal cases may show antitopoisomerase (Sci 70) antibodies, while a positive anticentromere pattern ANA is more suggestive of a CREST syndrome, with late noncutaneous involvement (**Table 17.3**).

Diagnostic Investigations

The principle clue to diagnosis is the clinical presentation—particularly of the skin signs. Unsurprisingly as a long-term condition, a normo-chromic, normocytic (chronic disease pattern) anemia will be noted, with ESR elevations—particularly in flares of activity. Characteristic vessel changes can be identified on nail bed vascular imaging. Serology can diagnose the condition by demonstration of elevated autoantibodies from the extractable nuclear antigen (ENA) class of epitopes. In particular, ENA Scl 70 (antitopoisomerase) and antinucleolar antibodies support systemic sclerosis, with an anticentromere positivity being diagnostic for CREST syndrome. ANAs may also be elevated but are not diagnostic. PM-Scl antibodies may indicate muscle involvement.

Radiological imaging can show calcium salts in hand skin, along with occasional distal

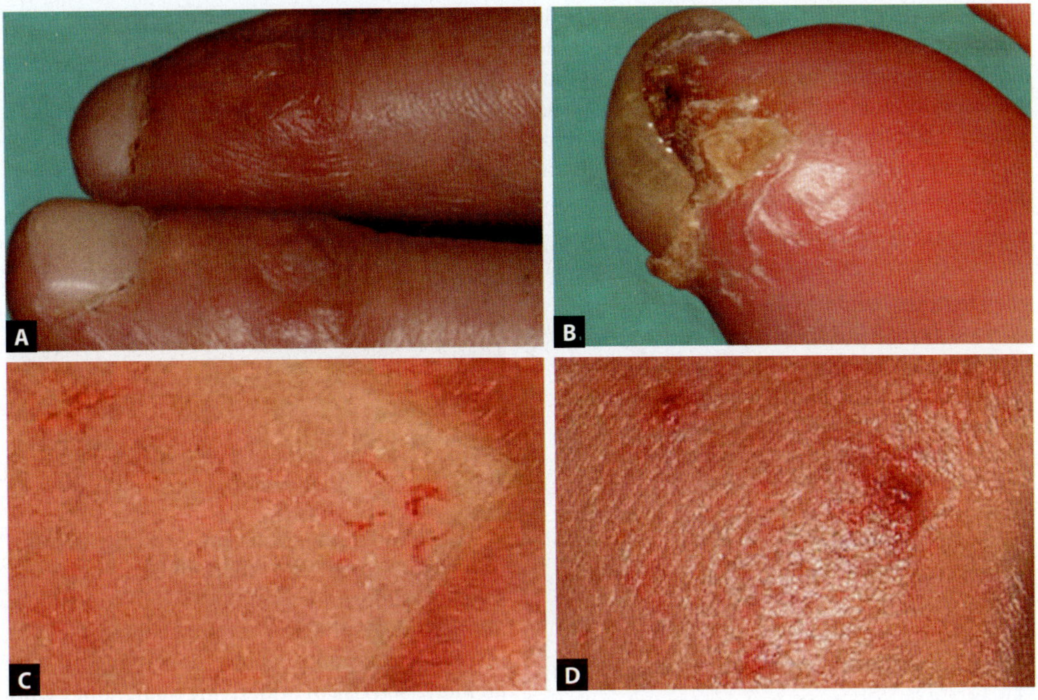

Figs 17.3A to D: The features of CREST. (A) Sclerodactyly—note the tightened scarred skin and damaged nail beds—aggravated by recurrent hypoxia of Raynaud's phenomenon; (B) Calcinosis cutis—the tight skin has puncture revealing a chalky deposit in the finger pulp, and telangiectasias; (C) Compressed under glass; (D) Fast refilling moments after removal of pressure

phalangeal erosion. High definition CT can show pulmonary fibrosis. Esophageal endoscopy may show sclerosis, marked reflux disease and possible Barrett's changes (premalignant) in the lower-third, while manometry will demonstrate hampered peristalsis and sphincter function.

Therapies

At present no specific therapies are known to combat the disease process. Esophageal surveillance, occasional dilatation of strictures and lung function testing are advisable. Hypertension control is essential to minimize renal damage progression—often using ACE inhibitors to counter renal disease too. Cyclophosphamide can be used for pulmonary fibrosis.

Outlook

In milder cases a 75 percent 10 years survival is expected, reducing to 50 percent in the diffuse disease group where more advanced visceral involvement occurs. Pulmonary disease is more likely to limit lifespan than renal disease and hypertension which are more amenable to medical management.

Oral Care Importance

Localized morphea over the malar region in childhood has been proposed as a cause of hemifacial atrophy, hampering TMJ function and secondary jaw growth. Beyond an unresponsive visage, perioral limitations lead to microstomia and tongue stiffening reduces function, hampering swallowing and routine dental care. In less than 1:10 cases, there is widening of periodontal ligament—a stable tooth is identified as having a widened but not periodontally diseased ligament space. Sjögren's syndrome may develop as a secondary condition to scleroderma—particularly if the patient also has primary biliary cirrhosis.

Box 17.3: Systemic sclerosis

Key features helpful in diagnosis

- Female predominance (F:M 8:1)
- Collagen scarring tightens epithelia—particularly limiting joint and organ movements (including lung and other viscera)—generalized and "skin only" patterns recognized

Associated with:

- **C**alcinosis **R**aynaud's **E**sophageal **S**tricture and telangiectasia to make (CREST) syndrome
- ANA centromere pattern (CREST) or nucleolar (Scleroderma)
- ENA Scl-70—organ involvement

Dermatomyositis and Polymyositis Group of Conditions

Dermatomyositis is an uncommon combination of a cutaneous rash and inflammation of the musculature. Absence of the rash confers a polymyositis diagnosis. Peak onset has bimodal distribution, arising in childhood and again in the 5th to 6th decades.

Etiology

The etiology remains unknown at present.

Signs and Symptoms

Difficulty with sitting, squatting, walking up stairs, rising from a chair and placing arms above the head are classical indicators of proximal pelvic and shoulder girdle weakness. Muscle tenderness and discomfort develop and in dermatomyositis cases, a characteristic heliotrope (purple) periocular rash **(Fig. 17.4)** develops along with a photosensitive scaling of the facial skin. Erythematous patches develop over the small joints and dorsum of the hands.

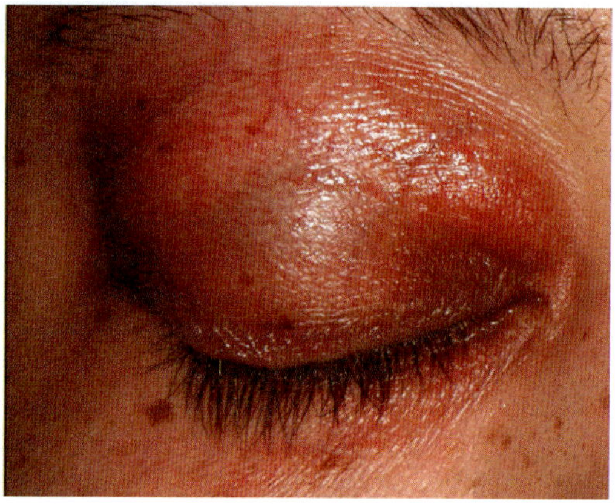

Fig. 17.4: Typical heliotrope (periocular) rash of dermatomyositis

Raynaud's phenomenon, arthralgias (pain only) and arthritis (inflammation, i.e. joint swelling, deformity or effusion) can supervene, along with dysphagia if esophageal muscles are involved. Cutaneous involvement may evidence an increased risk of underlying malignancy with increasing age.

Diagnostic Investigations

Muscle biopsy is diagnostic, showing necrosis and inflammatory infiltration and is supported by elevated serum muscle specific enzymes (creatinine phosphokinase and aldolase). Electromyography will similarly show characteristic changes and MRI can demonstrate muscle inflammation. ENA Jo-1 (antihistidyl tRNA synthetase) elevation in the serum is diagnostic.

Therapies

Management is confined to immunosuppression with steroid and steroid sparing agents such as azathioprine or methotrexate.

Outlook

Childhood onset carries a poor prognosis with approximately half of cases surviving beyond two years from diagnosis. The adult onset prognosis tends to be better unless associated with malignant tumor development.

Box 17.4: Dermatomyositis

Key features helpful in diagnosis

- Female predominance—bimodal presentation as child or 40–50s
- Classical heliotrope periocular rash
- Typical skin rash associated with inflamed muscles
- ENA Jo 1 positive

MIXED CONNECTIVE TISSUE DISEASE

A rare group of patients present with connective tissue disease symptoms not characteristic of any individual condition but seemingly a blend of symptoms and signs from the above conditions. "mixed connective tissue disease"—which includes common elements of two or more of these conditions is considered under the concept "overlap syndrome." Usually their outlook is good as CNS and renal involvement is rare. High ENA titers—particularly anti-RNP (antiribonucleoprotein) are often identified in this group who are managed both symptomatically and by immunomodulation if necessary (**Table 17.3**).

Sjögren's Syndrome

Although discussed in detail elsewhere in this book, the condition comprises a chronic auto-antibody mediated inflammatory destruction of exocrine glands—in particular salivary and lacrimal tissue, leading to the well-known oro-ocular dryness patterns also known as SICCA syndrome.

Arising in isolation, primary Sjögren's (often referred to as primary Sjögren's) is characterized by subjective and objective oro-ocular dryness, lymphocytic infiltration and acinar destruction in at least one foci in labial gland biopsy. It is also characterized by a positive ENA Ro and La in approximately 70 percent of patients. ANA and rheumatoid factor are also often positive in such cases. (Sjögrens—often formerly termed secondary Sjögrens) arises in association with another pre-existing) systemic condition—typically autoantibody mediated—most usually, rheumatoid arthritis, SLE or primary biliary cirrhosis (progressive intrahepatic bile duct inflammation and sclerosis leading to jaundice and cirrhosis, with serum antimitochondrial antibodies (AMA—isotype M2 elevated in 95% cases). Confusingly, some primary Sjögren's patients go on to develop arthritis, Raynaud's and renal failure blurring the boundaries between the arthritides, lupus and Sjögren's syndrome—leading to the development of the overlap syndrome philosophy. Philosophy and a recent trend to move away from primary and secondary nomenclature, particularly as a primary case would not be re-classified if a second condition such as rheumatoid arthritis developed later. Parotid swellings may often occur in Sjögren's syndrome but can also occur as part of and alcohol misuse but in HIV disease a CD8 lymphocyte predominated glandular swelling. Diffuse infiltrative lymphocytosis syndrome (DILS) can develop. Rheumatoid and ENA autoantibody titers are rarely elevated in this xerostomic condition.

Box 17.5: Sjögren's syndrome

Key features helpful in diagnosis

- Subjective and objective oral and ocular dryness
- Imaging positive—Sialogram (poss ultrasound)
- Lip gland biopsy (or parotid tail) focal lymphocytic inflammation focal lymphocytic infiltration around salivary acini rather than nonspecific diffuse pattern
- ENA Positive Ro and or La
- Particularly associated with lupus, primary billiary cirrhosis and rheumatoid

SYSTEMIC VASCULITIS

The term vasculitis describes inflammation of blood vessel walls and is a component of many conditions rather than a diagnosis in its own right. Accordingly, vasculitis may be seen in lupus, rheumatoid and polymyositic conditions. The "systemic vasculitides" defines a group of conditions in which the vasculitic reaction is the principle rather than an associated condition. Typically these conditions are characterized by the size of vessel involved. Major arterial involvement—aorta and branches can manifest as temporal (giant cell) arteritis and polymyalgia (giant cell arteritis is diagnosed by biopsy and high ESR), while medium sized vessel disease (main visceral supply) includes classic polyarteritis nodosa in adults and Kawasaki's disease in children. Of interest to oral care practitioners are the small vessel diseases, subdivided by the presence or absence of ANCA—Antineutrophil cytoplasm antibodies (ANCA).

Antineutrophil cytoplasm antibodies positive vasculitides include Wegener's granulomatosis (necrotizing vasculitis of mainly oral mucosae, upper airway, lung and kidney managed by systemic immunosuppression with cyclophosphamide) and Churg-Strauss syndrome (a rare triad of asthma, eosinophilia and vasculitis, responsive to systemic steroid and immunosuppression with azathioprine and cyclophosphamide).

The ANCA negative conditions include Behçet's disease; a rare multisystem disorder associated with circulating immune complexes—unknown antigens) elevated acute phase proteins and antibodies to intermediate filaments. The condition is characterized by recurrent refractory orogenital ulceration with associated eye involvement (uveitis and retinal vasculitis, optic atrophy and blindness), pathognomonic pathergy reaction (pustular eruption at injection sites) and cutaneous erythema nodosum patches and papulopustular rash development. Arthritis and myalgias can be associated, along with CNS involvement including confusional states, MS like conditions, brainstem lesions and encephalitides. Treatment is with immunomodulatory compounds such as colchicine, topical and systemic steroids and immunosuppressant agents such as azathioprine and cyclosporin. Henoch Schönlein purpura is also included in this group of conditions, featuring spontaneously recovering leg rashes associated with IgA immune complex deposition after recent upper respiratory tract infections.

Box 17.6: Systemic vasculitides

Key features helpful in diagnosis

Vascular inflammation drives disease hence elevated inflammatory markers ESR/CRP and some autoantibody associations:

Considered by vessel diameter involved:

Large	For example, temporal arteritis
Medium	For example, polyarteritis nodosa/ Kawasaki's
Small	For example, main oral association:

ANCA positive—Wegener's granulomatosis
ANCA negative—Behçet's disease

RAYNAUD'S DISEASE AND PHENOMENON

This phenomenon consists of three consecutive painful phases comprising cutaneous vessel constriction—leading to skin pallor, ischemia— leading to blue cyanosis, and finally vasodilatation resulting in erythema from reactive hyperemia. Typically hands and feet are involved and the events are triggered by exposure to cold. The triad of symptoms, when it occurs in isolation is known as Raynaud's disease, but the phenomenon can be associated with ß-blocker therapy, overuse of vibrating machinery, repetitive functions such as typing and the development of connective tissue disorders. Beyond maintaining peripheral warmth, smoking cessation and modifying hypertension control, interventional management includes, nifedipine, prostacyclin infusions and in extreme cases, localized sympathectomies to limit vasoconstriction.

HARD TISSUE DISORDERS/ARTHRITIDES

Osteoarthritis

Although not technically part of this group of conditions, a discussion of the most common painful joint disorder—osteoarthritis (OA) has been included here for comparison with the possible connective tissue disease differential diagnoses. OA is characterized by loss of articular cartilage with an osteoproductive response at the edge of the joint plateaus (lipping). While 10 percent of a total western population will show radiological changes, 60 percent of the populus over retirement age show such signs, although the black population is under represented and there is a 2:1 female predominance. Primary OA develops de novo, while secondary OA reflects a previous damaged joint, e.g. intra-articular fracture, congenital deformity or loading abnormality over a long period.

Etiology

Despite the commonly held belief that OA is the result of age and wear associated degeneration, modern thoughts suggest the etiology lies more with faulty reparative mechanisms. Accelerated wear from age, obesity, past-trauma and hereditarily deranged joints may accentuate the damage side of the equation, but faulty cartilage repair yields thinned or absent articular cartilage surfaces and subjacent local bone sclerosis, cyst formation and enhanced vascularity. Misdirected peripheral cartilage repair endochondrally ossifies to produce classic osteophytic lipping at joint edges.

Several hypotheses exist regarding the collagen break-down mechanisms (collagenase and lytic metalloproteinase levels elevated in the joints), perhaps stimulated by interleukin 1 and TNF α dependent processes? Deficiencies in growth factors such as insulin-like GF and transforming GF may further derange repair mechanisms. Background conditions may also be damaging cartilage such as hemochromatosis, Paget's disease and gout.

Signs and Symptoms

Joint pain is typically located in main weight bearing sites, hip, knee, ankle, and axial spine. In the hands the common sign is osteophyte formation at the distal interphalangeal joint (Heberden's node) and more rarely at the proximal interphalangeal joint (Bouchard's node)—mirrored by the metatarsophalangeal joints in the foot—In the great toe leading to lateral displacement—hallux valgus. Discomfort is provoked by movement and relieved by rest.

Diagnostic Investigations

In OA, FBC and ESR are usually normal, and rheumatoid factor is negative—although it can be low level positive as an incidental in the elderly anyway. Plain radiographic demonstration of loss of joint space (cartilage loss), sclerosis of the subchondral bone, osteophyte formation and cyst formation are all late signs, an MRI examination being more sensitive to early joint destruction. The lack of additional systemic involvements can assist further in the discrimination from rheumatoid damage, while elevated inflammatory markers are typically seen in inflammatory (and infective) arthropathies such as gout (Urate crystal deposition within involved joints) and pseudogout (pyrophosphate deposition) disease.

Therapies

The principle thrust of management is to re-establish comfort, by reducing joint loads (weight loss) and physiotherapy to establish better posture and loading patterns. Exercises, hydrotherapy and warmth can be useful. For pain relief, nonsteroidal anti-inflammatory drugs are preferred with an awareness of the risks of peptic ulceration and their mild anticoagulation effects. Intra-articular steroid placement can control acute exacerbations. Systemic therapy is generally avoided. Joint replacement surgery can facilitate full recovery if medical management has failed.

Oral Care Importance

Of interest to the oral care provider is the OA patient who presents with a seronegative Sjögrens syndrome pattern of subjective and objective oro-ocular dryness. A group of patients without iatrogenic (usually drug) etiologies can be considered as SOX syndrome cases—seronegative (RhF and ENA negative) osteoarthritic patients with xerostomia. Typically, lip biopsies fail to show more than non-specific sialadenitis in these cases but patients continue to suffer from Sjögren's like symptoms. Their long-term prognosis remains unclear at this stage.

Rheumatoid Arthritis

Unlike OA, rheumatoid arthritis is a chronic multisystem autoimmune disorder featuring a chronic symmetrical polyarthritis. Worldwide, approximately 2 percent of the population in the west (do you mean west and worldwide or should one be deleted?) will experience the condition,—although there is a 3:1 female predominance and a familial tendency among all races with an HLA DR4 tissue type association.

Etiology

Surprisingly, the etiology remains obscure but most consider an unknown antigenic triggering mechanism likely; allowing activation of T cells to promote an autoimmune inflammatory disease pattern in susceptible individuals (e.g. by gender or tissue type).

The principle lesion involves chronic inflammatory cell destruction of joint synovium (Lymphocytes, plasma cells and macrophages), driven by autoantibody and cytokine production (especially IL-8 and TNFα). Synovial angiogenesis allows recruitment of inflammatory cells to the region and synovial over-growth produces an erosive tissue mass called "pannus" which destroys articular cartilage and subchondral bone as it expands.

Rheumatoid factor—IgM class autoantibodies, which target human immunoglobulin (IgG usually) Fc portion are of unknown etiopathogenic role, but are commonly elevated in more aggressive disease (**Table 17.3**).

Box 17.7: Osteoarthritis and rheumatoid arthritis

Key features helpful in diagnosis

OA

- Seronegative joint pain and inflammation
- Aggravated by use and function (worsens during the day)
- Weight-bearing axial-skeleton and DIP (Heberden's) nodes in fingers hallux valgus of great toe
- Radiology—loss of joint space and lipping osteophytes

RA

- Female predominance (F:M 3:1) HLA DR4 association
- Characterized classically (but not universally) as rheumatoid factor positive
- Synovitis and worse joint stiffness on waking (takes time to loosen joints)
- Hands—ulnar deviation, Z thumb, Swan neck, Boutonniere's deformities and subluxed MCP and MTP joints (walking on pebbles)
- Radiographs show mousebite—mousebite peripheral erosions of joints indicating instability
- Watch for associated autoimmune conditions eg Sjögren's lupus, etc.

Signs and Symptoms

Morning pain in the hands and feet gradually settling on exercise is characteristic of this condition. In acute phases, aching, redness, tenderness and swollen joints with limited movement demonstrate the cardinal signs of inflammation and derangement—most typically of the metacarpophalangeal (MCP) and proximal interphalangeal (PIP) joints. Characteristically tapered digits, aggravated by muscle wasting around the swollen involved joints can resemble sclerodactyly. Instability at the carpus and MCP joints results in partial dislocation (subluxation) of the digits into the palm and deviation of the digits to the ulnar side of the wrist complex, while collapse of the carpus compensates by showing radial side deviation (**Fig. 17.2**).

Rupture of flexor and extensor tendons associated with the inflammation leads to digits adopting the classic Z thumb, swan neck and Boutonniere's deformity patterns. Progression includes wrist, elbows, shoulders, cervical spine, knees, ankles and feet (**Figs 17.5 and 17.6**). Joint effusions and wasting herald progression to subluxation, joint deformity and instability. One-third of patients develop cervical spine involvement.

Rarer presentations include sudden onset—explosive arthritis and relapsing—remitting and flitting larger joint (palendromic) disease.

Rheumatoid comprises a host of extra-articular features the most classic of which are the soft fleshy (rheumatoid) nodules which develop at the ulnar forearm adjacent to the elbow and in the hand, lung, pericardium and pleura in active disease. They share a common chronic inflammatory pathology—central necrosis surrounded by macrophages and fibrosis. Nodule positive cases generally are seropositive for rheumatoid factor.

Systemic indicators include soft? signs such as fever, weight loss and fatigue. Likewise reticuloendothelial involvement often produces regional lymphadenopathy (Note Felty's syndrome comprises RA, splenomegaly and neutropenia) and hematological screening often shows an anemia of chronic disease, aggravated by hypersplenism, hemolysis and a possible analgesic induced peptic ulcerative blood losses. Pulmonary and cardiac involvement can be asymptomatic but can include pleural effusions, fibrosis and small airways disease, pericarditis and pericardial effusions. Renal damage can result from analgesic abuse, and amyloid deposition in the

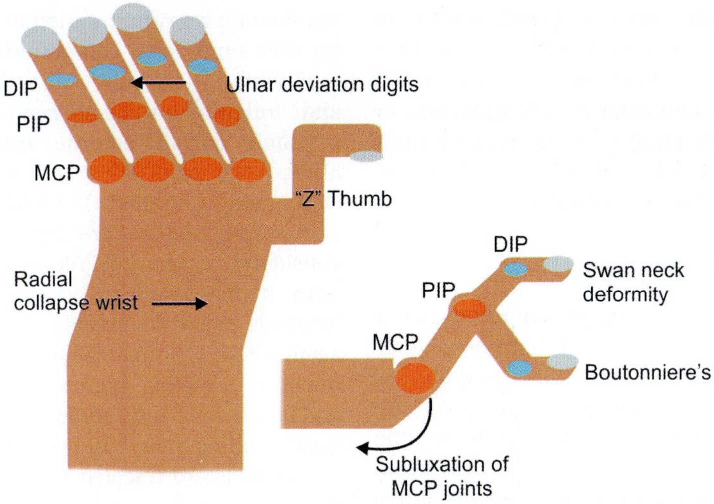

Fig. 17.5: Dorsum and lateral view of the left hand, showing changes in rheumatoid arthritis. Inflamed metacarpophalangeal (MCP) and proximal interphalangeal (PIP) joints are seen, with relatively uninvolved distal interphalangeal (DIP) joints. Radial wrist collapse with ulnar side digital deviation, palmar subluxation of the MCP joints and digit deformities—Z thumb, Boutonniere's and swan neck patterns are shown

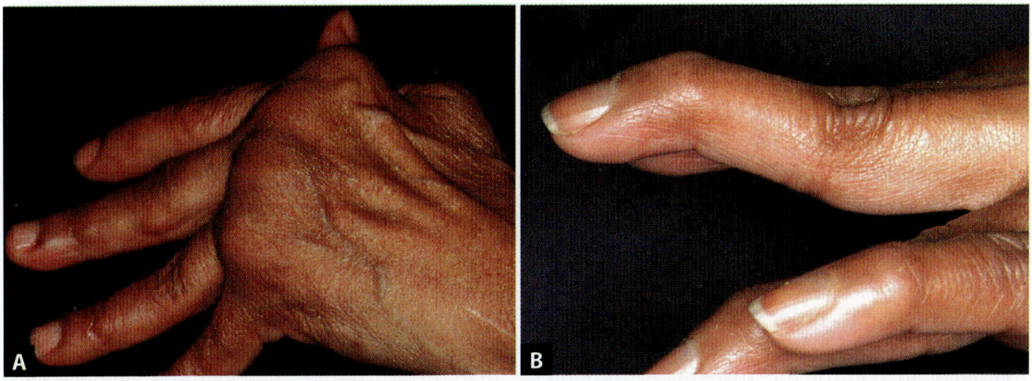

Figs 17.6A and B: Typical hand signs of rheumatoid. (A) MCP subluxation and ulnar deviation of the fingers, muscle wasting over the dorsum of the hand leaving tendon prominences and a Z-shaped thumb; (B) A swan neck deformity clearly in digits 3 and 5 with an early lesion developing in the 4th digit

face of the chronic inflammation. Joint damage can produce neurological complications—the most dramatic being atlantoaxial subluxation after C1-2 joint derangement, which threatens the spinal cord integrity by cord compression (of great importance under sedation and general anesthesia as muscle tone is reduced).

Wrist swelling can produce swelling on the palmar aspect of the carpus—compressing the carpal tunnel contents, particularly reducing grip power and palmar sensation. Vasculitis is also a feature of rheumatoid, typically (but not often) leading to leg ulceration, nail fold infarcts and in extreme cases peripheral end arterial obstruction, leading to tissue infarction and digit gangrene. Oro-ocular involvement can include inflammation and perforation of the sclera (scleritis and scleromalacia) and reduction or failure of the exocrine seromucous secretions manifests as secondary Sjögren's syndrome as discussed elsewhere in this volume.

Diagnostic Investigations

Clinical diagnosis is typically supported rather than categorically defined by investigations. A normochromic normocytic anemia of chronic disease is often seen with ESR and CRP titers reflecting disease activity at the time of sampling. Rheumatoid factor is positive in approximately three quarters of cases and a third will be ANA positive. If aspirated, synovial fluid will be sterile (unlike the infectious arthropathies, e.g. staphylococcal, tuberculous and gonococcal) and does not contain crystals (urate in gout and pyrophosphate in pseudogout). Likewise an absence of urethral irritation and conjunctival inflammation should exclude Reiter's seronegative reactive arthritis from the differential list. Seronegative psoriatic arthritis can be harder to distinguish if the articular disease has preceded the classical psoriatic skin scaling. Autoantibody screening is necessary and wise, particularly to assist in discrimination between rheumatoid joint pain and that associated with Lupus.

Therapies

A multisystem disorder commands a multidisciplinary care package, based around rheumatology to control the disease, orthopedics for joint repair and replacement, physiotherapy and occupational therapy to develop and maintain function while adapting environments as necessary.

In the past, early disease was maintained with prostaglandin inhibition via the nonsteroidal family of drugs. Good analgesia maintained function but failed to arrest disease progression.

The use of disease modifying agents (DMARDS):

The use of DMARDS aims to suppress disease progression at the earliest time possible to maintain maximum function for the longest possible time. Such compounds are immunomodulating (typically disturbing cytokine and inflammatory pathways). Methotrexate is often considered the drug of choice, along with penicillamine and azathioprine. Oral gold (auranofin) hydroxychloroquine, and sulphasalazine are less efficacious but considered safer. All require careful long-term hematoserological monitoring. TNF α blockade by blockade (etanercept) or antibody against TNF α (infliximab) can have significant impacts—arresting aggressive cases, but cost, and lack of long-term experience and expertise, is still limiting their worldwide use.

Steroids are injected to control local joint flares (up to per year to avoid aggravating damage processes). Systemic courses are avoided as high doses are necessary to gain good control—with major adverse (cushingoid) side effects.

Outlook

Overall prognosis has markedly improved; a quarter of cases having minimal adverse symptoms at 10 years while two-thirds will have some disability. A limited number of patients however do not respond to therapy, and become severely disabled in that time.

Oral Care Importance

The main difficulties for oral care arise from progressive loss of patient dexterity with advancing hand disease. Neck instability under sedation and general anesthesia presents significant but manageable risks. Occasional high dose steroid management is necessary and practitioners should be ever vigilant for increased fragility of the mucosa and skin, increased bruising and bleeding, as well as potential steroid insufficiency (Addisonian) crises during stress periods. Erosions and TMJ condylar head flattening may occur but is typically asymptomatic. The use of NSAIDs may aggravate bleeding and be associated with ulceration, as are methotrexate (with folate supplementation) and gold therapies. Antimalarials and penicillamine when used may yield lichenoid changes and the latter may also be associated with taste disturbances.

Juvenile rheumatoid arthritis typically develops in young girls, and is managed as for adult disease, but can involve most joints. The majority of cases are Rh factor positive. Sero- negative mild rheumatoid like damage is occasionally seen in association with psoriasis. Psoriatic arthropathy is generally mild, often focussed on the lower spine and sacroiliac joints and is typically controlled with NSAIDs, although occasional refractory cases may require methotrexate and folic acid cover.

In this chapter a group of conditions characterized by etiopathogenesis, and diagnosis with nontissue specific autoantibodies has been described, along with osteoarthritis for comparison and illustration of the difference in common arthritic conditions. The group is complex and the overlaps between pure line described diseases makes clinical diagnosis harder to achieve without the skilled interpretation of clinical, histopathological and serological assessments. The role of multidisciplinary care teams in such cases is paramount if the patient's holistic care needs are to be adequately met.

ACKNOWLEDGMENTS

The Author wishes to thank his friends and colleagues Dr Stuart Mceachen and Dr Helen McParland of King's College London Dental Institute for their invaluable assistance in the preparation of this chapter.

SELF-ASSESSMENT QUESTIONS

1. Provide a classification for connective tissue diseases affecting the orofacial region.
2. Describe the clinicopathological features and treatment of systemic lupus erythematosus.
3. Describe the key features and clinical importance of antiphospholipid (Hughes) syndrome.
4. Discuss the diagnosis of Sjögren's syndrome.
5. Describe the clinicopathological features and treatment of systemic sclerosis.
6. Provide a classification for the systemic vasculitides together with examples of each group which affect the orofacial region.
7. Describe the clinicopathological features of osteoarthritis
8. Describe the clinicopathological features of rheumatoid arthritis
9. Compare and contrast osteoarthritis and rheumatoid arthritis.
10. Discuss the dental relevance of a diagnosis of rheumatoid arthritis.

SUGGESTED READING

1. Dall'Era M, Wofsy D. Systemic lupus erythematosus clinical trials: an interim analysis. Nat Rev Rheumatol. 2009;5(6):348-51. Review
2. Daul P, Grisanti J. Monitoring response to therapy in rheumatoid arthritis—perspectives from the clinic. Bull NYU Hosp Jt Dis. 2009;67(2):236-42. Review.
3. Egner W. The use of laboratory tests in the diagnosis of SLE. J Clin Pathol. 2000; 53:424-32.
4. George D, Erkan D. Antiphospholipid syndrome. Prog Pr Cardiovasc Dis. 2009;52(2): 115-25. Review.
5. Kumar P, Clark M. Clinical Medicine, 6th edn. Elsevier Saunders Edinburgh, 2005.
6. Lafyatis R, York M. Innate immunity and inflammation in systemic sclerosis. Curr Opin Rheumatol. 2009 Jul 23.
7. Levesque MC. Translational Mini-Review Series on B Cell-Directed Therapies: Recent advances in B cell-directed biological therapies for autoimmune disorders. Clin Exp Immunol. 2009;157(2):198-208. Review.
8. Scully C, Cawson R. Medical Problems in Dentistry. Elsevier Churchill Livingstone, Edinburgh, 2005.
9. Shoenfeld Y, Meroni PL, Toubi E. Antiphospholipid syndrome and systemic lupus erythematosus: are they separate entities or just clinical presentations on the same scale? Curr Opin Rheumatol. 2009;21(5):495-500.
10. Web resources
http://www.lupus.org/newsite UK Lupus Society
www.rheumatology.org.uk/guidelines Guidelines for therapy
http://www.rheumatology.org/ Amrican College of Rheumatology
http://www.arthritis.ca/ The Arthritis Society

Chapter 18

Chronic Facial Pain

Andrew Sadler

Chapter Outline

INTRODUCTION

The treatment and management of those suffering from orofacial pain falls within the province of dental surgeons, oral and maxillofacial surgeons, otolaryngologists, neurologists, neurosurgeons, psychiatrists, psychologists and chronic pain physicians and anesthetists.

For most who experience pain it will be acute, and as the most common pain is around the mouth is odontogenic most patients will initially present to the dental surgeon. The numbers of people suffering from dentally related pain is vast and the dental, or oral and maxillofacial surgeon is privileged within the medical community in that he or she can relieve great suffering fairly easily. There can be few areas in medicine where a patient can present to a health care professional with severe debilitating symptoms and walk out of the surgery within an hour completely relieved. It is therefore frustrating for the clinician, as well as the patient, to find that chronic pain in the face or jaws is usually refractory to any of the operative techniques or medications which are usually so effective in the acute pain situation.

Dental pain easily falls within the concept of pain: an unpleasant sensation resulting from local tissue damage with the pain experienced being proportional to, and dependent upon, the local disease process. Most patients will relate to this concept as most will have experienced acute pain many times. After the injury has healed, the pain will have receded and probably been forgotten.

PAIN

Definition

This familiar concept of pain which was proposed by Descartes in the 17th century does not apply to the large number of people who suffer from chronic pain. The modern, internationally recognized, definition of pain is 'an unpleasant sensory and emotional experience associated with actual or potential tissue damage or described in terms of such damage'. This definition embraces chronic as well as acute pain. However, most sufferers of long-term pain will not understand that the unpleasant sensation they suffer is dependent on far more than simple tissue damage at the site they experience it to be; even less that any tissue injury may have passed or have not been there at all.

Pathogenesis

It is useful to understand some of the processes which may be involved in producing pain. This can be helpful in providing explanation to those suffering from chronic pain who present to us for our opinion and guidance as to how, or where, to get help.

Pain is an affective state which is usually perceived as unpleasant, it is a psychological experience with a strong emotional component but it is always invested with a local habitation in the body. It is usually experienced as a result of stimulation of peripheral nociceptive receptors as a result of structural or chemical change produced by tissue damage. However, it is affected by many factors including emotion and circumstances surrounding tissue damage. It has a different predilection between individuals so that what may be a painful sensation in one person may be quite different in another; this is especially so between members of different cultural or racial groups. Central to the experience of pain is the emotional component.

The pain perception pathway usually starts with nociceptive receptors in the tissues which respond to tissue damage and certain chemical mediators which have been shown to produce pain experimentally. These receptors fire small myelinated nerve fibers (known as Aδ fibers) which are fast conducting, have a high threshold and tend to be associated with sharp pain of short duration and also smaller non myelinated (C) fibers which respond to strong mechanical stimulation and are associated with a more intense burning pain which tends to fade gradually. Where these afferent fibers travel in spinal nerves they mostly terminate by synapse in the dorsal horn of the spinal cord. In the case of oro-facial pain the equivalent fibers traveling in the cranial nerves 5, 7, 9 and 10 and the first and second cervical nerves synapse in the spinal nucleus of the 5th nerve.

Damage to tissues can result in increased sensitivity of nociceptors, this is called peripheral sensitization. The receptors thus sensitized, usually in response to inflammatory mediators, may then exhibit lowered threshold or increased responsiveness to stimuli producing pain in response to a stimulus which would normally not be painful—Allodynia, or a pain disproportionate to the stimulus—Hyperalgesia. Together these are known as hyperesthesia.

There are more primary afferent neurones entering the central nervous system than there are second order neurones passing impulses forwards to higher centers, this is known as convergence and explains why pain may be felt in an area adjacent to where the injured tissues might be; primary afferent neurones from the injured area have converged onto second order neurones of an adjacent area. Furthermore, each primary afferent neurone branches and synapses with several second order neurones, this is known as divergence and explains why pain can appear to arise from a wider area than that which has been injured.

Thereafter the pain pathway passes by a circuitous route involving secondary and thence tertiary neurones. At each synapse the pain perception is modulated. The cerebral cortex is where pain is experienced at a cognitive level and in recent years functional magnetic resonance techniques, which are able to show differential blood flow in response to different stimuli, have facilitated neurobiologists to gain better, if incomplete, understanding of this. The temporal cortex is where the pain is remembered and the hypothalamus is where the visceral reflex effects of pain are mediated via the autonomic system, e.g. cardiovascular, gastro-intestinal and hormonal.

The traditional idea that pain perceived is directly proportional to the amount of tissue damage, which was proposed such a long time ago, is clearly not the case. The pain perceived by an individual varies according the emotional state, attitude, apprehension, time of day, suggestion and many other variables. Such observations were explained by Melzack and Wall's gate theory which proposed that peripheral nociceptive inputs must pass through a 'gate' in the dorsal horn of the spinal cord or in the case of orofacial pain the spinal nucleus of the trigeminal nerve. The 'gate' may be opened or closed by both peripheral afferent pathways (specifically Aβ mechanoreceptor fibers) or by efferent neurones passing from the central neuraxis. Thus, the ongoing transmission of nociceptive stimuli depends not just on the intensity of the stimulus but also upon modulating influences from higher and other peripheral influences such as touch. Similarly, the pain experience can be reduced by phasic down flow activity from the brain and is thus influenced by cognitive factors such as attention, anxiety and expectation.

In all types of pain a gate exists at all stages in the nociceptive pathway. Some factors such as tranquillity or anesthesia close the gate and reduce the awareness of pain whereas other cognitive influences such as anxiety or fear may potentiate it. Pain can therefore result not only from activation of excitatory neurones but also from loss of inhibitory control. We can, therefore, explain some of the techniques used by clinicians for reducing the pain experience. For example stretching and squeezing the tissues while injecting is widely used in routine dentistry to reduce pain of injection. This presumably closes the gate by stimulating Aβ afferents and manipulation of attitude and emotion may cause central modification of the gate.

Anxiety and its relationship to pain experience is of particular importance to surgeons, particularly to oral or dental surgeons who operate on awake patients. It is desirable that anxiety should be modulated, not only for its own sake, but because if it increase it can exacerbate the pain experience; cognitive factors such as anxiety, expectation and attention can change the phasic down flow from the cerebral cortex and modulate pain experience.

One of the most interesting pain phenomena is the influence of mood on pain experience, in particular the relationship between pain and depression and the concept of idiopathic pain which is not fully understood. Chronic pain is associated with depression. It is thought that chronic pain may be an important etiological factor in the causation of depression. It is less clear that it may be predisposed to by depressive illness.

After pain has been experienced for some time, a process of central sensitization or neuroplasticity can occur in which the second order neurones depolarize more readily; this then gives rise to the well recognized phenomena where pain occurs as a result of normally innocuous sensory input. Central sensitization is triggered by peripheral sensitization and this will trigger greater nociceptive input into the central nervous system. Repeated nociceptive input may produce a progressive increase in pain perceived by a patient.

CHRONIC PAIN

There is no generally agreed classification for chronic facial pain. Some pains have been difficult to classify into distinct groups of pains as they are unique to the orofacial region and have a poorly understood pathogenesis with considerable variation in opinion over causation.

However, a classification of pain (**Table 18.1**) is useful as it will help in management of the conditions and probably in prediction of prognosis. An attempt has been made to do this by the International Association of the Study of Pain.

NEUROPATHIC PAIN

Neuropathic pain is defined as a pain initiated by a primary lesion or dysfunction within the nervous system. In the facial region this may result from damage to a nerve as a result of nerve damage, trigeminal neuralgia or post herpetic neuralgia. Damage to a nerve can result from trauma or may be iatrogenic such as after orthognathic or third molar surgery. Trigeminal neuralgia is a neuropathic pain which frequently presents to the oral and maxillofacial surgeon. It occurs primarily in the elderly and is thought to result from demyelination of trigeminal sensory fibers in the nerve root, possibly due to looping of the superior cerebellar artery causing compression. Trigeminal neuralgia can be particularly refractory and occurs more commonly in those suffering from multiple sclerosis, itself a demyelinating disease. Post herpetic neuralgia occurs following a herpes zoster eruption. Viral damage to the afferent nociceptive fibers leads to peripheral and central sensitization so that the patients continue to experience excruciating pain up to six months after the viral lesions have healed. Found in a minority of patients who suffer from zoster. It is more common in the more elderly.

Table 18.1
Classification of chronic pain

1. Neuropathic pain
   - Trigeminal neuralgia
   - Postherpetic neuralgia
2. Vascular pain
   - Cluster headaches
3. Chronic idiopathic facial pain
   - Myofacial pain (facial-arthromyalgia)
   - Atypical facial pain
   - Atypical odontalgia
4. Burning mouth syndrome

Trigeminal Neuralgia

Trigeminal neuralgia is probably the best known chronic facial pain, although not the most common.

Clinical Features

Typically, it is a severe unilateral pain felt within the distribution of one of the peripheral branches of the trigeminal nerves, usually the second or third, rarely the first. Occasionally it may be bilateral.

Trigeminal neuralgia is often described as a severe lancing or electric shock-like pain and is commonly evoked by touch such that the patient may find eating, brushing teeth or shaving induces such severe pain that these functions are difficult or impossible, except in periods of remission which occur in this condition. Often there may be a dull background pain which lasts most of the time but it has severe short exacerbations, often lasting seconds, which characterises the pain and makes the clinical diagnosis. Most patients are elderly in their sixth or seventh decades and more women are affected than men. In younger patients it is associated with multiple sclerosis, in these cases the pain may be more intractable and difficult to manage.

Differential Diagnosis

Generally the diagnosis is easily made on the clinical features of a severe electric shock-like pain. Sometimes the pain is atypical, or there may be a prodromal pain which suggests atypical facial pain. Usually the symptoms mature into the typical clinical picture. The diagnosis is made clinically from the history, there are no special tests.

Patients should be examined for other orofacial disease, particularly for a tumor, including the cranial nerves. The teeth should be examined to exclude odontogenic pain. An MRI scan should be made of the posterior cranial fossa and the course of the nerve to look for a vascular compression of the root of the nerve which might be amenable to surgery or for a tumor causing compression. An MRI scan may show demyelination of multiple sclerosis. Most cases are responsive, at least in the initial stages, to a therapeutic dose of carbamazepine so that a positive response to this is helpful in confirming the clinical diagnosis.

Treatment and Prognosis

Simple analgesics such as Aspirin or Non Steroidal Anti Inflammatory Drugs are usually ineffective but anticonvulsants, particularly carbemazepine, are helpful in most patients. Unfortunately, the most effective drug carbemazepine becomes less effective with time and increasing doses are required, due to liver enzyme induction. Patients are more likely to cease medication due to side effects than because it is ineffective. It can cause ataxia, drowsiness, skin rashes and other allergic reactions and occasionally blood dyscrasias. Long-term treatment, particularly when higher doses are required, should be monitored with full blood counts and liver function tests to ensure there has been no marrow suppression or liver toxicity and plasma concentrations to check appropriate doses are being prescribed and taken at the optimal intervals. Oxcarbazepine is an alternative to carbemazepine when the latter is not tolerated but should be avoided in allergy as there is an approximate 25 percent cross reactivity. Gabapentine may be used where a patient has side effects or allergic reactions to carbamazepine. It is well tolerated but less effective and more expensive. Phenytoin, lamotrigine or baclofen can be used alone or in combination but there are no randomized controlled trials which give conclusive evidence of the best combinations.

Regardless of the absence of obvious side effects there is a small reduction in cognitive function with carbemazepine so medical management should be started in the knowledge that surgery can be curative, particularly when an MRI scan has shown a compression of the nerve. It is therefore desirable for TN patients to be offered a consultation with a neurosurgeon with a special interest in the subject to at least discuss the potential benefits of surgery.

The most effective surgical option for TN is microvascular decompression of the nerve in the posterior cranial fossa where a vessel has been shown by MRI scan to be causing a compression of the nerve root. Separating such a vessel from the nerve can be curative in patients with classical trigeminal neuralgia. Although complications from this type of surgery are low it has been reported that there is a very small risk of death. Alternatively, for medically higher risk patients radiofrequency thermocoagulation or balloon microcompression may be used to ablate the nerve. These give short-term pain relief but are less effective in the long-term and are likely to cause numbness of the face which itself might be painful (anesthesia dolorosa).

Stereotactic radiosurgery with a gamma knife has been introduced recently in a number of neurosurgery centers who have this facility. It has the advantage of safety for the very elderly who might be medically compromised and although short-term results are favorable, long-term results are yet to be fully evaluated. For all treatments the outcome for patients who have multiple sclerosis tend be worse but for patients with a short history the outcome tends to be better.

Postherpetic Neuralgia

Clinical Features

Postherpetic neuralgia is pain persisting for more than 4 to 6 weeks after the rash of reactivated varicella-zoster (shingles). The pain is felt as a severe constant pain most commonly in the second and third divisions of the trigeminal nerve. It occurs more commonly in women than men and is more likely in elderly patients with herpes zoster which is an affliction of the elderly. It occurs in about 15 percent of patients with herpes zoster but in those over 80 years of age it is over 35 percent.

Differential Diagnosis

Diagnosis is usually straight forward as the pain is typically severe in an elderly person who has had the rash of herpes zoster. However, it may be more difficult in a minority of patients who get viral reactivation without having a rash. Here the differential diagnosis will be from trigeminal neuralgia which may be further complicated by the fact that there can be an element of allodynia with post herpetic neuralgia.

Treatment and Prognosis

Many treatments have been tried including simple analgesics, opioids, hormones and nerve blocks. However, the most beneficial therapies seem to be Gabapentin and tricyclic antidepressants. The pain does tend to decrease with time and it is unusual for it to last more than 6 months.

VASCULAR PAIN

Cluster Headaches

Vascular pain affecting the face is known by a variety of names including migraneous neuralgia, histamine cephalgia, facial migrane and sphenopalatine neuralgia. The term cluster headaches has been adopted by the International Association for the Study of Pain as it tends to occur in clusters over a period of time with long periods of remissions between.

Clinical Features

The pain is severe, unilateral and principally in the ocular, frontal and temporal area over a period of a few weeks often with lacrimation, rhinorrhea or nasal congestion and sometimes photophobia. Incidence is rare and is less common in men. Peak incidence in men is during their fifth decade and seventh decade for women. Several studies have suggested a higher incidence in smokers.

Differential Diagnosis

Diagnosis is made on the clinical features. The main differential is with migrane but it may also be confused with atypical trigeminal neuralgia considering the severity of the pain. The age of the patient, the periodicity and the fact that it tends to stray outside the trigeminal area usually makes the differentiation. The pain occurs typically at night and may be induced by alcoholic drinks. The etiology of the pain is unclear but it has been suggested that vasodilatation plays a role.

Management and Prognosis

Acute attacks may be helped by oxygen delivered through a face mask or by sumatriptan administered subcutaneously rather than orally in order to gain a faster beneficial effect. It is contraindicated in ischemic heart disease.

Prophylaxis can be attempted during the cluster period and continued for two weeks after the last attack. Ergotamine is often used, combined with verapamil and is most useful for nocturnal attacks. Methylergonovine maleate has been reported as reducing the frequency of attacks by 95 percent. Sumatriptan is of limited use for prophylaxis due to its short half life.

Long-term prognosis is difficult to judge as remissions of pain last for varying periods between weeks or years. There is a variation from the episodic form of cluster headaches, which has no, or very short, periods of remission called chronic cluster headaches. Patients with this form tend to get less relief from medication.

CHRONIC IDIOPATHIC FACIAL PAIN

Chronic idiopathic pains of the face do not easily fall into classification with pain elsewhere in the body. In each case, there have been numerous theories about pathogenesis but no clear conclusion and consequently management is often unsatisfactory. It is, however, useful to differentiate them according to the clinical features as this does help with discussing the prognosis with a patient. In each case it is important to reassure the patient that there is no serious underlying disease present, particularly cancer.

Myofacial Pain

Clinical Features

Myofascial pain or myofacial pain as it is more commonly called in the face, can occur in any voluntary muscle in the body and is characterized by local and referred tenderness and trigger points. Myofascial pain may occur only on palpation of the muscles in which case it is referred to as 'latent'. When 'active' spontaneous pain is suffered, this can be described as an aching or tightening and may be deep in origin. Myofascial pain is usually poorly circumscribed. The patient may report a sensation of swelling and an exacerbation of pain in the cold. In the face the pain may be called myofacial pain or facial-arthromyalgia or temporomandibular disorder (TMD) when pain is felt in the temporomandibular joint. Muscular pain often accompanies internal derangement of the temporomandibular joint. This is a dysfunction in the relationship of the cartilaginous disc in the joint to the head of the mandibular condyle. Here pain is accompanied by obvious clinical signs, in addition to tenderness on palpation including painful clicking, locking of the jaw, limitation of opening and deviation of the mandible to the affected side. Internal derangement can occur at any age in either sex but is predominantly a problem in young women. Although some cases can become chronic with prolonged limitation of opening, which may, very occasionally need surgery, most cases resolve spontaneously with no invasive management.

As with myofacial pain elsewhere in the body, pain may be referred to other muscles without regard to the innervation. Thus there may be pain in the masseter (most commonly) referred to the temporalis, sternomastoid. Pain may also be felt in the posterior neck muscles and shoulders. This spread of pain may be due to central sensitization.

Differential Diagnosis

Patients with myofacial pain should have a thorough dental examination to exclude any odontogenic source of the pain although in most cases the differential diagnosis can easily be made on the basis of the clinical history and description of the pain. It is useful to differentiate those with myofacial pain, whose symptoms are limited to pain, from patients with symptoms and signs of internal derangement of the joint related to disc displacement. Diagnosis of myofacial pain may be confirmed with some confidence by being able to reproduce muscle pain and tenderness by palpation of the affected muscles, most frequently the masseters, by the examiner.

Treatment and Prognosis

Myalgic pain has been managed by a variety of methods including local application of heat, mild analgesics, topical analgesics, acupuncture, soft laser, ultrasound or low dose tricyclic medication, (which has been shown to be helpful for such chronic pain independent of its action on depression) or gabapentin. Botulinum toxin injection may be useful but has not yet been fully evaluated.

Patients with internal derangement (disc displacement) should be given a simple explanation of their symptoms in terms of the anatomy of the relationship of the disc to the mandibular condyle and reassurance of the usual benign course of the problem. Advice on resting and restricting extreme mouth opening may be useful. Resolution of symptoms in those with clinical evidence of internal derangement is usually much quicker than in those cases with only symptoms of muscle pain.

Atypical Facial Pain

Atypical facial pain (in recent years the preferred term has been "persistent orofacial pain") is generally described as a diagnosis of exclusion but its features are usually so recognizable that in practice it is an easy working diagnosis to make from the clinical history and exclusion of other causes by examination and imaging.

Patients are predominantly female and give a history of chronic dull pain which is present at some intensity most days. The pain may be described as 'liveable with' some of the time with exacerbations. Often the pain is described as following some event or other, sometimes dental treatment. The pain is usually felt in the mid face with varying locations, not related to the sensory innervation, and can move from the top to the bottom jaw area and from side to side. Patients frequently have, or have suffered, pain elsewhere such as headache, neck, shoulder or back pain.

Differential Diagnosis

Pain is usually easily distinguished from odontogenic pain by its chronicity, from trigeminal neuralgia by being less severe, its duller character and usually in a younger patient. The dull pain may be distinguished from myofacial pain in that it tends to be felt deeper and is not specifically related to the masticatory muscles.

A full oral and dental examination should be carried out clinically and radiographically as the patient may blame their teeth and a CT scan will help to convince them of the absence of cancer or sinus disease.

Treatment and Prognosis

The mainstay of management is a through explanation of the diagnosis and nature of chronic pain with reassurance of the absence of local disease where the pain is felt, followed by tricyclic medication which is used in small doses and whose response is independent of any depression. This can often help modulate the pain to the extent that the patient is able to cope with it. Anticonvulsants and mild analgesics may be used as secondary or adjuvant treatment. Other treatment strategies that may be used include transcutaneous nerve stimulation, acupuncture and psychological techniques to help the patient cope with the pain.

Surgical treatment, such as dental treatment, is often followed by a brisk placebo response with an apparent cure with great relief. Recurrence of more severe pain occurs a few weeks later with greater distress.

Atypical Odontalgia

Atypical odontalgia is not as uncommon as many authors have suggested. This is very similar to earlier described persistent oral facial pain except for the site is dentoalveolar. It is usually diagnosed from the clinical history which is typical of toothache, except from the chronicity with a patient at presentation, complaining of pain for many months or even years duration. As with atypical facial pain, patients are commonly female with pain being most frequent in premolars and molars of the maxilla. The pain may be dull or sharp, continuous or intermittent, severe or mild as can any odontogenic pain. The tooth where the pain is felt may be tender to percussion. At presentation the patient may have had attempts at endodontic treatment, surgical endodontics and extraction in one or several teeth. As with atypical facial pain operative interference often leads to a brisk placebo response followed by recurrence in an adjacent tooth. In some cases this may lead to multiple extractions followed by pain in the edentulous alveolus and the accusation that root fragments have been left behind.

Differential diagnosis is from odontogenic pain particularly cracked tooth syndrome. As with atypical facial pain it is often referred to as a diagnosis of exclusion but again the diagnosis is often immediately obvious if the patient comes with a clinical history involving multiple operative dental procedures. Etiology is unknown but it has been suggested that deafferentation resulting from minor trauma may be involved.

Treatment and Prognosis

Satisfactory management of atypical odontalgia is even more difficult than atypical facial pain.

This is possibly because the pain is so well localized to the teeth that the patient is sure that the cause is a tooth. Extraction usually produces a placebo response and when the pain recurs the patient may confidently rationalize this as a cure and recurrent pain as the same problem infecting another tooth or infected tooth fragments remaining.

Management depends on reassuring the patient that there is no local organic cause which may be difficult as the clinician may not be sure that there is not a cracked tooth and the patient is less likely to believe him. Tricyclic medication is recommended but a satisfactory response is less likely, phenothiazine may be added but there are no satisfactory clinical trials to prove effectiveness.

BURNING MOUTH SYNDROME

Burning mouth syndrome, also called oral dysesthesia, is a burning sensation in the oral mucous membrane. Patients are almost exclusively postmenopausal women and symptoms are chiefly in the tongue but the buccal mucosa is often involved and other surfaces may be affected. Frequently patients complain of dryness of the mouth.

In many cases a working diagnosis can be made from the clinical history of burning and dryness in an elderly woman, especially if there is a metallic taste.

The etiology of burning mouth is unknown. The obvious suggestion that it is due to the lack of hormonal influence on the oral mucous membrane following the menopause must be balanced by the observation that hormone replacement therapy does not reverse the symptoms. It has been suggested that it is due to salivary changes but if so these have not been identified.

Differential Diagnosis

Diagnosis must be distinguished principally from oral lichen planus by clinical examination; in burning mouth the oral mucosa is normal. Oral dryness may be present in diabetes which has not been diagnosed or Sjögren's syndrome. In primary Sjögren's the mouth may be very dry and be accompanied by salivary gland swelling, in secondary Sjögren's there will be a history of other connective tissue disease. Occasionally, oral candidiasis may lead to soreness, a feeling of dryness and altered taste so it may be productive to investigate for yeast with an oral rinse. Some clinicians test for serum iron and vitamin B_{12} levels as deficiencies have been implicated but there are no controlled trials to confirm this and replacement in deficiency is unrewarding. Allergies to dental materials are rare and would be expected to produce a viable mucosal reaction.

Treatment and Prognosis

Patients should be made to feel that their history has been carefully listened to and appropriately investigated. They should be told the diagnosis and that, having discounted any other disease process, the symptoms are not uncommon and do not signify any other underlying disease process. No treatment has been shown to cure burning mouth but patients may be told that symptoms often resolve. Tricyclic medication has been reported as being of possible help in those whose symptoms continue to be distressing; others have reported some success with zinc supplements, topical clonazepam, alpha-lipoic acid, selective serotonin release inhibitors, amisulpride or cognitive behavior therapy.

SELF-ASSESSMENT QUESTIONS

1. Discuss the various theories of the pathogenesis of pain.
2. Describe a classification for chronic facial pains.
3. Discuss the clinical features, investigation and treatment options for trigeminal neuralgia.
4. Give two examples of neuropathic pain and describe their clinicopathological features.
5. Describe the clinicopathological features of myofacial pain.
6. Discuss the differential diagnosis of atypical facial pain (persistent orofacial pain).
7. Compare and contrast atypical facial pain and atypical odontalgia.
8. Describe the clinical features, investigation and treatment of burning mouth syndrome.

SUGGESTED READING

1. Agostoni E, Frigenio R, Santoro P. Atypical facial pain: clinical considerations and differential diagnosis. Neurol Sci. 2005;26:S71-S4.
2. Bruggi G, Ferroli P, Franzini L, Galosi L. The role of surgery in the treatment of typical and atypical facial pain. Neurol Sci. 2005;26:S95-S100.
3. Feinman C and Madland G. The contribution of psychiatry and medicine to diagnosis and management of idiopathic orofacial pain: a multidisciplinary problem. Current Review of Pain. 1998;2:41-8.
4. Fredioni F. Pharmacological therapy of atypical facial pain: actuality and perspective. Neurol Sci. 2005;26:S92-S4.
5. Graff-Radford SB, Solberg WK. Atypical odontalgia. J Craniomandib Disord Oral Facial Pain. 1992;6:260-5.
6. Graff-Radford SB. Facial Pain. The Neurologist. 2009;15:171-7.
7. Graff-Radford SB. Myofascial Pain: Diagnosis and Management. Current Pain and Headache Reports, 8:463-467. Current Science Inc ISSN 1531-3432.
8. International Association for the Study of Pain. Classification of chronic pain. Description of chronic pain syndromes and definitions of pain terms. International Association for the Study of Pain. 1994. pp. 1-222.
9. Patton LL, Siegal MS, Benoliel R, De Laat A. Management of burning mouth syndrome: systematic review and management recommendations. Oral Surg Oral Med Oral Pathol Oral Radiol Endod. 2007;103(suppl):S39.e1-S39(e13).
10. Revant C, Patil R, Degwekar SS, Bhowate RR. Drug treatment of trigeminal neuralgia: a systematic review of the literature. J Oral Maxillfac Surg. 2007;65:40-5.
11. Zakrzewska JM. Cluster headache: review of the literature. Br J Oral and Maxillofacial Surgery. 2001;39:103-13.
12. Zakrzewska JM. The burning mouth syndrome remains an enigma. Pain. 1995;62:253-7.

Chapter 19

Temporomandibular Joint Disorders

Andrew J Sidebottom

Chapter Outline

INTRODUCTION

Temporomandibular joint (TMJ) problems are a common cause of morbidity with around 30 percent of the population complaining of problems related to the joint at some stage during their life. Approximately 10 percent of the population have one or more TMJ symptom or sign at any one time. Differential diagnosis can be confusing and patients are often considered to have "earache" and referred for ENT advice. This chapter will aim to guide in the differential diagnosis and primary management of TMJ disorders with advice when onward referral for specialist surgical advice is appropriate.

The most common form of TMJ disorder has various names from TMJ pain dysfunction, myofascial pain dysfunction, TMJ dysfunction syndrome, etc. This is really a spectrum of disorders of the joint and related masticatory muscles and is best defined as a spectrum from internal derangement (disk related disorder) to masticatory myofascial pain (purely muscle disorder). The majority of this chapter will deal with this spectrum, but will include the other less common disorders affecting the joint.

EPIDEMIOLOGY

TMJ disorders present in all age groups, but by and large in the under 40s there is little in the way of degenerative disease, unless the patient has been operated on or has suffered from significant trauma to the joint. In the over 40s there is increasing evidence of degenerative disease and remodeling of the joint although this may not be of significance in terms of dealing with the patients' symptoms. However, symptoms seem to be more prevalent in the under 40s.

In youths, acute restriction of opening is generally due to a reduction in lubrication within the joint—anchored disk phenomenon—and this can be dealt with effectively by arthrocentesis (see later). Additionally, acute muscle spasm secondary to clenching or grinding (particularly around the time of examinations) is common in this age group. This problem can also affect older age groups at times of stress as the balance of wear and tear to repair is switched towards the former by raised adrenaline levels causing increased muscle spasm, with induction of myofascial type symptoms.

Women seem to be affected more commonly than men with various ratios from 2:1 to 10:1 being reported. The rationale behind this seems to be a variance in estrogen joint receptors although the correlation of this is not fully clear.

Predisposing factors include previous trauma to the joint (macro-trauma) including previous open joint surgery, a history of a clicking joint (present in up to 30 percent of the population) and a history of clenching in particular, but also grinding (nocturnal bruxism) which cause recurrent microtrauma. There is no evidence for the role of occlusal/dental factors in induction of disease indeed the American Association of Orthodontists devoted significant research into this area in the late 1980s to show that orthodontic management did not induce or reduce the incidence of TMJ disorder or clicking during or after treatment. Subsequent Cochrane studies have shown no benefit for occlusal modification in the management of TMJ disorders, as most of the studies are case series, not randomized studies.

INITIAL CONSULTATION

History

The primary symptoms to be elicited from the history are:

1. Pain
2. Joint noises
3. Locking
4. Restriction of opening
5. Other joint disorders particularly rheumatological and hypermobility
6. Disturbance of the bite
7. Alteration in facial appearance.

Pain

Pain from TMJ disorders may be from the joint itself (TMJ pain) or the related muscles of mastication (myofascial pain). It is important from the history and examination to distinguish these two in terms of definitive management, although initial care is the same for both. Often both are interlinked giving a spectrum of disease from joint pain at one end to muscle pain at the other. Pain should be recorded using a reproducible pain score such as a 10 cm analog scale such that outcomes can be assessed.

Pain localized in front of the tragus of the ear, which can be pointed to with the finger, is likely to be TMJ pain. It is often made worse by function (eating and yawning), and may radiate to surrounding structures. Biting on a tongue spatula on the side of the pain induces the pain in the joint helping to confirm the diagnosis.

Myofascial pain is often a less well defined pain with a complaint of "numbness" or aching on the side of the face which is not well localized but often in the region of the ramus of the mandible or lateral cheek below the zygomatic process or into the temple. This tends to be worse in the mornings, due to clenching or grinding the teeth at night (which habit can sometimes be confirmed from the patient's partner), or after particularly "stressful" situations (e.g. a long drive through heavy traffic or around exam times).

Joint Noises

Clicking or cracking of the joint are common. Clicking is related to anteromedial displacement of the disk of the TMJ repositioning itself over the joint and predisposes to joint disease (*see* Internal Derangement). In itself it does not warrant any treatment other than reassurance that it will soften with time and does not lead to or indicate "arthritis of the joint". Cracking or crepitus again does not warrant treatment but suggests "scarring" or degeneration "within or around" joint. Again without any other symptoms the patient can be reassured, although occasionally it can be a presentation of arthritic conditions.

Locking

Locking is the inability to either fully open or fully close the joint. Inability to fully open the joint will often be overcome following massage with a click or crunch restoring full opening. This has been considered to be due to disk displacement with reduction (ADDR), although it may be due to acute muscle spasm of the lateral pterygoid muscle, which attaches to the anterior portion of the disk, or any of the other muscles of mastication (secondary to myofascial spasm). It may also be due to alteration in the lubrication of the joint (anchored disk phenomenon). Inability to fully close over a period of time is due to a joint effusion (synovial fluid) or blood (hemarthrosis). Both may be secondary to trauma although the former may also be secondary to the acute synovitis seen in rheumatoid diseases. Frequency of locking should be recorded.

Restriction of Opening

Normal range of mouth opening for an adult is above 35 mm inter-incisal distance (with upper and lower dentures in if present). An opening greater than 55 mm suggests hypermobility.

Muscle spasm and disk displacement can both cause restriction as can ankylosis of the joint, trauma or the spasm associated with cervicofacial infection. Opening less than 25 mm in a young adult without associated systemic illness suggests anchored disk phenomenon, due to loss of joint lubrication. This should be managed urgently by a maxillofacial specialist with an interest in TMJ disorders who will consider early arthrocentesis (joint washout under pressure) which is usually curative. Significant delay may lead to a permanent restriction.

Other Joint Disorders

The TMJ can be affected by rheumatoid joint diseases and hypermobility. Rheumatoid disease often presents with pain and ultimately can lead to joint collapse with a disturbance in the way the teeth bite together (occlusion). Ankylosing spondylitis may lead to joint ankylosis with pain and restriction of opening. Psoriatic arthropathy also may cause pain, restriction and occasionally joint collapse.

Joint Dislocation

Hypermobility can lead to joint dislocation. This occurs when the condyle of the mandible is displaced anterior and superior to the articular eminence. It tends to occur in two age groups—young adults with generally hypermobile joints and the elderly who have loose ligaments and overclosure of the jaw due to lack of teeth. The frequency of dislocations should be recorded. Often patients may complain of "dislocation" when in fact they are describing a click or locking.

Disturbance of the Bite

Collapse of the joint due to reduction in height of the ramus will cause a premature contact on the side of the collapse. This is because of loss of the joint surfaces causing reduction in height of the ramus. There may be associated centerline deviation of the chin or teeth towards the side of collapse. If both sides collapse the chin point will move backwards with bilateral loss of ramus height and an anterior open bite.

Clinical Examination

The aim of clinical examination is to determine the sites of tenderness and the degree of disorder present (**Figs 19.1 to 19.4**). The examination comprises:

1. Palpation of the joint for tenderness and noises/crepitus both closed and open, lateral and posterior (**Figs 19.1 and 19.2**).
2. Palpation of the masseter muscles for tenderness and areas of muscle tightness (**Fig. 19.3**).
3. Palpation of the temporalis muscles for tenderness and areas of muscle tightness (**Fig. 19.4**).
4. Use of a tongue spatula to bite between the teeth on each side.
5. Measurement of inter-incisal mouth opening in mm (**Fig. 19.5**).
6. Observation of the opening path of the mandible in relation to the maxillary centerline.
7. Assessment of left and right lateral deviation
8. Interdigitation of the teeth (Dental occlusion).

Palpation of the Joint

The TMJ is palpated just in front of the tragus of the ear (*see* **Figs 19.1 and 19.2**). Movement consists of rotation in the lower joint space and glide from the upper joint space over the articular eminence at the base of the zygomatic arch. Tenderness may be elicited over the lateral aspect of the joint whilst stationary or in motion. The posterior aspect of the joint can only really be felt in wide opening by palpating between the back of the joint and the tragal cartilage. Tenderness over a joint indicates inflammation in the joint related structures of capsule, synovium and bone.

Noises may be palpated and heard such as a click or crepitus (crunching). Often, due the close relation of the joint to the ear, the

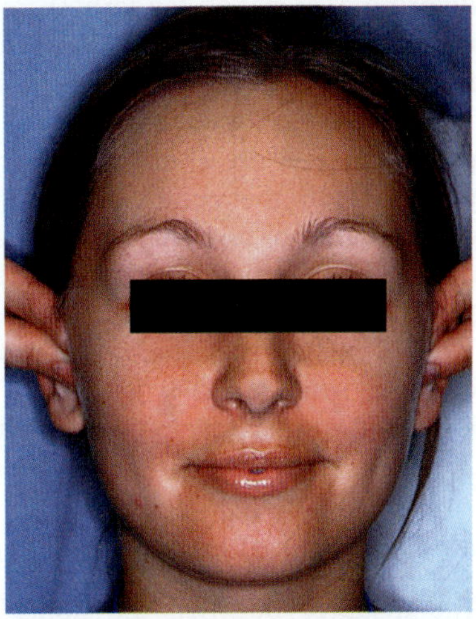

Fig. 19.1: Palpation of TMJ including side and back of the joints

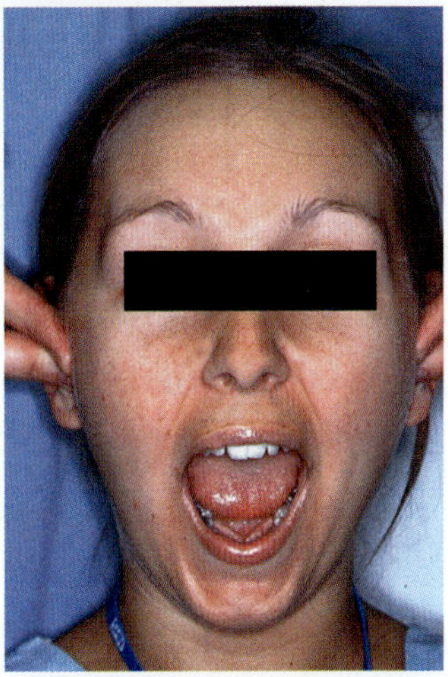

Fig. 19.2: Palpation of the TMJ for click and crepitus and examination for deviation on opening and degree of lateral deviation

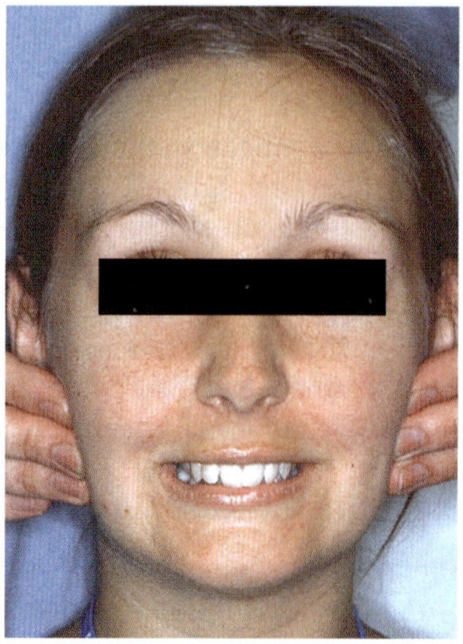

Fig. 19.3: Palpation of masseter muscles for tenderness and spasm

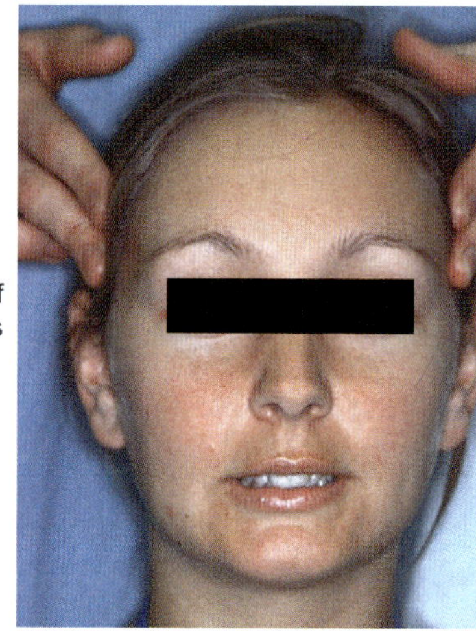

Fig. 19.4: Palpation of the temporalis muscles for tenderness and muscle spasm

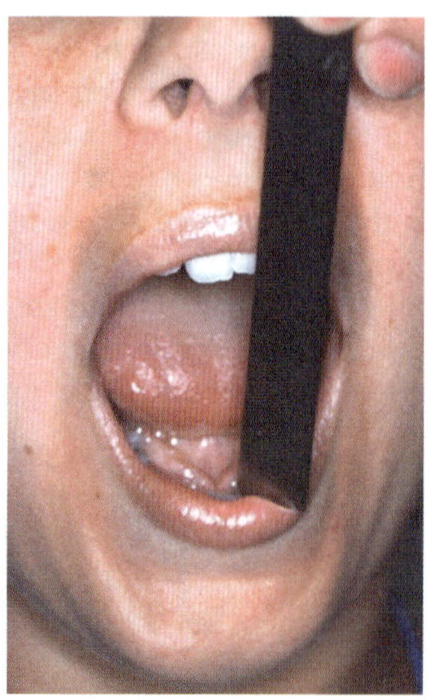

Fig. 19.5: Measurement of mouth opening in mm

patient will complain of noises which are either intermittent or cannot be palpated or heard by the examiner. Assume the noise is present if the patient complains of it. Tinnitus is not generally a symptom of TMJ disease.

Palpation of the Masseter and Temporalis

The masseter muscles lie over the vertical ramus of the mandible up to the base of the zygomatic arch. The temporalis lies above the zygomatic arch, extending behind and above the ear and onto the forehead below the hairline. **Figures 19.3 and 19.4** illustrate palpation of these muscles to elicit tenderness. Tenderness in a muscle during clenching or the palpation of tight bands of muscle indicate myofascial spasm and pain.

Use of a Tongue Spatula

It is relatively difficult and impractical to determine areas of tenderness in the other muscles of mastication and the author does not feel this is necessary in nonspecialist practice. They can be indirectly palpated by asking the patient to bite on a tongue spatula, with the pterygoid on the contralateral side of biting giving pain due to deviation towards that side due to its contraction. Pain on the ipsilateral side implies joint pain.

Headaches may be a symptom of TMJ disorder when there is associated muscle or joint tenderness, but alone are not indicative of TMJ problems.

Measurement of Interincisal Opening

The distance between the upper and lower incisors during maximal mouth opening gives a reliable and reproducible measure of loss of function and outcome (**Fig 19.5**). Ninety-seven percent of the population have an opening of greater than 35 mm and this provides a useful distance to aim to achieve in management. Some patients with opening greater than this will have subjective restriction and others with opening less than this will be normal. Improvement in opening following treatment gives a good measure of outcome.

Observation of Opening Path

Mouth opening tends to deviate towards the side of pathology. The early phase of opening is a rotation of the condyle of the mandible against the disk in the lower joint space. From about 25 mm opening continues with glide between the disk-condyle complex and the glenoid fossa of the temporal bone in the upper joint space. This latter causes the joint to move away from the side of the gliding. As much of the joint pathology causing restriction is related to upper joint space problems, muscle spasm restricting disk movement or muscle or joint pain restricting movement, the loss of glide is the most common outcome and therefore the "normal" joint glides causing the jaw centerline to deviate towards the other side. Looking for this loss of function aids confirmation of the side and site of the problem.

Interdigitation of the Teeth (Dental Occlusion)

The way the teeth bite together can be altered by joint collapse. If one joint collapses the fulcrum on that side moves superiorly causing

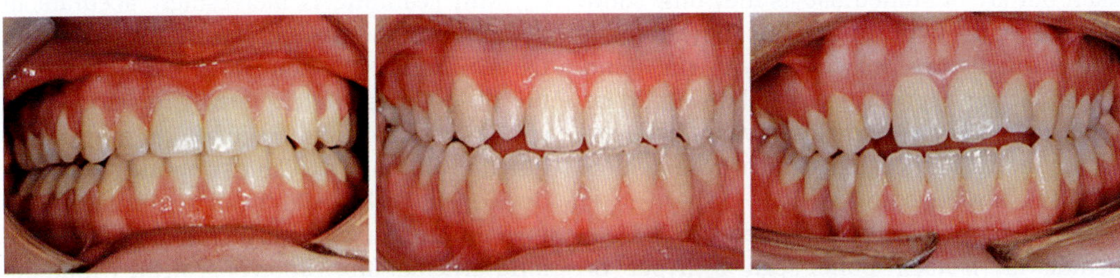

Gradual progression to anterior open bite with centerline deviation to the left following left sided joint collapse

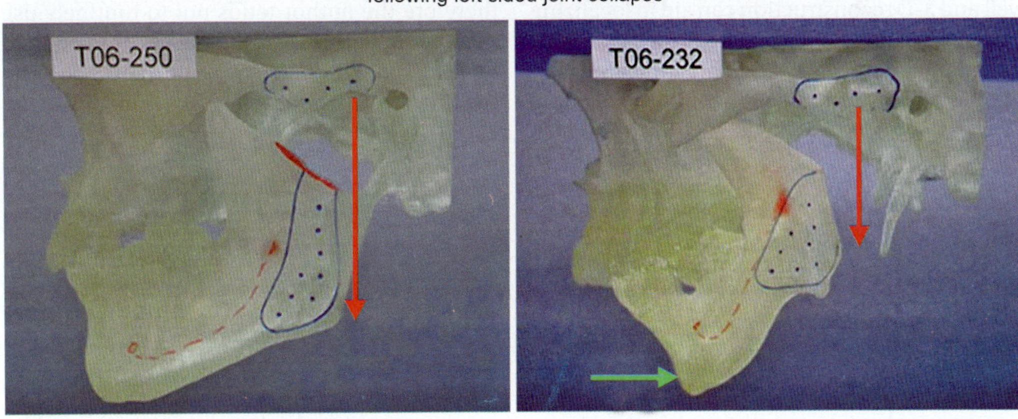

No vertical or horizontal collapse

Rheumatoid with horizontal and vertical collapse

Fig. 19.6: Change in jaw relationship and dental occlusion showing development of anterior open bite, loss of chin prominence (green arrow) and loss of vertical ramus height (red arrow) due to horizontal and vertical collapse of the TMJ in rheumatoid disease for example the posterior teeth to meet prematurely on that side and the centerline to deviate towards that side (**Fig. 19.6**). If both sides collapse the front teeth will not meet (anterior open bite), when the patient reports they previously did.

Conversely if there is an effusion (inflammatory fluid in the joint) or hemarthrosis (blood in the joint) the joint space increases lowering the fulcrum, preventing the posterior teeth on the side the effusion from meeting. Minor variances in the occlusion are usually clinically irrelevant.

Investigations

Plain radiographs form the mainstay of initial examination of the TMJ. Other pathologies should be excluded including dental pain, sinus problems, trigeminal neuralgia, etc. from the history, examination and often an OPG radiograph. This will help to eliminate dental pain. Plain radiographs of the joint are often taken but are of limited use as they only show a section of the joint surface and show nothing of the soft tissues associated with the joint. Transpharyngeal and transcranial views may be requested and open and closed views likewise, but they add little thorough clinical examination and OPG showing both TMJs.

Further investigations, where indicated, include an isotope bone scan if hyper or hypoplasia of the condyle is suspected. CT scanning of the joint shows the bony structures well and 3-D reconstruction can aid in localizing bony pathology particularly when joint resection and reconstruction are indicated. The soft tissues are best imaged with MRI scanning which will help to determine disk displacement, tears and disk movement (**Figs 19.7A and B**).

Isotope bone scanning involves injecting the patient with technetium 99m. This circulates the body and is taken up in bone which is actively turning over. Radiographs are taken 2 hours after injection. Uptake is increased in active bone and therefore will show as a "hot spot" in the condyle which is hyperplastic. It will also show where there is acute infection. The isotope is largely expelled within 24 hours. PET (Positron emission tomography) is often used at the same time and shows similar results.

CT scans are best placed to show the bony anatomy of the joint and surrounding structures. They are essential in planning for joint replacement, but of little use in assessing the joint soft tissues. The scan itself can be used to generate a 3-dimensional CAD-CAM model of the joint to aid planning and reconstruction (**Fig. 19.8**).

MRI scanning is increasingly accurate in determining the position and state of the soft tissues around the joint and the position of the disk. Unfortunately these are static scans in the most part and therefore do not look at function although dynamic scans are now being developed. Disk position can be displaced due to pain stopping the disk relocating, lack of intra-articular lubrication or scarring within the joint holding the disk in position. This cannot be differentiated by the MRI scanner and therefore the author tends not to routinely use this modality of assessment as it seems to add little to clinical diagnosis at present. Likewise, the accuracy of the scan lies in the quality of the

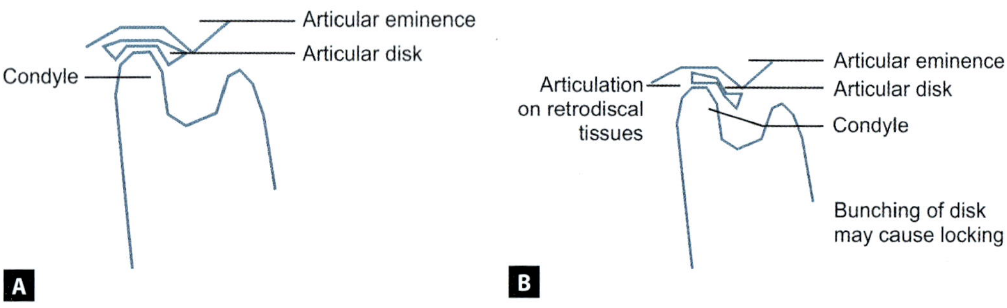

Figs 19.7A and B: (A) Schematic illustrations of the joint space with the disk; Normal disk relationship; (B) Anterior disk displacement

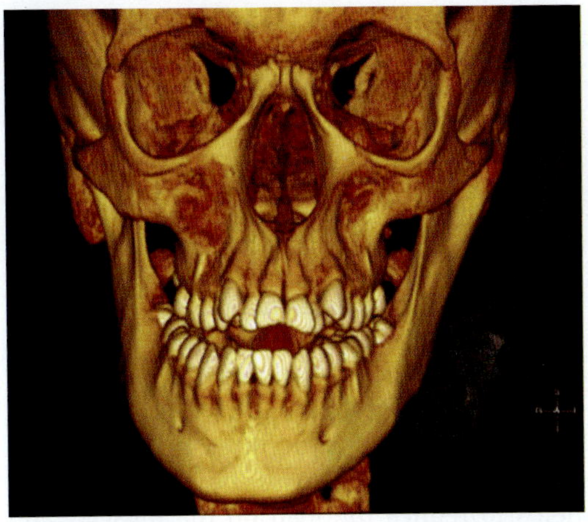

Fig. 19.8: Left condylar hyperplasia 3D CT scan showing cross bite on the contralateral side, centerline deviation away from the side of the pathology and anterior open bite. Bowing of the mandible suggests this has been long-standing

scan and the quality of the radiologist reading the scan. Even in the best hands under and over-diagnosis of disk related disease is made in around 50 percent of cases. The wise surgeon will manage a patient according to the clinical signs and symptoms and not based solely on radiological investigations, which add an aid to diagnosis (treat the patient not the X-ray!).

Arthroscopy, which will be discussed in more detail later, in good hands provides not only a significant aid to diagnosis, but also helps to relieve over 70 percent of patients of their symptoms.

Surgical exploration of the joint should only be considered as a last resort and there should be a specific pathology for which the surgical treatment is aimed to relieve. It should not be considered as a diagnostic aid.

Differential Diagnosis

Differential diagnosis of TMJ disorders follows the standard surgical sieve **(Table 19.1)**. Whilst there are numerous pneumonics for remembering this, the author finds Tinned Vim works (although the younger reader may not be aware of what Vim is!).

▪ Table 19.1
Conditions affecting TMJ

Congenital lesions
Acquired lesions

- Traumatic
- Inflammatory
- Infective
- Neoplasms
  - Primary
  - Secondary
- Nutritional
- Endocrine
- Degenerative
- Vascular
- Idiopathic
- Iatrogenic
- Miscellaneous

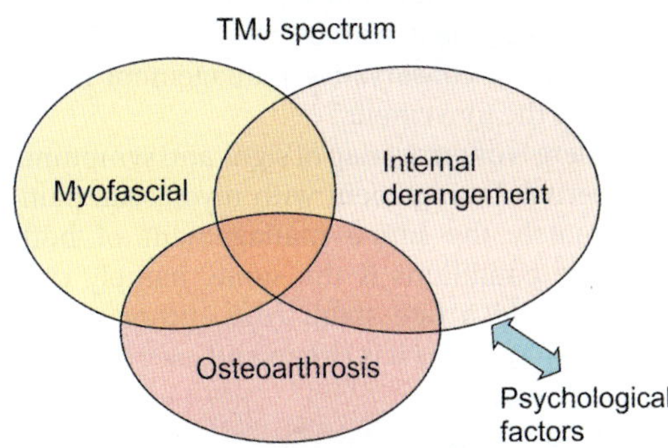

Fig. 19.9: TMJ spectrum-complex interactions of numerous disease processes in TMD

Whilst this surgical sieve is useful, the majority of patients presenting with TMJ symptoms have internal derangement, myofascial pain and degenerative disease. These can contribute to psychological factors **(Fig. 19.9)**. Internal derangement and myofascial pain will be dealt with first, followed by the standard surgical sieve.

MYOFASCIAL PAIN AND INTERNAL DERANGEMENT

This condition affects up to 1/3 of the population at some stage during their lives. Most patients suffer nothing more than a "clicking joint" and this is so common that some would say it is a normal variant. The clicking may be associated with pain, locking or restriction of movement. Clinical examination should determine if there is tenderness over the joints laterally and posteriorly, whether there is associated muscle tenderness and how much motion the joint can achieve by measuring the inter-incisal distance (normal greater than 35 mm) and lateral deviations. Where in the cycle the click occurs can be useful, but a determination of whether there is any glide (upper joint space movement) is more useful in determining whether there is physical restriction. Movements under 25 mm with no glide (loss of lateral deviation away from the affected side) suggest that the upper joint space is occluded, often by a lack of fluid and the joint spaces are sticking together due to lack of lubrication (anchored disk phenomenon). This can be simply dealt with by early arthrocentesis if 6 weeks of conservative management fail to improve the movement.

There is often overlap of signs and symptoms of internal derangement with myofascial pain. Fortunately the initial management of both of these conditions is the same, namely rest, NSAIDs and a bite splint (the author uses a lower soft splint as it is cheap and easy to fit) for at least 6 weeks.

Initial Management

The primary management of most TMJ disorders initially is reassurance that there is unlikely to be a significant underlying condition, it is unlikely to precede arthritis and the majority of patients can be managed with nonsurgical treatment. A significant proportion of patients will have some psychological input to their disease process, whether this is a primary cause or a secondary effect, and the reassurance will go some way to improving their symptoms. Also the placebo effect should affect a "cure" in around 40 percent.

Explanation of the disease process along the lines of a "sprain" of the joint with consequent joint pain due to inflammation and resultant muscle spasm will help to empower the patient and reduce the risk of following internet mis-advice. Initial rest with avoidance of chewy foods such as chewing gum, sticky toffees and tough foods (steaks and crusty bread) and restriction of wide mouth opening (occasionally the pain may have been induced by a long dental visit) will improve symptoms, but this regime must be persisted with for several weeks. The addition of topical nonsteroidal anti-inflammatory gels applied to the area of the joint 4 times daily for 4 weeks will give additional benefit in terms of pain relief and reduction of joint inflammation. Paracetamol as a simple analgesic can additionally be used.

A lower soft full occlusal coverage splint to wear at night should be provided. This helps to reduce the load on the muscles and joint overnight, particularly in those patients who have a clenching habit. It also will help to eliminate the habit. It may take a few nights for the patient to get used to the splint and it may take a few weeks for symptoms to start to improve. There is no benefit shown by occlusal adjustment of the teeth, although some dentists may feel this is the case. A Cochrane study (*see* Suggested Reading) has shown that doing nothing is just as effective and is much less harmful. Likewise no splint has been shown to be better than any other and since a full coverage lower soft splint worn part-time is unlikely to cause untoward occlusal effects, this method is used by the author. Hard splints should cover all the teeth and make a stable occlusion. They are more costly and time consuming to adjust, but are recommended by some restorative experts.

Although physiotherapy may be beneficial in the short-term there is no evidence of its long-term efficacy. Steroid injections to the joint should be avoided and left to a maxillofacial surgeon to decide whether these are indicated as their repeated use may cause joint collapse. Whilst exercises have often been prescribed there seems to be no good evidence that they are beneficial in internal derangement. Often the exercises are poorly explained and carried out inadequately by the patient, but it seems illogical to suggest that an injured joint should be exercised—imagine telling a patient with a sprained ankle they should run on it daily! Exercises may however be beneficial in mobilizing patients with acute muscle spasm secondary to myofascial pain.

▪ Table 19.2
When to refer for maxillofacial advice

- Acute severe restriction of opening
- Failure of simple conservative measures in conjunction with dentist over 2 months
- Associated rheumatological disease
- Recurrent dislocation of the joint
- Disturbance of the dental occlusion

Following a 2 month trial of these treatments, if there has been no significant improvement, or if the above measures cannot be instituted, or if there is acute severe restriction in opening then referral to a maxillofacial specialist, preferably with an interest in TMJ disorders should be considered (**Table 19.2**).

Management in Specialist Centers

Earlier intervention by means of therapeutic arthroscopy (examination and washout of the joint) or arthrocentesis (joint washout) is indicated in patients with restricted opening who fail to improve or in those with persistent locking. Around 80 percent will improve with this procedure. Additionally arthroscopy under GA gives a good idea of how much of the restriction is due to muscle spasm and pain and also whether there is any intra-articular damage (opening improves with the muscle relaxation of general anesthesia). Follow up physiotherapy gives added benefit.

Where there has been no improvement following arthroscopy, the joint was normal and mouth opening improved during anesthesia it is assumed that the majority of the problem is due to muscle spasm and a muscle relaxant medication may be suggested. Commonly a low dose tricyclic such as amitriptyline or dothiepin is indicated with doses starting at 10 mg and potentially rising to 75 mg titrated to symptoms and side effects. These medications take around three weeks to become effective and doses should be increased on a monthly basis until full pain relief is achieved or side effects prevent a further increase in dose. The pain relieving dose is maintained for 6 months and then the patient should be weaned off, according to recurrence of symptoms, over the next few weeks. Unfortunately no long-term studies have shown benefit from this management regime. Alternative therapy currently under investigation is the injection of botulinum toxin into the areas of muscle spasm, which is effective in around 70 percent of patients in the author's series of over 100 cases.

Other modalities which have been successfully used in myofascial pain include cognitive behavior therapy in which the patient receives psychological counseling to prevent the cause of the muscle hyperactivity. Acupuncture is also successful in dealing with the muscle spasm, but also the pain of internal derangement. It is however difficult to find a suitably trained specialist to manage the TMJ in particular. TENS (Transcutaneous electrical nerve stimulation) can also help in the management of the chronic pain associated with myofascial pain following failure of the other techniques.

Where arthroscopy has shown intra-articular problems these may be addressed with open joint surgery if symptoms do not improve. A variety of techniques have been used along orthopedic principles with ultimately joint replacement as the final option. The latter is not to be considered lightly and in the UK at present less than 100 total joint replacements are carried out each year by less than 10 recognized joint replacement surgeons. National guidelines have suggested when these may be indicated.

OTHER DISORDERS OF THE TEMPOROMANDIBULAR JOINT

Congenital

Congenital lesions of the joint are uncommon and will lead to facial asymmetry.

Hemifacial Microsomia

This is due to failure of the condyle to develop secondary to loss of the blood supply *in utero*. This causes associated undergrowth of the ear, ear canal, joint and fossa to varying degrees. This is a complex craniofacial disorder and should be managed in a supraregional cranio-facial center. The management involves craniofacial bone and soft tissue reconstruction in various stages throughout life. It may occur on both sides.

Condylar Hyperplasia

This is due to either overgrowth of the condylar growth center on one side before or during puberty, or continued growth after completion of puberty with cessation of growth on the contralateral side. The patient will present with progressive disturbance of the occlusion, usually with centerline deviation of the dental centerline and associated deviation of the chin point (hemimandibular hyperplasia) (**Fig 19.10**). It may also present with bowing of the mandible downwards and associated maxillary dentoalveolar compensatory growth with the occlusion developing a downward cant towards the side of the abnormality (hemimandibular hypertrophy). There is not usually associated pain, although in the adult onset version there may be limited translatory movement of the TMJ on the affected side.

Diagnosis is aided by seeing an elongated condylar neck on OPG (pubescent type) or an abnormal condyle (post-pubescent). Ongoing growth can be confirmed by an isotope bone scan using Technetium 99 or a PET (Positron emission tomography) scan. These will both show increased uptake on the affected side if it is still active. Management where there is increased uptake is to remove the growth plate by means of a condylar shave operation where the cartilage growth center is removed surgically. If the disease is burnt out or has been treated by condylar shave, the resultant deformity and centerline correction is managed by orthognathic surgery (jaw realignment). These procedures require referral to a maxillo-facial surgeon.

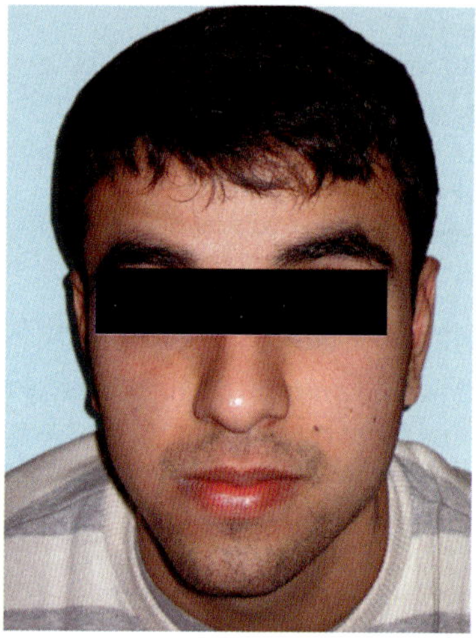

Fig. 19.10: Left condylar hyperplasia showing deviation of chin point to the right

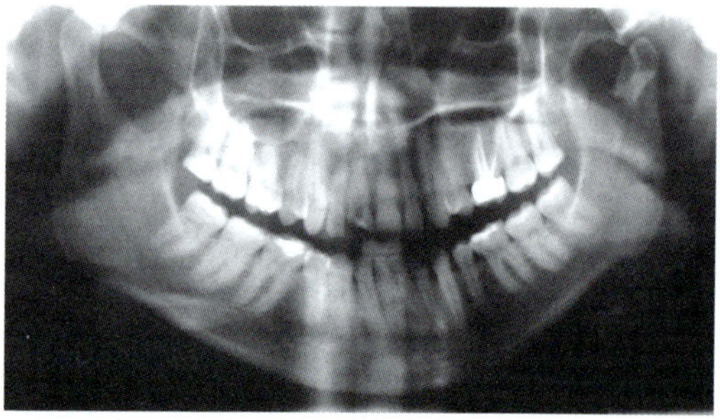

Fig. 19.11: Dental panarogram showing a fracture dislocation of left condyle with vertical collapse

Traumatic

Trauma to the TMJ is a common occurrence in fractures of the mandible. The majority of facial fractures in the UK are related to interpersonal violence. Condylar fractures are one of the more common mandibular fractures (**Fig. 19.11**) occurring in around 30 percent of cases. They may also occur bilaterally or be associated with fractures elsewhere on the bony mandible.

In children, fractures of the condyle tend to occur within the capsule and are difficult to treat surgically. Diagnosis is in a child following a direct blow over the joint or an indirect blow to the mandible elsewhere, particularly the chin. The child will complain of pain in the area, difficulty opening the mouth fully and sometimes inability to close the teeth together due either to bone displacement (contralateral open bite) or fluid within the joint (ipsilateral open bite) secondary to intra-articular soft tissue injury. There will be swelling and tenderness over the area of the fracture and the occlusion may be disrupted as above.

Initial management is often with mobilization and analgesia as this injury can affect the secondary growth plate in the condyle causing undergrowth, overgrowth or fusion of the joint surfaces (ankylosis). Intermaxillary fixation for a 2 to 4 week period, often with elastics may be considered where the occlusion is deranged. Occasionally internal fixation may be considered with resorbable plates.

Effusion or hemarthrosis should be managed with arthrocentesis (joint irrigation with isotonic fluid under pressure) to enable joint recovery.

The child should be monitored long-term to observe for growth abnormalities such that these can be treated at a stage when compensatory growth has not occurred to such an extent to make future management more difficult.

In the adult, the fracture pattern is often different. Extracapsular fractures are more common. Symptoms and signs are similar to those in children with pain over the site of the injury and on function, swelling and possible malocclusion. If the occlusion is normal then the fracture is managed conservatively with a soft diet for 4 to 6 weeks. Derangement of the occlusion warrants management either with intermaxillary fixation of some variety and in some cases open reduction and internal fixation with miniplates may be required. There is considerable controversy as to the best way of managing these fractures and the reader is referred to the standard maxillofacial trauma texts if they are interested in considering this further. Growth disturbances and ankylosis are much less common in adults.

Infective TMJ Disorders

Infection of the temporomandibular joint is an uncommon occurrence in the developed world. It does however remain a major source of morbidity.

Infection may be due to direct infection of the joint, from local spread from the surrounding structures or due to deposition from a distant site, usually from a polyarticular infective processes.

Primary infection may be of the intracapsular bone—osteomyelitis—or infection of the intra-articular soft tissues—arthritis. Both can be destructive of bone and soft tissues and lead to either joint collapse or ankylosis (fusion) of the joint. In childhood they will lead to secondary growth arrest with subsequent deformity. The usual organism is *Staphylococcus aureus* in immune competent individuals, with other staphylococci or unusual organisms where the host is immunocompromised.

The most common cause of infection is spread from neighboring structures of the ear, brain and nasopharynx. All of the organisms causing mastoiditis, otitis media and meningitis can be implicated, but again *Staphylococcus* is most likely to invade the joint. The effects of the infection long-term are similar to those from direct infection.

Hematogenous spread rarely occurs, but is occasionally secondary to enteric organisms (*Salmonella*) or systemic organisms causing a more generalized polyarthritis (syphilis, bacterial endocarditis, septicemia). Effects are similar to the other two causes, but often the systemic infective process carries more morbidity and risk of mortality.

Diagnosis is from a history of pain and swelling localized to the area of the joint, with acute onset limitation of movement. The patient will have generalized signs of an infective process with pyrexia, rigors, sweating (particularly night sweats) and malaise. They may also have signs and symptoms of other joint involvement. Locally there will be the signs of acute inflammation with tenderness over the joint, swelling, redness and heat. There may be additional cervical lymphadenopathy and tenderness over the mastoid if there is middle ear involvement.

The diagnosis can be confirmed with aspiration of pus from the joint and this should be sent for urgent culture and sensitivities. The patient should be admitted to hospital and broad spectrum intravenous antibiotics should be commenced with thorough arthrocentesis (washout of the joint) of at least 500 mL of isotonic solution or until the aspirate is clear. This should be repeated if necessary. The advice of a microbiologist should be sought for local sensitivities in guidance for antibiotic treatment. General systemic support would include antipyretic (paracetamol and NSAID) and adequate hydration, with management of the causative disease process. Systemic involvement with septicemia may require admission to intensive care.

Ultimate management may involve open surgical drainage. The long-term sequelae of the process may require further surgical input and early maxillofacial surgical advice is essential, in addition to long-term support. Reconstruction and rehabilitation may require open surgical procedures, osteotomies, rib grafts or joint replacement.

Inflammatory Disease

Many of the inflammatory arthropathies can affect the TMJ. Rheumatoid disease can occur in the child, adolescent and adult. It will usually present with the signs and symptoms of synovitis namely pain, swelling, heat and restriction of movement and therefore can be difficult to differentiate from infective causes. Progression can lead to joint collapse resulting in malocclusion with an anterior open bite and a retrusive chin (*see* **Fig. 19.6**). Usually other joints, particularly the hands and feet, will have been involved for some time, as rheumatoid disease is a polyarticular arthropathy tending to affect the smaller joints. Diagnosis can be confirmed serologically with a positive rheumatoid factor present in 80 percent. Seronegative arthropathy can occur with a similar clinical picture. In the head and neck there can be associated dry mouth, dry eyes (Sjögren's syndrome) and difficulty with oral hygiene due to involvement of the hands.

Management of the rheumatoid TMJ should initially follow the same principles as for most TMJ disorders. Rest, with a soft diet and avoidance of wide opening, NSAIDs (topical or systemic) regularly and a soft splint to "rest" the muscles which may be overactive and to offload the joint. Early consideration of arthroscopy and arthrocentesis will help to eliminate the inflammatory mediators from within the joint. If synovitis is active then steroid injection should be considered, although repeated injections, which calm down the inflammatory process, may lead to increased cartilage loss and joint collapse. End stage management of the collapsed joint is with total joint replacement (**Fig. 19.12**). A rheumatologist should be involved as they may instigate disease modifying medication.

Ankylosing spondylitis may initially present in the TMJ. The patients are mostly male and tend to have generalized signs with fixed kyphosis (flexion of the spine particularly the neck). Classically they are HLA B27 positive, although this is not exclusive to ankylosing spondylitis. The process leads to ankylosis of

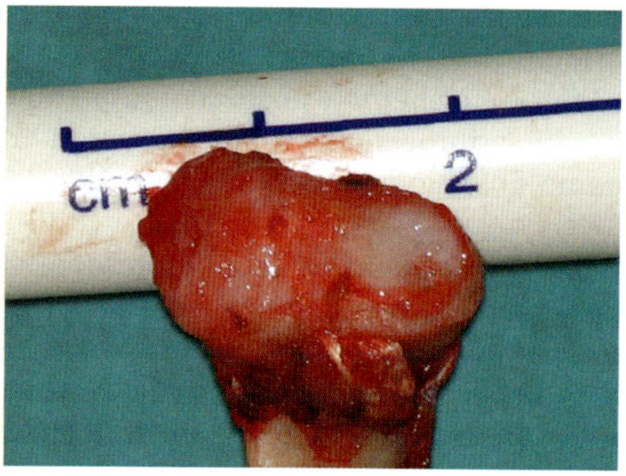

Fig. 19.12: Rheumatoid joint pannus of condyle

the TMJ and the restriction of mouth opening (**Figs 19.13A and B**) is made worse by the fixed flexion of the neck towards the chest wall. Release of the ankylosis surgically with joint reconstruction is required, optimally with total joint replacement to give a large enough gap to prevent re-ankylosis and enable adequate function.

Psoriatic arthropathy may affect the TMJ causing acute synovitis, joint collapse or ankylosis. The patients initially present with the skin condition of psoriasis, with involvement often of the larger joints in a degenerative type of arthropathy. Some patients may be HLA B27 positive and these tend to progress towards an ankylosis picture rather than the synovitis which often characterizes this disease process. Management of the synovitis is with rest, NSAIDs and bite splints. Arthrocentesis can help relieve symptoms as can steroid injections. Ultimately joint replacement may be required due to joint collapse or ankylosis.

All of the rheumatoid diseases may be managed by a rheumatologist with disease modifying medication which may have significant side effects on the oral mucosa and also interact with various other medications. One should be aware that bisphosphonates may be used particularly with osteopenic rheumatoid conditions and due diligence in general dental management with support to prevent disease to the oral structures is essential. Leucocyte inhibition medication may cause mild immunosuppression and aggressive management of infection is essential in these patients.

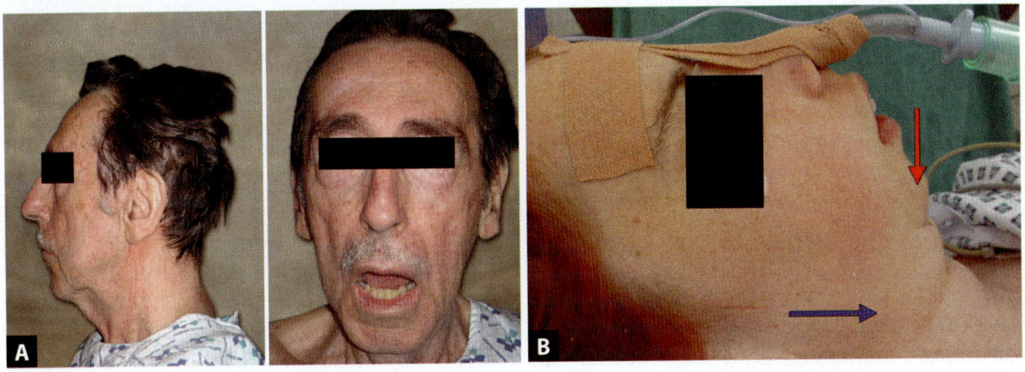

Figs 19.13A and B: (A) Ankylosing spondylitis with limited mouth opening and flexion of the cervical spine; (B) Rheumatoid arthritis—retrusion (red arrow) and loss of vertical height (blue arrow)

Neoplastic Disease

Neoplasms may be primary or secondary, benign or malignant.

Primary benign neoplasms of the TMJ are rare and include chondroma, synovial chondromatosis, osteochondroma and osteoma. Malignant neoplasms are even more uncommon and the condyle seems to be preserved when the mandible is invaded by squamous carcinoma. Chondrosarcoma, osteochondrosarcoma and osteosarcoma are extremely rare in the head and neck and even more so in the condyle. They are dealt with elsewhere in this textbook. The slightly anomalous pigmented villonodular synovitis behaves as a neoplasm with locally invasive tendency, but again is rare.

Benign neoplasms tend to slow growth (the commonest being osteochondroma) and therefore can present with pain, loss of movement and slowly progressive deformity with a lateral open bite on the side of the neoplasm. There is occasional centerline shift of the chin and dental centerline, but more commonly downward bowing of the lower border of the mandible occurs. Diagnosis is from clinical and radiological examination supported if necessary by open joint surgery to biopsy or excise the lesion and subsequent reconstruction and/or orthognathic correction of the resultant malocclusion and facial deformity.

Synovial chondromatosis is a rare condition which affects the joint often secondary to degenerative disease. Production of large amounts of small chondromata from the synovium occurs producing numerous millimeter size rounded loose bodies in the joint. These affect joint function and can induce pain. Management is with open washout as they are too large to pass through an arthroscope. This should allow the joint to function although there is often degenerative change which warrants surgical treatment in its own right. It is felt to be due to overproduction of cartilage by the synovium and therefore synovectomy is advocated.

Metastasis may occur to the condyle as to any other region of the mandible. The common neoplasms metastasizing to bone include breast, kidney, thyroid, and colon with osteolytic lesions and the prostate with osteosclerotic lesions. Diagnosis and management of the primary site is essential, but the metastasis should be managed symptomatically with either resection and reconstruction, radiotherapy or pain management.

Degenerative Disease (Osteoarthrosis)

This is the final common pathway for a number of TMJ conditions from trauma, infection, inflammation, neoplastic and iatrogenic (surgeon induced) causes. Primary degenerative disease can also occur but is much less common than involvement of the knee and hip. Internal derangement of the joint is a very common condition which does not usually lead to degenerative osteoarthrosis if the wear and tear component of this disease can be converted to repair by appropriate noninvasive interventions.

It is much less common than degenerative disease of the major joints as the load is significantly less in the TMJ. It tends to occur when the wear and tear in the joint overtakes the repair. Pain, swelling and restriction of movement are the common symptoms. Clinical examination reveals a tender joint with palpable crepitus and restriction of movement, with intermittent swelling.

Initial management is with conservative measures followed by arthroscopy, open surgery and ultimately joint replacement as above.

Iatrogenic/Idiopathic

The former use of open joint surgery for pain, restriction and joint noises has lead to the increasing frequency of degeneration of the joint from multiple operations, particularly in USA. Surgery for joint noise alone has now been accepted as inappropriate. However, less commonly these postoperated patients may have dysesthetic pain due to damage to the surrounding nerves. This is a debilitating type of pain which is difficult to manage. It may be of a shooting nature or dull background ache with acute exacerbations. Management under the direction of a pain team is indicated and is usually with low dose tricyclic medication, or some antiepileptic medication (carbamazepine, gabapentin, etc.).

SURGICAL MANAGEMENT

Surgery of the joint can be divided into closed and open surgery. Closed surgery comprises arthrocentesis and arthroscopy.

Arthrocentesis is the washing out of (usually) the upper joint space with isotonic solution under pressure (recommended 150 mm Hg) using around 200 mL of solution to eliminate inflammatory mediators and free radicals and to re-lubricate the joint initially with the solution, but allowing the lubricant producing cells to recover. Usually two needles are used to carry out this procedure—inlet and outlet. Whilst in Europe and the Rest of the World this is often performed under local analgesia potentially with sedation, in the UK patients will often require general anesthesia. It is a day case procedure and has been shown to be successful in 70 to 80 percent of cases of locking, restriction and pain. The advantage of carrying out the procedure under GA is that the patient can be examined with the muscles relaxed giving a good idea of the degree of restriction due to muscle spasm.

Arthroscopy is a similar procedure, although a small scope is inserted into the joint rather than two needles. A needle is still used as the outlet. The scope size varies from internal diameter of 2.1 mm, although disposable scopes of 1.2 mm are now available. There is some debate regarding the advantage of arthroscopy over arthrocentesis as by its nature the insertion of a larger scope should carry more morbidity. The rationale behind inserting a scope is to aid in diagnosis, not outcome. The outcomes are similar for arthroscopy and arthrocentesis, but arthrocentesis does not see into the joint and will miss diagnoses of disk damage, joint surface damage, scarring and synovitis. There have been no comparisons of complications with arthrocentesis and arthroscopy and long-term no obvious detrimental affects of arthrocopy, other than a small risk of temporal branch weakness of the facial nerve occurring temporarily in less than 1 percent. Other rarer complications have been described.

Open joint surgery follows the principles of orthopedics. The joint is approached via a pre-auricular approach (**Fig. 19.14**) staying close to the cartilaginous auditory meatus to avoid damage to the temporal branch of the facial nerve. If there is damage to the disk this is removed and may or not be replaced with temporalis muscle flap or auricular cartilage, although there has not been any benefit shown to providing this replacement. Damage to the joint surfaces can be adjusted using eminoplasty (modification of the articular eminence) or condylar shave (modification of the condylar head).

Severe degeneration of the joint with associated pain and restriction of opening, ankylosis (**Fig. 19.15**) or inflammatory joint disease with joint collapse warrant joint replacement. Whilst this was often with a costochondral graft (rib) recently alloplastic joint replacement has become the mainstay of treatment using a combination of cobalt-chrome and titanium or all titanium on high molecular weight polyethylene

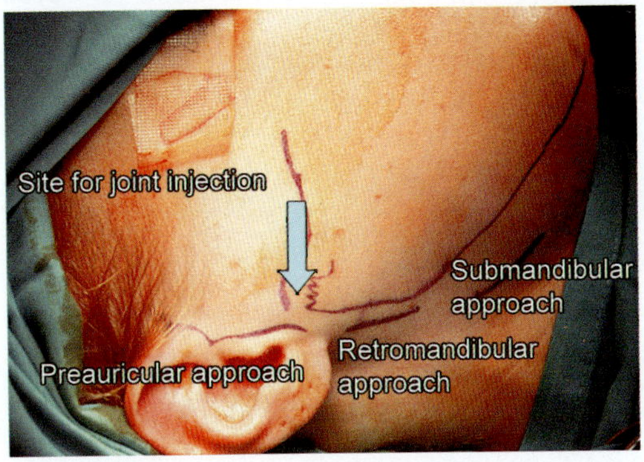

Fig. 19.14: Markings for surgical approaches to TMJ, periaricular approach is preferred

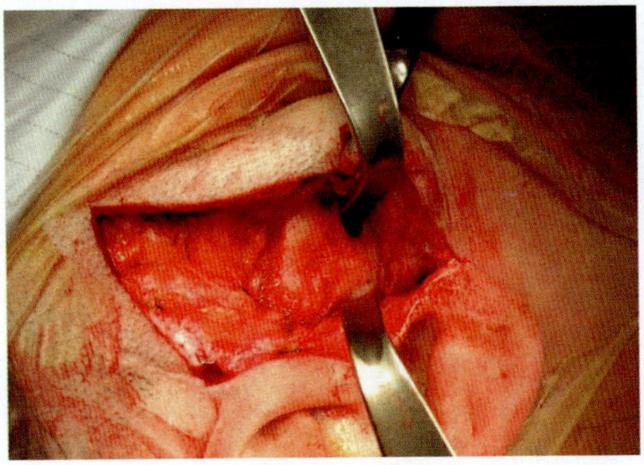

Fig. 19.15: Ankylosed TM joint

for replacement (similar to total knee replacement). Outcomes of 90 percent survival at 15 years are reported with improvement of dietary scores and pain of 90 percent at one year and improvement in mouth opening. The frequency of use of this procedure warrants at present the surgery only being carried out in limited numbers by a few high volume operators, although the indications seem to be increasing. For this reason NICE guidelines have suggested indications for this line of management.

CONCLUSION

Temporomandibular disorders are a common cause of morbidity in dental practice, although most can be managed with simple measures, such as reassurance that joint noises do not require any form of management and do not necessarily lead to degenerative joint disease. The final common pathway of a number of conditions is degenerative disease and arthroscopy followed by surgery. Surgery should be considered as a last resort.

SELF-ASSESSMENT QUESTIONS

1. Give an account of the epidemiology of temporomandibular joint disorders.
2. Describe the primary features of temporomandibular joint pain and their significance.
3. Outline a protocol for the clinical examination of a patient presenting with a history of temporomandibular joint symptoms.
4. Diskuss the use of radiological investigations in the diagnosis of temporomanibular pain.
5. Describe the possible nonsurgical interventions available for temporomadibular joint pain.
6. Describe two congenital disorders resulting from derangement of condylar growth.
7. Describe the causes, clinical features, investigation and treatment of infective diseases of the temporomandibular joint.
8. Give an account of inflammatory diseases which may affect the temporo-mandibular joint.
9. Describe the neoplastic diseases which may affect the temporomandibular joint.
10. Diskuss the role of surgical intervention in the management of diseases of the temporomandibular joint.

SUGGESTED READING

1. Koh H, Robinson PG. Occlusal adjustment for treating and preventing temporomandibular joint disorders. Cochrane Database of Systematic Reviews 2003, Issue 1.
2. NICE Guidelines. IPG 329. Total prosthetic replacement of the temporomandibular joint. Guidance, December 2009.
3. Sidebottom AJ. Guidelines for the replacement of the TMJ in the UK. Br J Oral Maxillofac Surg. 2008:46:146-7.
4. Sidebottom AJ. Leading Article. Current thinking in TMJ management. Br J Oral Maxillofac Surg. 2009;(47):91-4.

Chapter 20

Oral Manifestations of Systemic Disease

Anwar R Tappuni, WM Tilakaratne

Chapter Outline

INTRODUCTION

The importance of oral examination as a part of the full medical examination is well-established, as many systemic conditions affect the mouth. The accessibility of the oral cavity for examination and biopsy taking allows for early and convenient detection of such disorders. The severity of the oral manifestations is often reflective of the activity of the systemic disease and therefore can be used as a tool for determining disease progression and treatment efficacy.

Many diseases have nonspecific presentation in the mouth such as mucosal pallor in anemia, and a yellowish-green hue as a result of jaundice in liver disease. Other conditions, such as some of the dermatological and gastroenterological diseases, have very specific and well-established oral signs and symptoms.

The remit of this chapter is to describe the oral manifestations of the more common systemic conditions. However, some of these have been described already in other chapters.

GASTROINTESTINAL DISEASES

Crohn's Disease

Crohn's disease was first described in 1932 by Crohn, Ginzberg, and Oppenheimer, who reported the predilection of this condition to the terminal segment of the small intestine. Subsequent publications demonstrated that although the most common sites are the ileocecal region followed by the colon, this chronic inflammatory bowl disorder may affect any part of the GI tract from the mouth to the anus.

Crohn's disease seems to be increasing in prevalence and incidence especially in northern altitude countries. Incidence rates in America and Europe are higher than Asia and Africa and range from 0.7 to 9.8 cases per 100,000 persons. CD is reported to have a higher prevalence in urban areas and in upper socioeconomic classes. Studies report that both sexes are affected equally by CD, with the most cases presenting in the first three decades of life. However, it appears that CD has a bimodal distribution with the second peak being between the ages of 60 to 80.

Crohn's disease is a long-standing condition characterized by intermittent flares and remissions. Medical therapy is more effective in its early stages. The chance of death and complications increases the longer the duration of the illness. The 15-year survival rate is about 94 percent.

Box 20.1: Crohn' disease

Key features helpful in diagnosis

- Crohn's disease is a chronic inflammatory bowel disease usually presenting in the first three decades of life.
- Orofacial symptoms of the disease (Crohn's orofacial granulomatosis) are common and characterized by swollen lips, mucosal tags and cobblestoning.
- Early dizgnosis and treatment improve disease outcome.
- Crohn's disease is a chronic disease that is characterized by periods of flare and remission.

Etiology

It is believed that the signs and symptoms of CD are precipitated by a transmural inflammatory process caused by a disparity between pro- and anti-inflammatory mediators. The exact etiology as to why this disparity occurs is unknown. The role of diet, the environment, microbes, immunological factors and genetics have been explored. Current theories favor an interaction between genetics and external provoking factors.

Studies have shown that mononuclear cells in the lamina proporia of OFG patients have increased production of cytokines, which activate Th1 cells (IL-12 and IL-18). Th1 cells in turn trigger the macrophages to produce proinflammatory cytokines and chemokines which increase the inflammatory reaction and contribute to the damage of the endothelial membrane of the intestine.

Clinical Features

Crohn's disease is the most common inflammatory bowel disease (IBD), besides ulcerative colitis. Abdominal pain is the most common symptom of CD, especially in the lower right area. Symptoms of malabsorption are common in CD, manifesting as diarrhea, malnutrition, weight loss, vitamin deficiency and dehydration. In children, it may cause stunted growth and delayed puberty and development. Anal fissures, perianal fistulae or abscesses are seen in about a one-third of CD cases.

The severity and range of symptoms in CD varies. Extraintestinal manifestations of the disease are not unusual. The most common are inflammatory joint diseases, which may precede other symptoms by several years and may persist even after remission of the disease. CD associated rheumatological conditions are seronegative autoimmune-relateddisorderscausingjoint,hipand back pain. They include ankylosing spondylitis, psoriatic and reactive arthritis and sacroiliitis.

Skin manifestations include erythema nodosum and pyoderma gangrenosum. Acrodermatitis enteropathica manifesting as psoriatic erythema is seen due to zinc deficiency caused by malabsorption. Ocular manifestations of CD include recurrent iritis and uveitis. Their severity usually reflects the bowel disease activity. They usually subside when the disease is under control.

Involvement of the liver in CD varies from simple abnormal liver function tests to benign autoimmune chronic active hepatitis and cirrhosis. Urinary system involvement includes nephrolithiasis due to calcium oxalate stones and renal amyloidosis due to acute phase reaction proteins.

Compared with the general population, patients with inflammatory bowel disease are at higher risk of having thromboembolism, antiphospholipid antibody syndrome and cholelithiasis.

Oral Manifestations

Intraoral signs and symptoms are seen in about 10 percent of CD patients. They may be the presenting symptom of the condition. If CD is suspected, full evaluation and investigation of intestinal involvement including colonoscopy and histopathological examination are warranted. Early recognition and treatment of CD increase the likelihood of remission. The severity of the oral manifestations of CD reflects the systemic disease activity and has been used as a marker for disease progression.

The oral manifestations of CD are rare. The most common facial manifestations are labial swelling (**Figs 20.1A and B**) (granulomatous cheilitis) and angular cheilitis. This feature is often reported by patients as the most distressing symptom of the disease as it is painful and affects aesthetics.

Nonspecific signs of the disease include gingivitis and aphthous-like oral ulcers which may make eating difficult, exacerbating the nutritional deficiency secondary to the malabsorption. Specific intraoral signs of the disease include noncaseating granulomas, mucosal tags (**Fig. 20.2**), fissures and hyperplasia giving the classical appearance of cobblestoning of the mucosa.

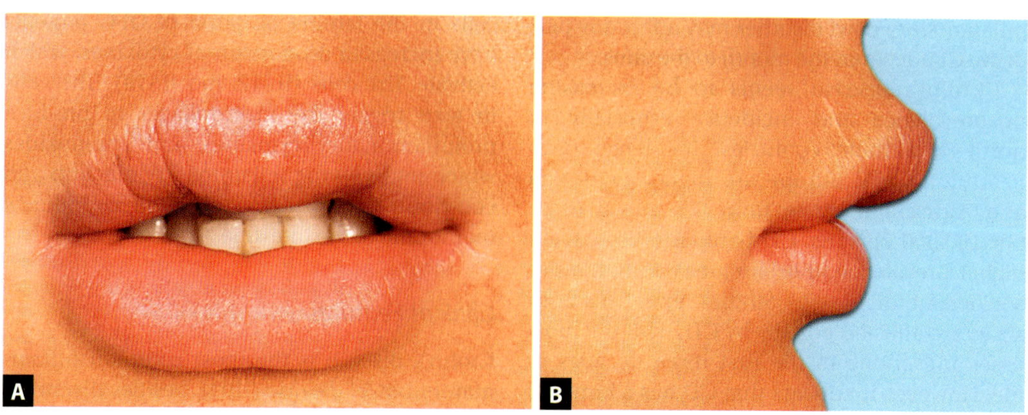

Figs 20.1A and B: Crohn's disease. Enlargement of lips is a common feature

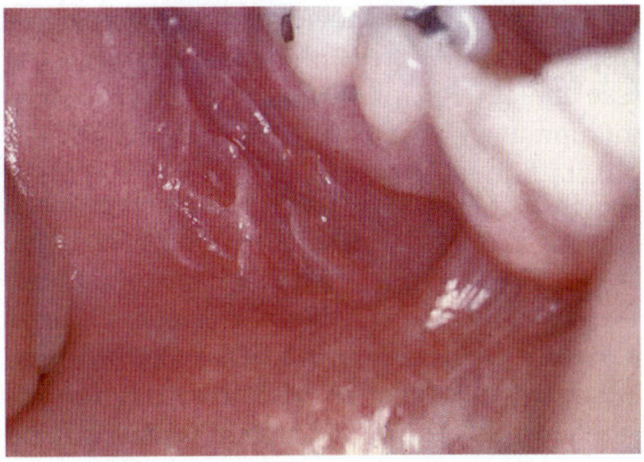

Fig. 20.2: Crohn's disease. Mucosal tags in the lower buccal sulcus

Histopathological Features

Crohn's disease in the intestines causes hyperemia and edema affecting segments of the mucosa at the initial stages. This may progress slowly into a chronic form of ulcerative lesions and thickening of the intestinal wall, giving rise to the characteristic cobble stone appearance of the mucosa. The inflammatory condition affects the whole thickness of the mucosa, unlike ulcerative colitis in which only the superficial layers are affected. Advanced CD is complicated by intestinal obstruction and fistulization, microperforation and abscess formation.

The microscopic appearance of an intestinal biopsy depends on the stage of the disease. In the early stages, a focal inflammatory infiltrate around the crypts is seen. Later in the disease, superficial ulceration and villous blunting, inflammatory cells in the deep mucosal layers and noncaseating granulomas through the thickness of the intestinal wall are seen. The latter is characteristic and pathognomonic of CD but their absence does not exclude CD. Histopathological features of oral lesions are similar to those seen in an intestinal biopsy. Well formed granulomas are found in the majority of established cases. Early cases may show a mixed inflammatory infiltrate without organized granulomas. However, in some cases granulomas are difficult to identify and deep biopsies are frequently required. The epithelium is usually hyperplastic.

Treatment

Crohn's disease is characterized by intermittent flares and remissions. Acute attacks are usually managed with aminosalicylates and corticosteroids to reduce symptoms and control the inflammatory process. Alternative medications used for nonresponsive cases include azathioprine, cyclosporin and infliximab. Supplementary treatment is frequently necessary, e.g. antibiotics for infections, vitamin supplements to treat nutritional deficiencies and anti-diarrhea medication for symptomatic relief. Hospitalization may become necessary in particularly severe attacks and surgical removal of the affected intestinal segments has been reported necessary in up to 80 percent of patients, although recurrence elsewhere remains a possibility.

Orofacial Granulomatosis

The currently used description of orofacial granulomatosis (OFG) was introduced by Wiesenfeld in 1985. The pathological features of OFG include lymphoedema and multiple noncaseating giant cell granulomata in the perioral and oral region (**Fig. 20.3**). This definition encompassed what was known previously as cheilitis granulomatosa (Miescher's cheilitis) and a subgroup of patients with facial nerve palsy previously termed Melkersson-Rosenthal syndrome. OFG is a

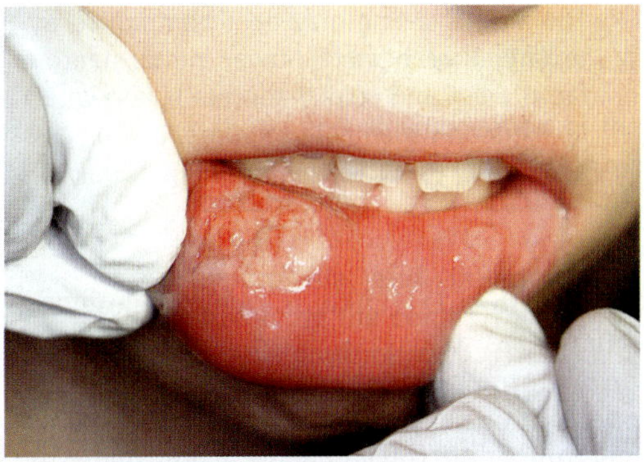

Fig. 20.3: Orofacial granulomatosis. Granulomatous lesions in labial mucosa

rare condition that affects males and females equally with a predilection to younger age groups. It is worthy to note here that the term 'orofacial granulomatosis' is sometimes also used to refer to the oral manifestations of other granulomatous disorders including sarcoidosis and tuberculosis.

Strictly speaking, the term OFG should be applied to patients, who have disease manifestations in the oral and perioral region only. Further, all the known granulomatous conditions should be excluded before arriving at the diagnosis of OFG. If patients manifest gastrointestinal signs and symptoms in addition to the oral manifestations, then the term CD should be used.

Orofacial granulomatosis may be the presenting feature of CD or may precede the intestinal symptoms by months or years. Therefore, periodic intestinal examination in OFG patients may be deemed necessary, especially if there are symptoms of abdominal pain and diarrhea.

Box 20.2: Orofacial granulomatosis

Key features helpful in diagnosis

- Orofacial granulomatosis is characterized by lymphoedema and multiple noncaseating giant cell granulomata affecting the oral and perioral region.
- The manifestations are limited to the head and neck area with no evidence of systemic involvement.
- The clinical presentation is similar to orofacial Crohn's.
- The facial swelling may be accompanied by unilateral or bilateral lower motor-neuron facial palsy and scrotal tongue is known as Melkersson-Rosenthal syndrome.

Etiology

Similar to CD, OFG is a granulomatous inflammatory disease of unknown etiology. An abnormal immune reaction in genetically predisposed individuals is implicated. Several environmental triggers have been suggested. These include infections, medication, allergy to dental materials and food substance such as cinnamon aldehyde and benzoates.

Studies have shown that the immune response in OFG resembles that found in CD (see etiology of Crohn's disease). It appears that inflammatory activity in OFG is mediated by a Th1 immune response leading to over activity of cytokines and chemokines.

Clinical Features

The most striking clinical feature of OFG is the enlargement of one or both lips. This usually starts as an episodic painless, soft swelling of one of the lips, more commonly the lower. Early episodes may last hours or days. If not treated, the condition will progress and the severity and frequency of the swellings will increase. Eventually one or both of the lips become permanently enlarged and feel firm and rubbery. The lips appear thickened and lobulated and are predisposed to median cheilitis (midline fissuring) and angular cheiltis (**Fig. 20.4**). Other regions of the face, such as the periorbital areas and the chin may be affected by similar swellings. Patients, especially teenagers, find these facial features disfiguring and very distressing.

Intraorally, the granulomata affect the buccal and labial mucosa giving a characteristic lobulated and corrugated appearance, often described as a 'cobblestoned' mucosa. The gingiva appears erythematous and hyperplastic. There is altered taste sensation and reduced salivary flow. The sublingual folds and submandibular duct orifices are prominent and firm. Mucosal tags may be found in the buccal

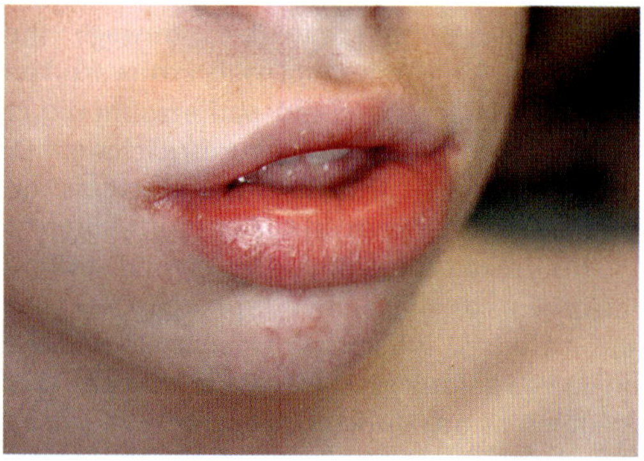

Fig. 20.4: Orofacial granulomatosis. Enlarged lower lip with signs of angular cheilitis

and labial sulci and retromolar areas. Mouth ulcers are also seen in OFG. These can either be recurrent resembling aphthous ulcers or present as long standing deep linear ulcers of the buccal sulci.

Up to 2 percent of OFG patients form a subgroup presenting with recurrent lower motor-neuron facial palsy accompanying the facial swellings. This condition was referred to previously as Melkersson-Rosenthal syndrome. The facial palsy may progress to become permanent and may be unilateral or bilateral.

Histopathological Features

When a biopsy is performed in early disease, edematous corium and perivascular lymphocytic infiltration without proper granuloma formation can be found. Lymphatics can be dilated and may contain macrophages causing granulomatous lymphangitis. Noncaseating granulomas are evident in the more advanced disease (**Fig. 20.5**). Granulomas may present in the corium, or in some cases within the muscle layer. Therefore, a deeper biopsy is always indicated.

Treatment

There is no known cure for OFG. The treatment is mainly symptomatic, aimed at controlling the acute episodes of the disease and to restore function and esthetics. The response to therapy is often slow and incomplete. Complete remission of OFG is very rarely achieved.

It has been suggested that using compression devices for several hours daily may lead to a reduction in the labial swelling. Diet exclusion of cinnamon and benzoate, has been shown to cause significant improvement of the lip edema, especially if implemented early in the disease.

The most common class of drugs used for OFG is corticosteroids. In mild cases, topical steroids in the form of ointments, mouthwashes and inhalers are used to control the intraoral granulomata and ulcer formation. Intralesional corticosteroid injections given periodically have been shown to reduce swelling, albeit temporarily. Severe cases are treated with systemic corticosteroids.

Several other medications are used in treating OFG, such as long-term antibiotics, tacrolimus, clofazamine, azathioprine, dapsone and thalidomide. None of which however, have strong clinical evidence supporting their efficacy. Surgical intervention is used for treating severe and disfiguring swellings but is rarely successful unless it is supported by other forms of treatment such as radiation or postoperative periodic intralesional steroid injections.

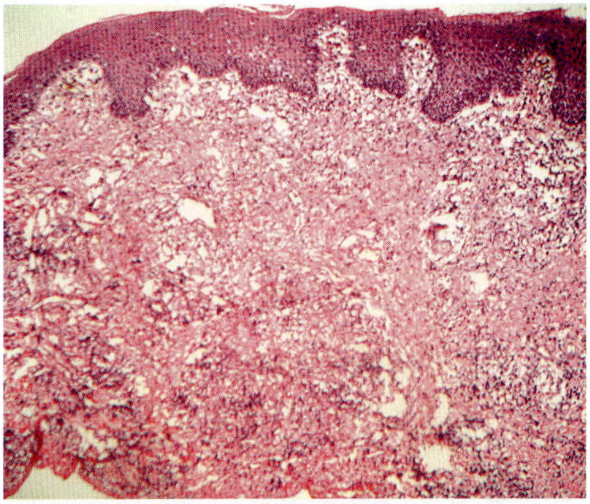

Fig. 20.5: Orofacial granulomatosis. Granulomas containing epithelioid macrophages, lymphocytes and few giant cells. The corium shows marked edema

Ulcerative Colitis

Ulcerative colitis (UC) is an idiopathic chronic inflammatory bowel disorder of part or the entire colon. The rectum is almost always involved in active disease. Ulcerative colitis is similar to CD in many aspects but also has its own distinct characteristics. In UC, the inflammatory changes are confined to the colon, unlike CD where the condition may affect any part of the gastrointestinal tract. Ulcerative colitis effects are usually restricted to the mucosa and submucosa whilst CD affects the full thickness of the intestine. UC is seen more frequently in white people with a slight increased incidence in females and has a bimodal distribution with the first peak at the age of 15 to 25 and a second peak at age of 55 to 65.

Box 20.3: Ulcerative colitis

Key features helpful in diagnosis

- Ulcerative colitis is an inflammatory bowel disorder of the mucosa and submucosa of the colon.
- Bacterial antigen and diet have been implicated in the etiology of UC.
- The oral mucosa affected by UC appears erythematous with scattered pustules, hemorrhagic ulcerations and abscesses.
- Pharmacotherapy can be effective but colectomy may be necessary in severe cases.

Etiology

Autoimmunity has been associated with the etiology of UC, although not as strongly as it is with Crohn's disease. There seem to be enhanced intestinal reactivity in UC against bacterial antigens of normal intestinal bacterial flora and certain dietary items such as milk. The role of genetics in UC is supported by the fact that positive family history is associated with a higher risk for this condition. Environmental factors may be involved but smoking has been shown to be negatively associated with ulcerative colitis, unlike CD which has been reported to show a positive association with smoking.

Clinical Features

Similar to CD, UC has intermittent pattern of acute episodes. The characteristic features are bloody diarrhea and abdominal pain. There are associated nutritional deficiencies, weight loss and failure to thrive in children. Extraintestinal signs and symptoms include finger clubbing, iritis and uveitis. The joints may be involved manifesting as arthritis, ankylosing spondylitis and sacroiliitis. Cutaneous signs include Erythema nodosum and pyoderma gangrenosum, which may be very painful.

Oral Manifestations

Oral and perioral lesions in UC are less common than in CD. The oral lesions may precede the intestinal disease. When present simultaneously, the extent of the oral lesions reflects the severity of the disease affecting the colon. The oral mucosa in UC looks generally erythematous with scattered pustules, hemorrhagic ulcerations and abscesses. Pyostomatitis vegetans may be seen as an oral manifestation of UC presenting clinically as multiple friable pustules, with varying degrees of severity and pain.

Histopathological Features

Microscopically, the changes in UC do not usually reach the muscular layer and are limited to the mucosa and submucosa. The crypts are shortened and branched. The cellular response seen microscopically may be similar to that seen in CD. There is intense infiltration of neutrophils, eosinophils, plasma cells, mast cells and lymphocytes.

Oral lesions of UC, pyostomatitis vegetans shows epithelium with areas of ulceration or necrosis. The epithelial hyperplasia may be florid amounting to pseudoepitheliomatous hyperplasia in some cases. Eosinophil abscesses are found at the tip of the connective tissue papillae and within the epithelium. Mixed inflammatory infiltrate is present in the corium (**Fig. 20.6**).

Treatment

Most cases of UC are controlled with medication although patients may continue to experience

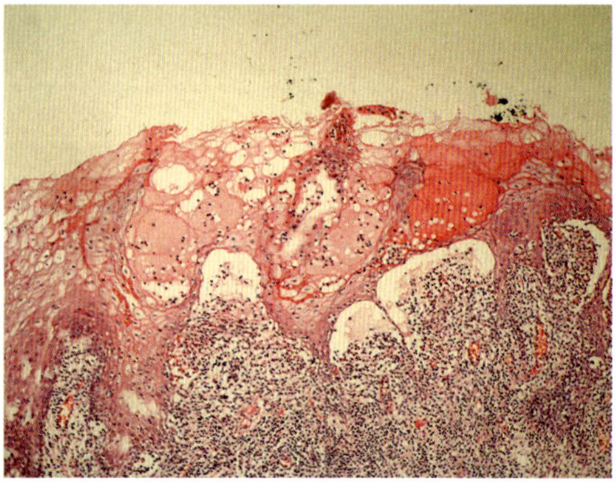

Fig. 20.6: Pyostomatitis vegetans. Epithelial hyperplasia with prominent eosinophils in the epithelium

intermittent acute phases. In severe cases, removal of the large intestine is curative. Patients with UC are at higher risk of colorectal cancer therefore, regular surveillance with colonoscopy is indicated.

No specific dietary restriction has been shown to be beneficial in UC. However, many patients have concurrent lactose intolerance and would benefit from avoiding milk. Pharmacotherapy depends on the severity of the disease. It is aimed at reducing symptoms and preventing progression. Aminosalicylates have an anti-inflammatory effect and are used regularly in treating mild-moderate UC. Antibiotics have had demonstrable benefit in active UC. Corticosteroids are usually used in acute phases to induce remission. Other medications that are effective in controlling UC include tumor necrosis factor (TNF) inhibitors, infliximab and immunomodulators such as azathioprine and cyclosporine. Failure of pharmacotherapy indicates refractory disease and colectomy usually cures the disease.

Celiac Disease

Celiac disease is a chronic inflammatory disease of the gastrointestinal tract. It is also known as celiac sprue, nontropical sprue or gluten-sensitive enteropathy. Patients affected by this condition suffer from intolerance to gluten, specifically the alcohol-soluble part, gliadin. Ingestion of food stuff containing gluten such as wheat, rye and barley, trigger signs of enteropathy, malabsorption and indigestion.

Celiac disease runs in families and therefore should be suspected in relatives of patients known to have this condition. The concordance for this condition is about 30 percent in first-degree relatives and 75 percent in monozygotic twins. Celiac disease has a slightly higher incidence in females. Like Crohn's disease and ulcerative colitis, it has a bimodal age distribution. The first is in infancy at 8 to 12 months and the second at 20 to 40 years.

Celiac disease is debilitating but rarely fatal, unless patients develop a malignancy. It is considered as a premalignant condition for the development of lymphoma or gastrointestinal carcinoma, which usually have poor prognosis.

Box 20.4: Celiac disease

Key features helpful in diagnosis

- Patients suffer from intolerance to the alcohol-soluble part of gluten, gliadin.
- There is strong association between celiac disease and HLA haplotypes DQ2 and DQ8.
- The gastrointestinal symptoms in celiac may lead to impaired digestion, malabsorption and cause weight loss and multiple nutritional deficiencies.
- Oral ulcers similar to aphthous ulceration may be the presenting symptom.
- The risk of adenocarcinoma of the oropharynx and esophagus is increased in celiac patients.

Etiology

The etiology of this gluten intolerance is not fully understood but it is believed that genetic factors play a role in an interaction between immunological responses to an environmental factor (gliadin). A strong association has been found between celiac disease and two human leukocyte antigens (HLA) haplotypes; DQ2 and DQ8.

In patients with celiac disease, ingesting glaidin triggers an immunologically mediated inflammatory response which causes damage to the intestinal lining. The immunological process is driven by the conversion of the glutamine in gliadin to a negatively charged protein which induces interleukin 15 in enteric epithelial cells. The production of the latter stimulates proliferation of natural killer cells and intraepithelial lymphocytes. Large numbers of CD8+ T lymphocytes are present in the intestinal epithelium suggesting that cell-mediated immune responses are also important in driving the inflammatory process in the pathogenesis of this disease.

Clinical Features

The disease affects multiple body organs and can be debilitating. The clinical signs and symptoms are generally as a consequence of the indigestion and malabsorption due to the damage of the intestinal mucosa. In some cases, the symptoms are very mild or even absent (silent celiac disease). This leads some experts to believe that celiac disease is underdiagnosed in the general population.

The most common gastrointestinal symptom is diarrhea. The stool is characteristically oily with a foul smell. Intestinal bacteria will grow on undigested food material causing excessive gases and abdominal bloating. Nutritional deficiency causes weakness and fatigue and may cause delayed development and failure to thrive in children.

Skin manifestation of celiac disease is called dermatitis herpetiformis and presents as itchy stinging small papules on the skin of the elbows, knees, sacral, buttocks, scalp, neck, and shoulder areas. The distribution of the papules is usually symmetrical.

The impaired digestion and absorption may cause weight loss and deficiency in several nutrients such as iron, folate, B_{12}, vitamin D and magnesium. Patients may have a bleeding tendency caused by prothrombin deficiency due to impaired absorption of the fat-soluble vitamin K. Hypocalcemia may cause muscle weakness and paresthesia.

Oral Manifestations

Oral ulceration similar to aphthous stomatitis is seen in celiac patients (**Fig. 20.7**). Some experts include a celiac screen as part of the routine investigation of recurrent oral ulcers, in an attempt to capture the 'silent' form of the disease. There is no strong clinical evidence to justify this practice at present.

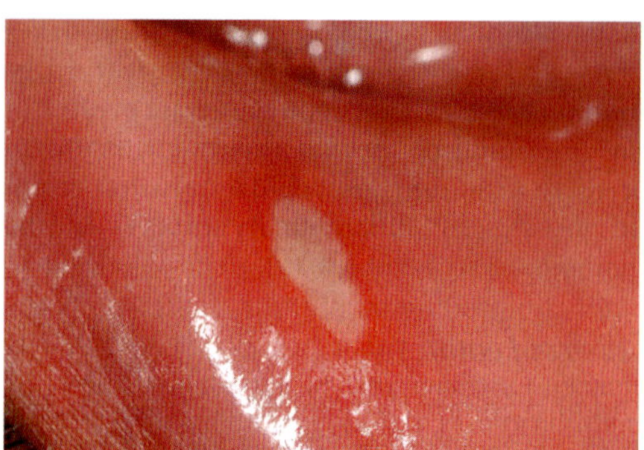

Fig. 20.7: Celiac disease. Oral ulcers similar to recurrent aphthous stomatitis may be the presenting feature in celiac disease

Other oral signs and symptoms of celiac disease are generally a reflection of the malabsorption and nutritional deficiency. These include glossitis, depapillation and fissuring of the tongue. Patients are at risk of oral candidiasis and may show intraoral signs similar to dermatitis herpetiformis.

It is of importance to note that the risk for malignancy of the head and neck is increased in patients with celiac disease namely, adenocarcinoma of the oropharynx and esophagus. Therefore, clinical monitoring is paramount.

Histopathological Features

The effects of the disease are seen more prominently in the jejunum rather than in the ileum. The villi are flattened and sometimes completely absent. The crypts become elongated which helps in maintaining the overall thickness of the disease mucosa as normal, despite the atrophic villi. Celiac primarily involves the mucosa, usually sparing the submucosa, muscularis, and serosa. Oral ulcers in patients with celiac disease show the same features of aphthous ulcers due to any other reason.

Treatment

Barium studies and endoscopy are helpful in diagnosing celiac disease. The most common test used for confirmation of the diagnosis is immunoglobulin A (IgA) antibodies to smooth muscle endomysium and tissue transglutaminase. The titer correlates with the degree of intestinal damage and therefore may be helpful in instigating treatment and evaluating compliance. IgA antiendomysial antibody often becomes undetectable in the serum after 6 to 12 months of gluten withdrawal. Constant serum antibodies for 12 months usually indicate poor compliance with a gliadin-free diet.

The primary treatment of celiac disease is dietary restriction. Elimination of gluten from the diet is essential, albeit difficult to achieve and maintain. For those, who do not respond to gluten-free diet, corticosteroids might be helpful. 5 to 10 percent of patients are refractory to treatment. Poor response to gluten-free diet and corticosteroids indicate poor prognosis of the condition. Patients with celiac disease are at increased risk for complications and malignancy development and should be monitored regularly.

GRANULOMATOUS DISEASES

Tuberculosis

Tuberculosis (TB) is an infectious and potentially fatal disease. TB is the leading infectious fatal disease worldwide responsible for 6 percent of deaths globally. In 1882, Robert Koch discovered the principal causative agent of TB, *Mycobacterium tuberculosis* which is a member of the group *Mycobacterium tuberculosis* complex. This group also include *M. bovis* and *M. africanum*.

Improved knowledge and the introduction of streptomycin in the 1940s, lead to a reduction in the transmission rates and an improvement in the survival rate of patients. However, the emergence of drug-resistant strains of *M. tuberculosis* has increased the risk of mortality in this disease. Furthermore, there was resurgence in the infection rate of TB during the mid 1980's due to the spread of HIV infection and the emergence of acquired immune deficiency syndrome (AIDS). HIV positive patients are at a high risk of acquiring TB due to their compromised immunity. There is also a risk of reactivation of TB in a subgroup of HIV patients, who start antiretroviral therapy, as a manifestation of immune reconstitution inflammatory syndrome (IRIS).

The World Health Organisation (WHO) estimates that 30 percent of the world population are infected by TB. India has the largest worldwide patient load. The WHO is leading a worldwide campaign to slow the spread of the disease and eventually eradicate it. However, TB remains a challenge and continues to be widespread and endemic to many parts of the world. Each person with active TB transmits the causative bacilli *M. tuberculosis* to 10 to 15 people on average every year (WHO report 2010). Contaminated airborne droplets can linger in the atmosphere, spreading the disease hours after release. The transmission rate increases in heavily populated and deprived communities. Vulnerable and immunocompromised patients catch the disease readily from sharing the same space with active TB patients via inhaling infective droplets.

Inhaled bacilli can either be overcome by the immune system, or they populate the terminal airspace of the lungs and grow in the intracellular environment. The infection has potentially one of three outcomes:

1. May be eradicated by the immune system,
2. Cause primary TB,
3. Remain dormant and asymptomatic (latent infection).

Patients, who have acquired the bacteria (primary TB or latent infection) are at risk of reactivation of the disease at a later stage.

The Mantoux tuberculin intradermal skin test has replaced the heaf test as the standard method for determining *M. tuberculosis* infection. Other diagnostic aids include the acid-fast stain for the bacilli, which is a reliable and relatively easy test, and polymerase chain reaction for M. tuberculosis. The Bacillus Calmette-Guérin (BCG) vaccine is used world-wide for the prevention of TB. It is prepared in the lab from attenuated (weakened) live bovine tuberculosis. The effectiveness of the vaccine is variable and at best offers 80 percent protection from TB infection for 15 years. The BCG vaccine has been employed since 1984 without serious side effects. It requires single intradermal inoculation and can also be given orally. At present, the WHO recommends that BCG is given to all children born in TB endemic countries.

Box 20.5: Tuberculosis

Key features helpful in diagnosis

- Tuberculosis is the leading infectious fatal disease in the world.
- The infectious agent in TB is *Mycobacterium tuberculosis* complex, the most prevalent of which is *M. tuberculosis*.
- The transmission is via airborne droplets contaminated with *M. tuberculosis*.
- The dental setting poses an environment conducive for transmission by aerosols.
- Caseating granuloma is the whole mark of TB.
- Tuberculosis can manifest in the head and neck as a persistent lump, an enlarged lymph node or an ulcer.

Etiology

M. tuberculosis is the principal causative bacteria for TB. It is a weak gram-positive rod-shaped bacterium that has no flagellum or capsule, does not form spores nor produces toxins. Exposure to *M. tuberculosis* causes infections in high risk patients such as heavy smokers and immunocompromised or malnourished patients.

M. tuberculosis reaches the lung via contaminated droplets. The bacilli are intracellular pathogens that primarily infect the pulmonary system. If not immediately eliminated by the immune system, they grow into localized lesions called tubercles. Cellular immunity comes into play 4 to 6 week postinfection which leads to the elimination of most of the bacilli and ending the primary infection, commonly without any clinical symptoms. In such patients, residual calcified lung lesions may be evident on subsequent radiographs.

Bacilli that are not destroyed by the immune system eventually become established in the lungs causing TB infection. The infection may remain dormant in the lung macrophages inside the tubercles. At this time, the host's immune system is activated against the bacteria. However, this host defense mechanism is also the cause of tissue damage in TB through granuloma formation and necrosis. TB-associated granulomas are a consequence of CD4-mediated delayed-type hypersensitivity reaction within parenchymal tissues.

Clinical Features

Pulmonary TB is the most common type presenting in 85 percent of TB patients, typically with chest pain, fever, hemoptysis, anorexia and fatigue. Untreated infection progresses to tuberculous pneumonia in the lower and middle lobes of the lung. Patients have a productive cough with purulent exudates which contain large numbers of acid-fast bacilli. Extrapulmonary disease is seen in lymph nodes, meninges, skin and the GI tract. Meningitis TB causes fever, seizures, persistent headache and muscle weakness. Tuberculous pericarditis is found in approximately 1 percent of autopsied TB cases. The infection causes thickening of the pericardium and eventual heart failure. Skeletal TB usually involves the spine causing back pain and lower limbs paralysis. Tuberculosis arthritis can affect any joint but most commonly found in the hips and knees.

Genitourinary TB may manifest as a scrotal mass in men and mimic pelvis inflammation in women. It may lead to sterility. Gastrointestinal TB can cause persistent ulcers in any part of the digestive tract from the mouth to the anus. These are symptomatic and may lead to pain, diarrhea and malabsorption. Gastrointestinal TB can cause a mass to form in the intestine which is frequently mistaken for cancer. TB may affect the lymph node especially the neck, causing TB lymphadenitis. Advanced cases may suppurate and form a draining sinus. If the bacilli are directly inoculated into skin, it causes an ulcer or wart-like lesion which is contagious and spreadable to the lymph nodes.

Miliary TB (disseminated TB) is a complication of about 2 percent of all TB cases. It occurs when the bacteria enters the blood stream and disseminate to infect any number of organs including bone marrow, lungs, liver and spleen. Miliary TB is always fatal in the absence of prompt treatment.

Oral Manifestations

Orofacial TB is often a secondary disease, disseminated from the lungs. It manifests as ulcers, lymph node enlargement, salivary gland or bone involvement. Tuberculous ulcers are usually deep punched out ulcers with marked periulcer swelling and erythema (**Fig. 20.8**).

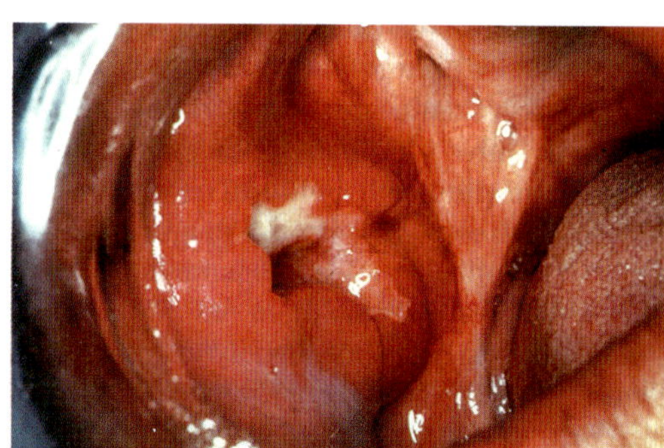

Fig. 20.8: Oral tuberculosis. A deep punched out ulcer on the buccal mucosa

Although any site of the oral mucosa can be affected, in most patients tongue and gingival lesions are common. TB should be on the differential diagnosis list of any persistent ulcer and enlarged lymph node, especially in high-risk groups such as immunocompromised patients. TB in the head and neck area may prove difficult to diagnose.

Lupus vulgaris has frequently been reported as the most common type of cutaneous TB. It is caused by lymphatic and blood transmission of tuberculous foci to the skin. About 90 percent of lupus vulgaris cases affect the head and neck region, mostly around the nose, eyelids, lips and ears. Cartilage (nose or ear) affected by TB lesions will be completely destroyed. Lesions are usually painful, solitary, well demarcated red papules that progress to form chronic atrophic plaque. Reappearance of nodules within atrophic lesions is characteristic. The associated mucosa such as oral, nasal and conjunctival may also be affected but the underlying bone is usually spared.

Histopathological Features

The characteristic histological lesion of TB is known as a tubercle and it occurs as a result of cell mediated hypersensitivity. The area of infection shows a well-circumscribed collection of epithelioid macrophages with multinucleate giant cells (Langhans giant cells) and peripheral part of the lesion contains lymphocytes. Central caseous necrosis is present in most granulomas (**Fig. 20.9**). Demonstration of *M. tuberculosis* within the lesion using Ziel-Neelsen acid fast technique is helpful for diagnosis. However, failure to demonstrate organisms does not rule out the diagnosis. PCR is the more reliable method to identify organisms.

Treatment

Treatment of TB aims to shorten the clinical course of the disease and prevent complications. Successful treatment prevents latency and reduces the risk of transmission.

The standard regime for treating TB is a combination of antimycobacterial drugs for 6 months. For drug resistant TB, it may be necessary to continue the therapy for upto 24 months.

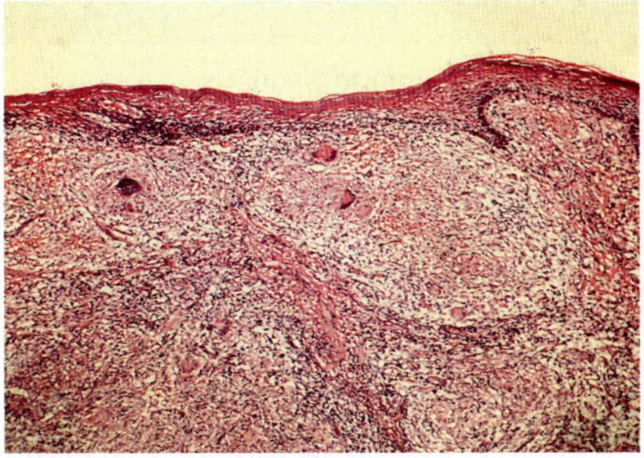

Fig. 20.9: Oral tuberculosis. Multiple granulomas containing epithelioid macrophages, Langhans type giant cells with early caseous necrosis

If hospitalized, patients with TB should be placed in appropriate isolation and their sputum tested weekly for *M. tuberculosis* until it becomes negative. There is a particular high-risk for transmission of TB in dental surgeries because of the presence of aerosols during dental treatment. High standards of infection control measures are paramount such as high speed aspirators, wearing surgical masks and visors.

Sarcoidosis

Sarcoidosis is a multisystem granulomatous disease. It mainly affects the lungs and lymph nodes but may involve any organ. Sarcoidosis usually progresses slowly and the symptoms may be very subtle. The resolution of the condition is usually spontaneous and may take a few months to a few years but relapse is common. Sarcoidosis is incapacitating in about 10 percent of patients. Mortality is mostly due to respiratory failure and associated heart failure. Sarcoidosis is seen more commonly in the African race compared with caucasians. The incidence is twice as high in males compared with females.

Box 20.6: Sarcoidosis

Key features helpful in diagnosis

- Sarcoidosis is a multisystem granulomatous disease.
- The pathogenesis of sarcoidosis is triggered by an interaction of environmental and genetic factors, and driven by immune dysregulation.
- Oral sarcoidosis presents as multiple asymptomatic submucosal indurated nodules or ill-defined radiolucency in the alveolar bone.
- The salivary glands are involved in up to 30 percent of sarcoid patients.

Etiology

Sarcoidosis is of unknown etiology. Studies using twins have shown that genetic factors increase the susceptibility to this disease. However, it is believed that the trigger for sarcoidosis is an interaction between a yet unidentified environmental factor and genetic determinants. It is widely accepted that the immunological process in sarcoidosis is not an autoimmune process but rather driven by alteration or dysregulation of the immune system. There is an increase in macrophages and CD4 helper T-cell activation but paradoxically the immune response to antigens is reduced. It is believed that the regulatory T-lymphocytes in the sarcoid granulomas suppress IL-2 secretion, which prevents antigen-specific memory responses and causes anergy (reduction or lack of an immune response to a specific antigen). This reduction in the immune response has been implicated as a risk factor for increased rate of infections and cancer in sarcoidosis patients.

Clinical Features

Sarcoidosis is a multisystem disease that may present clinically with nonspecific symptoms such as fever, loss of appetite, tiredness and cough. Other specific symptoms depend on the organ involved and the severity of the disease. Many of the signs and symptoms are attributed to the effect of the granulomas on the surrounding tissues. The most common system-specific symptoms are respiratory related and include cough, dyspnea and chest pain. A characteristic skin manifestation of sarcoidosis is lupus pernio which are chronic, indurated papules or plaques usually affecting the skin of the mid-face, especially the alar of the nose. Other cutaneous lesions include erythema nodosum and skin rash. Granulamatous uveitis and conjunctival lesions may lead to blindness. There is a significantly increased risk of hypothyroidism, hyperthyroidism and thyroid autoimmune disease in sarcoidosis, especially in women. Sarcoidosis has also been associated with increased level of vitamin D and celiac disease. Other vital organs such as the heart may be affected causing heart failure and death.

Oral Manifestations

The oral manifestations of sarcoidosis usually follow the systemic symptoms. They include multiple asymptomatic submucosal nodules in the palate, buccal and labial mucosa. On the gingivae and tongue, the disease manifests as indurated swellings. In the floor of the mouth the presentation resembles a ranula. Lesions of the jaws are seen as ill-defined radiolucencies in the alveolar bone.

Salivary glands may be involved leading to long-term swellings (**Fig. 20.10**). Studies have reported parotid gland swellings in 5 to 30 percent of sarcoid patients. The usual presentation is bilateral, painless swelling of the

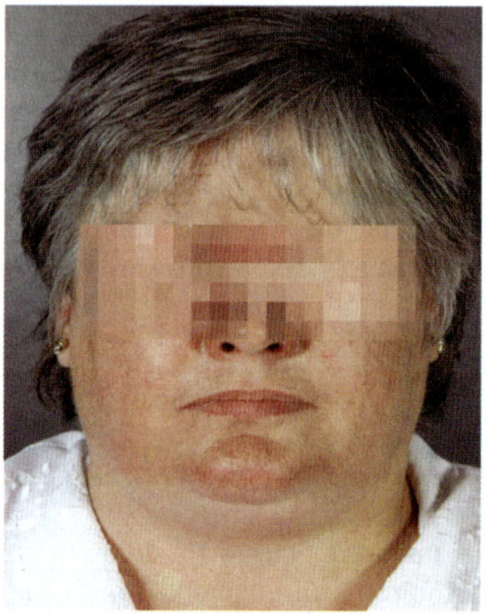

Fig. 20.10: Sarcoidosis. Bilateral parotid gland swelling

parotid gland with or without xerostomia. This may be the initial presentation of the disease. Sarcoidosis patients may develop Heerfordt syndrome (uveoparotid fever) which comprises of parotid gland swelling, xerostomia, uveitis, and facial nerve palsy.

Histopathological Features

Although investigations for this disease include serum calcium levels and a chest radiograph, definitive diagnosis requires a biopsy in the most cases. The main histopathological finding is the presence of noncaseating granulomas containing multinucleate giant cells and lymphocytes (**Fig. 20.11**). Calcified bodies are present in some cases. Rarely, cases with a few foci of caseation may mimic the appearances of tuberculosis.

Treatment

Usually symptomatic treatment in the form of anti-inflammatory drugs will suffice. However, in some cases disease-specific treatment may be necessary as in chronic pulmonary disease. Steroids are used as long-term therapy. Recently, steroid-sparing immune modulators such as methotrexate, azathioprine and choloroquine are being used more frequently.

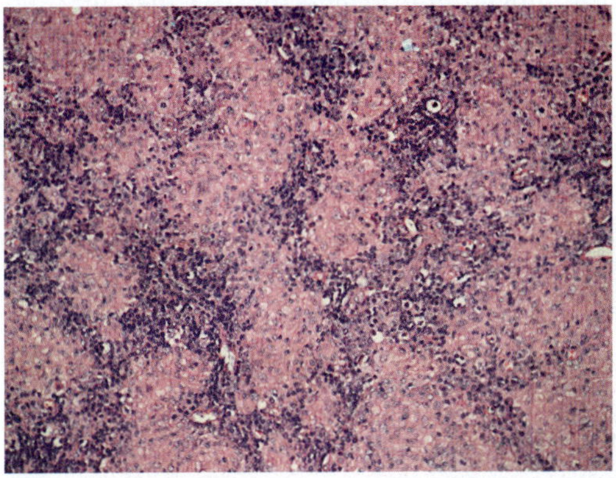

Fig. 20.11: Sarcoidosis. Noncaseating granulomas containing numerous epithelioid macrophages and lymphocytes

Lung transplantation is the only option to improve long-term survival in cases of reduced vital lung capacity due to advanced pulmonary sarcoidosis and lung fibrosis.

Wegener's Granulomatosis

Wegener's granulomatosis (WG) is a rare necrotizing vasculitis with distinct clinical and histopathological features affecting the small-to-medium sized vessels and associated with necrotizing granulomas. It is one of the antineutrophil cytoplasmic antibody (ANCA)-associated vasculitides. In 1936 Wegener reported three patients with distinct clinical and histopathologic findings showing systemic symptoms, joint symptoms, proptosis, upper respiratory tract inflammation leading to saddle nose deformity and glomerulonephritis. The definitive description of WG however was established by Goodman and Churg in 1954 as a condition with a triad of features including systemic necrotizing angiitis (inflammation of lymph and blood vessels), necrotizing granulomatous inflammation of the respiratory tract, and necrotizing glomerulonephritis.

WG has a wide spectrum of clinical presentation. It is considered as a 'limited' disease when the clinical findings are restricted to the upper and lower respiratory tracts. This type of disease is not generally considered life threatening. If there are additional significant multisystem manifestations the condition is classified as severe WG. Limited WG may later progress to the severe form.

WG is rarely seen in children and usually presents at the age of 35 to 55 years. About 90 percent of WG patients are of northern Europeans descent. It affects males and females equally although women are more likely to have limited disease.

Untreated WG has a very high mortality rate of more than 90 percent within two years. The most common causes of death include pulmonary and renal failure, malignancy, severe infections and cardiovascular disease. Early diagnosis of this disease may prevent irreversible kidney damage and improve morbidity and mortality rates.

Box 20.7: Wegener's granulomatosis

Key features helpful in diagnosis

- Wegener's granulomatosis is a rare necrotizing granulomatous disease affecting the small-to-medium vessels.
- The characteristic granulomas are formed as a result of a cellular immunity reaction to an environmental trigger such as respiratory tract infection or allergies.
- Strawberry gingival hyperplasia is a classic presentation of WG in the mouth and is pathognomonic of WG.
- Specific histological features and the presence of ANCA are diagnostic for WG.

Etiology

The etiology of WG is largely unknown. The pathogenesis is not fully understood but is thought to be driven by a complex interaction of the immune system with an environmental trigger, in the presence of a genetic predisposition. Both cellular and humoral immunity are thought to be implicated. The current theory is that an environmental factor such as respiratory tract infection or allergies triggers a cellular immunity reaction, which leads to the formation of the characteristic granulomas. It is accepted that the humoral autoimmunity plays a role in the pathogenesis of this condition. This is supported by the presence of ANCA in most patients with WG.

Clinical Features

Wegener's granulomatosis has a spectrum of nonspecific symptoms including fever, night sweats, lethargy, arthralgia and loss of appetite. Ocular involvement is very common, including conjunctivitis, scleritis, uveitis, optic nerve vasculitis, proptosis and nasolacrimal duct occlusion. Chronic sinusitis is the most common presenting symptom of WG. Patients also suffer from epistaxis and rhinitis. The shape of the nose becomes deformed due to collapse of nasal support. Serous otitis media may cause hearing loss in some patients. Pulmonary symptoms include cough, hemoptysis, dyspnea, stridor and wheezing.

Less than 20 percent of patients have renal disease when they first present with WG, usually manifesting as glomerulonephritis with haematuria. The skin is involved in about half of WG patients due to vasculitis manifesting as purpura and skin ulcers. The vasculitis may also affect the nervous system leading to focal motor and sensory complaints or cranial nerve abnormalities. Other organ specific manifestations include pericarditis and splanchnic vasculitis.

Oral Manifestations

The classic presentation of WG in the mouth is granular enlargement and erythema of the gingivae, termed as 'strawberry gingival hyperplasia' or "strawberry gingivitis" (**Figs 20.12A and B**). This is pathognomonic of WG. It starts on the interdental papillae as red/purple friable papules and then spreads to other sites. The lingual and palatal mucosa may become involved eventually (**Figs 20.12A and B**). It commonly causes bone resorption and tooth loss. Painful or painless ulcers may affect the buccal mucosa and/or palate.

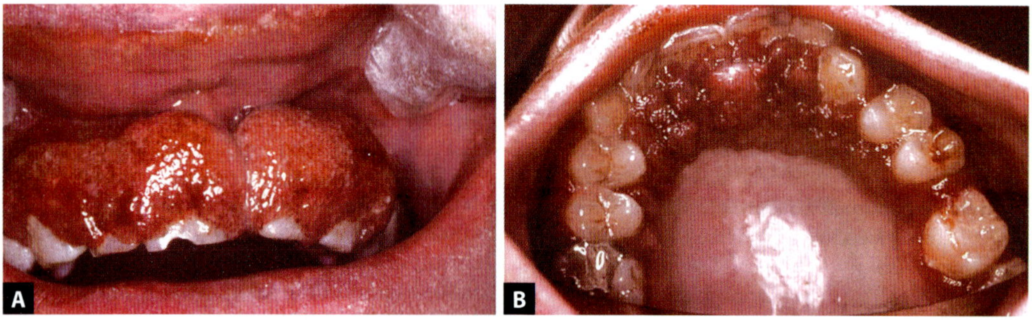

Figs 20.12A and B: (A) Wegener's granulomatosis. Strawberry gingival hyperplasia; (B) Granular hyperplasia with erythema of the palate

Recognizing the oral lesions of WG may initiate running the appropriate tests and lead to an early diagnosis and management, therefore improving prognosis and preventing further damage. Clinicians use the oral and skin manifestations as a measure of disease activity as their severity correlates with the progression of systemic disease.

Histopathological Features

The histological features of a gingival biopsy are not pathognomonic. However, there is granulomatous inflammation without discrete granuloma formation. Eosinophils, neutrophils, lymphocytes and occasional giant cells are present in the background. Vasculitis cannot be properly demonstrated in oral biopsies. Pseudoepitheliomatous hyperplasia and micro-abscess formation is evident in most cases. The presence of relevant histological features in a biopsy and positive ANCA results are diagnostic for this condition.

Treatment

The introduction of a combination of corticosteroids and cyclophosphamides as treatment for WG in the 1970's improved the survival rate dramatically. Complete remission is achieved in approximately 75 percent of the patients although more than a third experience at least one relapse. To maintain remission, azathioprine has been shown to be safer than, and as effective as cyclophosphamide. Methotrexate has been shown to have a similar efficacy to azathioprine in maintaining remission and stabilizing WG.

Surgical intervention is not a primary treatment but may be necessary to repair the damage caused by the severe inflammatory process causing tissue necrosis and fibrosis in the nose, trachea, and bronchi, or to open up the obstructed nasolacrimal ducts.

HEMATOLOGICAL CONDITIONS

Amyloidosis

Amyloidosis is a fatal disease caused by deposition of extracellular and/or intracellular insoluble amyloid interfering with normal function of the affected tissue. The terms "primary" and 'secondary' amyloidosis are no longer used. Based on a chemical classification, amyloidosis is classified into subtypes, referred to with a combination of letters. The first is capital letter A (for amyloid) followed by an abbreviation for the fibril protein. For example, AL is amyloidosis with the fibril protein being immunoglobulin light chain or light chain fragment which includes most cases that used to be referred to as primary amyloidosis or myeloma-associated amyloidosis. When the deposited protein fibrils consist of the transport protein transthyretin (TTR), amyloidosis is referred to as ATTR. Most of the latter used to be termed as familial amyloid polyneuropathy (FAP).

Up to 20 percent of patients with multiple myeloma have been reported to have amyloidosis. Therefore, myeloma should be investigated in patients with amyloidosis.

Box 20.8: Amyloidosis

Key features helpful in diagnosis

- Amyloidosis is a serious condition caused by deposition of extracellular and/or intracellular insoluble amyloid in body tissues.
- Nephritic syndrome is the most common clinical presentation of amyloidosis.
- The characteristic oral feature of amyloidosis is macroglossia.
- Myocardial insufficiency is the most common cause of death in amyloidosis patients.

Etiology

Twenty-three different fibril proteins have been described and implemented in amyloidosis. These proteins either arise locally from proteins expressed by the cells, or deposited systemically after production at a local site causing systemic effect. The theories explaining the pathophysiology of amyloidogenesis include nonphysiologic or defective physiologic proteolysis, mutations involving changes in thermodynamic or kinetic properties, and pathways that are not yet fully understood.

Clinical Features

Many body organs may be affected by amyloidosis including skin, joints, heart, kidneys, liver, bowels and lungs. The symptoms are a result of abnormal functioning of the affected organ. The diagnosis of amyloidosis is often delayed as the presenting symptoms are usually vague and include fatigue, weight loss, shortness of breath, lack of appetite, numbness and enlarged tongue.

One of the most common organs affected by amyloidosis is the kidney, causing signs and symptoms of nephritic syndrome. Skin amyloidosis characteristically presents with waxy papules or plaque on the anogenital area, neck, behind the ear or on the eyelids (**Fig. 20.13**). Other skin manifestations include petechiae and ecchymoses on the eyelid. Purpuric lesions are found periorbitally and in skin folds such as axilla, neck and nasolabial folds. The nails become dystrophic and brittle.

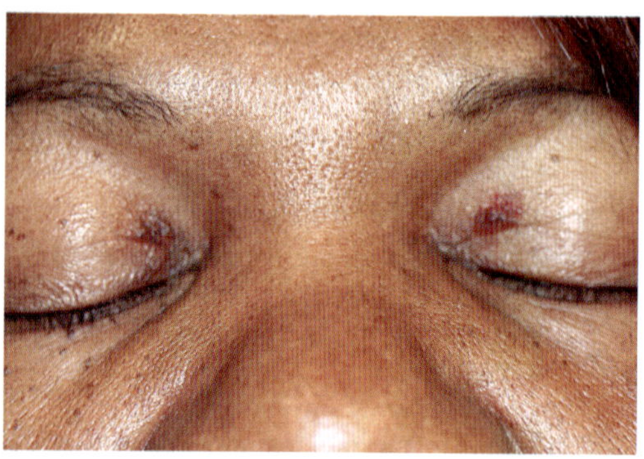

Fig. 20.13: Amyloidosis. Extraoral features of the disease

Oral Manifestations

The deposition of amyloid in the oral cavity often presents as localized, soft, elastic papules. The classical oral manifestation of amyloidosis is macroglossia, occurring in about 20 percent of patients. The enlarged tongue extrudes through the gaps between the teeth and present with lateral ridging due to teeth indentation (**Figs 20.14A and B**). The condition is often asymptomatic but patients may complain of large firm tongue that is less mobile. Dysgeusia and hyposalivation have also been reported. Amyloid deposition in the salivary glands may result in submandibular swelling. This coupled with enlargement of the tongue may lead to respiratory obstruction.

Histopathological Features

The capillaries in the subcutaneous fat are often involved in patients with amyloidosis. Therefore, immunostaining and amino acid sequence analysis of subcutaneous fat biopsy may be sufficient and avert the need for a biopsy of the organ. For example, when cardiac amyloidosis is suspected, a specific diagnosis is often made by taking a subcutaneous fat aspiration instead of endomyocardial biopsy, thereby avoiding an invasive procedure.

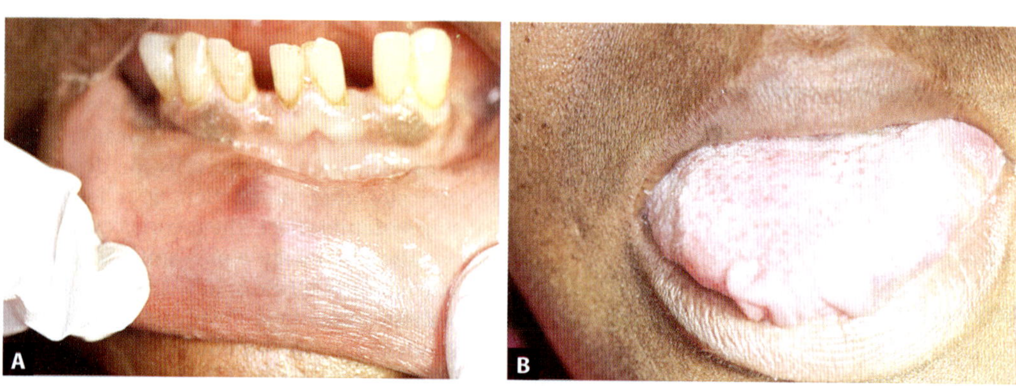

Figs 20.14A and B: Amyloidosis. Deposits of amyloid in the lip and tongue

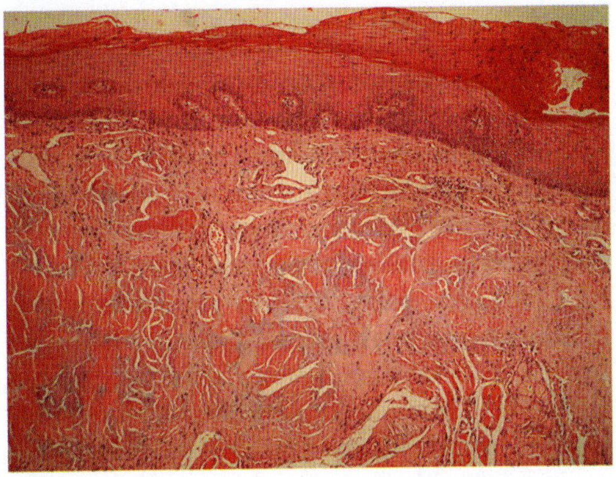

Fig. 20.15: Amyloidosis. Characteristic amorphous fissured appearance of amyloid replacing muscles

In some cases, the subcutaneous fat aspiration biopsy does not provide enough information and an organ biopsy is necessary to confirm the diagnosis. The microscopical appearance of amyloidosis is distinctive on electron microscopy and characterized by the ability to bind to Congo red and Thioflavine T. Immunostaining of the biopsy specimen is necessary to identify the type of deposited protein, which determines the most effective clinical management.

Microscopic features of a tongue biopsy include the classical amorphous fissured appearance of amyloid replacing muscles (**Fig. 20.15**). The overlying epithelium may become atrophic with advancement of the disease and loss of vascularity. When the salivary glands are affected, deposition of amyloid is seen in both periductal and periacinar areas leading to acinar atrophy. Polarized light microscopy shows apple green birefringence in tissue stained with congo red.

Treatment

The treatment depends on the type of protein being deposited and its effect on body organs and function. At present, there is no known cure for amyloidosis. The current treatment is symptomatic and aims to limit further production of the protein.

Although amyloid is a protein, dietary protein intake has no link to amyloidosis. However, diet restriction is necessary in some instances to control symptoms. For example, if the heart or kidneys are affected, a low-salt diet is advised in order to limit fluid retention.

Peripheral stem cell transplantation and chemotherapy is the basis of the treatment for the most common forms of amyloidosis. Aggressive treatment may be necessary to slow the disease progression and improve the patient's quality of life.

ENDOCRINE ABNORMALITIES

Addison's Disease

Addison's disease is now considered an autoimmune disease. The destruction of the cortex of the adrenal glands is due to autoimmunity or rarely an infection (TB) and results in insufficient production of steroid hormones (glucocorticoids and often mineralocorticoids).

Addison's disease is most commonly diagnosed in patients aged 30 to 50 years and is a life-long condition that can be treated by replacement therapy.

Addison's disease should not be confused with the acute form of adrenaline insufficiency termed adrenal crisis. The latter occurs in patients with a history of prolonged steroid use. It is precipitated by physiological stress such as severe trauma or surgical intervention. Adrenal crisis is recognized as one of the medical emergencies that might occur in the dental environment. Therefore, dental surgeons are expected to have full and upto date knowledge of its physiology and management.

Etiology

Addison's disease is due to a damaged adrenal gland and reduced steroid hormones. The destruction of the gland is caused by autoantibodies and cytotoxic T lymphocyte and precipitated by infection, trauma or neoplasia. Due to the negative feedback loop, the reduction in the adrenaline output will stimulate the hypothalamus and anterior pituitary gland to produce adrenocorticotropic hormone (ACTH) and melanocyte-stimulating hormone (MSH). The latter causes the classic hyperpigmentation seen in Addisonian patients.

Clinical Features

Signs and symptoms occur once the destruction of the adrenal cortex is more than 90 percent. The deficiency of adrenaline, the stress 'flight or fight' hormone causes a range of clinical symptoms including light-headedness and dizziness when standing for a long time, anxiety, fatigue, weight loss, gastrointestinal symptoms, headache and sweating. Mood and personality changes including irritability and depression are common. There is hyperpigmentation of the skin which makes patients look tanned.

Oral Manifestations

Hyperpigmentation of the mucous membrane is pathognomonic of Addison's, appearing in upto 95 percent of patients. Pigments are seen on the skin in the perioral area and intraorally affecting buccal mucosa, gingiva and palate. The oral soft tissue appears dry and there is reduced salivary flow in these patients due to dehydration.

Treatment

The treatment is mainly is by replacement therapy to reduce morbidity and to prevent mortality. Prednisolone or hydrocortisone sodium succinate is used as replacement for glucocorticoid hormone replacement. Prednisolone is longer acting when compared with hydrocortisone with a biologic half-life of 18 to 36 hours. Hydrocortisone is also used for steroid replacement in acute adrenal crisis. Its biologic half-life is 8 to 12 hours.

Gigantism and Acromegaly

Gigantism and acromegaly are growth abnormalities due to excess production of insulin-like growth factor-I (IGF-I), causing robust growth of the musculoskeletal system and internal organs. Hypertrophy of the soft tissues makes the patients susceptible to potential fatal diseases like respiratory infections and heart failure. Patients also suffer from debilitating joint deformities and vision problems. The mortality rate is significantly higher in gigantism and acromegaly when compared with the general population. The most common causes of death in this group of patients are cardiovascular abnormalities and respiratory diseases. Normalization of IGF-I levels improves life expectancy.

Gigantism is a term used when the standing height of a person is more than 2 standard deviations above the mean for the person's sex, age, and physical development stage (Tanner stage). This rare condition occurs when there is excess secretion of the growth hormone (GH) while the epiphyseal growth plates are open during childhood.

Acromegaly is more common than gigantism and is a result of IGF-I hypersecretion after the epiphyseal plates are fused, usually in the third decade of life. It affects both sexes equally.

Etiology

The over production of IGF-I action is always due to GH-secreting pituitary adenoma or hyperplasia. The tumor is usually distinctly

Box 20.9: Gigantism and acromegaly

Key features helpful in diagnosis

- Excess production of insulin-like growth factor-I in childhood leads to gigantism, and in adulthood causes acromegaly.
- The mortality rate in gigantism, and acromegaly is significantly higher than in the general population.
- Patients affected by these conditions classically have coarse features and exaggerated growth.
- The most common causes of death in this group of patients are cardiovascular abnormalities and respiratory diseases.
- About 20% of patients with gigantism have McCune-Albright syndrome (pituitary hyperplasia or adenoma).
- Oral features in these conditions include macroglosia, macrognathia and macrodontia.

within the anterior lobe of the pituitary gland. However, in some cases the tumor spreads outside the sella and invades surrounding structures including the optic nerves and brain. Less commonly, gigantism and acromegaly are due to certain rare pancreatic islet-cell, and bronchial neoplasms.

Gigantism

The over-secretion of the IGF-I in children causes dramatic linear growth that is usually noticed and diagnosed promptly. Compared with acromegaly the changes are more in the musculoskeletal system rather than in the soft tissues. All growing tissues are affected but not necessarily symmetrically, causing disfigurement. There is exaggerated growth resulting in large and high stature. The rib cage becomes bigger and barrel shaped. There is macrocephaly with frontal bossing and coarse facial features. The skin thickens, hair darkens and the sebaceous and sweat glands become overactive causing hyperhidrosis and body odor. Joints become painful and deformed eventually leading to crippling degenerative arthritis. The soft tissues and internal organs are enlarged and may compress nerves causing neuropathy or loss of vision, particularly in the outer field. Vital internal organs are also affected such as the heart and the brain causing heart failure and severe debilitating headaches respectively.

Puberty is delayed and the menstrual cycle is irregular. The most common type of GH-secreting cells involved in this condition is mammo-somatotrophs. Therefore, hyperprolactinemia in gigantism is common. Other associated conditions include endocrinopathies such as hypogonadism and diabetes mellitus.

Approximately 20 percent of patients with gigantism have McCune-Albright Syndrome, which is pituitary hyperplasia or adenomas with the triad of early puberty, café-au-lait skin spots and fibrous dysplasia.

Acromegaly

Changes due to GH hypersecretion in adulthood are subtle and slow and may go on for some time before they are diagnosed. The presentation is usually that of coarse facial features and peripheral edema including bigger hands and feet. Patients notice that they need bigger hats, shoes and rings. Unlike gigantism, the general stature and linear height is not changed significantly. The skin and hair change to become more coarse and dark. Joint disease may become crippling if not treated.

Acromegaly is associated with irregular menstrual periods in women and erectile dysfunction in men. There is galactorrhea in women even if they are not breast feeding due to increase GH production or increase in prolactin production.

Enlargement of internal tissue and organs may cause impaired sensation and function such as neuropathy, heart failure and loss of vision. Acromegaly puts patients at higher risk of developing other systemic conditions such as diabetes mellitus and hypertension. Some experts believe that there is an increased risk of cancer, especially intestinal tumors in untreated acromegaly.

Oral Manifestations

Generally increased GH secretion causes all the oral-related structures to become larger than normal in gigantism and renews the growth of small bones in acromegaly. Oral features include macroglossia which causes the tongue to protrude out of the oral cavity or to be pressed against the teeth causing indentation on the lateral borders. The mandible increases in length and in thickness causing class III malocclusion and macrognathia. Intraoral and extraoral soft tissues of the head and neck are also affected. The lips appear thick and there is hypertrophy of the soft palate and epiglottis. The major salivary glands may be enlarged. The voice becomes deeper due to thickening of the vocal cords.

Radiographically, there are features of hypercementosis and a larger condyle. Characteristically there is cortical thickening of the skull bones including the mandible, enlargement of the frontal sinuses and enlargement and erosion of the sella turcica.

Treatment

The aim of the treatment is to stop, or dramatically reduce the overproduction of GH. This cannot be achieved easily and may necessitate a combination of surgery, radiation therapy and drug therapy.

At present, the first line treatment for acromegaly is removal or reduction of the tumor surgically. This has an immediate effect on reducing the level of the GH, often without causing deficiency of other pituitary hormones. A follow-up radiotherapy may be necessary for the treatment of large tumors.

Medical therapy has an important role in treating gigantism and acromegaly, if surgical intervention is not possible or has failed. Recently, long-acting somatostatin analogs and dopamine agonists have been developed. These have been shown to improve adherence and efficacy, as they are given once a month and they are well-tolerated. With the available treatment modalities at present, normalisation of GH levels can be achieved in more than 90 percent of patients, therefore, decreasing the mortality rate significantly.

HUMAN IMMUNODEFICIENCY VIRUS INFECTION

Human immunodeficiency virus (HIV) is a lentivirus (a member of the retrovirus family) that infects and compromises the immune system. If untreated, this infection progresses to cause the potentially fatal disease, acquired immunodeficiency syndrome (AIDS). The main causes of death in AIDS are opportunistic infections and malignancies.

HIV was first recognized in the early 1980's. Since then more than 26 million people have died as a result of AIDS. Most of these deaths are in developing countries. The availability of HIV treatment in the developed world meant that the death rate from the disease has reduced dramatically and the quality of life and life expectancy of HIV-positive patients increased significantly.

The main route of transmission of HIV is exchange of body fluids that contain the virus. Free viral particles and intracellular HIV are present in blood, saliva, semen and vaginal fluid, and breast milk. Horizontal transmission is mainly via sexual intercourse and contaminated needles. Vertical transmission occurs from mother to child at birth or during breastfeeding.

Etiology

HIV mainly infects helper T cells expressing CD4 (CD4+), macrophages, and dendritic cells.

The virus affects the CD4+ T cells by directly killing the cells or increasing the rate of apoptosis. CD8 cytotoxic lymphocytes recognize infected cells and attack them hence reducing the number of CD4+ cells even further. The cycle of infection and cell death continues and eventually leads to a critically low CD4+ T cells number and a breakdown in the cell-mediated immunity. This leads to a range of opportunistic infections. The significance of these opportunistic infections depends on their severity and the organ involved.

Box 20.10: Human immunodeficiency virus infection

Key features helpful in diagnosis and management

- HIV is mainly transmitted sexually and infects CD4+ cells, macrophages and dendritic cells eventually leading to a fatal immune deficient state.
- The oral manifestations in HIV positive patients can be the presenting clinical symptom and are used to evaluate the progression of the disease.
- HIV-related opportunistic infections that manifest in the head and neck area include: Candidiasis, oral hairy leukoplakia, HIV-related periodontal disease, Kaposi's sarcoma, Non-Hodgkin's lymphoma and HPV infection.
- The implementation of modern regimes of combination retroviral therapy has significantly improved mortality and morbidity rates in HIV positive patients.
- Severely immunocompromised patients who respond dramatically to antiretroviral therapy may exhibit immune reconstitution inflammatory syndrome.

Oral Manifestations

Oral manifestations (OM) of HIV can be the presenting symptom of HIV due to the accessibility of the oral cavity and the fact that the HIV-related oral lesions are recognized reasonably easy. The OM have been used to diagnose HIV infection and assess the disease progression and the need for treatment. The presence of OM is indicative of the immune-deficient state and is inversely related to the CD4+ cell count. Therefore, in patients who are already on treatment, the manifestation of opportunistic infections in the mouth indicates treatment failure.

Knowledge of the classification and the clinical presentation of the OM of HIV are imperative for good clinical management of HIV infection. In this chapter, we include the description of the group of the OM that are strongly associated with HIV infection according to the most widely used classification (EC Clearing House classification, 1993). This group of lesions include oral candidiasis, hairy leukoplakia (HL), specific forms of periodontal disease such as necrotizing ulcerative gingivitis and necrotising ulcerative periodontitis, Kaposi's sarcoma (KS) and non-Hodgkin's lymphoma (NHL). The strength of the association between these OM and HIV infections is variable. Oral candidiasis and periodontal disease are relatively common and are frequently seen in HIV-negative patients. However, HL and KS occur almost exclusively in immunocompromised patients and are indicative of HIV infection in the absence of other reasons for profound immunodeficiency such as severe combined immunodeficiency disease or organ transplant treatment.

In addition, human papilloma viral infection in relation to HIV infection is also included as it is ubiquitous and increasing in prevalence.

ORAL MANIFESTATIONS STRONGLY RELATED TO HIV

Candidiasis

Candidal infection is one of the most frequent opportunistic infections in HIV positive patients.

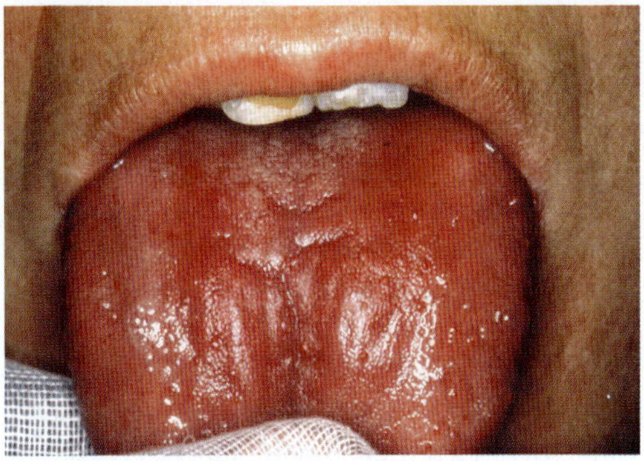

Fig. 20.16: Erythematous candidiasis of the tongue

However, it has been repeatedly reported in the literature, that the prevalence of oral candidiasis has decreased with the advent of antiretroviral therapy (ART).

Pseudomembranous Candidiasis (Thrush)

This is characterized by a creamy white soft layer that if scraped off, will reveal an oozing erythematous surface. It can be localized or florid, affecting more than one oral mucosal surface. Lesions may be transient/intermittent or long-standing. In immunocompromised patients, it can be recurrent or refractory to treatment.

Erythematous Candidiasis

This condition can be acute or chronic. It manifests as intermittent, or long-standing atrophic patches of the oral mucosa. The most common sites are the palate and the dorsum of the tongue. It may be asymptomatic or may cause mild to moderate burning pain. This lesion usually appears intermittently, but may be long-standing (**Fig. 20.16**).

Angular Cheilitis

This is a mixed *Candida* and *Staphylococcus aureus* infection of the lip commissures. It manifests as cracks or fissures at the corners of the mouth and can cause pain when opening the mouth.

Chronic Hyperplastic Candidiasis

A white adherent lesion. The most common site is the anterior region of the buccal mucosa. It is mostly long-standing and asymptomatic.

Oral Hairy Leukoplakia

Oral hairy Leukoplakia (OHL) is associated with the Epstein-Barr virus (EBV) and occurs mostly, but not exclusively in HIV positive patients. The incidence of OHL has been shown to decrease with ART. OHL has been suggested as an indicator for disease progression and therapy failure in HIV patients.

Of the oral manifestations that are strongly related to HIV, OHL is probably the one that is most under-reported. It can present a challenge to capture as it can be asymptomatic and the signs can be subtle and transient (see Chapter 12 for differential diagnosis).

OHL usually appears as a white adherent lesions on the lateral border of the tongue but may extend to the ventral and dorsal surfaces (**Fig. 20.17**). It usually exhibits vertical corrugations, which can range in size and in intensity. HL is mostly asymptomatic but may cause mild burning sensation. Histopathological features are characterized by the upper prickle cells of the epithelium showing enlarged cells with finely granular or glassy eosinophilic cytoplasm. There is a prominent perinuclear halo in those cells with clumped chromatin at the periphery. Superficial layers of the epithelium shows candidal hyphae. However, there is no immune reaction in the upper corium (**Fig. 20.18**). The diagnosis can be confirmed by demonstrating the presence of Epstein-Barr virus in the epithelium.

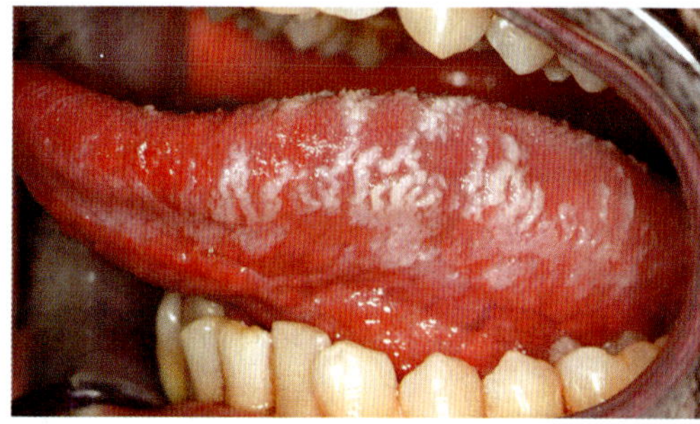

Fig. 20.17: Oral hairy leukoplakia. White lesion with vertical corrugations on the lateral border of the tongue in an HIV positive patient

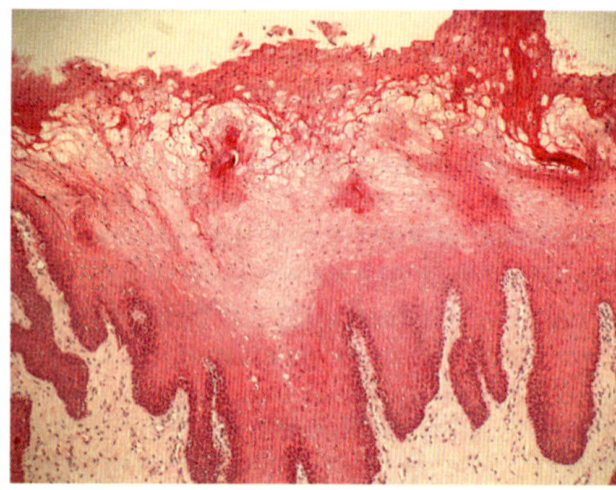

Fig. 20.18: Oral hairy leukoplakia. The upper prickle cells of the epithelium showing enlarged cells with finely granular or glassy eosinophilic cytoplasm

HIV-related Periodontal Disease

Necrotizing Ulcerative Gingivitis

Necrotizing ulcerative gingivitis (NUG) is characterized by ulceration and eventual destruction of one or more interdental papillae. In the acute stage the patient presents with moderate to severe pain, oral ulceration, gingival bleeding and characteristic fetid odor. The onset is usually sudden with rapid progression.

Necrotizing Ulcerative Periodontitis

This is a progression of NUG. It is characterized by irreversible soft tissue and alveolar bone loss. The teeth may become mobile. It is associated with moderate to severe pain in the acute stage. If this is untreated and in the presence of progressive HIV infection, it may cause severe bone destruction and develop into necrotizing stomatitis (**Fig. 20.19**).

Kaposi's Sarcoma

Kaposi's sarcoma (KS) is the most common neoplasm that occurs in patients with AIDS. Typically, the first lesions noticed are red, purplish, flat or macular lesions on the skin

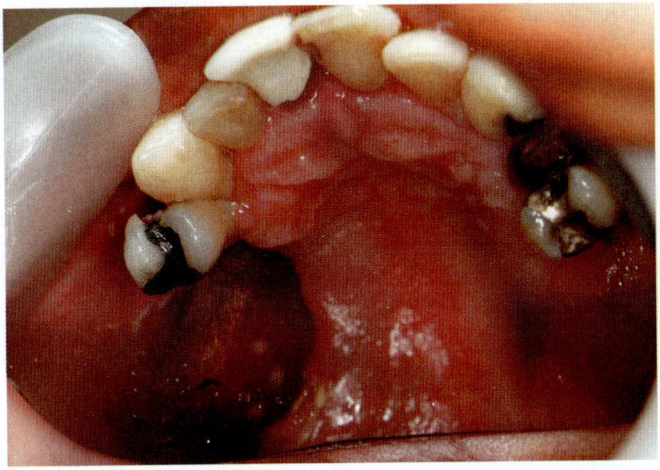

Fig. 20.19: Necrotizing ulcerative periodontitis progressing to necrotizing stomatitis and causing oro-antral fistula in an HIV-positive patient

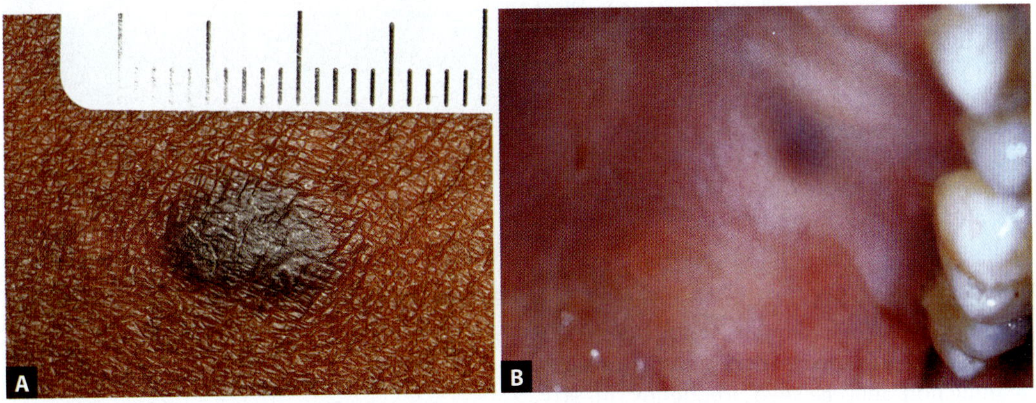

Figs 20.20A and B: Kaposi's sarcoma. Early cutaneous (A) and oral lesions (B) are flat macules

(**Figs 20.20A and B**) or intraorally (**Figs 20.20A and B**). If untreated, the lesions increase in number and size (**Figs 20.21A and B**). The most common sites in the oral cavity affected by KS are the palate and the gingivae. At the early stages, KS is asymptomatic but pain may be experienced with larger lesions, KS is believed to be caused by Kaposi's-sarcoma-associated herpes virus/human herpes virus 8 (KSHV/ HHV-8). It arises as a cancer of lymphatic endothelium and forms vascular channels, which are filled with blood, giving the tumor its characteristic bruise-like appearance. KS is an AIDS-defining malignancy and one of the oral manifestations that are strongly related to HIV infection. Recently, the incidence of KS, especially in the western world has decreased due to the instigation of ART. However, some patients experience emergence or relapse of KS after the initiation of anti-HIV treatment. (Please refer to Chapter 8 for histopathological features).

Non-Hodgkin's Lymphoma

The head and neck are the two most common sites for extranodal Non-Hodgkin's lymphoma (NHL). Waldeyer's ring and specifically, the

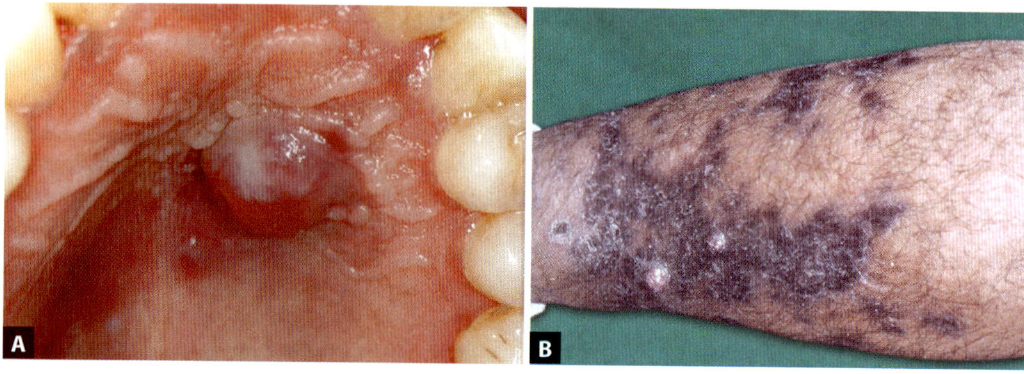

Figs 20.21A and B: Kaposi's sarcoma. Nodular palatal lesion and disseminated cutaneous lesions

tonsils are the most frequently involved areas. NHL manifests as a firm, elastic, reddish swelling with or without ulceration (**Fig. 20.22**). Like many other malignant tumors, NHL is usually asymptomatic at the early stage but pain may develop later in the disease. Patients usually present with signs and symptoms very similar to squamous cell carcinoma of the head and neck. It is therefore of particular importance that oral biopsy samples from patients at risk should specifically be submitted for evaluation by appropriate immunohistochemical and molecular biological investigations.

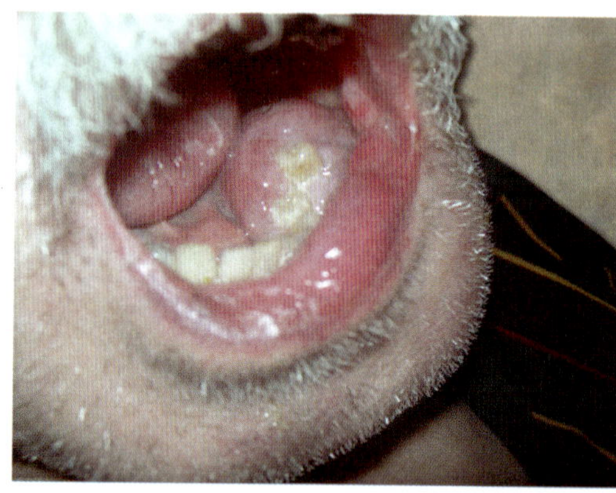

Fig. 20.22: Non-Hodgkin's lymphoma. Large gingival lesion with both intra- and extraoral swelling

Human Papillomavirus Infection

Human papillomavirus (HPV) is an opportunistic infection that is seen frequently in HIV infected individuals. It is the most common sexually transmitted virus and ubiquitous in the general population but the rate of infection is higher in HIV positive patients. Over eighty subtypes of HPV have been recognized, some of which have been identified as oncogenic. Recently, studies have shown a strong link between oral HPV infection and oropharyngeal cancer among subjects with, or without the established risk factors of tobacco and alcohol use.

The most common clinical manifestation of HPV infection is warts (condyloma, condylomata acuminata) affecting skin, genitals and oral mucosa (**Figs 20.23A and B**). Ninety percent of oral warts are caused by HPV types 6 and 11. Histopathological features of these warts are very similar to squamous cell papilloma (Please refer to Chapter 8).

Although HIV seems to promote HPV infection, treating HIV infection does not seem to have a significant effect on HPV infections, precancer and cancer, even after immune restoration. In fact, there is evidence that HPV infection may persist or occur well after the initiation of ART. In contrast to other oral manifestations of HIV, several publications have reported an increased prevalence of oral warts in patients on ART. Furthermore, oral warts in this group of patients appear to be proliferative and refractory to treatment.

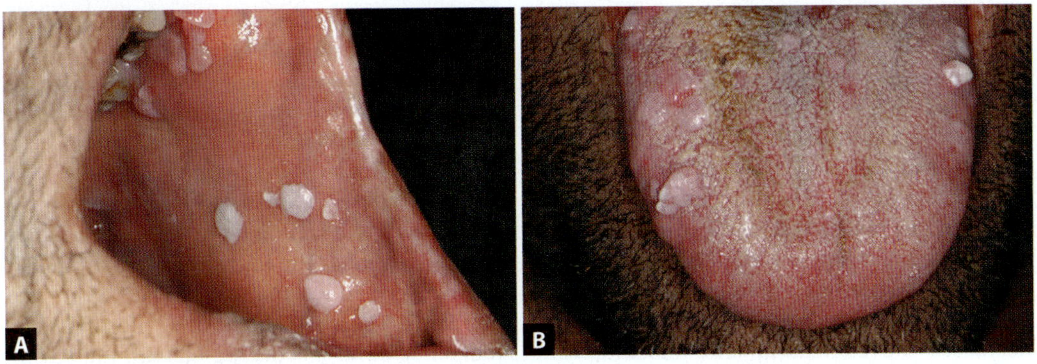

Figs 20.23A and B: Intraoral human papilloma virus infection. Multiple warty lesions on buccal and lingual mucosae in HIV-positive patients

Treatment of HIV

Currently, there is no cure for HIV infection. The available treatment aims at reducing the viral load and improving the immune system. Successful therapy slows the disease progression and reduces mortality and morbidity.

The first ART, zidovudine was developed in the 1990's and represented as a significant breakthrough in AIDS therapy that changed the natural history of the disease. Since then several classes of drugs have been developed.

- Nucleoside reverse transcriptase inhibitors
- Non-nucleoside reverse transcriptase inhibitors
- Protease inhibitors
- Integrase inhibitors
- Fusion inhibitors
- Chemokine receptor antagonists.

Each class of drug targets a different stage of the viral life cycle increasing the efficacy of the treatment and reducing the likelihood of developing resistance. The recommended therapy in the developed world is a combination of the above drugs. This regime is potent and has many side effects. Patients, who are severely immunocompromised and are put on an effective ART may show signs of exuberant reaction associated with the recovery of their immune system. This phenomenon is termed immune reconstitution inflammatory syndrome.

Immune Reconstitution Inflammatory Syndrome

Immune reconstitution inflammatory syndrome (IRIS) is caused by an overwhelming inflammatory response to a viable, dormant or nonviable antigen in patients with rapidly recovering immune systems. The clinical presentation of IRIS involves the unmasking of covert infections or worsening of overt conditions. IRIS is described as a 'paradox' because it manifests as worsening of clinical symptoms in patients whose immune system is improving.

Clinical Features

The clinical presentation is usually atypical. The manifestations depend on the trigger antigen, which can be an infective agent (viable or nonviable), a host or a tumor antigen. Most IRIS cases are self-limiting but in few cases it can be overwhelming and life-threatening, hence early recognition is important. In most cases, there is no need to discontinue the ART, though in the more severe cases, other clinical interventions may be necessary. The clinical presentation is widely varied and can involve any system.

Pathogenesis of IRIS

The pathogenesis of IRIS is poorly understood but in recovering HIV patients its initiation and progression seems to be linked primarily to increased CD4+ T-helper and CD8+ T-suppressor cell count, a reduction in T-regulatory cells (TREG), all endorsed by exaggerated cytokine release and activity. The immune suppression in HIV positive patients impairs the body's ability to detect and respond to antigens. Therefore, an infection that may normally cause symptoms in an immune competent individual may remain undetected (subclinical) in an HIV-positive patient. Effective ART in HIV positive patients decreases the circulating and infecting viral load, enhances lymphocyte proliferation and improves the quantity and function of immune cells. The recovery of the immune system leads to an awakening of the normal immune responses to a variety of dormant antigens.

Several causes and pathways have been suggested, most recognizing an inflammatory flare component occurring in the context of rapid immune reconstitution. In HIV-infected patients, IRIS occurs inadvertently as the consequence of a successful ART and is affiliated with improvement of the immune function, complicating the course of the disease and presenting treatment challenges to clinicians.

Although IRIS usually occurs in patients starting ART for the first time, it can also occur in patients changing their treatment regime to a more potent one. IRIS has a broad spectrum of clinical manifestations as it can be activated by a wide range of antigenic stimuli. The literature describes manifestations ranging from the common dermatological and respiratory conditions to the unusual neurological manifestations, splenic rupture and severe skin rash reaction to a ten-year-old tattoo.

Viral infections are one of the most common conditions that have been reported to flare up with anti-HIV treatment. The incidence of these infections especially herpes simplex and herpes zoster have been reported to be on the increase. HPV infection may be seen to become more severe after the initiation of ART. This has been described in the literature as IRIS-related papilloma (**Figs 20.24A and B**). Recently, the incidence of KS has decreased with the advent of ART. However, some patients experience emergence or relapse of KS after the initiation of anti-HIV treatment. The only oral neoplasm that has been reported to deteriorate with immune reconstitution after ART is KS. IRIS-related oral KS has been reported in the literature, including a remarkable and life-threatening case of a rapidly increasing palatal mass **(Figs 20.24A and B)**.

CONNECTIVE TISSUE DISEASES

Connective tissue disorders are presented in detail in Chapter 17. A brief summary is given below:

Systemic Lupus Erythematosus

Systemic lupus erythematosus (SLE) is an inflammatory connective tissue disease that affects multiple body organs. SLE is a debilitating and potentially fatal disease. The most common causes of death in SLE patients

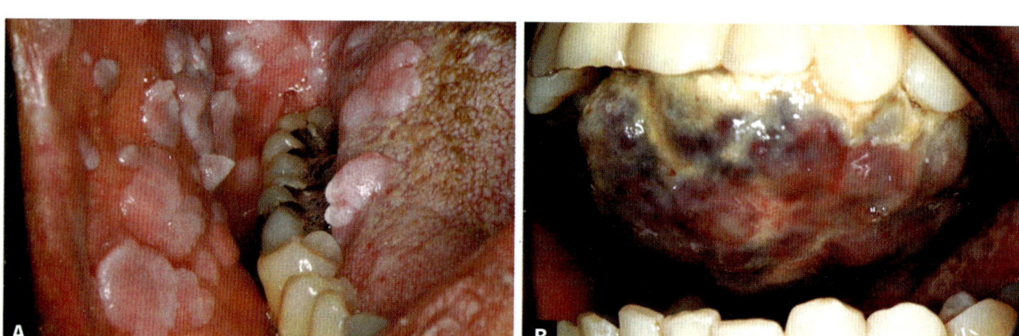

Figs 20.24A and B: Immune reconstitution inflammatory syndrome. Florid human papillomavirus infection (A) and Kaposi's sarcoma (B) as manifestations of Iris (*Photos Courtesy*: Tappuni 2011)

▪ Table 20.1
Classification criteria for the diagnosis of systemic lupus erythematosus

Criteria	*Description*
1. Malar rash (Butterfly rash)	Flat or raised erythema over the nose and cheeks, sparing the naso-labial folds
2. Discoid rash	Raised and circular erythematous skin patches with adherent keratotic scaling and folliculr plugging. May cause scarring
3. Photosensitivity	Skin rash caused by exposure to sunlight
4. Ulcerations	Oral, nasal or pharyngeal
5. Arthritis	Nonerosive arthritis of two or more peripheral joints, with tenderness, swelling, or effusion
6. Serositis	Pleuritis or pericarditis documented by ECG or rub or evidence of effusion
7. Renal condition	Proteinuria >0.5 g/d or 3+ by dipstick or cellular casts
8. Neurological disorder	Seizures or psychosis
9. Hematological abnormalities	Hemolytic anemia, leukopenia, lymphopenia or thrombocytopenia
10. Immunological disorder	Anti-dsDNA, anti-Sm, and/or anti-phospholipid
11. Antinuclear antibodies	Abnormal titer of ANA by immunofluorescence or an equivalent assay at any point in time

are central nervous system disease, renal failure and concurrent infections. With modern treatment, the survival rate has improved to about 80 percent. The worldwide prevalence of SLE is 50 to 100 cases per 100,000 population. SLE has a higher incidence in the Caribbean, China and Southeast Asia. The condition is about ten times more common in females than in males. Females are more prone to SLE in their childbearing years (16-55). SLE rarely starts after the age of 50. Patients diagnosed with SLE at an advanced age have better prognosis than those patients, who have the disease at a young age.

Box 20.11: Systemic lupus erythematosus

Key features helpful in diagnosis

- Multisystem autoimmune inflammatory disease that may be fatal.
- High titer of double-stranded de-oxyribonucleic acid (DNA) antibody.
- Malar rash (butterfly rash) on nose bridge and cheeks.
- Female:male ratio is about 10:1.
- May be triggered by sunlight or medication.

Etiology

The etiology of SLE remains unknown, although the involvement of autoantibodies is well-established. In SLE the blood vessels, kidneys, connective tissue and skin are damaged due to the deposition of immune complexes and a range of autoantibodies, particularly antinuclear antibody (ANA), which trigger organ-specific inflammatory response. In susceptible patients, SLE may be triggered by sunlight or the use of antihypertensives, antiarrhythmic, antiemetics, anticonvulsants and antibiotics.

Clinical Features

The diagnosis of SLE is made if patients fulfil four out of the eleven criteria in **Table 20.1**. SLE presents with nonspecific symptoms such as fatigue, weight loss, fever and weakness. The most common symptoms in this group of patients are rheumatological and include symmetrical inflammatory arthritis and arthralgia. Photosensitive skin rash typically appears on the face and the extremities. SLE is associated with classic malar rash, known as butterfly rash affecting the skin over the cheeks and nasal bridge, with the nasolabial folds characteristically spared. Other skin symptoms may be present such as telangiectasis, urticaria and vesicular lesions. Palmar erythema and Raynaud's phenomenon are frequently present. The eyes may be affected by dryness and conjuctivitis or episcleritis.

Heart function and circulation problems are features of SLE including myocarditis, endocarditis, pericarditis and atherosclerosis. Other systems that may be affected are pulmonary, gastroenterology, genitourinary and neurology. SLE-associated antiphospholipid syndrome causes abnormal clotting and leads to deep venous thrombosis and migrainous headaches.

The clinical course of SLE may be complicated by the presence of other autoimmune conditions such as thyroid disease, limited scleroderma or CREST syndrome. The latter is an acronym of the five main features of this condition: calcinosis, Raynauds phenomenon, esophageal dysmotility, sclerodactyly and telangiectasia.

Antinuclear antibody titer is higher than 1:80 in the vast majority of SLE patients. The most specific laboratory test for active SLE is high titer of double-stranded deoxyribonucleic acid (DNA) antibody. Other abnormal laboratory tests include high ESR, abnormal liver and kidney function tests.

Oral Manifestations

Signs and symptoms of discoid lupus may be present in SLE patients (Refer to discoid lupus erythematosus section).

Treatment

There is no known cure for SLE. The clinical management aims to reduce signs and symptoms, induce remission and decrease morbidity. A multidisciplinary approach is necessary in the management of SLE. Systemic steroids are employed to control the progression of SLE and control the active flare ups. Nonsteroidal anti-inflammatory drugs are used to control the musculoskeletal pain. Local steroid therapy administered as an injection into affected joints has been shown to give remission in arthritic pain. Long-term use of steroids compromises the immunity and put patients at higher risk of infections such as tuberculosis, fungal infections and herpes zoster. To avoid the debilitating side effects of high dose, long-term steroid therapy, alternative medications are steroid-sparing therapy, such as methotrexate, azathioprine and cyclophosphamide.

Discoid Lupus Erythematosus

Discoid lupus erythematosus (DLE) is an inflammatory skin and oral condition rarely occurs in the head and neck area. DLE may manifest in patients with SLE. DLE patients rarely fulfil four of the classification criteria for SLE. However, about 5 percent of patients with DLE progress to develop SLE. Careful history taking is important in all DLE patients to ascertain whether they have any symptoms of SLE. DLE is usually diagnosed between the ages 20 to 40 years with a female to male ratio of 2:1. DLE in children has similar history to the adult form but is less photosensitive and is more likely to progress to SLE.

DLE is slightly more prevalent in dark-skinned people compared with whites. Patients may complain of pruritus.

Box 20.12: Discoid lupus erythematosus

Key features helpful in diagnosis

- discoid lupus erythematosus can be localized, affecting the head and neck area only or generalized, spreading to the chest and upper limbs.
- The skin rash is photosensitive and painful.
- The lesions heal with scarring which may be disfiguring and lead to alopecia.
- discoid lupus erythematosus is not life-threatening.
- The oral lesions may manifest as ulcers or lichenoid reactions.

Etiology

Genetic predisposition to DLE has been suggested but no exact genetic association has been found yet. In susceptible patients, DLE is activated after exposure to environmental triggers such as sunlight. The pathophysiology is not fully understood but some studies have shown that ultraviolet light may induce a heat shock protein in the keratinocytes which may attract gamma (delta) T-cell-mediated epidermal cell cytotoxicity. Toll-like receptors possibly contribute to the pathogenesis of DLE by activating the immune cells.

Clinical Features

The lesions in DLE are erythematous papules or plaque. The rash is photosensitive and painful. The lesions are severe and cause scarring and hair loss. Classically the skin rash appears as a red and inflamed patch with lighter colored center. DLE can be localized affecting the skin of the head and neck area, typically the scalp, bridge of nose, cheeks, lower lip and ears. Less commonly, DLE can be generalized affecting the skin of the thorax and the upper limbs in addition to the head and neck area. Generalized DLE patients are more likely to have serological abnormalities and progress to SLE

The lesions may become hypertrophic forming verrucous or wart-like lesions or develop a scaly surface and become hypopigmented in the center. These lesions heal with atrophy or scarring. When the scalp is affected, permanent alopecia may result. DLE rarely causes systemic problems or becomes fatal.

Oral Manifestations

One of the most common features of DLE is oral ulcers (**Fig. 20.25**). The severity of the ulceration reflects the general disease activity. The oral ulcers will settle if the lupus is well-controlled. During severe flare ups adjunct therapy with topical medication may be necessary such as antiseptic mouthwashes or steroid rinse.

The intraoral lesions may appear very similar to the skin rash, or may appear similar to lichenoid reaction/lichen planus. Oral lesions of DLE may appear in isolation and in the absence of any skin manifestations.

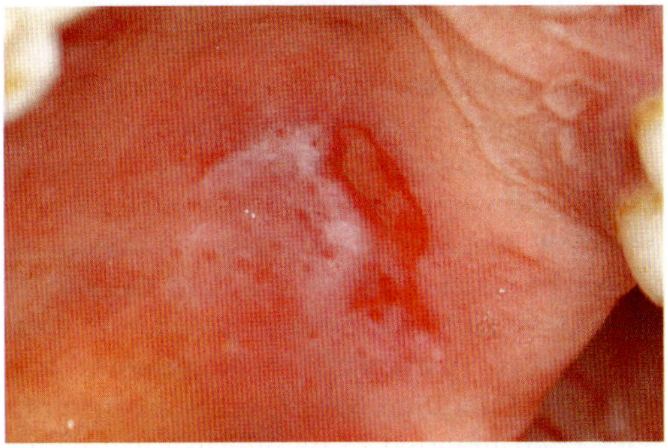

Fig. 20.25: Discoid lupus erythematosus. Ulcerative lesion with a white background in the palate

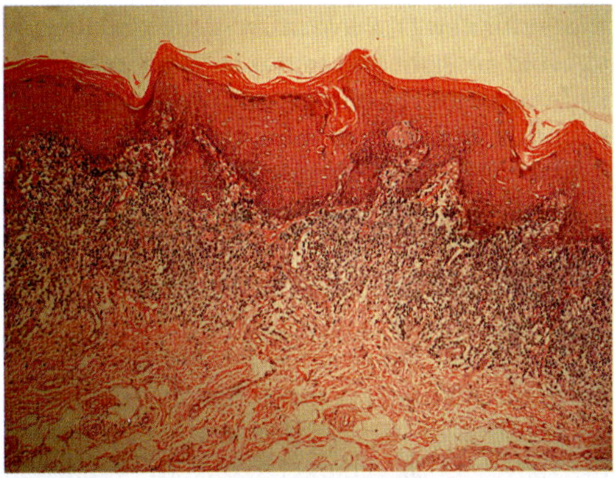

Fig. 20.26: Discoid lupus erythematosus. Flame-shaped retes with dipping keratinization and containing a lymphocytic infiltrate in the upper corium with associated apoptosis of basal cells

Histopathological Features

Histopathological features of DLE overlap significantly with that of lichenoid reaction and lichen planus. Although the epithelium shows generalized atrophy, the rete processes have the characteristic short and spiky appearance or more importantly flame-shaped configuration. True keratin plugging is not evident in oral lesions but V- shaped indentations on the surface (dipping keratinization) are usually found. Lymphocytic infiltrate with associated basal cell destruction and apoptosis are observed similar to that of lichen planus or lichenoid reaction (**Fig. 20.26**). Approximately 90 percent of patients with DLE have a positive direct immunofluorescence (DIF) test on lesional skin.

Treatment

DLE treatment is palliative and preventative of new flare ups. The management of DLE aims to prevent new attacks and control existing ones to limit scaring and to improve the patient's quality of life. Steroid (intralesional injections, topical or systemic) is the standard therapy for DLE. Other DLE treatments include antimalaria medication, particularly chloroquine and hydroxychloroquine. Several other medications have been reported to be effective in treating DLE such as azathioprine, thalidomide and mycophenolate mofetil. In severe cases of scarring, surgical excision or laser treatment is employed to improve aesthetics.

As ultraviolet light has been identified as a trigger for new DLE lesions, patients are advised to avoid sunlight and to use sunscreen creams. Patients should be counseled and monitored for the possibility of developing systemic disease.

SYNDROMES

Behçet's Disease

Behçet's syndrome (BS) or Behçet's disease (BD) is a multisystem condition, first described by the Turkish dermatologist Hulusi Behçet's in 1937. BS is characterized by recurrent oral ulcers, genital ulcers, and uveitis. The disease activity is intermittent, each attack usually lasting for several weeks or months. The frequency of the attacks decreases with the progression of the disease. Over the years, the affected organs may become damaged, causing chronic morbidity including vascular thrombosis, arthralgia and blindness. Rarely, BS can cause death due to complications such as neurological involvement, cardiovascular disease or intestinal perforation.

BS is seen more frequently in what is termed as the 'silk route' countries, which include the Mediterranean region, Middle East, and Far East. The estimated prevalence is 1:10,000 persons. The male:female ratio depends on the geographic region but generally BS is seen more frequently and more severely in men. It can occur at any age but is more prevalent between the ages of 20 to 30 years.

Box 20.13 Behçet's syndrome

Key features helpful in diagnosis

- Behçet's syndrome is a multisystem disease that may cause morbidity and mortality.
- The incidence of BS is highest in the "silk route" countries.
- The diagnosis of BS is established in the presence of oral aphthous-like ulcers and at least 2 other features (The International study group for Behçet's disease).
- The disease is characterized by alternating flare-ups and acquiescence periods.
- Typically, patients have positive pathergy test.

Etiology

The etiology of BS has been studied extensively but still is not completely understood. Factors such as genetics and immune dysregulation have been implicated. Bacterial and viral infections have been investigated as a cause for BS but the real trigger remains elusive.

The association of HLA-B51 or its B101 allele with BS has been established in Japan, Korea, Turkey, and France and with ocular manifestations in Britain. Single nucleotide polymorphism of the gene encoding protein tyrosine phosphatase type 22 (PTPN22 620W), which is genetically linked to autoimmune diseases, has been shown to have an inverse relationship with BS. Tumor necrosis factor-alpha (TNF-alpha) has been shown to be significantly elevated in BS and lead to the deployment of TNF-alpha blockers as therapy.

Cross-reactivity between microbial agents and oral mucosal antigens has been investigated as a trigger for BS, along with viral and bacterial infection, especially herpes simplex virus (HSV) and streptococcal infection. HSV DNA has been isolated from the saliva, genital and intestinal ulcers of BS patients.

Several immunological markers are found to be elevated in BS especially during the active stage, including Th1 cytokine interferon (IFN), interleukin (IL)-12 and Th2 cytokine IL-6. The proinflammatory cytokine vascular endothelial growth factor, is significantly higher in the plasma of patients with BS.

The underlying pathophysiology of some of the symptoms of the disease can be explained such as the presence of vasculitis and vascular symptoms due to the high levels of thrombomodulin and the increased thrombosis risk due to high level of Thrombin activatable fibrinolysis inhibitor. However, the real etiology and trigger of BD is yet to be explained fully.

Histopathological Features

Histopathological features of BD are not specific for the diagnosis. The ulcers present in the disease show very similar histopathology of aphthous ulcers. However, deep perivascular infiltrate of lymphocytes may indicate BD. Most frequently described histological feature in these patients is the leukocytoclastic vasculitis. Ulcerated areas show invasion of small sized blood vessels by neutrophils with surrounding fibrinoid necrosis.

Clinical Features

Behçet's syndrome patients may present with a variety of non-specific symptoms such as malaise, weight loss, headaches, lymphadenopathy, arthralgias and recurrent upper respiratory tract infections. The diagnosis of BS is frequently missed or delayed due to the absence of a pathognomic laboratory test and the clinical symptoms being nonspecific. The major features of the disease are:

- Recurrent aphthous-like oral ulceration (**Fig. 20.27**), (see Chapter 14)
- Skin lesions such as erythema nodosum (**Fig. 20.28**), subcutaneous thrombophlebitis, folliculitis, acne-like lesions and hypersensitivity (**Fig. 20.29**)
- Eye lesions (Iridocyclitis, chorioretinitis, retinouveitis)
- Genital ulcers—Minor features include: Arthritis, gastrointestinal lesions, vascular lesions and central nervous system symptoms

According to the international study group for Behçet's disease, the diagnosis of BS is established in the presence of oral aphthous like ulcers and at least 2 of the following: genital ulcers, eye lesions, cutaneous lesions, positive pathergy test (**Table 20.2**).

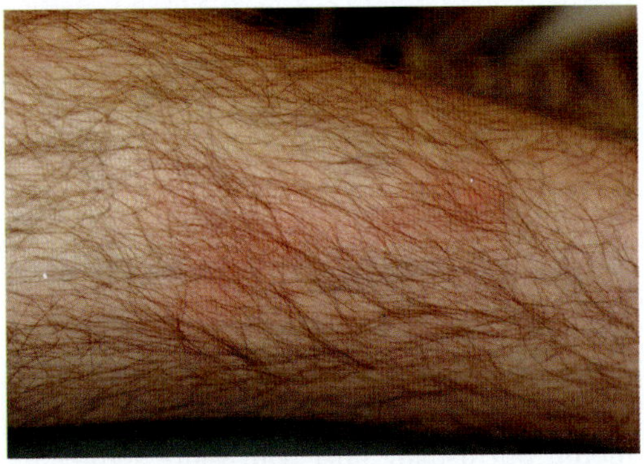

Fig. 20.28: Behçet's disease. Erythema nodosum in Behçet's syndrome

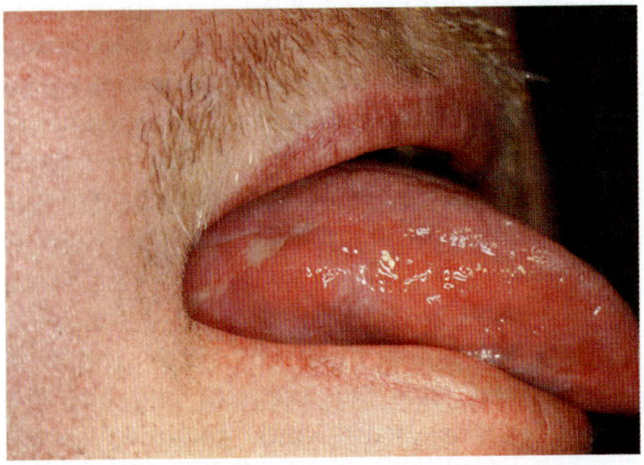

Fig. 20.27: Behçet's disease. Aphthous-like ulceration on the lateral border of the tongue

Fig. 20.29: Behçet's disease. Acne-like lesions on the back

▪ Table 20.2
International criteria for classification of Behçet's disease (1990)

Recurrent oral ulceration	Minor aphthous Major aphthous or herpetiform ulceration Recurrent at least three times in one 12-month period. (Observed by a physician or reported reliably by patient) Plus two of
Recurrent genital ulceration	Recurrent genital ulceration or scarring (Observed by a physician or reliably reported by patient)
Eye lesions	Anterior uveitis Posterior uveitis Cells in vitreous on slit lamp examination or retinal vasculitis (Observed by ophthalmologist)
Skin lesions	Erythema nodosum-like lesions (Observed by physician or reliably reported by patient) Pseudofolliculitis Papulopustular lesions or acneiform nodules consistent with Behçet's disease (Observed by a physician and in postadolescent patients not receiving corticosteroids)
Positive pathergy test	An erythematous papule, >2 mm, at the prick site 48 hr after the application of sterile needle, 20-22 gauge, which obliquely penetrated avascular skin to a depth of 5 mm: (Read by physician at 48 hrs.)

Ulcers in the genital and perianal areas are very common and resemble those seen in the mouth but usually heal with more significant scarring. They occur on the vulva, vagina, cervix and groin in females and on the penis, scrotum and groin in males.

Ocular symptoms are reported in more than half of BS patients. Posterior uveitis (Retinal vasculitis) is specifically related to BS. However, other eye lesions are seen regularly in BS patients such as anterior uveitis, scleritis, keratitis, vitreous hemorrhage, optic neuritis and conjunctivitis. The visual acuity decreases, usually secondary to glaucoma or cataract. The ocular symptoms pose a serious threat to patients' health as they are a major cause of morbidity and may lead to blindness. There have been reports of blindness ensuing within 4 years of diagnosis or even sudden blindness due to retinal or cerebral venous thrombosis. Another complication of this condition is the vascular and perivascular changes which may lead to varices, aneurysms and arterial or venous occlusions. Arterial stenosis leads to avascular tissue necrosis and hypertension.

The skin manifestations of BS appear in the majority of patients and include erythema nodosum, acne, papulopustular eruptions, erythema multiforme-like lesions, thrombophlebitis, pyoderma gangrenosum and lesions resembling those seen in sweet syndrome. Classically, patients will have positive pathergy test (nonspecific skin inflammatory reaction to trauma).

About half of Behçet's disease patients develop joint problems and about 10 percent present with gastrointestinal problems. One of the most debilitating effects of this disease is the development of neurological symptoms, seen in less than 5 percent of patients. The manifestations vary and include severe headaches, multiple sclerosis-like illness and stroke. These occur usually within 5 years of the onset of the disease and may be fatal.

Oral Manifestations

The presence of oral ulceration is a prerequisite for the diagnosis of BS. The oral ulcers are aphthae-like and can resemble major, minor or herpetiform aphthous stomatitis. The oral ulceration vary from mild, limited and singular to severe, extensive and wide-spread ulceration with a punched-out appearance. The recurrence frequency also varies from weeks to months. They may affect anywhere in the oral cavity but the tongue, labial and buccal mucosa are the most common sites.

Treatment

Behçet's syndrome is a multisystem disease that is best managed by a multidisciplinary approach. The treatment is symptomatic and governed by the course of the disease. Topical therapy is used for the oral and genital ulceration, and eye problems. The standard topical treatment for the oral symptoms is a steroid mouthwash of betamethasone 500 mcg tablet in 10 mL of water or a triple mouthwash of 500 mcg prednisolone, 250 mg tetracycline and one ml of 100,00 U/mL nystatin suspension, in 10 mL of water. This mouthwash is used for 2 to 4 minutes, 2 to 3 times per day. Other useful preparations include hyaluronic gel, 2 percent lidocaine and 5 percent amlexanox.

Systemic therapy is frequently necessary in the management of BS. The treatment of choice depends on the manifestations of the disease but steroids are considered as the first line therapy, especially during acute phases of the disease. To spare patients, the side effects associated with long-term steroid therapy, they are frequently replaced by other agents such as nonsteroidal anti-inflammatory, immunosuppressives and immunomodulators. These include levamisole, colchicine, dapsone, azathioprine, chlorambucil, and cyclophosphamide. Thalidomide is used only in limited, severe recalcitrant conditions because of its teratogenic side effects.

Gardner's Syndrome

This is an autosomal dominant defect on chromosome 5. Frequently, the oral manifestations are the presenting signs of this potentially fatal condition. It is characterized by supernumerary or unerupted teeth in the incisor and premolar area with associated compound odontoma in some patients. The bony exostoses cause focal protuberance on the jaw bones and head. Multiple osteomas are seen intraorally on the palate, upper alveolar process and lower jaw buccally and lingually (**Figs 20.30A and B**). Epidermoid cysts may also be seen. Gardner's syndrome is associated with intestinal polyposis with a very high-risk of malignant transformation into colonic adenocarcinoma.

The presence of unexplained bony exostoses in the jaw and skull should trigger investigation for Gardner's syndrome therefore appropriate screening for bowel polyposis and adenocarcinoma can be commenced. Family

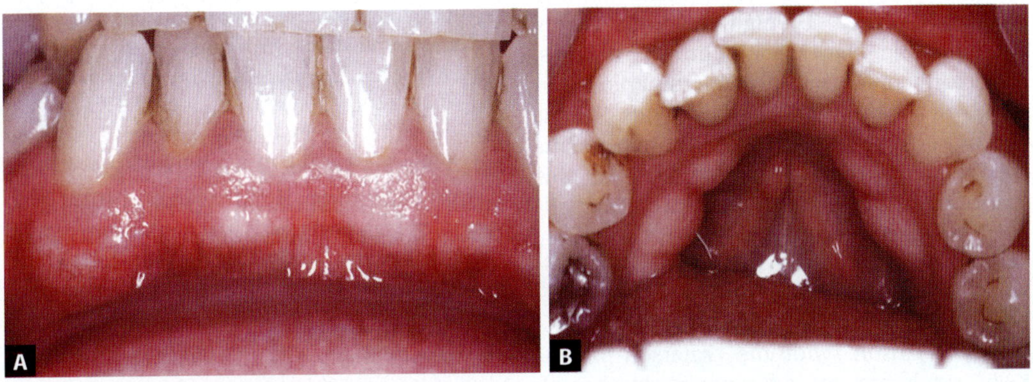

Figs 20.30A and B: Gardner's syndrome. Lower jaw and palatal multiple osteomas

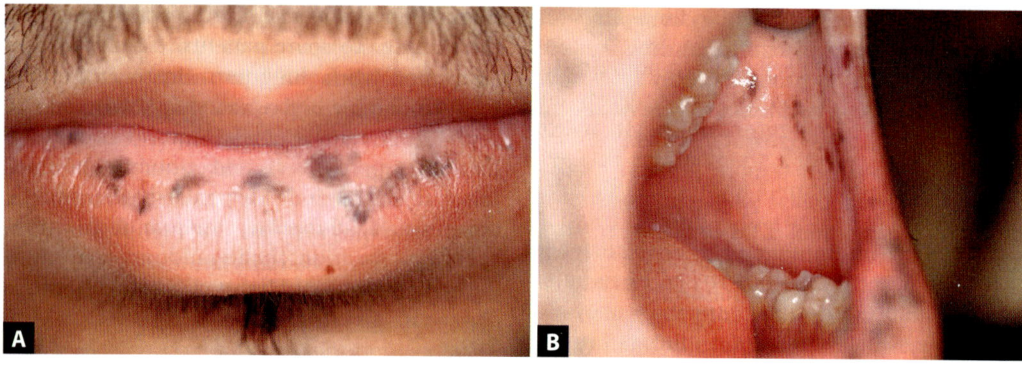

Figs 20.31A and B: (A) Peutz-Jegher's syndrome. Labial pigmentation; (B) Intraoral pigmentation

members of patients with proven Gardner's syndrome should be investigated for this syndrome and put under surveillance.

Peutz-Jegher's Syndrome

This is either an inherited condition (autosomal dominant) or occurs as a result of mutation of the LKB1 gene. The syndrome was first described in 1921 by Jan Peutz. Subsequently in 1949, Harold Jeghers established the definitive description of the syndrome. The syndrome is characterized by the coexistence of intestinal hamartomatous polyps and mucocutaneous melanocytic macules. Patients with Peutz-Jegher's syndrome (PJS) have a 15-fold increased risk of developing intestinal cancer compared with the general population.

The freckles are seen perorally on the surrounding skin and the lips (**Figs 20.31A and B**). Intraorally, the pigmented macules can affect the tongue, buccal and labial mucosa (**Figs 20.31A and B**). The pigmentation is usually asymptomatic flat, bluish brown patches. Hyperpigmentation is seen microscopically in the melanocytes and the keratinocytes. Similar to Gardner's syndrome, the oral manifestations are frequently the presenting sign of this syndrome and allow early diagnosis and surveillance for gastrointestinal cancer.

Plummer-Vinson Syndrome

Plummer-Vinson syndrome (Paterson-Brown-Kelly syndrome or sideropenic dysphagia). This syndrome is caused by iron deficiency as a result of poor diet or blood loss. It tends to affect middle aged women. The presence of post-cricoid esophageal web is characteristic. The web is 2 to 3 mm wide and contains mucosa and submucosa as an extension of the esophageal tissue. The web is considered premalignant and may lead to carcinoma of the esophagus or postcricoid carcinoma. Patients present with pagophagia (compulsive consumption of cold drinks and ice), koilonychia (spoon-shaped nails), dysphagia, anemia and angular cheilitis. Intraorally, the oral mucosa appears atrophic and pale with occasional keratotic patches. The filiform papillae are atrophic and give the tongue a smooth erythematous appearance. Replacement and maintenance of iron levels is necessary to treat this condition.

SELF-ASSESSMENT QUESTIONS

1. Give the differential diagnosis for a patient with recurrent oral ulceration and associated gastrointestinal symptoms.
2. What are the classification criteria for the diagnosis of systemic lupus erythematosus?
3. Describe the erythematosus most common oral manifestations of human immunodeficiency virus (HIV) infection.
4. Describe the etiopathological process underlying immune reconstitution inflammatory syndrome.
5. Describe the clinical and pathological features of amyloidosis.
6. Describe the histopathological features of an intestinal and an oral biopsy in Crohn's disease.

7. Outline the management of a patient suspected of having Gardner's syndrome.
8. What is the pathophysiology of Addison's disease?
9. Describe the clinicopathological features of sarcoidosis.
10. Describe the oral manifestations of Wegener's granulomatosis?

SUGGESTED READING

1. Kalantzis A, Scully C. Applied Medicine and Surgery. Oxford University Press; 2010.
2. Cawson RA, Odell EW. Cawson's Essentials of Oral Pathology and Oral Medicine, 8th edn. Churchill Livingstone; 2008.
3. Color Atlas of Oral Diseases, 3rd edn. Laskaris, George, Thieme; 2003.
4. C Scully. Medical Problems in Dentistry, 6th edn. Churchill Livingstone; 2010.
5. Dimmitt S, Crawley WA. Medicine for Dentists -A Problem Based Approach. University of Western Australia Press; 2003.
6. Gandolfo, Sergio, Scully, Crispian, Carrozzo, Marco. Oral Medicine, Churchill Livingstone; 2006.
7. Soames JV, Southam JC. Oral Pathology, 4th edn. Oxford University Press; 2005.
8. Regezi, Joseph A, Sciubba, James J, Jordan, Richard CK. Oral Pathology: Clinical pathologic correlations, 5th edn. Saunders/Elsevier; 2008.
9. Macleod Iain, Crighton, Alexander, Wilson, Nairn HF, Meechan, JG. Practical Oral Medicine, Quintessence; 2005.
10. Tappuni AR. Immune Reconstitution Inflammatory Syndrome. Ad Dent Res. 2011;23(1):90-6.
11. Tilakaratne WM, Freysdottir J, Fortunre FJ. Orofacial grnulomatosis; review on aetiology and pathogenesis. Oral Pathol Med. 2008;37:191-5.

Chapter 21

Forensic Dentistry

Induwara Goonerathne

Chapter Outline

INTRODUCTION

Definitions

The English dictionaries define the term "forensic" as 'used or applied in the investigation and establishment of facts or evidence in a court of law'. As the definition implies, the term "forensic" inherently is associated with courts of law as a means in the investigation and establishment of facts or evidence.

The term "odontology" literally means the scientific study of teeth. Hence, the term forensic odontology means the "scientific study of teeth in the establishment of facts or evidence in a court of law.

The extensive scientific study of teeth is carried out in the discipline of dentistry. Therefore in a broader sense, forensic odontology is a synonym for forensic dentistry. The nature and the scope of dentistry have evolved exponentially over the years. Dental Science is in a highly advanced milieu today and involves the scientific study of not only teeth but also the entire mouth, jaws and the face. Parallel to these advancements in the study and scope of dentistry, the scope of forensic dentistry too has evolved and developed to include the scientific study of the teeth, mouth, jaws and face towards investigation and establishment of relevant facts or evidence in a court room for legal purposes.

To illustrate the use of forensic dentistry for legal purposes assume that there is an allegation in a court of law, alleging the accused "X" of biting the victim "Y" causing bodily harm. Causing bodily harm is a crime. The scientific study of the victim's alleged injury and the careful investigation of the accused's teeth could lead to scientific evidence to establish relevant facts concerning issues such as " is the alleged injury a "bite" caused by human teeth?", When could the "bite" have occurred? How could it have occurred? Who could have made the "bite"? The use of forensic dentistry is crucial in this scenario and dental evidence is essential in incriminating the accused for the crime.

Keiser-Nielsen and others define forensic odontology, or forensic dentistry as the branch of odontology/dentistry which in the interest of justice deals with the proper handling and examination of dental evidence and with the proper evaluation and presentation of dental findings to courts or other legal authorities.

The scope of the domain of forensic dentistry includes all aspects of dentistry that involves a legal issue or a justice issue. Therefore, the practice of forensic dentistry involves courts of law or other legal authorities. The key issues where forensic dentistry involves include:

- Identification of victims and wrong doers
- Analysis and interpretation of dentofacial trauma for legal purposes
- Bitemarks analysis
- Estimation of age for legal purposes
- Lip print analysis
- Dental fraud, ethics and dental negligence cases.

The nature of forensic dentistry is different and unique from any other branch in dentistry in the sense that forensic dentistry practice involves court proceedings and police or other law agency proceedings. The practice of forensic odontology involves living people as well as dead. The dead victims include putrefied, fragmented, charred or mutilated bodies. The forensic dental practice inherently involves victims of a crime or suspects of a victim crime (instead of victim). Unlike any other branch of dentistry, forensic dentistry involves field visits, scene visits, visits to courts to give evidence, postmortem examinations, team work hand-in-hand with other members of a crime investigation team. This discipline like any other scientific discipline requires rigorous specific training, commitment, integrity, long working hours, team spirit, variable work environments such as hospital clinics, mortuary, crime scene, exhumation site, mass disaster site, etc. Anyone aspiring to become a forensic dental practitioner need to understand the scope and the nature of the work it involves.

Apart from forensic dentistry, other major forensic branches include forensic medicine, forensic science, forensic ballistics, and forensic toxicology.

The Roles of a Forensic Odontologist

The main function of a forensic odontologist is to assist in identification of victims and wrong doers based on dental and facial evidence. The cases include burnt or charred victims, victims of mass disasters, skeletonized and fragmented bodies, putrefied or mutilated bodies. Other roles include:

- Bitemarks analysis
- Dental and facial trauma analysis for legal purposes
- Assist in the estimation of biological age using dental evidence
- Provide opinions regarding dental fraud or negligence cases
- Lip print analysis.

Forensic Dentistry Training and Career

There is a growing demand for forensic dentistry as a career. Essentially, all forensic odontologists need to possess a dental degree and dental license. Before enrolling in postgraduate forensic dental programs, one must have at least one year of clinical experience.

To function as a forensic odontologist one must possess a sound knowledge, skills and attitude in dentistry, related law, ethics, jurisprudence, medicolegal issues, criminal investigation procedures and medicolegal practice, etc. Often forensic odontologists work as members of a large team including police, court officers, forensic medical practitioners, forensic scientists, etc.

A Few Famous Cases Involving Forensic Odontology

Below are some cases described briefly to demonstrate the relevance of forensic dentistry in the medicolegal practice.

Ted Bundy Case

Theodore Robert Cowell also known as "Ted Bundy" is an American serial killer who committed about 30 murders who was active in the mid 70s. He was convicted for murder by a court of law and was executed by electric chair by the State of Florida in 1989.

Bundy would assault and rape his victims and strangle them to death. In his brutal sexual attacks, he used to engage in biting his victims. This serial killer was finally convicted with the use of bitemarks evidence that were found in one of the victim's buttocks. If not for the bitemarks evidence, Bundy would not have been convicted.

Savitri Case

A seven-year-old girl was brought to a dental hospital for fracture of anterior teeth. On examination, it was revealed that there was a large bruise on her lip and a fracture of the mandible in addition to injuries to teeth. The parents were of the opinion that it was a fall from a chair. However, the history did not match the injury pattern. The medical records indicated that there were similar injuries in the past and evidence of bone healing at different ages. The case was suspected to be of child abuse and referred for further medicolegal analysis. Later, it was found that the child was repeatedly physically abused by the father.

Tsunami Identifications

Almost all American and British citizens who died in Sri Lanka due to tsunami in 2004, were positively identified using forensic dental approaches. Later, their identity was confirmed using DNA evidence. Due to this, bodies have been handed over to relatives at a minimum cost.

History of Forensic Dentistry

The use of dental information in medicolegal purposes dates back as far back as 66 AD at the time of Nero. As the story goes, Nero's mother, Agrippina, had her soldiers kill Lollia Paulina, with instructions to bring back her head as proof that she was dead. Agrippina, unable to positively identify the head, examined the front teeth and on finding the discolored front tooth confirmed the identity of the victim.

The first forensic odontologist in the United States was Dr Paul Revere who identified the body of Dr Joseph Warren, a revolutionary who fought against the British in 1775, through a dental bridge of silver and ivory that he had constructed two years previously.

Dental evidence was first accepted in the United States court in the Webster-Parkman case. Dr JW Webster allegedly stabbed and dismembered the victim Parkman on November 23rd, 1849 in Boston. Charred fragments of mineral teeth fused to gold were recognized as those of the deceased. This evidence was enough for the jury to provide a verdict of guilty of premeditated murder against Dr Webster who was subsequently hung.

Parallel to other sciences, forensic odontology has also developed and expanded its scope, nature and methods. Today, this discipline is a recognized science. Forensic dental opinions are considered an important and integral part of contemporary crime investigations. Forensic odontology has been useful in recent mass disasters such as Tsunami disasters and Hurricane Katrina and others, towards victim identification. In addition, bitemarks analysis, lip print analysis, dentofacial trauma analysis by forensic dental officers are increasingly used in administration of justice.

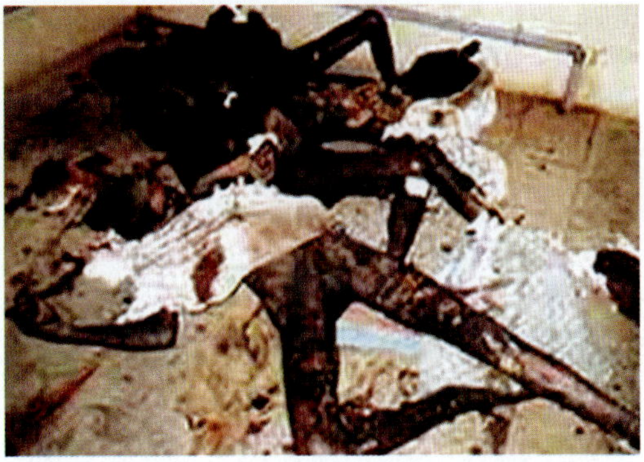

Fig. 21.1: Illustratrtion of burnt and charred bodies. As teeth and dental restorations are resistant to heat, forensic odontologic method will be very useful in identifying the victims. It may not be possible to extract DNA in some cases as DNA is heat sensitive

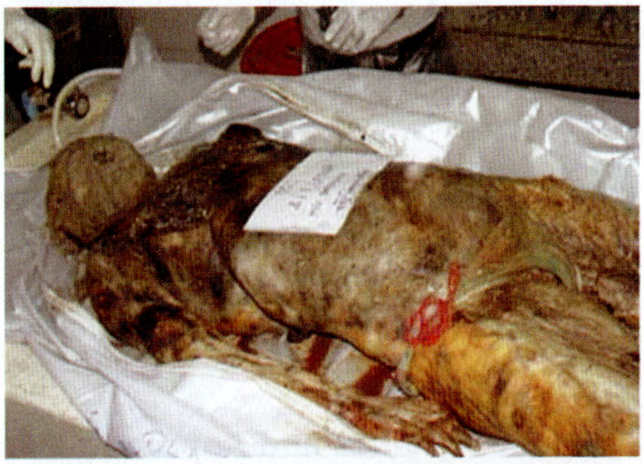

Fig. 21.2: Putrefied body which needs scientific method of identification

IDENTIFICATION

Definitions and the Theoretical Framework

Definitions

In medicolegal contexts, "identification" means the exact fixation of the "identity" of the individual. This includes victims and wrongdoers identification. However, in practical contexts the medicolegal process of identification is more focused on victim identification.

The need for "Identification" arises in many medicolegal contexts. This includes living victims/individuals or already dead individuals. Examples/indications for identifying a living individual include instances of interchanges in baby units, missing individuals, elderly who have forgotten their whereabouts due to psychiatric conditions.

The need for identification arises amongst dead victims whose bodies are putrefied, mutilated or fragmented. These include cases of drowning, bomb blast, plane crash, mass disasters burn, etc. (**Figs 21.1** and **21.2**).

The identification of individuals is important in two aspects, namely from a legal stand point and the other from a psychosocial aspect. If a victim is not identified accurately, then it is impossible for the law to believe that this person is actually dead. Therefore his family will not be able to claim for his property, finances and others. Also, when someone is dead, the families need to have the real body or body parts for funeral functions. Therefore, from a legal and a psychosocial stand point, identification becomes very important.

Theoretical Framework

In day-to-day life when we want to identify a person, we instantly look at visible features of the individual and try to compare those features with the image of the person we have in mind. For example, if you want to recognize a friend whom you had not seen for years, when you meet them after a long time, you involuntarily compare the features that had already been recorded in your brain from earlier encounters, with that of what you would see now. In the medicolegal process of identification too, we apply the same theoretical approach. We compare what has been recorded earlier with what is available now. However, the difference in the scientific approach is that we use reliable scientific data for comparison. The courts would want reliable scientific evidence to confirm the identity of the individual.

Identification is a process that involves many professionals. It essentially has a team approach. Those involved include a forensic dental expert, forensic anthropologist, police, forensic medical expert and DNA expert.

In the scientific approach of identification, it is important to record all data/information and evidence available. There are two main aims of the activity: to identify the person and to identify how he has died. The forensic medical officer is involved primarily in answering the second question: how the individual died. Others engage in identifying who the person is.

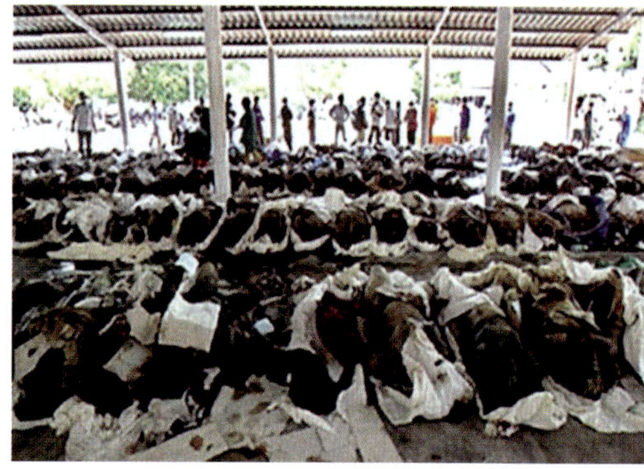

Fig. 21.3: Illustration of a collection of putrefied bodies recovered in a Tsunami disaster. These warrant scientific method of identification

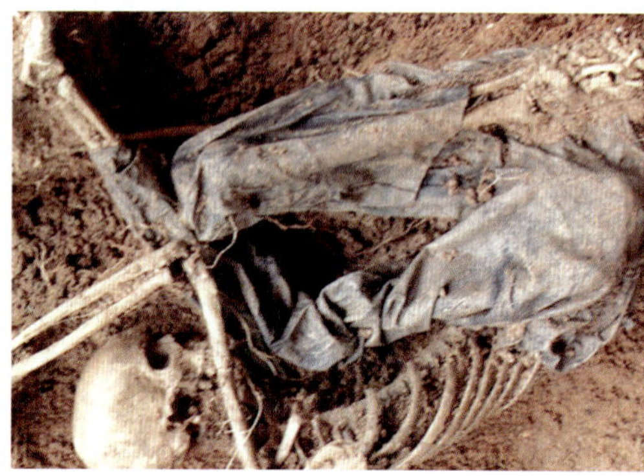

Fig. 21.4: Skeletonized fragmented specimens which warrant identification

Different Scenarios and Approaches to Identification

Scenarios

- Mass disasters and bodies found in natural disasters (**Fig. 21.3**)
- Putrefied bodies found in forests, etc. (**Fig. 21.2**)
- Skeletal remains found (**Fig. 21.4**)
- Burnt bodies (**Fig. 21.1**), bodies found in bomb blasts and charred bodies
- Bodies with severe animal attacks that has disfigured the body
- Road traffic accidents that had severe injuries disfiguring the body/face
- Bodies found in plane crashes.

Approaches to Identification

The first approach employed is to examine the clothes, ornaments and accessories that are found with the body. At the postmortem examination such clothes, accessories, jewelries, etc. that were found will be verified with the victim's family. Although these findings are not confirmatory, such evidence is useful as presumptive evidence of identification.

The victim's family is in an emotionally disturbed moment and it is very likely that mistakes can happen. There have been instances of foul play and false claims; therefore one has to be very sure about the identity of the victim. If the facial features are intact, then relatives can be called and asked if they could identify. If the facial features are distorted which is more often the case, the scientific approach has to be employed.

If the soft tissues of the body are intact, then the forensic pathologist could assess the victim's sex/gender, age, stature and time since death which are important in the identification process. In this process, it is very likely that the forensic pathologist will obtain an opinion from the forensic odontologist with regards to the age and identity.

If the soft tissues are deteriorated or skeletonized, then the forensic anthropologist and odontologist examine the body and provide an opinion with regards to the age, sex, stature and time since death which are useful in the identification process.

Then the forensic odontologist performs an autopsy on the victim (subsequent to the pathologist's postmortem examination determining cause of death) and attempts to establish positive identification.

Parallel to this, DNA fingerprinting can be employed to confirm identity where necessary.

Other ancillary procedures such as photographic superimpositions, facial reconstructions and radiological examinations can also be performed.

Forensic Odontology Method of Identification

The fundamental theory underpinning the forensic odontological method of identification of victims is that "Antemortem dental data of the victim should be scientifically compatible with postmortem dental data of the victim. If they are not compatible, it means that the two do not match: in other words, two different persons".

In this approach, it is believed that all dental data of the victim are entered into a computer system or into official clinical records. Also, it is believed that all dental data of the victim are accurately recorded by the clinician in the past. It is also believed that such dental records are readily available. When antimortem dental data are not available or when antemortem dental data are not accurately entered, this method cannot be employed in a scientific manner.

The other theory behind this approach is that the more antemortem dental data are available, the better and more accurate the opinion is. As there are 32 teeth in most adults the availability of dental data (as variables) are high and in-turn reliability is better.

This method of identification is widely accepted in worldwide jurisdictions. To engage in such an activity one needs to have a rigorous training in forensic odontology.

Dental evidences that are useful in the forensic odontological method of identification:

- The availability of permanent or deciduous dentition
- The morphology of teeth, abnormalities of teeth
- Occlusion and variations in occlusion
- Rotation of teeth, malaligned teeth
- Caries pattern in the dentition
- The degree of periodontal disease and loss of attachment
- Restorations
- Dental prosthesis
- Tattoos in the mouth, tongue rings, etc.
- Lip print patterns
- Orthodontic measurements such as cephalometrics, facial measurements, skeletal relationship and incisor relationship
- Previous oral surgeries, healed fractures of jaws
- Anatomical variations of face and teeth
- Other relevant dental information.

Method

In a routine identification process a request for dental identification will be made to the relevant forensic dental officer by the respective legal authority (coroner, magistrate or police depending on the jurisdiction). As has been emphasized above, identification is a result of teamwork.

When a death occurs, then there are two important medicolegal issues to be solved; the cause and manner of death and the identity of the victim. The cause of death is dealt by the forensic pathologist with the support of many other experts and identification is dealt with by other experts to which the medical expert could also contribute.

A forensic dental officer plays a key role in the identification process. At postmortem examination, once all ornaments, accessories, clothes and photographs are collected and subjected to a postmortem examination to identify the cause of death by the medical examiner. Subsequent to this the forensic odontologist starts his postmortem examination. He records all external features that are helpful in identification. He performs an extraoral and intraoral examination. In his intraoral examination, he looks at pathologies of the mouth and teeth and also evidence that are helpful in identification. Due to postmortem changes, it may be practically difficult to open the mouth for examination. In this instance the forensic odontologist performs an autopsy and dissects the jaws. The jaws are taken to the laboratory for analysis. It is better to obtain all orthodontic and facial measurements of the victim. All such parameters are recorded in the especially designed record sheet.

For dental charting and recording of dental parameters, one can use any recommended dental chart forms. The jaws are examined well and all dental abnormalities, caries, fillings, prosthetics, pathologies and occlusion features are recorded in the prescribed dental record chart.

Then the radiographs of the jaws are taken and the findings are documented. The radiological findings and postmortem clinical findings are collated and entered into a computer. There are recommended computer programs for automated comparisons. With the use of these computer entries, if the antemortem dental records of the victim are known, then they can be compared and assessed for the compatibility. A careful scientific examination is done and an opinion is forwarded indicating whether the victim's antemortem dental records are matched or not matched with the postmortem victim's dental data.

In examining a body at postmortem, there are a few important things that the forensic dental officer needs to do in addition to other things. Among them are taking photographs, taking dental impressions, taking radiographs, dental charting and resection of the jaws preferably by using inframandibular dissection technique. Photographs taken properly can provide more detailed data than a written description. All photographs should be labeled properly with all details and stored for reference. Facial dissection and jaw resections should be done where necessary to observe total intraoral examination. However, the approval of the coroner should be sought for this.

In dissecting the mouth, the following has to be considered.

- Intraoral incision of masticatory muscles, with or without fracture of the condyle
- Breaking the rigor with bilateral leverage on the jaws in the retromolar regions
- Waiting until the rigor subsides
- Inframandibular dissection with or without mandibular resection.

Removal of the larynx and tongue at autopsy may facilitate the visual examination of the teeth and/or placement of intraoral films. Again, the removal of these tissues should only be performed after the autopsy and with concurrence of the pathologist/coroner. These tissues should either be retained by the pathologist or replaced with the body. When dissecting putrefied or burnt bodies one needs to be careful not to damage any valuable dental evidence.

While most morgues have the standard autopsy equipment, the forensic odontologist may wish to assemble his own forensic kit to include mouth mirrors, explorers, camera equipment, anatomic dental charts, impression materials, etc. Postmortem dental examinations utilize anatomic dental charts, photographs, radiographs, models, tape recordings and/or narrative descriptions. The data collected should be comprehensive in scope since antemortem records are commonly not discovered until days, weeks or even years later.

A universal tooth numbering system should be used whenever possible. The record should reflect any missing dental structures or jaw fragments as well as those present and available for evaluation.

The chart should illustrate as graphically as possible the following:

- Configuration of all dental restorations (including prostheses), caries, fractures, anomalies, abrasions, implants, erosions or other features for all teeth.
- Materials used in dental restorations and prosthetic devices, when known.
- Periodontal conditions, calculus, stain.
- Occlusal relationships, malpositioned teeth; anomalous, congenitally missing and supernumerary teeth.
- Intraoral photographs should be used to show anatomic details of teeth, restorations, periodontium, occlusion and lesions.

If there are no victim or relatives claiming for the deceased, then the postmortem dental data can be given to the law enforcement agency. The agency send the postmortem dental data to all practicing dental surgeons in the country and request that patients with similar antemortem and postmortem records be supplied. These will be further investigated and compared.

The antemortem data for comparisons may include dental radiographs, written records and models. The collection of antemortem records is the responsibility of the investigative agency that has access to missing person's reports at local or national level (Ref. ABFO manual).

Dental Features Useful in Identification

Teeth

- Teeth present
- Erupted
- Unerupted/impacted

Missing Teeth

- Congenitally missing
- Lost antemortem
- Lost perimortem/postmortem

Tooth Type

- Permanent
- Mixed dentition
- Retained primary teeth
- Supernumerary teeth
- Tooth position
- *Malpositions:* Facial/lingual version, rotations, supra/infra positions, diastemas, other occlusal discrepancies
- Crown morphology
- Size and shape of crowns
- Enamel thickness
- Location of contact points, cementoenamel junction
- *Racial variations:* Shovel-shaped incisors, Carabelli cusp, etc.
- Crown pathology
- Caries
- Attrition/abrasion/erosion
- *Atypical variations:* Peg laterals, fusion/gemination, enamel pearl, multiple cusps
- Dens in dente
- Dentigerous cyst
- Root morphology
- Size, shape, number, dilaceration, divergence of roots
- Root pathology
- Root fracture
- Hypercementosis
- External root resorption
- Root hemisections
- Pulp chamber and root canal morphology
- Size, shape, number
- Secondary dentin
- Pulp chamber and root canal pathology
- Pulp stones, dystrophic calcification
- *Root canal therapy:* Gutta percha, silver points, endopaste and retrofill procedures
- Internal resorption
- Apicectomy
- Periapical pathology
- Periapical abscess/granuloma/cyst
- Cementoma
- Condensing osteitis
- Dental restorations
- *Metallic restorations:* Amalgams, gold or non-precious metal crowns/inlays, endoposts, pins, fixed prostheses, implants
- *Non-metallic restorations:* Acrylics, silicates, composites, porcelain, etc.
- Partial and full removal prostheses
- Periodontium
- *Gingiva:* Morphology/pathology
- *Contour:* Gingival recession, focal/diffuse enlargements, interproximal craters
- *Color:* Inflammatory changes, physiologic or pathologic pigmentations
- Plaque and concretions, oral hygiene status, stains, calculus
- *Periodontal ligament:* Morphology/pathology
- Thickness
- Widening
- Lateral periodontal cyst
- Alveolar process and lamina dura
- Height/contour/density of crestal bone
- Thickness of inter-radicular alveolar bone
- Exostoses, tori
- Pattern of lamina dura (loss, increased density)
- Periodontal bone loss

- Trabecular bone pattern osteoporosis, radiodensities
- Residual root fragments, metallic fragments.

Maxilla and Mandible

- Anatomical landmarks/pathology
- *Maxillary sinuses:* Size, shape, retention cyst, antrolith, foreign bodies, oral antral fistula
- Relationship to adjacent teeth, anterior nasal spine, incisive canal, median palatal suture, incisive canal size, shape, cysts
- *Pterygoid hamulus:* Size, shape, fracture
- *Mandibular canal/mental foramen:* Diameter, anomalous (bifurcated) canal, relationship to adjacent teeth
- *Coronoid and condylar process:* Size and shape
- *Temporomandibular joint:* Size, shape, hypertrophy/atrophy, ankylosis, fracture, arthritic changes.

Other Pathologic Processes/Jaw Bones

- Developmental/fissural cysts
- Hemorrhagic (traumatic) bone cyst
- Salivary gland depression
- Reactive/neoplastic lesions
- Metabolic bone disease
- Other disorders inducing focal or diffuse radiolucencies or radiopacities
- Evidence of orthognathic surgery or prior evidence of trauma (e.g. wire sutures, surgical pins, etc.) (Ref. ABFO manual).

In addition, facial measurements, craniometry, cephalometry and other orthodontic measurements are also relevant. The examining forensic dental officer is not in a position to verify the accuracy of the antemortem dental records that are presented. Therefore in writing the report, he must indicate that his opinion is based on the evidence available.

In routine forensic dental examination, there are four opinions that can be provided to the law enforcement depending on the evidence available.

1. *Positive identification:* This opinion can be made when antimortem and postmortem data match significantly and sufficiently to establish that they are from the same individual. Also there should be no unexplainable discrepancy.
2. *Possible identification:* In this situation, there is consistency with the antemortem and postmortem data. However, due to poor quality of the evidence either antemortem or postmortem, it is not possible to establish the identity accurately.
3. *Insufficient evidence:* The available evidence is insufficient to make a conclusion.
4. *Exclusion:* It is possible to exclude the identity of the person concerned with the available evidence. A DNA test can be made if one requires a further confirmation of the identified victim. If there is no computer package available, the forensic dental expert has to do the comparison manually.

There are a few practical concerns that need discussion in respect to the dental identification process. One such concern is that many developing countries do not keep up to date dental records in archives for various reasons. Therefore it is impossible to perform a scientific comparison and provide a positive opinion. However, all developed countries have a structured organized way of keeping dental and medical records so that in a victim identification process, it is going to be very useful. The other practical issue is that many developing countries do not have forensic dental experts. Consequently, either the authorities have to give up the forensic dental approach or they have to rely on foreign experts. There is a growing demand for this discipline and it is time that developing countries think about training and implementing this discipline.

BITEMARKS ANALYSIS

Bitemarks are imprints made by teeth on inanimate (**Fig. 21.5**) or animate (**Fig. 21.6**) objects. First of all when such a mark is suspected to be a bitemark, a forensic dental expert has to confirm that it is in fact is a 'bitemark'. There can be many types of imprint marks on animate or inanimate objects that can look like bites.

Bitemarks analysis from crime scenes and on victims has been useful in solving scenes. For example, in the Ted Bundy case explained

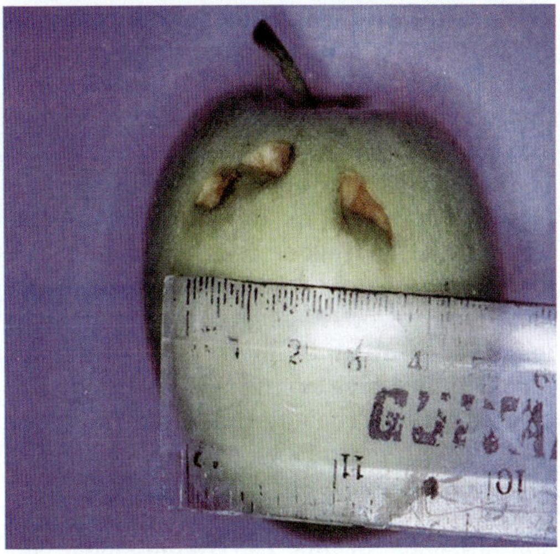

Fig. 21.5: Illustration of a visible bitemark on a fruit. The bitemark shows remarkable indentations which will be useful to identify the biter

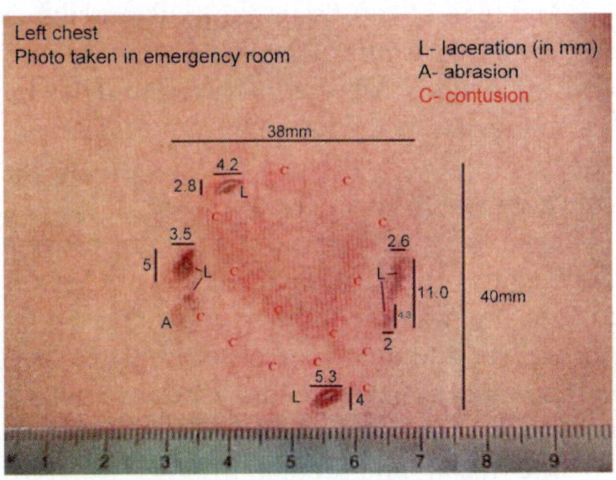

Fig. 21.6: A bitemark appeared in a victim's left chest.
Note: The appearance of a human bite

above, if not for bitemarks evidence, the serial murderer would never have been convicted. There have been many cases in which bitemarks on victims, especially on rape and murder cases, has been critical and very useful. Bitemarks studies have been useful in child abuse cases where parents, guardians, etc. had bitten their children. There are many instances where bitemarks evidence found on fruits, cheese and cigarettes have been used to incriminate the suspect.

In analyzing, the bitemark certain standards and quality need to be maintained.

In practice, it is not the forensic odontologist who observes the bitemark first. It could be a clinician, general practitioner or a judicial medical officer. Later, it will be referred to a forensic dental officer for further examination.

When examining the bitemark, the forensic odontologist must ensure that a swab from the injury has been taken for DNA analysis. If the judicial medical officer or the crime scene investigation team has not obtained a swab from the alleged bitemark, then the forensic dental officer who examines it must take a swab. It may be relevant for the forensic dental officer to take a swab from the suspected bite anyway. In taking a swab, it is highly recommended that forensic odontologists use the double swab technique, then label and preserve the specimen properly. It may be necessary that a buccal swab or a blood sample be taken from the victim as a control for future DNA tests.

Later in analyzing a bitemark the following procedures are important in establishing quality expert evidence:

1. Accurate and complete photograph of the bite should be taken with ABFO "L" scale. When the scale is used it should be used in the same plane as the injury. The scale should be close to the injury. Proper case number/ID number in the picture is also useful.
2. Impressions of the bite injury should be taken with recommended materials whenever it is relevant.
3. In the deceased the tissue specimen of the bite can be preserved as this may provide valuable information.

The principle aim of bitemarks analysis is to ascertain if the dentition of the suspect could produce the bite in question beyond a doubt. In other words, could anybody else with a reasonable probability make the same bite pattern? To answer these questions, the bitemark in question will have to be compared scientifically. The impressions and casts of the suspect's dentition should be taken for comparison and analysis. Before taking the impressions, or examining the suspect, the forensic odontologist should have a proper legal request/order to examine for medicolegal purpose. Even with a request, informed consent of the suspect must be taken for examination and impressions. The suspect has to be informed that the examination findings will be reported to the courts. If the suspect does not provide consent, the odontologist must inform the relevant court of law.

When taking impressions it is recommended to take 2 impressions from each arch, accurately labeled, with a suitable material.

Then sample bites have to be taken from the suspect. The sample bite can be taken to a suitable material to simulate the bite under study.

Then the study casts must be made in recommended materials.

A buccal smear from the suspect can also be taken if DNA studies are to be performed.

It will be mandatory that the bite injury is described properly for medicolegal purposes. In this regards, location of the injury, site, size, shape, color, injury type, and all other relevant data are required.

In analyzing and comparing the bites, several method combinations are used.

- Overlays
- Test bites
- Transillumination studies.

More recently some concerns have been raised with reference to convicting someone solely on bitemark evidence. When traumatised skin will react with an acute inflammatory response distorting the surface marks and patterns. It is therefore prudent while presenting the evidence to courts to also explain the limitations.

MEDICOLEGAL ASPECTS OF DENTAL AND FACIAL INJURIES

Medicolegal examination analysis and interpretation of dental and facial injuries should preferably be performed by a forensic odontologist. In doing this the forensic odontologist should have undergone rigorous training in forensics, dentistry and medicolegal aspects of orofacial traumatology.

The face is a common target of assault and accidents. The upright position of the human and the forward projection of the face, make it more vulnerable. Additionally, the face being a vital area of concern for the human, psychosocially face and mouth is a common target of assault. The causes for facial and dental injuries vary from accidents to violence such as assault.

Dental and facial injuries can be categorized broadly into two types. They are the soft tissue injuries and hard tissue injuries. In almost all jurisdictions hard tissue injuries to face and teeth are categorized as grievous or serious in nature. Depending on the severity of the soft tissue injuries, they too can fall into the grievous category. The face being an important projection in terms of personality and appearance of a person, damages to facial features or its appearance could be considered very serious and grievous in the law. Additionally, the injuries to face and teeth could lead to the death of the person and can endanger a person's life. Therefore proper medicolegal management of dentofacial injuries is important.

Any type of soft tissue injury is possible in the face. Abrasions, lacerations, cut injuries and contusions are commonly found in soft tissue injuries to the face and mouth. Stab and gunshot injuries to the face and mouth are also common due to violence.

The face and mouth contains several important structures such as salivary glands, tongue, temporomandibular joint and important nerves and blood vessels. Damage to these structures can make the injury more serious in the medicolegal sense.

The facial and dental injuries will have their respective long-term and short-term complications. Therefore, it is relevant that the patients are reviewed in prescribed intervals for medicolegal examinations.

Scars on the face, teeth loss, nerve damage and facial deformities will cause serious psychosocial impact for the patient, therefore such injuries will be considered serious in the medicolegal milieu.

The hard tissue injuries to the face include jaw fractures, dental fractures and dislocations of teeth (**Fig. 21.7**) and other facial bone fractures and dislocations. It is not the intention of this chapter to provide details of dental or facial injuries but to provide the medicolegal impact and considerations regarding them. The

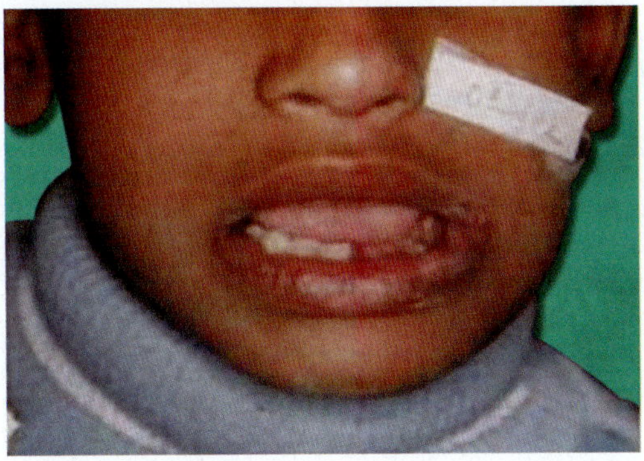

Fig. 21.7: Illustration of soft and hard tissue injuries in the face and teeth. There were several dental fractures, dental evulsions, and a fracture of the mandible. Around the lip note contusions and abrasions. This case was investigated for child abuse

readers are encouraged to refer a standard book on dentofacial injuries for further details.

Medicolegal Aspects of Facial Injuries

Fractures and dislocations of the facial bones are grievous and serous in nature from a medicolegal stand point.

Postmortem facial fractures or distortions could be to hide identity of the victim

All medicolegal examinations of facial or dental injuries will require a medicolegal written report and expert opinion.

Dental injuries include injuries to teeth, gums and supporting tissues. Even a fracture of the enamel is considered to be grievous in nature in a court of law.

As per medicolegal aspects in relation to dental injuries the following points are important and relevant.

- The compatibility of the injuries with the history; people will try to hide a crime or attempt malingering.
- The reconstruction of the event; as to how and in what context the dental injuries could have occurred.
- What weapons could have been used to cause the injury?
- The volatile activity of the person.
- Time of the injury
- The nature of the injury; is it simple, grievous or endangering life?
- Describing the type of dental injury: if it is a crown fracture, root fracture, complicated fracture, luxation, crown-root fracture dislocation, etc.

The law on tooth injuries is insensitive to the severity of the injury, However, the expert opinion will help the court to estimate damages or punishments.

In deciding the time, since the injury it may be relevant to observe radiological and clinical evidence such as healing of the socket, healing of bone, complications of injury and histology.

For medicolegal reasons, the following may be considered to evaluate the seriousness of the dental injury:

- Pain and discomfort
- Possibility of tooth becoming nonvital or loss
- Chances of periapical lesions
- How extensive the restoration and the cost involved?
- The social background/profession of the victim
- Treatment effects
- How long did the victim suffer without normal work?

Sometimes the medicolegal examination of dental injuries will be referred to the practicing forensic dental officer directly via police or courts. Other times, they will be referred by hospital authorities or Judicial Medical Officers.

In reporting dental and facial injuries for medicolegal contexts, it is important to obtain an accurate history giving emphasis to medicolegal aspects. It is important to clinically examine the patient with a detective mind. It is mandatory to read and record all relevant notes of the attending clinician. All investigation findings such as radiographs are important evidence to establish and medicolegally manage the case.

DENTAL FRAUD

Fraud is defined literary as, deliberate misinterpretation and misappropriation of money, services, etc. Dental fraud means such misinterpretations that occur in dentistry. The dental surgeon, dental products, dental drug companies, etc. can be held responsible. In many instances, when the patients face a dental fraud, depending on the jurisdiction, the patients takes administrative or legal actions against the dentist or the dental product. In these situations, a dental expert's inputs are necessary to clarify matters to the inquiry board. As forensic dental officers often deal with legal cases, forensic dental practitioners are often called for evaluation of such a dental fraud claim by the police. Therefore, a forensic dental practitioner should have a sound training in all aspects of dentistry.

ILLEGAL DENTAL PRACTICE

The term illegal dental practice is synonymous with the term quackery. This entity includes unqualified persons practicing dentistry without a due license. In each country, there are laws to prosecute such people and the law enforcement agencies take actions against them. When such inquiries take place, then there may be instances where an expert opinion is required to estimate compensations, damages or punishments. Therefore, forensic odontologists can be called upon to provide expert opinions.

DENTAL NEGLIGENCE AND DENTAL MALPRACTICE

Negligence is the failure to exercise a reasonable degree of skill and care in the management of patients. In other words, commission of an act which a reasonable and a prudent dental surgeon would not commit is defined as negligence. In cases of dental negligence, a forensic dental expert can be summoned to courts to enlighten courts on the science of dentistry and to provide an expert opinion regarding the issue in court.

Dental malpractice is unprofessional conduct of the dental practitioners. Usually, these instances deal with moral conduct of the dental practitioner. These cases are generally dealt by the dental licensing authority to see whether the practitioner has carried out his professional duties in accordance with the moral conduct expected. In such cases, a forensic practitioner could be called upon to provide an opinion to the inquiring authority on a dental or a moral aspect. Forensic dental officers are expected to follow dental ethics and jurisprudence deeper than any other dental practitioner.

AGE ESTIMATIONS

The age estimations are required in many respects in medicolegal scenarios. One main indication for age estimation is in the process of identification. Other indications include:

- *Sexual offenses:* There is a minimum age, a girl can consent for sex. At times, there are instances where deliberately or not, birth details of the child or suspect concerned are missing. In such instances, it is important to assess the biological age using scientific means.
- There are age limits to employment. It may be necessary to assess age when issues of age arise in employment.
- When there are issues about age in children assessed for criminal capacity
- In criminal abortion and infanticide cases where the age of the infant and the separate existence is an issue.

General Identification Purposes

The basis of dental methods of age estimations is the chronological development of teeth. Since humans have a large number of teeth (variable), the opinion based on a large number of variables (teeth) is more reliable. In odontological methods, teeth eruption times, crown development and root development and completions are generally taken in to account (**Fig. 21.8**). As there are two sets of teeth for

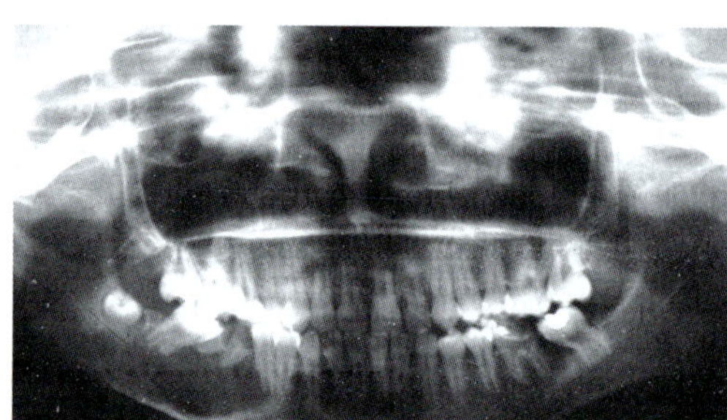

Fig. 21.8: An orthopantomogram used in estimation of age. Observe crown completion, root completion and mixed dentition in different chronological stages

humans, namely deciduous and permanent, it is relevant to have these chronological data for both sets for specific populations.

It must be noted that the chronological data can vary depending on many factors such as ethnicity, social status/nutrition, other medical conditions, genetic factors, etc. Therefore, it is recommended that data should be based on at least ethnic type and socioeconomic status.

In establishing the age both clinical and radiological dental examinations should be done. The estimate of dental age should be compatible with the age estimated using other parameters such as long bone ossification, general examinations, sexual maturation and mental maturity.

Other than the dental eruption and development chronological data of teeth, there are several other dental methods that are used. The attrition of teeth, and the Gustafson method are amongst them. In addition to these, a rough idea about the age can be obtained by examining the alveolar bone loss, the position of dental attrition, fusions of palatal sutures, position of the mental foramen, etc. in a skeletonized body.

DENTAL SURGEON AS AN EXPERT WITNESS

Dental Surgeons undergo a rigorous academic and clinical training in dentistry for years. All jurisdictions in the world accept dental surgeons as expert witnesses on matters pertaining to the field of dentistry. Forensic odontologists, who are essentially dental surgeons, undergo a further specialized training in forensic dentistry. Therefore forensic odontologists are specialists in medicolegal matters pertaining to dentistry. The court generally in the adversarial system considers evidence of ordinary witnesses such as eye witnesses and expert witnesses. Apart from these, the courts rely on productions such as weapons, documents, etc. as documentary/production evidence.

An expert witness has specialized knowledge in a field. In courts, they are able to provide facts they have identified and also to provide opinions. Their opinions have to be evidence based.

Expert witnesses can be summoned for prosecution and/or defense.

As a forensic practitioner, it is important to keep records of all patients examined. After examining the patients the forensic practitioner will have to send a medicolegal report to courts or other legal authorities. In addition, he will have to appear in courts personally and provide oral evidence when summoned to court. In court, the prosecution attorneys and judges ask questions. In addition, the defense lawyer cross examines and asks tricky questions.

When writing reports and answering questions in court, a forensic practitioner should maintain professional standards. When appearing in court an expert must dress appropriately and act professionally.

FORENSIC DENTAL EXTENSIONS

In this section, some applications are discussed which are not exactly in the field of forensic dentistry but it has some links to dentistry. Some forensic dentists engage in these studies and practice based on other extended additional trainings.

Saliva analysis has been in use for decades in crime scene investigations. In this context saliva has been analyzed for its blood grouping, proteins and chemical components which had been useful in the crime scene.

With the advent of DNA technology crime scene investigations increasingly use DNA from various biological samples. In rape and murder cases, where bitemarks present, a smear taken from the victim had matched DNA evidence from the suspect which was very helpful in incriminating the suspect (**Fig. 21.9**).

Lip print analysis has a growing demand in the forensic dental sciences. The principle behind the analysis of lip prints is the same as fingerprint analysis. However, the markers that are looked at in lip prints and fingerprints are different. Lips show a wide variety of print patterns among human individuals and analyzing a lip print found on an object such as a glass, cloth, etc. had been useful to incriminate a suspect (**Fig. 21.10**).

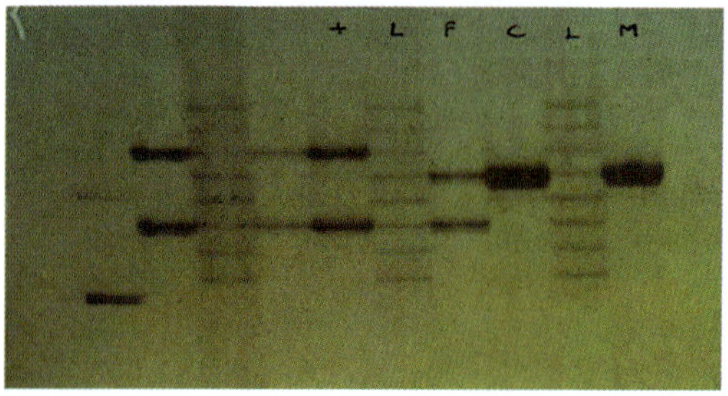

Fig. 21.9: The DNA extracted from teeth especially from skeletonized remains or burnt/charred bodies had been useful to establish the positive identity of the victim. An Illustration of a short tandem repeat (STR), DNA analysis used in forensic practice

Fig. 21.10: Illustration of different lip print patterns. *Note:* The lip print differences in each other

Photographic superimposition is a technique that is used to superimpose an unidentified skull with a suspected victim's photograph. Here the methodology principle is to enlarge the photo to the natural size and superimpose it with the natural size photo of the skull concerned. There will be comparisons of standard facial anthropometry between skull and photograph. In video superimpositioning, the same principles are applied.

Another technique often used in forensic identification is the facial reconstruction. This method is based on the principle that the facial skeletons have individual and ethnic specific features. Here the face is reconstructed manually with clay or via 3D computer techniques with the use of population facial soft tissue thicknesses and then using individual facial characteristics.

As dental surgeons study the anatomy and anthropology of the face in detail, a lot of forensic odontologists tend to engage in photographic superimpositioning and facial reconstruction work for forensic purposes.

Another aspect that a forensic odontologist can engage in is wild life forensics, especially when teeth of endangered species are used illegally. In this regard, the most common aspect is the use of ivory or ivory substitutes. As ivory is of dental origin, a forensic odontologist can analyze the morphology, radiography, chemistry and histology of an ivory in question and provide an opinion regarding its origin.

Another aspect is to determine the sex using dental and facial characteristics especially in skeletonized bodies. It is possible to provide an opinion regarding the race, sex, age, socio-economic state and possible stature by analyzing the dental and facial skeleton. Also in clinical and forensic practice, Barr body detection is done using a buccal smear to determine the sex. It is possible to determine the sex by DNA analysis of a buccal smear taken from a person.

SELF-ASSESSMENT QUESTIONS

1. Briefly explain the nature and the scope of forensic dentistry.
2. What are main roles of a forensic odontologist?
3. What are limitations in forensic dental practice?

4. List the steps involved in the analysis of a bitemark found on a victims thigh.
5. List medicolegal issues stemming out from a dental injury.
6. What is the theoretical basis of dental method of identification? What are its limitations?
7. What constitutes dental negligence? How can dental negligence be minimized in a clinical set up?
8. How does child abuse related to dental practice?
9. What are dentofacial determinants of gender?
10. What is the basis of lip print analysis?

SUGGESTED READING

1. Adams C. The role of forensic dentistry in forensic science: issues and validity. Faculty Dental Journal. 2012;3:199-201.
2. Pretty IA. Forensic dentistry: I Identification of human remains. Dent Update. 2007;34:621-2;624-6; 629-30.
3. Pretty IA. Reliability of bitemark evidence. In Dorian RBJ (Ed). Bitemark evidence. New York. Marcel Dekker; 2005. p. 543.
4. www.abfo.org.

Chapter

22

Laboratory Investigations and their Interpretation

Helen McParland

Chapter Outline

INTRODUCTION

A large number of special investigations and procedures are available for the diagnosis of oral disorders and conditions that may manifest in the oral cavity, some associated with systemic disease. These tests are carried out for screening, to aid diagnosis of an unidentified condition, or to confirm a specific diagnosis. They can also be useful and to monitor progress and assess response to treatment. Special investigations for particular conditions have been discussed in previous chapters but it is helpful to provide an overview of the more routine tests available to the clinician separately in this chapter. Most hematological and biochemical testing is now fully automated and so although average values for all indices will be used throughout it should be noted that reference ranges for specific tests can vary from laboratory to laboratory and between populations. A hemoglobin estimation, count of blood cells and blood film used to be considered sufficient, but now it is recognized that minor changes in the blood can cause oral symptoms at latent stages of hematological disease before showing up in these general indices. So the majority patients attending the clinic will require a full hematological examination: full blood picture, serum ferritin, serum or red cell folate and Vitamin B_{12} estimation. This is especially important in patients complaining of:

- A persistent sore or burning mouth
- A depapillated tongue
- Chelitis, glossitis, mucositis or stomatitis
- Oral ulceration including aphthous stomatitis
- Patients with acute or chronic candidosis
- Those with oral lesions resistant to treatment.

The information in this chapter has been divided into four sections and some information is presented in tabulated form to allow quick reference. In the first three sections the clinical relevance of routine hematological investigations and clinical biochemistry will be explained as well as some aspects of immunological tests relevant to maxillofacial medicine. Blood monitoring to assess toxicity of some of the more commonly used potent drugs in the practice of Oral Medicine is covered in last section.

HEMATOLOGY

Hematology is the study of the blood and the blood forming tissues. Hematological laboratory studies are frequently used when screening patients as they play an important role in understanding the well-being of the patient. The most commonly ordered test is a full blood count. The indices (normal ranges) obtained by performing a FBC are given in **Table 22.1**. The use of these tests is explained separately in the text which follows.

Blood Film

A blood film is made using a peripheral blood sample smeared on a glass slide and by staining the cells (**Table 22.2**). It allows for the examination of physical characteristics of all blood cells by microscopy (**Table 22.2**). Additionally, it helps to detect any parasites in blood or any abnormal cells.

Hemoglobin

Hemoglobin (Hb) is a protein pigment which gives blood its color. It is responsible for the transport of oxygen. Each hemoglobin molecule is composed of four globin chains; two alpha

▪ Table 22.1
The main indices in a full blood count

Indice	*Value*
Hemoglobin (Hb)	13.0–18 g/dL male 12–16 g/dL female
Hematocrit or packed Red cell volume (PCV)	40–54% male 38–47% female
Red cell count (RBC)	4.6–6.2 x 10^{12}/L
Mean cell volume (MCV)	80–98 fl (fl = 10^{-15} liters)
Mean corpuscular hemoglobin (MCH)	26–32 pg
Mean corpuscular hemoglobin concentration (MCHC)	32–36%
Red cell distribution width (RDW)	11.6–14.6%
White cell count (WBC)	4–10 x 10^9/L
Platelets	150–400 x 10^9/L

▪ Table 22.2
Reported hematological features in a blood film and their significance

Description of blood cell	*Explanation*	*Significance*
Microcytic	Small	Iron deficiency anemia
Macrocytic	Large	Pernicious anemia Folate deficiency
Megalocytic	Very large >12 μ	Pernicious anemia Folate deficiency
Anisocytosis	Variation in size	Most anemias
Poikilocytosis	Variation in shape	Most anemias
Spherocytic	Spherical	Congenital anemias-hemolytic
Hypochromic	Pale staining	Iron defiency anemia
Hyperchromic	Densely staining	Pernicious anemia
Target cell	Concentrically stained	Chronic anemias
Reticulocyte	Reticulated	Active response of marrow to demand for more red blood cells
Erythroblast-normoblast	Nucleated, normal size	Excessive red cell production, e.g. hemorrhage, anemia or leukemia
Erythroblast-microblast	Nucleated, small size	As above
Erythroblast-megaloblast	Nucleated, large size	Excessive red cell production, e.g. in pernicious anemia or following gastrectomy
Myelocytes		Primitive cells seen in myeloid leukemia
Myeloblasts		Acute myeloid leukemia
Lymphoblasts		Lymphocytic leukemia

(α) and two beta (β), each of which envelopes a haem molecule which contains a central atom of iron (**Fig. 22.1**). Haem and globin are synthesized in two very different ways and each pathway is precisely controlled. Both processes require certain nutrients, minerals and amino acids to be available. Deficiencies of these micronutrients and minerals can lead to a reduced number of total red cells or a reduced amount of hemoglobin.

The level of hemoglobin is measured as grams per every 100 mL of blood (g/dL). Normal values differ between sexes, 13.0 to 18 g/dL for males and 12 to 16 g/dL females, and are lower in childhood (11 g/dL) and pregnancy (11 g/dL). Normal ranges are a guide and not absolute.

Hemoglobin values, in healthy individuals within a population, show a normal distribution, therefore, a certain number of healthy individuals may fall below a given cut-off point. Also, genetic differences exist between populations regarding hemoglobin levels, e.g. the prevalence of low Hb concentrations is

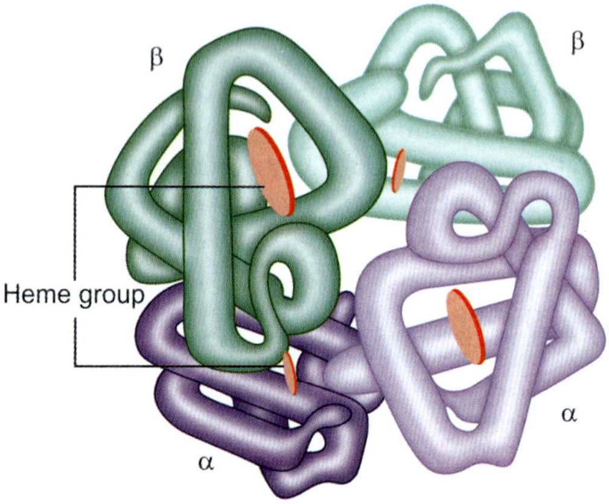

Fig. 22.1: Hemoglobin molecule

higher among African Americans than Caucasian Americans. Furthermore, the hemoglobin level may vary because of a person's biological constitution and the surrounding environmental conditions. In addition to age, gender, and pregnancy additional factors such as smoking and altitude may lead to an increase in the hemoglobin level of healthy individuals.

Disorders of Hemoglobin

Anemia

When the Hb level falls to below normal the patient is said to have anemia. The type of anemia depends on what factor is responsible for the low Hb level. Anemias are more common in people with chronic blood loss, e.g. through menstruation, multiple pregnancies and in the tropics due to hookworm infestations. Anemia is also a feature of some chronic autoimmune diseases, e.g. rheumatoid arthritis.

The most common cause of low levels of hemoglobin is due to nutritional deficiency of iron and to a lesser extent vitamin B_{12} and folic acid. These deficiencies are therefore more common in the middle and low income countries where diet and nutrition is poor, and in strict vegetarians particularly who do not consume regular supplements of minerals and vitamins. Tests to examine hematinics and other blood indices to differentiate anemias will be discussed later in the chapter in the biochemistry section.

Anemia, whatever the cause, can give rise to many general signs and symptoms, the severity of which will depend on two factors; the stage of the anemia and the speed of onset. Patients with mild anemia, Hb > 10 g/dL may have no symptoms, while those with severe anemia, Hb < 6 g/dL invariably do. Those who develop anemia quickly, e.g. as a result of blood loss are more likely to have symptoms than those who develop anemia more slowly as in anemia of chronic disease or in the elderly.

As we will see later, using the other indices in a full blood picture investigation, in addition to Hb, helps us to diagnose anemia and to ascertain its cause. For example:

- Measurement of RBC and PCV help to identify anemia but do not help to distinguish between the causes of anemia.
- Measurement of MCV, and RDW along with microscopic features of the red cells (in the blood film) helps to identify the cause of the anemia. Using the MCV result, we can classify anemia into 3 types: microcytic (low MCV), normocytic (normal MCV), macrocytic (high MCV).
- Microcytic anemias are usually as a result of iron deficiency or thalassemia. To help distinguish between the two we can look at the RDW. This is normally raised in iron deficiency but normal in thalassemia.
- Anemia of chronic disease, e.g. rheumatoid arthritis, malignancy, hemolytic anemia and aplastic anemia are associated with a normocytic picture. The RDW in chronic disease is typically normal but is raised in hemolytic anemia so this can be helpful to distinguish the two.
- Macrocytic anemias are caused by vitamin B_{12} and folate deficiency and tests to help distinguish between the two are discussed later in the chapter.
- A blood film (**Fig. 22.2**) indicates an alteration of cell size as well as color, i.e. whether the RBCs are microcytic or macrocytic (by their cell size) and hyperchromic or hypochromic (by their color) (**Figs 22.3A and B**).

There are also several hereditary disorders that may affect the hemoglobin level. The most common of these are thalassemia and sickle cell anemia. Because they are hereditary disorders, the resulting anemia is not correctable, but early detection can significantly reduce complications and genetic counseling can control inheritance. If a hereditary disorder is suspected additional investigations such as electrophoresis may be indicated to examine the hemoglobin molecule in detail.

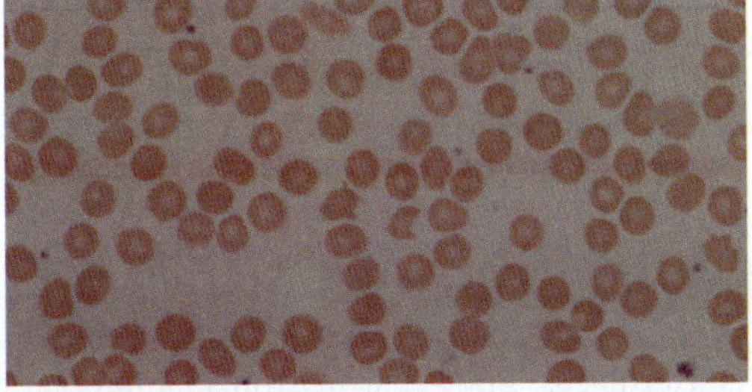

Fig. 22.2: A blood film showing normal red cells

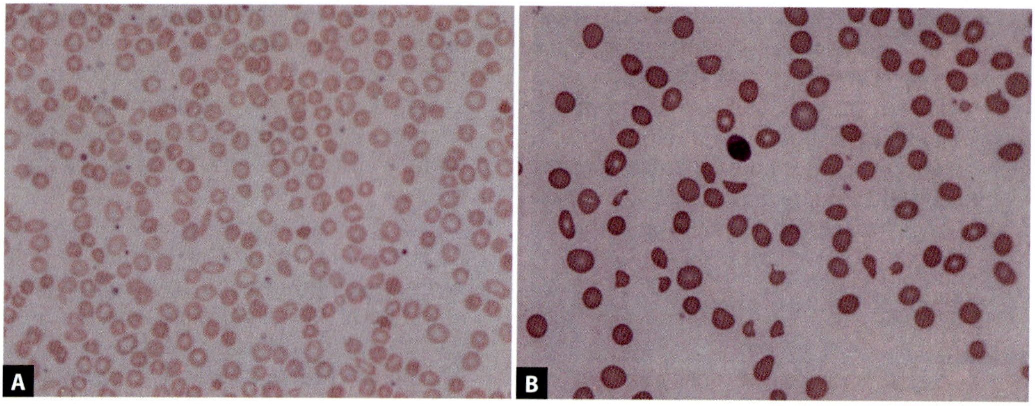

Figs 22.3A and B: Red cells (erythrocytes) showing. (A) microcytosis (large pale areas within RBCs); (B) Macrocytosis (Large RBCs, some oval shaped)

Thalassemia

Thalassemia is a group of inherited disorders in which there is deficient synthesis of either α or β globin chains (*see* **Fig. 22.1**). The result is a low hemoglobin (Hb) value causing a microcytic anemia in the presence of normal iron levels. Over 150 genetic defects have been identified.

Thalassemia is most prevalent in parts of Africa, Mediterranean countries, the Middle East, Indian subcontinent and South East Asia. Depending on which chain is affected thalassemia can be divided into β thalassemia or α thalassemia.

β-Thalassemia Minor

When a defective β globin chain is inherited from only one parent the patient is said to have β thalassemia minor or trait. As the patient also has normal β globin chains, synthesis of normal Hb is increased to help to maintain a normal Hb. Affected women are at risk of anemia during pregnancy.

β-Thalassemia Major

When defective β chains are inherited from both parents severe anemia develops shortly after birth. Repeated transfusions are needed to prevent death. Iron overload from the treatment is a problem. Bone marrow transplantation is another treatment option.

α-Thalassemia

The defect in α thalassemia is caused by impaired production of α globin chains and the degree of severity depends on how many α globin chains are missing. The severest form in which 4 α chains are missing is incompatible with life. Less severe cases cause anemia in varying degrees.

Laboratory findings for all thalassemias:

- MCV low
- MCH low
- Hb normal or low
- Normal test for iron
- RDW normal.

Sickle Cell Anemia

In sickle cell anemia a gene defect causes the production of abnormal hemoglobin HbS with two normal α globin chains and two abnormal β globin chains. HbS makes the red blood cells deform at low oxygen tensions into the familiar sickle shape that gives the condition its name (**Figs 22.4A and B**).

If the gene is inherited from just one parent, over half the hemoglobin synthesized will be normal HbA. This is named sickle trait and sufferers may not necessarily be anemic although care is needed during general anesthesia.

In sickle cell disease both parents pass on the faulty gene and most of the hemoglobin is

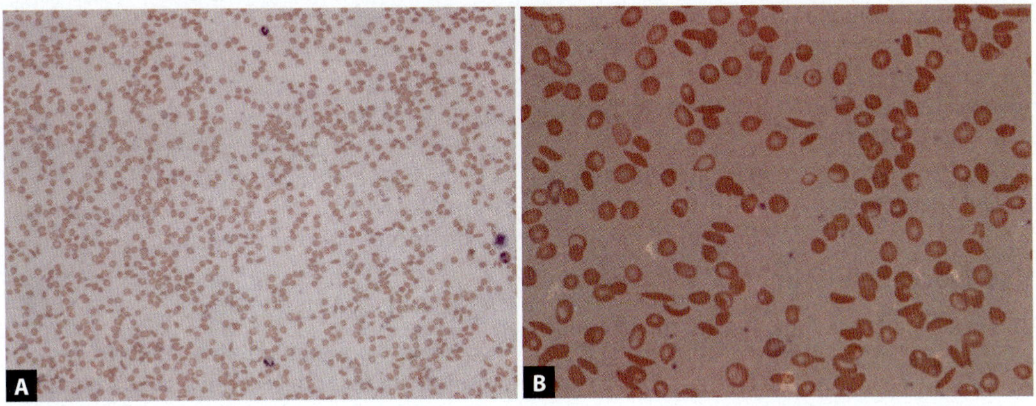

Figs 22.4A and B: A blood film showing sickle cells in a patient with sickle cell disease (HbSS)

abnormal HbS. The expression of the disease varies greatly from one individual to the other with some dying in childhood, while others lead a relatively normal life. In between are those who suffer from hemolytic anemia with periods of good health interspersed by periods of painful sickle cell crises. Sickle cell disease is most commonly found in Africa, West Indies, the Middle East and India.

Porphyria

This rare inherited or acquired disorder, named from the Greek word porphyria—meaning purple—is not a single disease but a group of disorders caused by defects in enzymes needed at the various stages of haem synthesis. Each porphyria is caused by a slightly different enzyme deficiency with a different pattern of resulting symptoms. They are mostly inherited as autosomal defects.

Porphryias can be clinically classified into acute, affecting the liver/nervous system, non-acute affecting the skin, and mixed forms.

King George III of England was thought to have porphyria, having been reported to have had symptoms of abdominal pain, rashes, purple urine, and psychotic episodes that are consistent with the condition. Whether the King had porphyria or not, is now a topic for debate.

Urine porphyrin studies are the mainstay in the diagnosis of acute porphyria attacks. Blood tests for specific porphyrins may be useful in non-acute conditions. The genetic defects causing porphyria have all been identified and testing is available to check carrier status in the family members of those who are affected. Porphyria can present with orofacial anomalies, and developmental anomalies of teeth can be pronounced.

Some drugs are absolutely contraindicated in porphyria. These include many general anesthetic agents, carbamazepine, tricyclic antidepressants, azole antifungals, doxycycline, erythromycin, flucloxacillin and sulfonamides. For local anesthesia bupivacaine is considered safe; lidocaine and prilocaine can be used with caution. Midazolam is considered safe but other benzodiazepines are contraindicated.

Hematocrit or Packed Cell Volume

This is the volume of red cells as a proportion of the blood, measured after the blood is centrifuged.

A low hematocrit may indicate anemia, blood loss, over-hydration or nutritional deficiency. It may also be seen in bone marrow failure, leukemia, multiple myeloma, and rheumatoid arthritis.

A high hematocrit may indicate dehydration (for example, due to burns or severe diarrhea), eclampsia (a serious condition that can occur during pregnancy) or polycythemia.

To properly interpret the packed cell volume (PCV) however, you also need to know the mean cell volume (MCV) and red blood cell count (RBC). For example, if the PCV is high, the question arises: is this secondary to an increased amount of red cells (high RBC), larger cells (high MCV) or both?

Normal range: Males 40 to 54 percent, females 38 to 47 percent.

Red Blood Cell Count

The red blood cell (RBC) is the total number of red cells, in every liter of blood measured in 10^{12}/L. Low numbers of red blood cells may indicate anemia as a result of blood loss, bone marrow failure, malnutrition, e.g. iron deficiency, or over-hydration with IV fluids. Abnormally high numbers of red blood cells may be seen in congenital heart disease, some lung diseases, dehydration, kidney disease or polycythemia.

Polycythemia

Polycythemia can be primary or secondary depending on the cause of the increase in red cell numbers. It is worth noting that a contraction in blood volume can cause apparent or relative polycythemia.

Primary Polycythemia

Primary polycythemia, or polycythemia vera as it is sometimes known, is a rare condition with peak incidence between 50–70 years. Males are slightly more affected than females. It is a malignant disease of the bone marrow causing marked overproduction of red cells (white cell and platelet numbers may be also raised). Symptoms of polycythemia vera (PV) are often insidious in onset and are due to the huge increase in red cell numbers which causes the blood to become more viscous. This leads to many symptoms including hypertension, headaches, dizziness, vertigo, visual disturbances, angina and intermittent claudication. Patients are at risk from venous thrombosis and stroke. The increase in red cell numbers result in a characteristic ruddy complexion and redness of the palms, nail-beds, mucosa, and conjunctiva. Splenomegaly is also present in many patients.

Laboratory findings

- High Hb
- High PCV
- High platelet count
- High WBC (particularly granulocytes)
- Low level erythropoietin (EPO)
- Increased red cell mass (tested in nuclear medicine—rarely carried out).

Secondary Polycythemia

Secondary polycythemia is defined as an absolute increase in red blood cell mass that is caused by enhanced stimulation of red blood cell production. It can be congenital for example in cyanotic heart disease where blood is less oxygenated due to defects or malformations in the heart, or acquired due to the following:

- Living at high altitude where the air has less oxygen
- Chronic lung disease
- Cigarette smoking, due to the presence of carbon monoxide in the blood which displaces oxygen from hemoglobin
- Erythropoietin-secreting tumors especially of the kidney.

Symptoms and clinical findings in secondary polychythemia will depend on the cause of the disease but again are caused by increased blood viscosity, similar to primary polycythemia. Slenomegalogy is rare.

Laboratory findings

- High Hb
- High PCV
- High platelet count
- High white cell count (particularly granulocytes)
- High level erythropoietin (EPO)
- Increased red cell mass (tested in nuclear medicine by labeling red cells—rarely carried out).

Treating the underlying cause, if possible, is the treatment of choice but phlebotomy or bloodletting is the mainstay of treatment for primary and secondary polycythemia. The object is to remove the excess cellular elements, mainly red blood cells, from the blood to improve the circulation and reduce blood viscosity. Unfortunately the effect of phlebotomy is only transient and so has to be repeated regularly. Patients with PCV values of less than 70 percent may be bled twice a week to reduce the hematocrit (PCV) to the range of less than 45 percent. The frequency may have to be increased for severe cases.

Mean Cell Volume

This is the average volume of red cells. The size of cells is a useful indicator when evaluating anemia or when monitoring a secondary effect of drugs.

The mean cell volume (MCV) will be reduced when the size of the red cells decreases, e.g. in iron deficiency anemia when the cells become smaller than normal (microcytic) (*see* **Fig. 22.3A**). A low MCV may also be present in pregnancy, in a hemoglobinopathy such as thalassemia, and in anemia due to blood cell destruction or bone marrow disorders.

In anemia of chronic disease, e.g. rheumatoid arthritis or Sjögrens syndrome the MCV will be normal (normocytic) or low.

A high MCV may indicate anemia due to nutritional deficiencies for example vitamin B_{12} or folate deficiency. These will be discussed in more detail later on in the chapter. It may also be a sign of bone marrow abnormalities, liver disease, alcoholism, and chronic lung disease. Therapy with certain medications can cause a raised MCV; for example Dapsone, used in the treatment of vesicullobullous disease. Dapsone can cause hemolysis of blood cells which triggers the early release of immature red blood cells, reticulocytes, into the blood. Because they are larger than mature red cells, the MCV rises.

Normal values: 80 to 98 femoliters (fL = 10–15 liters) for both males and females.

Mean Corpuscular Hemoglobin and Concentration

The mean corpuscular hemoglobin (MCH) is the hemoglobin content of the average red cell. The mean corpusular hemoglobin and concentration (MCHC) is the average hemoglobin concentration in a given volume of packed red cells. These indices are two ways of expressing the average amount of hemoglobin in a red cell and are useful in the investigation of anemia.

The MCH may be low in types of anemia where the red blood cells are abnormally small (e.g. in iron deficiency anemia) or high in other types of anemia where the red blood cells are enlarged (for example, as a result of folic acid or vitamin B_{12} deficiency).

The MCHC is low in iron deficiency, blood loss, pregnancy and anemia caused by chronic disease.

Normal values: MCH 26 to 32 pg, MCHC 20 to 35 percent.

Red Cell Distribution Width

Red cell distribution width (RDW) is a measurement of the variability of red blood cell size. It is expressed as a percentage and higher numbers indicate greater variation in size. The RDW can be useful when there is a wide variety of cell sizes which could make the overall average look normal.

Normal value: 10 to 15.

White Blood Cells (Leukocytes)

White cells, like red cells, are derived from stem cells in the bone marrow. Their total numbers tend to increase for physiological reasons, i.e. stress, extreme cold or heat or exercise and pregnancy, as well as in infection, inflammation, trauma or after hemorrhage, and in leukemia and other malignancy.

A reduction in white cells (leukopenia) is less common and can imply a reduction in the ability to fight infection. A low white cell count can occur spontaneously but can also be caused by drug therapy (**Table 22.3**) (e.g. azathioprine causes suppression of T lymphocytes), some autoimmune diseases, viral infections, and diseases of the bone marrow (such as marrow aplasias and widespread disseminated bony metastases). Total WBC count is a rough approximate screening tool; it is often useful to have the relative numbers of the different white cells (differential white cell count) (**Table 22.4**).

The white cell population is made up of 5 morphologically and functionally different cells

▪ Table 22.4
Systemic medications which may affect the white cell count (WBC)

Drugs that may increase WBC count	*Drugs that may lower WBC count*
Allopurinol	Antibiotics
Aspirin	Anticonvulsants
Chloroform	Antihistamines
Corticosteroids	Antithyroid drugs
Epinephrine	Arsenicals
Heparin	Barbiturates
Quinine	Chemotherapy drugs
Triamterene	Diuretics
	Sulfonamides

comprising neutrophils, eosinphils, basophils, monocytes and lymphocytes (**Figs 22.5A to D**). The total white cell count (WBC) is the number of all the white cells. Normal values are shown in **Table 22.4**.

Neutrophils

Neutrophils are the most common blood cells comprising between 40 to 70 percent of the total white cells. Their function is to enter tissues and kill invading bacteria, usually by phagocytosis. Their numbers rise and fall in similar circumstances to the total white cell count. In those with neutrophil counts less than 0.5×10^9 there is risk of serious uncontrolled bacterial infection. Some Afro-Caribbeans have a low neutrophil count as a racial variant.

Eosinophils

Eosinophils comprise only 0.2 to 5 percent of the total white cell counts. They are important in targeting foreign material too large for normal phagocytosis, for example parasitic worms. They are involved in inflammation caused by allergy and are found in large numbers in the airways of those who suffer from asthma or hay fever. Their numbers are also increased in lymphoma and some skin diseases.

Basophils

Basophils go rapidly to the tissues where they mature to become mast cells so are rarely seen in a blood film. Mast cells, when activated, produce inflammatory mediators to attract neutrophils, histamine to dilate blood vessels,

▪ Table 22.4
Differential white cell count and observed changes in infective and other disorders

	Normal range	*Increased*	*Decreased*
Neutrophils	2.5–7.5 x 10^9/L	Acute bacterial infections Acute inflammation, e.g. Rh arthritis Tissue damage: Surgery, burns, MI Solid tumors, e.g. lung cancer Physiological: Exercise, pregnancy Chronic myeloid leukemia(CML)	Viral infection, e.g. (HIV, hepatitis) Severe bacterial infection Aplastic anemia Acute leukemia
Eosinophils	0.04–0.44 x 10^9/L	Parasitic worm infections, e.g. tape worm Allergic disease, e.g. hay fever, asthma Hodgkins lymphoma (not always)	
Basophils	0.01–0.10 x 10^9/L	Rare Raised in CML	
Monocytes	0.2–0.8 x 10^9/L	Rare bacterial infections, e.g. TB	
Lymphocytes	1.5–4.0 x 10^9/L	Infectious mononucleosis Viral infections, e.g. early HIV infection Chronic bacterial infections Miscellaneous infections, e.g. toxoplasmosis Ch lymphocytic leukemia Non-Hodgkin's lymphoma	AIDS SLE Acute inflammation Influenza Burns, trauma, surgery Congenital disorders Drug-induced

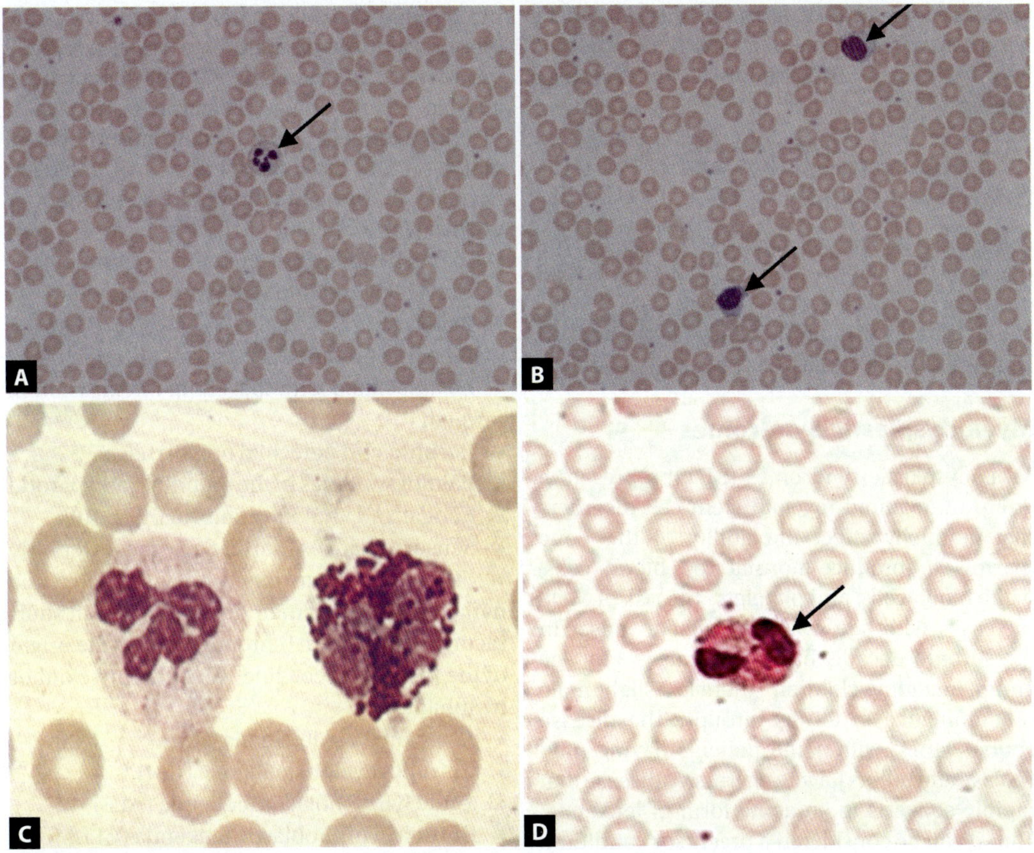

Figs 22.5A to D: White blood cells. (A) Neutrophil; (B) Lymphocytes; (C) Basophil; (D) Eosinophil

and heparin needed in the early stages of the repair process.

Monocytes

Monocytes are the largest cells in the white blood cell population and comprise 1 to 5 percent of the total number. In the tissues they mature to macrophages which are involved in phagocytosis in a similar way to neutrophils. They have a second important function in the presentation of antigens to T lymphocytes in cell mediated immunity. Their numbers are increased in infection, granulomatous disorders, e.g. sarcoidosis, collagen diseases and malignancy.

Lymphocytes

Lymphocytes comprise between 20 to 40 percent of the total white cells. They are derived in the bone marrow, and are the second most abundant white cell. Approximately 70 percent of the lymphocytes are processed in the thymus, (which along with bone marrow is primary lymphoid tissue) and become T lymphocytes. Most of the remaining lymphocytes are named B lymphocytes. They complete their maturation as they leave the bone marrow and go to the secondary lymphoid tissue (spleen and lymph nodes), a tiny proportion called natural killer (NK) lymphocytes are non-B and non-T lymphocytes. Lymphocytes are required for mounting immunity to infection which they do by recognizing and reacting to antigens. Total numbers of lymphocytes fall in some infections, with HIV, and with drug therapy. A severe reduction in lymphocytes leads to opportunist infection by viruses, fungi and bacteria and can be life threatening as seen in AIDS. Lymphocyte numbers will rise in some infections (e.g. in response to a viral or bacterial threat) and in lymphoid types of leukemia. Different subsets of lymphocytes are discussed in the immunology section.

White Blood Cell Count and Differential Count

Differential white cell count is helpful in the diagnosis of infective and other disorders and observed changes are given in **Table 22.4**. A WBC count should be immediately performed if leukemia is suspected as a cause of oral ulceration.

Myelodysplastic Syndromes

Myelodysplastic syndromes (MDS) represent a group of acquired myeloid stem cell disorders that gradually affect the ability of the bone marrow to produce normal red blood cells, white blood cells, and platelets. The risk of MDS increases with age, with the median onset in the seventh decade, but may occur in any age group, including children. There is a slight male predominance in all age groups. The disease course varies, with some patients having mild disease and others having aggressive disease that rapidly converts to an acute form of leukemia. Thus it can be considered a precursor condition.

Myelodysplastic syndrome (MDS) can be classified as primary (no known exposure) or secondary following treatment with radiation, alkylating agents, or topoisomerase II inhibitors, and in those heavily irradiated before bone marrow transplants.

The majority of patients with MDS present with fatigue due to anemia, but sometimes the diagnosis is made as a result of unexplained macrocytosis or pancytopenia. Patients may also present with petechiae, ecchymoses, and nose or gingival bleeding as a consequence of severe thrombocytopenia (platelet count $<10 \times 10^9$/liter) or, when neutrophils counts drop to $<1 \times 10^9$/liter, with infections, e.g. bacterial pneumonia or skin abscesses.

Leukemia

Leukemia is a malignant disease of the bone marrow in which there is unrestrained proliferation of one clone of immature white blood cell at the expense of normal blood cell production. The resulting pancytopenia causes anemia because of a reduction in red cells, bleeding tendency due to lower numbers of platelets, and an increased risk of infection because of the reduction in the number of normal white cells.

Oral manifestations of leukemia include:

- Cervical lympadenopathy
- Pallor
- Bleeding and ulcerated gingivae, which may be associated with loosening or extrusion of teeth
- Purpura and petechial hemorrhages
- Painful swellings in the mandible and parotid
- Fungal and viral infections of the mouth
- Sensory changes (particularly the lower lip)

There are four main types of leukemia named by whether their disease course in short (acute) or long term (chronic), and by the origin of the malignant cell line, i.e. either myeloid or lymphatic:

- Acute myeloid leukemia (AML)
- Chronic myeloid leukemia (CML)
- Acute lymphoblastic leukemia (ALL)
- Chronic lymphoblastic leukemia (CLL).

Leukemia is diagnosed by FBC, differential WBC and examination of a blood film. **Table 22.5** shows the main features of the different leukemias and the expected features of the blood results of each.

Tests of Clotting Function

For normal hemostasis to occur it is essential to have adequate numbers of normally functioning platelets and an intact blood clotting cascade.

The clinician may wish to check clotting function in patients who report, or present with:

- Excessive bleeding following past extractions
- Excessive bruising
- Oral purpura
- Spontaneous hemorrhage from the gingivae
- Petechial hemorrhages in the skin
- Patients taking anticoagulants, e.g. warfarin before surgery.

▪ Table 22.5
Comparison of the symptoms, changes noted in the blood picture and possible oral manifestations in different types of leukemias

	AML	*CML*	*ALL*	*CLL*
Age of onset	Most common acute leukemia. Rare in childhood incidence increases with age	15–20 percent of all leukemias, most common 40–60 years	Mostly occurs in childhood with peak incidence at 4 years	30 percent of all leukemias, occurs in patients over 50 years
Main symptoms	Tiredness due to anemia, fever, bleeding tendency	Slow progress of disease, fatigue, breathlessness due to anemia, bleeding, night sweats	Acutely ill; tiredness due to anemia, fever, bleeding, headaches and vomiting due to CNS involvement	Either symptomless or fatigue, breathlessness due to anemia, bleeding, night sweats
Blood picture	Pancytopaenia WBC: Normal or Blast cells, ↑ Auer rods* Normocytic anemia Platelets ↓	WBC ↑ Neutrophils ↑ Myelocytes ↑ Basophils ↑ Normocytic anemia Platelets normal/ or ↑	Pancytopenia WBC: Normal or Blast cells Normocytic or Macrocytic anemia Platelets ↑	WBC ↑ Isolated lymphocytes Anemia Hypogammaglobulinemia (2/3 monoclonal IgM) Platelets normal/or ↓
Oral manifestations	Oral bleeding (spontaneous) Mucosal pallor Gingival swelling—localized or general ulceration of mucosae or gingivae	Oral bleeding Mucosal pallor Liability to infections *Swelling:* Lacrimal and salivary glands Rarely granulocytic sarcoma of jaws	Oral bleeding Mucosal pallor Gingival swelling Ulceration Pericoronitis lympadenopathy Infections: *Herpes zoster* *Candida* Gram-negative Swellings: mandible, parotids extrusion of teeth	Oral bleeding Mucosal pallor Gingival swelling Ulceration *Infections:* *Herpes zoster* *Candida* *Swellings:* Palate (sumucosal leukemic nodules)

*Auer rods are clumps of granular material that form elongated needles seen in the cytoplasm of leukemic blasts.

A brief summary of clotting function and the relevance of laboratory tests to check clotting function will now be discussed.

Platelets

Platelets like red and white blood cells are produced in the bone marrow but are smaller (1–2 um) and have no nucleus. Their main function, following vessel injury is to plug "holes" in damaged vessel walls by adhering to them. Von Willebrand's factor, released from the blood vessel walls, facilitates this process. Platelets also secrete substances necessary for the clotting cascade (explained below). Platelet numbers are included in a FBP or FBC.

Normal values: 150–400 × 10^9/L (Critical values: ≤ 40 × 10^9/L or ≥ 1000 × 10^9/L).

Reduced Platelet Numbers

Since platelets are required for hemostasis, a severe reduction in their numbers can lead to excessive hemorrhage. Clinically spontaneous

Table 22.6
Factors I–XIII involved in the blood clotting cascade and their origins

Factor	*Name*	*Pathway*	*Notes*
I	Fibrinogen	Common	Glycoprotein made in the liver
II	Prothrombin	Common	Proenzyme made in the liver
III	Tissue factor	Extrinsic	Protein present in tissue
IV	Calcium	All pathways	Ion cofactor needed for conversion of prothrombin to thrombin and for activation of factor X
V	Labile factor	Common	Cofactor needed for conversion of prothrombin to thrombin
VI	*Does not exist now*		
VII	Proconvertin stable factor	Extrinsic	Proenzyme made in the liver
VIII	Antihemophillia factor	Intrinsic and extrinsic	Protein cofactor needed for activation of factor X
IX	Christmas factor	Intrinsic	Proenzyme made in the liver
X	Stuart factor	Intrinsic and extrinsic	Proenzyme made in the liver
XI	Plasma thromboplastin	Intrinsic	Proenzyme
XII	Hageman factor/contact factor	Intrinsic	Proenzyme
XIII	Fibrin stabilizing factor		Proenzyme

bleeding can occur if numbers fall below 40 × 109/L and can be fatal if numbers fall below 5 × 109/L. The causes of a reduction in platelets are as follows:

- Reduced production in the bone marrow as in aplastic anemia, acute leukemia, radiotherapy and chemotherapy, in advanced cancer and to a minor extent in vitamin B_{12} or folic acid deficiency.
- Increased platelet destruction; immune thrombocytopenic purpura (ITP) is the most common cause which can arise in healthy or secondary to other conditions, e.g. SLE, HIV or chronic lymphatic leukemia, and as a result of viral illness.
- Increased rate of consumption, for example, in disseminated intravascular coagulation (DIC) which is a complication of many severe diseases including septicemia, cancer, major trauma or surgery, obstetric disorders, incompatible blood transfusions, or as a side effect of drugs, e.g. anti-inflammatories, antibiotics (sulfonamides, penicillin) and some diuretics (frusemide and acetazolamide).

Blood Clotting Cascade

While platelets aggregate at the site of injury, fibrin is produced by the blood clotting cascade. In this cascade, clotting factors, which are mainly pro enzymes named in roman numerals in the order they were discovered are activated in sequence (**Table 22.6**). There are two pathways an intrinsic pathway and an extrinsic pathway which lead to activation of factor X (**Fig. 22.6**). This activated factor X is necessary for the final common pathway in which fibrinogen is converted to fibrin. Some factors act as cofactors within the cascade e.g. factor VIII, factor V and factor IV.

A range of clotting function tests should be included for the purpose of investigating the potential for a bleeding disorder, or for monitoring anticoagulation therapy. The most commonly ordered tests are prothrombin time (PT), activated partial thromboplastin time (APTT) and thrombin time (TT) (**Table 22.7**). They all test the ability of the blood to make a fibrin clot via the clotting cascade. The PT test specifically measures the extrinsic and common

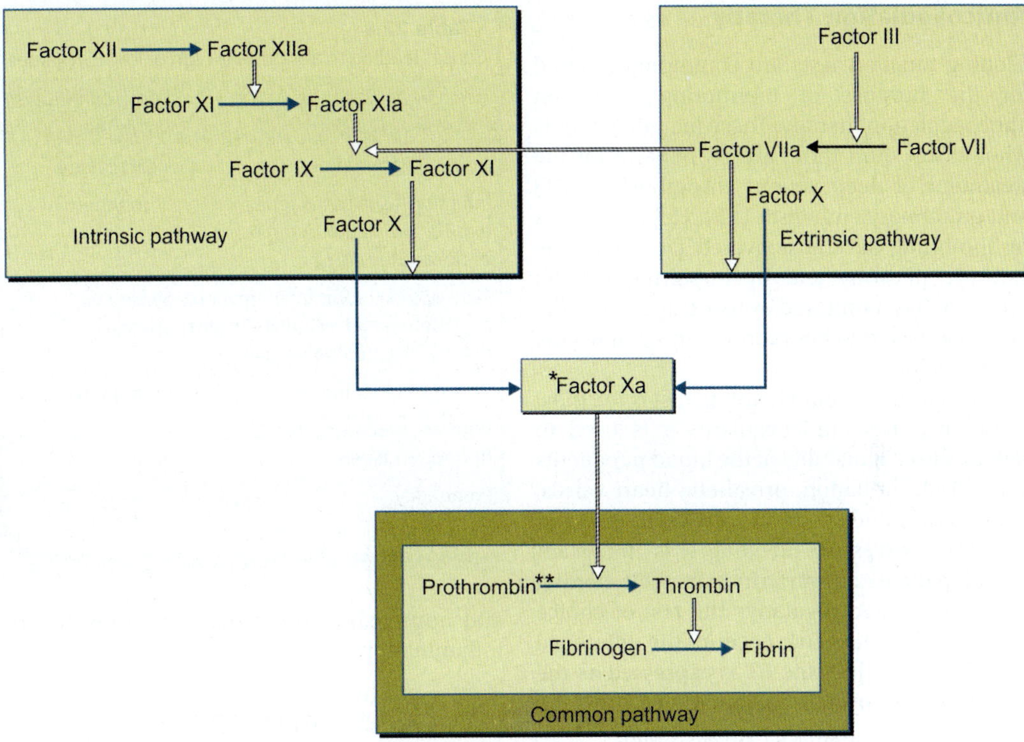

*Cofactors VIII and IV (calcium) are required for activation of Factor X.
**Cofactors V and IV (calcium) required for the activation of prothrombin to thrombin.
The letter (a) after factor denotes activation.

Fig. 22.6: The blood clotting cascade involved in the generation of fibrin

pathways. The APTT is a measure of the intrinsic and common pathways. Finally TT measures the final stage in the common pathway.

An increase in PT, APTT or TT indicates a deficiency in one or more of the clotting factors. The deficiency can be inherited as in hemophilia A where the deficiency is Factor VIII, or Hemophilia B also known as Christmas disease, in which there is a deficiency of Factor IX. More commonly the deficiency is acquired as the result of mainly liver disease. The clotting cascade is dependent on a normally functioning liver since many of the factors are synthesized there, so many liver diseazes, e.g. acute or chronic hepatitis and cirrhosis affect clotting. PT, APTT and TT can all be raised in liver disease but PT is the most sensitive marker.

Vitamin K is also required for the synthesis of some factors. It is derived from dietary sources and also synthesized by bacteria in the gut so a normally functioning gastrointestinal tract is also essential. Deficiency of Vitamin K is associated with a rise in PT and APTT; TT is normal.

PT, APTT and TT are all raised in DIC and after massive blood transfusion.

▪ Table 22.7
Tests useful in assessing normal/abnormal blood clotting

Test	*Normal value*	*Critical value*	*Clotting pathway*
PT	10–14 seconds	>30 seconds	Extrinsic and common
APTT	30–40 seconds	>78 seconds	Intrinsic and common
TT	14–16 seconds		Common

Anticoagulation Therapy

Clotting function tests are commonly ordered for the purpose of monitoring those on anticoagulation therapy. These include patients who, in the short term, are on heparin for the treatment of deep venous thrombosis (DVT) and pulmonary embolism (PE). Heparin works by inhibiting several activated factors in the extrinsic pathway and by impairing platelet function. It is monitored by using the APTT. The dose is adjusted to between 1.5 and 2 times the normal value.

Warfarin, a vitamin K antagonist is the most commonly used anticoagulant. It is used to reduce the coagulability of the blood in patients with atrial fibrillation, prosthetic heart valves, antiphospholipid syndrome, DVT, etc. In order to prevent excessive bleeding it is important that all patients on warfarin have their clotting function checked regularly. The test of choice is the PT but to take into account the difference in laboratory values the PT is expressed as the International Normalized Ratio (INR).

$$\text{INR} = \frac{\text{Patient's PT (in seconds)}}{\text{Mean normal PT (in seconds)}}$$

Most patients are maintained between 2.0 to 3.0, and keep a record of their INR in a book given to them for the purpose. If a dental extraction or minor oral surgery is planned, warfarin should be continued because the risk of a thromboembolic incident outweighs the risk of bleeding which can be controlled by local measures. The INR should be tested within 3 days of the surgery, ideally on the same day, and should be 4.0 or below.

Erythrocyte Sedimentation Rate

When uncoagulated blood is placed in a long narrow test tube the red cells settle at the bottom leaving a fluid level above. The measurement from the top of the sedimented blood to the top of the fluid is called the ESR and is expressed in mm. Normal values are 15 mm/hour in men and up to 20 mm/hour in women. The rate of fall is influenced by the ability of red cells to agglutinate (clump together). Factors that cause an increase in agglutination cause the ESR to rise (**Table 22.8**). The test is nonspecific and nonsensitive but remains a useful test of inflammation.

Table 22.8
Causes leading to abnormally high or low ESR values

The ESR tends to rise in the following situations	*Some conditions lower the ESR*
Acute inflammation	Heart failure
Infection usually bacterial, e.g. TB, sub acute bcterial endocarditis	Polycythemia
Flare ups in chronic inflammation, e.g. rheumatoid arthritis, Crohns disease, SLE, ulcerative colitis	Sickle-cell anemia
In response to injury	Cryoglobulinemia
With an increase in blood fibrinogen levels	
Pregnancy	
Neoplastic conditions	

CLINICAL BIOCHEMISTRY

Clinical Biochemistry is concerned with the measurement of chemicals (inorganic ions, carbohydrates, lipids, hormones and enzymes, etc.) in the blood to aid with diagnosis and monitoring of disease. Other body fluids, e.g. urine, feces, cerebrospinal fluid are also sent for biochemical analysis and are beyond the scope of this chapter but testing of urine in the clinic will be covered at the end of the section.

In an oral medicine clinic commonly ordered tests in addition to full blood count, include those to check hematinics, renal and liver function (particularly important if the oral physician is considering the use of systemic drugs), endocrine function (for diabetes and thyroid function) and metabolic bone disease. Utility of these tests are presented below:

Hematinics

Iron, vitamin B_{12} and folate are collectively known as the hematinics. These micronutrients are essential for the production of healthy red cells. Many patients in the oral medicine clinic will be tested for deficiencies in the hematinics as well as a full blood picture.

▪ Table 22.9
Serological tests for measuring iron status

Tests	*Normal value*	*Notes*
Serum ferritin	12–300 μg/dL	A level below 12 μg/dL signifies iron deficiency. Serum ferritin is raised in iron overload and also in anemic/normal subjects if there is liver damage or disease.
Serum iron	50–150 μg/dL	Measures the amount of iron bound to transferrin
TIBC measures the capacity of transferrin to bind iron	240–360 μg/dL but decreases in people over 70 years to 250 μg/dL	TIBC increases in iron deficiency as the transferrin has more available binding sites. Levels may be normal in chronic disease or malnutrition so this is a drawback of TIBC and it is now rarely assayed
Transferrin saturation	20–40% saturation is highest in the morning	This is not measured but is a ratio of the serum iron and TIBC. It is low in iron deficiency $\% \text{ transferrin saturation} = \frac{\text{Serum iron}}{\text{TIBC}} \times 100$

Iron

Each day 20 to 25 mg of iron are needed for hemopoiesis. It is essential for hemoglobin production and function. As we have seen, iron deficiency causes microcytic anemia with small hypochromic cells seen on a blood film. Iron is present in meat, whole grain cereals, leafy green vegetables and pulses. The amount of iron absorbed each day is affected by the type of iron in the diet, other foods eaten concurrently that may chelate iron, the gastric acidity, the activity of the bone marrow and the existing iron stores. It is absorbed in the small intestine mainly in the duodenum and upper jejunum, and is then transported to the blood. Defects of the small intestine (e.g. coeliac disease Crohn's disease, or following surgery) will affect iron absorption.

Sixty-five percent of the total iron in the body is present in hemoglobin, in circulating red cells. About 25 percent is stored as ferritin and hemosiderin in the liver, spleen and reticulo endothelial cells.

Several serological tests can be undertaken to assess iron status (**Table 22.9**). A small amount of ferritin is present in the plasma, and measurement of this is a reliable indicator of total body stores.

Just 0.1 percent circulates bound to the transport protein transferrin. It is this bound portion of iron that is measured by the test serum iron.

Vitamin B_{12} and Folate

Although tests for Vitamin B_{12} and folate will be discussed separately, it is wise to check for deficiencies in both folate and vitamin B_{12} at the same time as there are potential interdependencies between the two because:

- Deficiencies in either of them can cause MCV to be raised if deficient
- Either or both can cause an increase in homocysteine levels
- Decreases in folate can cause decreased levels of vitamin B_{12} because of metabolic blocks.

Vitamin B_{12}

Vitamin B_{12} is required in the synthesis and breakdown of amino acids and in the synthesis of DNA and RNA. It is therefore needed to build new cells, e.g. blood cells. It is synthesized in nature by microorganisms, and is readily available to humans in meat and dairy products. No reliable plant sources have been found so vegans are particularly at risk from deficiency from a dietary cause.

The most common cause of vitamin B_{12} deficiency however is malabsorption. Vitamin B_{12} is absorbed from the terminal ileum only when bound to intrinsic factor—itself produced and released by the parietal cells in the gastric epithelium. It follows that patients can suffer vitamin B_{12} deficiency in atrophic gastritis, or

▪ Table 22.10
Tests for assessing vitamin B_{12} status

Tests	*Normal value*	*Notes*
Serum vitamin B_{12}	200–900 pg/mL	Reduced in vitamin B_{12} deficiency
Active B_{12} Methymelonic acid (MMA)	25–108 nmol/L	Elevated level of MMA indicates B_{12} deficiency: as B_{12} is needed for its metabolic pathway. Can confirm a low B_{12} for a specific patient (disadvantage—may be raised in genetic disorders of hydroxycobolamine synthesis and renal disease so will not be an accurate marker of vitamin B_{12} deficiency in some patients)
Homocysteine	<6.5	Elevated level if B_{12} is low as B_{12} is needed for its metabolic pathway (disadvantage-affected by folate level also) Raised homocysteine levels are a risk factor for progression of atherosclerosis and MI
Holotranscobolamin Holo TC	<37 pmol/L	30 percent of circulating B_{12} is attached to TC in the blood and in this form can enter cells

following gastrectomy for malignancy, but the most common cause is pernicious anemia. Patients with Crohn's disease and ulcerative colitis can also be at risk when inflammation of the colon causes terminal ileitis. B_{12} is stored in the liver and stores are sufficient to last several years on a B_{12} low diet.

Several tests can be used to investigate vitamin B_{12} deficiency status (**Table 22.10**).

Pernicious Anemia

The most common cause of failure to absorb vitamin B_{12} is in pernicious anemia, an autoimmune condition in which intrinsic factor (IF) is not produced due to damage to the stomach parietal cells. The stomach lining becomes atrophic and also ceases to produce acid. The disease was named pernicious anemia because it was fatal before treatment became available. Although this is no longer the case, the name has remained for historical reasons. Patients with pernicious anemia have a 2- to 3-fold increased incidence developing gastric carcinoma, and often have other autoimmune diseases, which include thyroid disorders, type 1 diabetes mellitus, ulcerative colitis, and Addison's disease.

Pernicious anemia probably has a genetic predisposition as it tends to run in families and is associated with human leukocyte antigen (HLA) types A2, A3, and B7, and type A blood group.

The Schilling test was used for many years to establish a diagnosis of pernicious anemia but has now largely been replaced by tests to check the presence of antiparietal cell antibodies (occuring in 90 percent of patients with pernicious anemia), and antibodies to IF. Results are more accurate if both tests are carried out.

Schilling Test

The Schilling test is performed by administering radioactive cyanocobalamin in a glass of water to a fasting patient. Two hours later, the patient is injected with 1 mg of unlabeled vitamin B_{12}. A 24-hour urine sample is collected, and the radioactivity in the specimen is measured and compared to a standard. If abnormally low values are obtained, a stage II Schilling test is performed. The test is repeated and this time the patient is also given 60 mg of active hog intrinsic factor to see if this enhances the absorption of vitamin B_{12}. If poor absorption of vitamin B_{12} is normalized, the patient has pernicious anemia.

Folate

Folate, like vitamin B_{12} is required in the synthesis and breakdown of amino acids and in the synthesis of DNA and RNA. It is therefore needed to build new cells, e.g. blood cells. Rich sources include leafy green vegetables and liver. Most breakfast cereals are fortified

▪ Table 22.11
Tests of folate status

Test	*Normal value*	*Notes*
Serum folate	3–20 ug/L	Most commonly used assay
Red blood cell folate	150–700 mcg/L	This test is theoretically more accurate as it is not affected by dietary factors but lab difficulties make it less reliable
homocysteine	< 37 pmol/L	Elevated level if folate is low as folic acid is needed for its metabolic pathway (disadvantage-affected by B_{12} level)

with folate. The daily requirement is 150 mcg. Folate is absorbed in the upper small intestine and is transported free or bound to albumin to the bone marrow and other tissues. It is stored in the liver but stores are only sufficient to last a few months. Folate level can be estimated in both serum and red cells (**Table 22.11**).

Blood Glucose Measurement

Blood glucose is used to check for diabetes and to monitor the condition. It is an important test in those complaining of oral dysesthesia or those with chronic candidosis. Random blood glucose should be less than 11.1 mmol/L and can be affected by sugary meals so an abnormal value should be repeated. Normal fasting blood glucose should be less than 7 mmol/L. Patients with random blood glucose greater than 11.1 mmol/L and/or fasting blood glucose greater than 7 mmol/L are said to have diabetes. A drop of blood can be taken from the thumb in the clinic and be tested instantly or a tube of blood can be sent to the lab in the normal way. The latter tends to be more accurate.

HbA_{1c} (glycosylated hemoglobin) and fructosamine testing give a better idea of the blood glucose levels over longer periods so are more useful than blood glucose when checking diabetic control. Another advantage of these tests is that fasting is not required. The HbA_{1c} test, which gives an idea of diabetic control over the previous months, is more popular and widely accepted. A level of 6.5 percent corresponds to a fasting glucose of 7 mmol/L or a random glucose of 11 mmol/L. New units to help standardize this test are being introduced so HbA_{1c} of 6.5 percent will be 48 mmol/L. It should be noted that false readings can occur in conditions which affect the life span of red cells and therefore the hemoglobin glycosylation, e.g. false positives after splenectomy and false negatives in hemolytic anemia. Blood samples from patients with certain hemoglobinopathies may, with certain assay techniques, give false readings also.

The fructosamine test, because it measures blood sugar over weeks rather than months can be more useful when evaluating the effectiveness of diabetic drugs new to a patient, in pregnancy where control is more crucial, and in situations where the there are abnormalities in red blood cells or loss of blood, e.g. in hemolytic anemia or after hemorrhage, which would make the HbA_{1c} test unreliable. In practice fructosamine testing is rarely requested.

Urea and Electrolytes (Us and Es)

Us + Es stand for urea and electrolytes, and are the most frequently ordered blood test. They comprise tests for sodium, potassium, bicarbonate, urea and creatinine, and are important to gauge the electrolyte balance of the body (between potassium and sodium), and renal function. The most common tests included in Us and Es together with other tests of renal function, e.g. glomerular filtration rate (GFR), are shown in **Tables 22.12** and **22.13.**

▪ Table 22.12
Staging of kidney damage using the (estimated) glomerular filtration rate (GFR)

Kidney damage stage	*Description*	*GFR mL/minute*
1.	Normal or minimal kidney damage with normal GFR	90+
2.	Mild decrease in GFR	60–89
3.	Moderate decrease in GFR	30–59
4.	Severe decrease in GFR	15–29
5.	Kidney failure	<15

▪ Table 22.13

Urea and electrolytes (Us and Es); Possible explanations for raised and lower values observed in test results

Index	*Normal range*	*Raised*	*Lower*
Urea	3.3–6.7 mmol/L	Renal failure, dehydration and in old age	Liver disease, nephrotic syndrome, low protein diet, pregnancy because of increased GFR
Sodium	135–145 mmol/L	Cushing's and Conn's syndromes, lithium therapy dehydration, chronic renal fever, diabetes insipidus	Acute renal failure, Addison's disease, edema in cardiac failure and cirrhosis, untreated diabetes, diuretic therapy
Potassium	3.5–5.0 mmol/L	Renal failure, severe tissue damage (trauma/major surgery), Addison's disease, test tube error	Vomiting, diarrhea, malabsorbtion, diabetes, diuretic therapy, Cushing's syndrome, Conn's syndrome
Creatinine	0.06–0.11 mmol/L	Renal failure, renal obstruction	Pregnancy, muscle mass decrease
GFR	127 mL/min (male) and 118 mL/min (female)	Pregnancy	Renal disease, in old age

Sodium and Potassium

Sodium is necessary for conduction in nerve cells and also in bone formation; its main function however, is the maintenance of the water balance by keeping osmolality constant. Sodium is mainly present in extracellular fluid (plasma and interstitial fluid), while potassium is present within the cells. The maintenance of differing levels of each cation inside and outside the cell is achieved by active transport (the sodiumpotassium pump). The balance of water in the body is inextricably linked to the levels of sodium in particular. Potassium is required for nerve impulse transmission, muscle contraction and for the action of many metabolic enzymes. Both sodium and potassium are absorbed in the intestine and regulated in the kidney so require normal renal, gastrointestinal, and normal adrenal gland function (for secretion of aldosterone), to keep their levels constant. Common causes of raised and abnormally low levels are given in **Table 22.13**.

Normal values: Sodium 135 to 145 mmol/L, potassium 3.5 to 5.2 mmol/L.

Critical values: Sodium <120 mmol/L or >160 mmol/L, potassium < 2.5 mmol/L or > 6 mmol/L.

Urea and Creatinine

Urea is a waste product of protein synthesis. It is synthesized in the liver from ammonia via the urea cycle. Creatinine similarly is a waste product of muscle metabolism. Both urea and creatinine are transported via blood to the kidney where they are excreted in urine. The levels of urea and creatinine in blood depend on how the rate of their synthesis (in the liver and from muscles) compares with the rate of their excretion. Thus anything which affects either of these processes will cause changes in blood levels, e.g. if renal function is compromised and the glomerular filtration rate (GFR) falls then blood levels of each will rise.

Estimated Glomerular Filtration Rate and Creatinine Clearance

The estimated GFR can be determined, with no extratesting, using the same sample of blood sent for a creatinine measurement. It is the best overall index of kidney function and is usually automatically calculated by the laboratory every time a creatinine test is done. It is a better indication of renal function than creatinine alone. Many formulae for calculation of GFR exist. A useful calculation is the MDRD Study equation which takes account of age, sex, and body size and race which are all known to affect GFR:

$186 \times (\text{Creat}/88.4)^{-1.154} \times (\text{Age})^{-0.203} \times (0.742$ if female) $\times$ (1.210 if black)

The creatinine clearance test provides an actual GFR. This test requires a 24-hour timed urine collection for urine creatinine measurement in order to compare blood and urine creatinine concentrations and to calculate the clearance. It is therefore more costly but may be more reliable in some cases, e.g. in those over 75 years when muscle mass has significantly decreased. Normal values for GFR: 127 mL/min (male) and 118 mL/min (female) assuming standard body mass.

An estimate of the extent of kidney damage based on the GFR value is shown in **Table 22.12**.

Tests of Liver Function

The liver profile is measured by liver function tests (LFTs) a combination of tests that may vary from laboratory to laboratory. They usually include measurement of serum bilirubin, albumin and the levels of certain enzymes usually found within the liver cell that leak out when hepatocytes are damaged, such as alanine transaminase (ALT), aspartate amino-transferase (AST), gamma-glutamyl transferase (GGT) and alkaline phosphatise. Alkaline phosphatise is also included in the bone profile as a measure of bone metabolism or disease.

The normal LFT values and the significance of abnormal results are outlined in **Table 22.14**.

Bilirubin

Bilirubin is the breakdown product of the hemepart of the hemoglobin molecule. Bilirubin (unconjugated) is bound to albumin and carried in the blood to the liver, to be excreted from the body in bile. To enter the liver cells the bilirubin is released from albumin and joined with glucuronic acid to make it water soluble (conjugated bilirubin). Conjugated bilirubin then passes from hepatocytes into bile canaliculi. It is then transported in bile to the duodenum where it converted to the brown pigment stercobilinogen and then stercobilin, and mostly excreted from the body as feces.

High levels of bilirubin in the blood, i.e. greater than 50 μmol/L, cause jaundice. Bilirubin levels can be used to monitor the progression of jaundice and help discover its cause. If the conjugated bilirubin is high there may be some kind of blockage of the liver or bile duct (e.g. gallstones or cancer of the head of the pancreas) or liver disease (e.g. hepatitis, cirrhosis), trauma, a drug reaction, or long-term alcohol abuse. If the unconjugated bilirubin is increased, hemolysis (undesirable breakdown of red blood cells) may be the cause. An isolated raised bilirubin in the absence of disease may be due to an inherited abnormality (Gilbert's, Rotor's, DubinJohnson, or Crigler-Najjar syndromes). To further elucidate the causes of jaundice or increased bilirubin, it is wise to check other liver function tests.

Alkaline Phosphatise

Alkaline phosphatase (ALP) is an enzyme located mainly in the liver and bones. Normal ranges vary greatly during childhood and periods of bone growth and female values are slightly higher than males. Abnormally high levels can result from liver and biliary tract disease, bone disease and to a lesser extent intestinal disease. Regarding liver and biliary tract disease, the highest levels of ALP are seen in diseases that obstruct the flow of bile (gallstones and carcinoma of the head of the pancreas). More moderate rises of ALP occur in cirrhosis and liver cancers, and values may be normal in acute hepatitis. ALP from the liver, bone and intestine can be distinguished by electrophoretic techniques and this may prove useful when assessing the significance of a solitary raised ALP level.

Alanine Transferase and Aspartate Transferase

These liver aminotransferases, are enzymes that are present in the hepatocytes. They leak into the blood stream when liver cells are damaged so are a good measure of liver inflammation (their values are usually high in hepatitis).

▪ Table 22.14
Liver function tests (LFTs) and their relevance

Test	*Normal range*	*Relevance*
Bilirubin	1–17 mmol/L	• Increased with any cause of intra-and extrahepatic biliary tract obstruction including gallstones, liver damage and hepatitis • Increased in hemolytic anemia
ALP	30–110 IU/L	• Marker of posthepatic disease, e.g. bile duct obstruction from stones or carcinoma of the head of the pancreas • Also raised in pregnancy and puberty • Decreased in hypothyroidism, hypophosphatasia and malnutrition
ALT	3–60 IU/L	• Increased in liver disease, excessive alcohol consumption • Viral illnesses, such as the common cold, can also cause a temporary rise in levels
AST	3–40 IU/L	• Increased in liver disease, e.g. hepatitis, heart disease or damage (e.g. myocardial infarct), biliary disease, excessive alcohol, drugs
GGT	5–42 IU/L	• Raised in liver disease, MI, pancreatitis, diabetes, renal disease, drugs, alcohol excess and roughly correlates with alcohol intake, can be temporarily elevated during generalized viral illnesses
Total proteins: Albumin and globulin	62–80 g/L	• Raised in liver disease, connective tissue diseases, sarcoidosis and myeloma • Decreased in pregnancy, malnutrition, nephritic syndrome, renal failure and lymphoma
Albumin	35–55 g/L	• Raised in liver disease, connective tissue diseases, myeloma, malabsorption and nephritic syndrome • Decreased in dehydration and in proteinlosing enteropathy
Globulin	7–2 g/L	• Raised in liver disease, sarcoidosis, connective tissue diseases • Decreased in dehydration

The ALT value is more specific to the liver than the AST value. The AST value may also give an indication of heart or other muscle damage elsewhere in the body. The ALT level in health is usually higher than the AST but this situation is usually reversed in alcoholic liver disease and in cirrhosis.

Gammaglutamyl Transferase

Gammaglutamyl transferase (GGT) is an enzyme which occurs mainly in the liver, but is also present in the kidneys and pancreas. It is a very sensitive indicator of liver damage. Nearly all forms of liver and biliary disease will be associated with a raised GGT. These include:

- All obstructive lesions of the biliary tree, whatever the site
- Alcoholic liver disease especially indicative if it is very high relative to the transaminases (AST, ALT) or alkaline phosphatase
- *Infectious disease:* Mild rise only
- Drug-induced liver inflammation/toxicity.

Total Proteins

Tests for total proteins (globulin and albumin) can help to assess synthetic function, immunity and the adequacy of dietary intake. Of the total protein level noted in serum, the globulin fraction reflects B cell immune function—totally or fractionated by antibody class, while the albumin level comprises the remaining fraction of the assay, itself reflecting the synthetic function and thus health of the patient's liver at the time of the test.

▪ Table 22.15
Estimation of bone profile using serological markers

Index	*Normal range*	*Raised level*	*Low level*
Calcium	2.2–2.6 mmol/lL	• Metastatic cancer with bony metastases (breast, lung, kidney, stomach and prostate) • Renal failure, hyperparathyroidism myeloma, sarcoidosis • Artefactual due to prolonged venous stasis with tourniquet	• Vitamin D deficiency due to poor diet/malnutrition • Renal failure • Hypoparathyroidism (eg post thyroid surgery)
Phosphate	0.8–1.5 mmol/L	• Bone disease, renal failure, hypoparathyroidism • Hypervitaminosis D	• Hyperparathyroidism • Rickets, malabsorbtion syndrome
Alkaline phosphatase	30–110 IU/L	• Page's disease, osteomalacia, fibrous dysplasia, bone malignancy, liver disease	
Albumin	35–55 g/L	• Dehydration	• Liver disease, connective tissue diseases, myeloma, malabsorbtion and nephrotic syndrome

Bone Profile

A routine bone profile includes an estimation of calcium, phosphate, albumin, alkaline phosphatase (**Table 22.15**) and is ordered when patients are suspected of having metabolic bone disease, or when there is disease of those organs controlling the levels of calcium and phosphate in the body (parathyroids, kidneys and gastrointestinal tract). It is also routinely measured in the critically ill and in those patients suffering with malignant disease.

▪ Table 22.16
A comparison of serological results of the bone profile in osteoporosis, osteomalacia and Paget's disease of bone

Osteoporosis	*Osteomalacia*	*Paget's disease of bone*
Calcium normal	Calcium low or normal	Calcium normal (but may be elevated with immobility)
Phosphate normal	Phosphate low or normal	Phosphate normal
ALP normal	ALP mildLy raised	ALP raised

Some conditions where the bone profile is useful in diagnosis are given in **Table 22.16**.

C-reactive Protein

C-reactive protein (CRP) is produced by the cells in the liver. It is a nonspecific marker for inflammation, infection and trauma and rises in the same instances as the ESR with a few exceptions. In SLE and in ulcerative colitis although the ESR is significantly raised, CRP is usually normal. This can be used to help distinguish between disease-related joint swelling and joint swelling caused by infection in patients with SLE. It can also be used to distinguish between ulcerative colitis and Crohn's disease which can give similar symptoms. In the latter ESR and CRP are both raised.

C-reactive protein measurement has advantages over ESR and is now preferred for the following reasons:

- C-reactive protein rises and falls more quickly than the ESR (within hours as opposed to days and weeks)
- C-reactive protein is more sensitive
- C-reactive protein is not affected by red cell numbers unlike ESR.

Thyroid Function Tests

The thyroid, situated in the neck, is responsible for the production and secretion of two hormones, throxine (T4) and triiodothyronine (T3). These hormones increase the speed of many cellular metabolic reactions, e.g. the metabolism of fat, protein and carbohydrates, and are essential for normal growth and development. Iodine, present in a normal diet, is essential for their manufacture. The levels of T3 and T4 in the blood are controlled by thyroid stimulating hormone (TSH) released from the pituitary gland. The release of TSH is in turn controlled by thyrotropin releasing hormone (TRH) secreted by the hypothalamus. Both TSH and TRH are secreted in a control back mechanism dependent on blood concentrations of T3 and T4.

The oral medicine specialist may decide to test thyroid function in patients with visible signs of exophthalmus or goiter, those complaining of fatigue and weight gain, or in patients complaining of burning or enlargement of the tongue.

The most commonly requested tests to measure thyroid function (**Table 22.17**) and their normal values are given below:

- TSH 0.3–4.5 mU/L
- Free T4 (FT4) 9–26 pmol/L
- Free T3 (FT3) 3–9 pmol/L.

When thyroid function is low the patient suffers from hypothyroidism. Conversely hyperthyroidism occurs when there is an overproduction of thyroid hormones. The problem can be primary if the thyroid itself is not functioning normally or secondary when the problem is a result of abnormal function of the pituitary gland or hypothalamus.

▪ Table 22.17
Tests of thyroid function and their interpretation

Hyperthyroidism		*Hypothyroidism*	
Primary	*Secondary*	*Primary*	*Secondary*
TSH always reduced	TSH raised	TSH always raised	TSH reduced
FT3 raised	FT3 raised normal, if disease mild		
FT4 usually raised	FT4 raised normal, if disease mild	FT4 reduced	FT4 reduced

Thyroid Antibody Tests

Thyroid antibody testing may be performed as a follow-up when other thyroid test results such as T3, T4, and/or TSH show signs of thyroid dysfunction to help distinguish an autoimmune thyroid disease from other forms of thyroiditis. Thyroid antibody tests may also be ordered if a person with a known nonthyroid-related autoimmune condition, e.g. SLE develops symptoms that suggest thyroid involvement. There are three main antibodies tested:

- Thyroid peroxidase antibody (TPOAb) usually ordered when a patient has symptoms of hypothyroidism but is also present in Hasimoto thyroiditis and Graves disease
- Thyroglobulin antibody (TgAb) present in Hasimoto thyroiditis and thyroid cancer
- Thyroid stimulating hormone receptor antibody (TRAb) present in Graves disease.

Angiotensin Converting Enzyme (ACE)

The serum ACE (SACE) test is normally used to determine the presence of sarcoidosis and will be elevated in 50 to 80 percent of patients with the disease. ACE is synthesized by sarcoidotic granulomas. It can also be used to monitor disease activity. Sarcoidosis is an uncommon chronic granulomatous multisystem disease of unknown etiology. The lungs are the most commonly affected organ but sarcoidosis may present first in the head and neck with symptoms of xerostomia and cervical lymphadenopathy. Other oral manifestations include nontender well-circumscribed brownish red swellings or submucosal nodules of the buccal mucosae, tongue or floor of mouth and erythematous swellings of the gingivae. The presence of a raised ACE alone does not confirm sarcoidosis; a chest radiograph and biopsy (e.g. of the lung or minor salivary glands) is often carried out to confirm diagnosis of the condition. Conversely a negative result does not exclude the disease because in subacute disease ACE levels can be normal.

Normal ranges for this test are laboratory-specific but can range from 8 to 57 U/mL for patients over 20 years of age. (People under 20 years of age normally have very high ACE levels). Elevated ACE levels are also found in a number of other conditions, including disorders of fat metabolism and leprosy. Decreased levels may be seen in hyperlipidemia, hypothyroidism, and in patients with bronchogenic carcinoma. Decreased levels may also be seen in those taking ACE inhibitors for hypertension.

Dipstick Urine Testing

In contrast to all the tests previously described, dipstick urine testing is usually carried out immediately after a sample has been produced by the patient, on the clinic. The test is carried out by placing a commercially available plastic strip containing absorbent pads with reagents that test for a number of constituents in urine. Not all strips are the same; some test simply for the presence or absence of a substance while others give a semiquantitative assessment by means of a graded color scale. The more important constituents of urine detectable by dipsticks, and their significance if found, are detailed in **Table 22.18**.

IMMUNOLOGY

Clinical immunology tests are carried out mainly for the diagnosis and monitoring of autoimmune disease. In this section, following

Table 22.18
Dipstick urine testing on the clinic

Test	*Normal result*	*Significance if detected*
Glucose	Negative	• Suspect diabetes but must be confirmed with a blood test • Rarer causes include Cushing's disease, acromegaly, pheochromocytoma and hyperthyroidism. Sometimes found in pregnancy due to lowering of renal threshold. Excess vitamin C in the diet can cause a false positive
Bilirubin	Negative	Either liver disease (e.g. hepatitis, cirrhosis, primary billiary cirrhosis, liver cancer) or obstruction to bile flow (e.g. bilestones, carcinoma of the head of the pancreas)
Urobilinogen	Positive	Suspect obstruction of the bile duct, if not detected. If very high levels are detected suspect liver disease or hemolytic anemia
Ketones	Negative	Found in ketosis and is worrying in a diabetic patient; confirm with a blood test. Can also be detected in late pregnancy, dehydration and alcoholism
Nitrite	Negative	Screening test for urinary tract infection (UTI); nitrates in the urine means bacteria are present. Early morning sample preferred to avoid false negative results
White blood cells	Negative	Screening test for UTI; neutrophils are present as a result of infection.
Blood	Negative	UTI is the most common cause, rarely can be a sign of serious renal or urological disease (e.g. bladder cancer)
Protein	Negative	Mild proteinuria can be brought on by UTI, strenuous exercise and fever and is usually transient. Persistent proteinuria would suggest renal disease and or hypertension
pH	Normal 5.5–6.5	Can vary with diet (vegetarians have more alkaline urine) and infections (high pH). There is a high pH in alkalosis, low pH in acidosis. Measurement Important in patients with kidney stones and renal tubular acidosis
Specific gravity	1.001–1.035	A measure of the level of hydration of a patient; the lower the value the more dilute the urine

a short summary on the principals of immunity and autoimmunity some of the more commonly ordered tests in oral medicine will be explained.

B Lymphocytes (B Cells)

When B cells are exposed to antigens they differentiate into antibody secreting plasma cells. Antibodies bind to the antigens and, together with other molecules and cells of the immune system, can destroy them. Individual B cells make their own particular antibodies.

Some B cells becomes memory cells, and when they are exposed to the same antigen in the future they rapidly become activated and produce antibodies at a much faster rate than the initial response (acquired immunity). Antibodies (also known as immunoglobulins, abbreviated Ig) are part of the gamma globulin fraction of serum proteins. There are five classes with differing functions (**Table 22.19**).

IgA, IgG, and IgM are frequently measured simultaneously. Evaluated together, they can give important information about the functioning of the immune system, especially relating to infection or autoimmune disease.

Checking for the presence of specific immunoglobulins can be helpful in diagnosing or ruling out certain illnesses, e.g. in Herpes Simplex infections, IgG is elevated in secondary viral exposures while IgM is elevated more often in primary exposures.

Immunoglobulin levels can help to diagnose immunodeficiencies which can be congenital or acquired through infection, disease, malnutrition, burns, or as a side effect of medications. They are also used as part of an evaluation for autoimmune conditions such as rheumatoid arthritis, lupus erythematosus, celiac disease and Sjögren's syndrome.

T Lymphocytes (T Cells)

T lymphocytes (T cells) do not make antibodies; when they react with antigens they release cytokines which regulate the function of other lymphocytes. Some T cells express molecules on their cell surface, which are important to their function. For example T-helper cells express CD4 molecules on their surface. These cells help B cells by secreting cytokines which promote their growth, differentiation and activation. T-suppressor cells express CD8 molecules on their surface. They act to counterbalance the effect of T-helper cells and to suppress immune responses. The measurement of relative levels of CD4 and CD8 and their ratio has become important clinically in indicating changes in the functioning of the immune system. For example in AIDS low levels of CD4 and high levels of CD8 are found in the peripheral blood leading to a compromised immune system.

▪ Table 22.19

Five classes of antibodies (also known as immunoglobulins, abbreviated Ig); their differing functions are listed

Ig class	*Function*
IgG	This is the most abundant type of antibody. Found in all body fluids, it protects against bacterial and viral infections. (seen to rise in subsequent/second meetings of infectios, e.g. HSV recurrences
IgM	Effective in the blood and lymph fluid as the first defense against a new infection. (seen to rise in primary exposure to antigen e.g. first meeting of *Herpes simplex)*
IgA	Protects mucous membranes from attack, particularly those lining the respiratory passages and gastrointestinal tract, found also in saliva and tears in secretory form (dimer plus S chain link) may bind antigen to transport to gut associated lymphoid tissue as part of immune system surveillance
IgD	Exists in minute amounts in the blood and is the least understood antibody, but is thought to have a role in lymphocyte function
IgE	Associated mainly with allergic reactions, it is found in the lungs, skin, and mucous membranes. It also protects against intestinal parasites

Natural Killer Lymphocytes

Natural killer (NK) cells are large lymphocytes (**Fig. 22.7**) which have 3 main functions: to destroy virus infected cells, to destroy some tumor cells, and to control the growth of stem cells in bone marrow.

Autoimmunity

Autoantibodies (against self) are made as a normal part of the immune system and it is unclear what leads them, in some individuals, to target one or many organs causing damage. Genetic predisposition and environmental factors (perhaps viral or other infections) no doubt play their part. It is generally thought that improper activation of T cells is central to the initiation of some autoimmune diseases. Damage can be caused by the build up in the tissues of antigen-antibody complexes, or by delayed sensitivity reactions. Autoantibodies can target a specific organ as in thyroid disease or target many organs as in systemic lupus erythematosus (SLE). Laboratory tests that detect autoantibodies in the blood sera of affected patients are a valuable tool for the diagnosis of various autoimmune diseases. They support the attending physician in finding the right diagnosis and in monitoring therapy outcome. Some of the more commonly ordered tests to diagnose autoimmune diseases with relevance to oral medicine are described below.

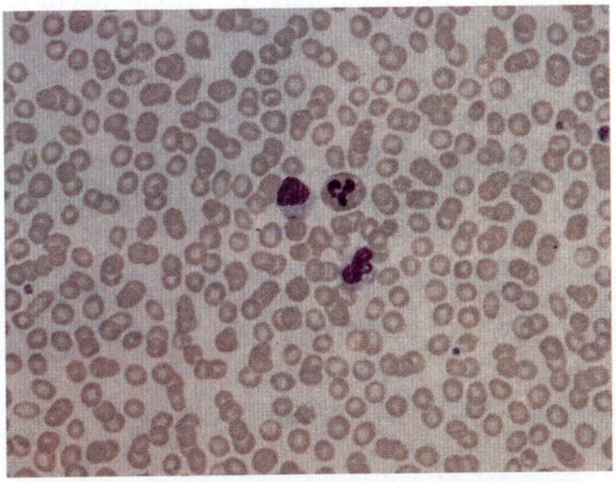

Fig. 22.7: Illustration of a natural killer lymphocyte (A large T cell)

Antinuclear Antibody Test

The antinuclear antibody (ANA) test detects the presence of antibodies in the body which target components of a cell nucleus. It is typically ordered when the clinician suspects an autoimmune disease. Testing for ANA is carried out using the immunofluorescence (IFA) technique or enzyme-linked immunosorbent assay (ELISA). The ANA test is not specific for a particular disease, but different staining patterns in the nucleus or cytoplasm of reagent cells used in the test, can help to differentiate between different autoimmune conditions results may be misleading, as the staining pattern of certain antibodies can prevent detection of others (**Table 22.20**).

The ANA test result is expressed as a titer, which is a measure of how much the blood sample can be diluted before the activity of the antibodies can no longer be detected. Everyone has auto-antibodies in low levels; a normal titer

Table 22.20
Descriptive patterns of antinuclear antibodies (ANA) and their associations with some immunological disease status

Descriptive features of a positive ANA test	
Homogeneous	This pattern is associated with dsDNA, ssDNA and histone antibodies. The dsDNA antibodies are of greatest importance. They are primarily associated with SLE but can be positive in other connective tissue diseases. Histone antibodies may be present in drug-induced lupus
Speckled	This pattern is predominantly associated with antibodies to SSA (Ro), SSB (La), Sm and ribonucleoprotein (RNP)
Centromere	This pattern is particularly associated with limited systemic sclerosis (CREST syndrome) but may also be present in some patients with Sjögren's syndrome or primary biliary cirrhosis
Nucleolar	This pattern may be found in patients with systemic sclerosis, SLE, primary Raynaud's sisease or polymyositis

of ANA is 1:40. Although results vary from lab to lab it is generally accepted that a value of 1:80 is positive.

A positive ANA is seen in most patients with systemic lupus erythematosus (*see* Chapter 17) but, in addition to clinical signs and symptoms, further antibody tests against purified nuclear proteins (dsDNA) and Smith (Sm) can help support the diagnosis. Antibodies to dsDNA occur in 60 to 80 percent of patients with SLE but are highly specific (97%) for the disease. Antibodies to Sm are specific to SLE but occur in only 10 to 40 percent of patients.

Lupus can also be caused by certain drugs (including chlorpromazine, methyldopa, isoniazid, lithium, hydralazine, procainamide, anticonvulsant drugs e.g. Dilantin, some antibiotics including isoniazid, penicillin and tetracyclines, some diuretic and some oral contraceptives). This condition can be associated with the development of autoantibodies to histones in cell nuclei and is detected by an antihistone test. Drug-induced lupus usually resolves when the drug is withdrawn.

A positive ANA can also be seen in other immune diseases including rheumatoid arthritis (30–40% of patients), Sjögren's syndrome (40–70%), scleroderma (60–90%), mixed connective tissue disease, polymyositis, Raynaud's, disease, antiphospholipid syndrome, autoimmune thyroid disease, primary biliary cirrhosis and autoimmune hepatitis. Further tests to define nuclear antigens can help in the diagnosis.

Extractable Nuclear Antigen Test

The extractable nuclear antigen (ENA) blood test screens for antibodies against the following nuclear components:

- Ro, also known as Sjögren's syndrome-A (SS-A)
- La, also known as Sjögren's syndrome-B (SS-B)
- Ribonucleic protein RNP
- Smith (Sm)
- Scleroderma-70 (SCL-70)
- Jo-1.

The blood sample is first screened for reactivity to all the ENAs in a combined test. If this test is negative then no further tests are performed. If positive then antibodies to the individual ENAs are tested. Disease associations with these autoantibodies are shown in **Table 22.21**.

Table 22.21
Types of extractable nuclear antibodies and findings associated with immunological and connective tissue disorders

Ro antibody	Associated with Sjögren's syndrome and SLE. Of particular relevance during pregnancy as presence may be associated with neonatal lupus (70%) and congenital heart block (90%).
La antibody	Generally present with Ro antibody, associated with Sjögren's syndrome and SLE
Sm antibody	Pathognomonic of SLE but only occurs in a minority of patients
RNP antibody	Particularly associated with SLE, and with mixed connective tissue disease if this alone has a high titer
SCL 70 antibody	Particularly associated with scleroderma
Jo 1 antibody	Found in a small number of patients with polymyositis

Of most interest to clinicians of Oral Medicine are antibodies against Ro and La, which are used in the diagnosis of Sjögren's syndrome (SS) in those with sicca symptoms. Earlier studies suggested antibodies to Ro are found in 75 percent of patients with primary Sjögren's syndrome but only in 10 to 15 percent of patients with secondary SS. Antibodies to La occur in association with Ro in 40 to 50 percent of those with primary SS.

Recent International multicenter studies indicate that any distinction between primary and secondary forms of SS may be obsolete. Finding of positive serum anti SSA/Ro and/or Anti SSB/La however, remains one of the three objective criteria for diagnosis of SS in individuals with signs/symptoms suggestive of SS.

Antineutrophil Cytoplasmic Antibody Test

The antineutrophil cytoplasmic antibody (ANCA) test is carried out by separating out

▪ Table 22.22
Antineutrophil cytoplasmic antibodies (ANCAs) against antigens in the cytoplasm of neutrophils and monocytes associated with systemic vasculitis

Position of fluorescing granules in neutrophils	*Name given*	*Significance*
Cytoplasm (90% accurate in severe cases 50%t accurate in mild cases)	C-ANCA	Suggests Wegners granulomatosis (WG)
Perinuclear Small proportion of WG stain in this way	P-ANCA	Suggests CSS or MPA
Cytoplasm and perinulclear, i.e. diffuse	Positive mixed ANCA	Suggests vasculitis but further tests necessary to aid diagnosis

neutrophils which are then examined with an immunofluorescent technique to determine the pattern of the fluorescing granules. The test is highly specific for autoimmune disease affecting blood vessels, e.g. Wegener's granulomatosis, [now known as Granulomatosis with polyangiitis—(GPA)] Churg-Strauss syndrome (Eosinophilic granulomatosis with polyangitis—EPGA) and microscopic polyangiitis (MPA). Abnormal values range from 1:16 to 1:32 with some laboratory variations.

Table 22.22 shows the results that may be expected, and their significance in diagnosis if the ANCA test is positive.

Tests for the Diagnosis of Celiac Disease

Celiac disease is caused by a reaction, in certain individuals, to the protein gliadin in wheat, (and similar proteins found in barley and rye). Upon exposure to gliadin, an enzyme tissue transglutaminase modifies the protein, and causes an immune inflammatory reaction in the small-bowel tissue. If a patient has symptoms, or is at risk of having celiac disease (e.g. oral ulcers with a positive history of GI problems or a family history of celiac disease) the following blood tests may help with diagnosis (in practice they are usually ordered together as a panel):

- *IgA antigliadin or IgG antigliadin:* This antibody against gluten is useful in young children and in those with IgA deficiency. Adherence to diet can be monitored by this test.
- *Endomysial antibodies (EMA):* This autoantibody test is the gold standard but may be falsely negative in young children, in patients with IgA deficiency and requires blood examination by a clinician so is subject to human error.
- *Tissue transglutaminase antibodies (tTGA):* A very accurate and automated test but can also be falsely positive in other autoimmune disease, e.g. diabetes.

It is important for patients to continue having a normal gluten-containing diet before considering diagnostic tests for celiac disease to avoid false negative results. If the diet has been modified, foods that contain gluten should be eaten in at least one meal everyday for at least six weeks before testing. A positive result with blood tests should be confirmed by small bowel biopsy.

BLOOD TESTS IN MONITORING TOXICITY TO DRUG TREATMENT

During oral medicine practice a number of drugs are prescribed for oral administration when topical treatments have been unsuccessful in controlling disease. The medications are themselves not without hazard but careful baseline screening and blood monitoring during treatment reduces risk of unwanted side effects. A full blood picture and white cell differential is necessary to check the well-being of the patient and for any signs of anemia. It is

▪ Table 22.23

Systemic drugs used in oral medicine practice and guidelines for monitoring for toxic effects

Name of drug	*Use in oral medicine*	*Base line blood tests required*	*Blood tests required in monitoring*
Azathioprine*	For immunosupression in Ulcerative LP MMP Pemphigus Erythema Multiforme SLE/DLE Wegener's granulomatosis Behçet's disease OFG	TPMT FBC Diff WBC LFT Us and Es	Weekly FBC for 1 month then every 3 months. Expect with an initial drop in lymphocytes is noted. Caution required. Monitor renal and liver function monthly and then 3 monthly
Colchicine	Behçet's disease Major RAS	FBC Us and Es LFT	FBC monthly
Dapsone	MMP Pemhigus Behçet's disease	G6PD FBC Reticulocytes Us and Es LFT	Weekly FBC and reticulocytes for 1 month, then monthly for 3 months, then 3–6 monthly. Monitor renal and liver function monthly and then 3 monthly
Glucocorticosteroids, e.g. predisolone	For immunosuppression in Ulcerative L P MMP Pemphigus Erythema multiforme SLE/DLE Wegener's granulomatosis Behçet's disease	FBC Us and Es LFT Glucose	After 1 month then 2–3 monthly Us and Es glucose urinalysis (BP and weight monitoring, bone density scans for those on long term steroids)
Hydroxychloroquine	Fatique and joint pain in Sjögren's syndrome SLE C. Tissue disease	FBC Us and Es LFT Eye examination before (treatment and then yearly)	
Mycophenolate mofetil*	For Immunosuppression in Ulcerative LP MMP Pemphigus Erythema multiforme SLE/DLE Wegener's granulomatosis Behçet's disease	FBC Us and Es LFT	Weekly FBC for 1 month then fortnightly for 2 months then monthly for the first year
Sulphamethoxypyridazine	MMP Pemphigus Linear IgA disease	G6PD FBC Reticulocytes Us and Es LFT	FBC and urinalysis monthly for 6 months and then every 3 months for 1 year. Then after 6 monthly. Monitor renal and liver function monthly and then 3 monthly

*Before prescribing drugs that cause immunosuppression BAD Guidelines advice screening for HIV, Hepatitis B and C, TB (by Chest X-ray) and immune status to *Varicella zoster*

also important to check renal and liver function prior to starting systemic therapy since most drugs are processed in the liver and excreted by the kidney. Any impairment in hepatic or renal function can lead to higher levels of the drug in the bloodstream and therefore toxicity. Those with hepatic or renal impairment may require lower doses of the selected medication.

Some commonly used drugs and the blood tests recommended prior and during therapy are listed in **Table 22.23**. The intervals for monitoring of blood are guidelines only and many vary from hospital to hospital. The immunosuppressive drugs Azathioprine, Dapsone and Sulphamethoxypyridazine (SMP) require further blood testing, in addition to the base lines tests already mentioned, prior to starting therapy, and are dealt with separately in **Table 22.23**.

Azathioprine

Azathioprine, a prodrug of 6-mercaptopurine (6-MP), requires the enzyme TPMT for its metabolism. The quantity of TPMT produced is governed by the copy number of TPMT gene: most people have two copies of the normal TPMT gene that produces sufficient enzyme. People who produce an intermediate amount of TPMT may be heterozygous for the abnormal normal gene. Those who produce little or no TPMT typically are homogeneous for an abnormal TPMT gene. If a patient has little to no detectable TPMT activity, they are at risk of

▪ Table 22.24
Sample collection for hematological, biochemical and immunological studies

Tests	*Bottle color*	*Size*	*Lab*
Autoantibodies	Yellow	8 mL	Biochemistry
B_{12}	Yellow	8 mL	Biochemistry
Coagulation screen (INR)	Light blue	5 mL	Coagulation/Hemostasis
CRP	Yellow	8 mL	Biochemistry
ESR	Black—thin tube	Thin sedatainer tube	Hematology
FBP	Purple—EDTA	5 mL	Hematology
Ferritin	Yellow	8 mL	Biochemistry
Folate	Yellow	8 mL	Biochemistry
Glucose	Gray	5 mL	Biochemistry
HLA typing	Purple—EDTA x 2 or Pink EDTA—k3 x 1	5 mL x 2 6 mL x 1	Tissue Typing
Immunofluorescence	Yellow	8 mL	Immunofluorescence
LFT	Yellow	8 mL	Biochemistry
Lymphocyte subsets	Purple—EDTA	5 mL	Hematology
Mercury—Blood Mercury—Urine	Pink Universal—10 mL urine	8 mL	Biochemistry
Thrombophilia	Light blue x 4 Yellow x 1	5 mL x 4 8 mL x 1	Coagulation/Hemostasis
TPMT	Purple—EDTA	5 mL	Purine
TSH	Yellow	8 mL	Biochemistry
U+Es	Yellow	8 mL	Biohemistry
Viral screen – HSV + EBV + Toxoplasmosis + CMV	Yellow	8 mL	Virology

developing severe side effects to azathioprine and related drugs. A few patients may have high levels of TPMT activity. It is thought that this decreases the effectiveness of therapy so higher doses may be needed. It is recommended that a blood test to check TPMT status is carried out in a purine laboratory before commencing treatment with Azathioprine.

Dapsone and Sulfamethoxypyridazine

Dapsone is a sulfone drug, chemically related to sulfonamide, sharing its antibacterial mechanisms of action. It is useful in the management of mucous membrane pemphigoid.

The most frequent adverse effects of dapsone are dose-related hemolytic anemia and methemoglobinemia. Hemolysis occurs in most patients receiving 200 mg or more of dapsone daily. Hemoglobin level is generally decreased by 1 to 2 g/dL and the reticulocyte count is increased to 2 to 12 percent. These adverse hematologic effects occur in most patients, but are most severe in patients with G6PD (Glucose-6-Phosphate Dehydrogenase) deficiency. Sulpha Methoxy Pyridazine is often used as a second line drug when treatment with Dapsone fails, or a first line treatment in patients in whom Dapsone is considered unsuitable. A baseline G6PD, if not already carried out, is also recommended before using this drug.

Table 22.24 gives a summary of the different blood tests and the blood bottles used for sample collection in clinical practice.

ACKNOWLEDGMENTS

Dr Deepti Radia is acknowledged for providing illustrations for this chapter and Professor Timothy J Peters (formerly Clinical Biochemistry, King's College London) for his constructive criticisms.

SELF-ASSESSMENT QUESTIONS

1. Describe the common congenital conditions that may lead to an abnormal hemoglobin level.
2. List those conditions in which hematinic assays should be taken in addition to a full blood picture.
3. Describe the value of a white cell differential count in diagnosis.
4. Define a reticulocyte and describe the situations in which the reticulocyte count should be monitored.
5. Compare and contrast C reactive protein and erythrocyte sedimentation rate.
6. Describe the value of liver function tests in clinical dental practice.
7. Describe the role of autoantibody assays in the diagnosis of orofacial disease.
8. Describe the hematoserological diagnosis of Sjögren's disease.
9. Compare and contrast the value of a blood glucose test and an HbA_{1c} assay.
10. Define the International Normalized Ratio (INR) and describe its value in clinical dental practice.

SUGGESTED READING

1. Oral Diagnosis: Handbook of Modern Diagnostic Techniques Used to Investigate Clinical Problems in Dentistry. Pergamon Press.
2. Pagna KD, Pagna TJ. Mosby's Diagnostic and Laboratory Test Reference, 11th edn. Elsevier Press.

Chapter

23

Imaging for Diagnosis of Oral and Maxillofacial Diseases

Jimmy Makdissi

Chapter Outline

INTRODUCTION

The use of imaging modalities in the diagnosis of oral and maxillofacial conditions has been at the center of clinical practice for many decades. Imaging is continuously evolving with a multitude of newer imaging modalities coming into practice. With the increasing availability of multiple and more advanced imaging modalities to the practicing clinician, it is important to understand the operating principles of each of these modalities and fully appreciate the advantages and limitations of each.

Understanding the radiographic technique provides the clinician with a good appreciation of the anatomical structures and frequently occurring artefacts. This in turn allows better radiological interpretation of abnormal findings. While physics and radiographic technology might come across as 'boring' to the clinical team, it certainly underpins the solid foundation of diagnostic radiology.

When considering an imaging modality, it is vital to justify the exposure by obtaining a thorough history and carrying out a comprehensive clinical examination. Any radiographic examination is expected to provide new information and likely to alter the management of the patient. Once an exposure has been justified, the radiation dose should be optimised by keeping it as low as reasonably achievable.

The purpose of this chapter is to provide the clinical team with an overview of the available imaging modalities and an insight into the operating principles, the key advantages and limitations of each.

PLAIN RADIOGRAPHS

Periapical Radiography

Periapical (PA) radiography remains the most common dental imaging modality in use within dental practices and hospitals. It is predominantly used to provide high resolution images of the teeth and their supporting structures. The ideal periapical radiograph is expected to cover the crown, the root, the apex and at least 5 mm of the surrounding apical tissues. The image should be an accurate representation of the tooth of interest. It is therefore important to achieve correct horizontal and vertical angulations. Beam aiming devices are used to provide good alignment of the beam with the film or digital sensor to achieve good geometric accuracy and minimal distortion.

The resultant dose is approximately in the region of 1 to 8.3 μSv. The variation is caused by multiple factors some of which are film speed, exposure factors, (kV, mA, time) and the use and type of collimation (circular or rectangular). The clinical applications of periapical radiographs are:

- Diagnosis and monitoring of caries
- Assessment of periodontal bone levels
- Assessment of periapical granuloma and small radicular cysts
- Assessment of traumatic injuries to the teeth and the alveolar bone
- Assessment of teeth and retained roots prior to extraction
- Assessment of working length and obturation in endodontics
- Assessment of unerupted teeth
- Assessment of root resorption.

Many of these radiographic features and assessments are illustrated below (**Figs 23.1 to 23.5**).

While conventional periapical radiographs are readily available and have high image resolution (approximately 120 lp/mm), they are only able to show a limited area in 2 dimensions. Information in the buccal lingual dimensions is not provided.

Bitewing Radiography

Bitewing radiography is often used in dental practice usually with the aid of beam aiming devices. This ensures no distortion of the horizontal angulation and therefore no overlapping of teeth.

The main applications (**Figs 23.6A to C**) of bitewing radiography include:

- Assessment and monitoring of inter-proximal caries
- Assessment of recurrent caries
- Assessment of periodontal bone levels.

Usually, a pair of bitewing radiographs is sufficient to cover the full arch. This delivers a low dose of approximately 2 μSv if standard

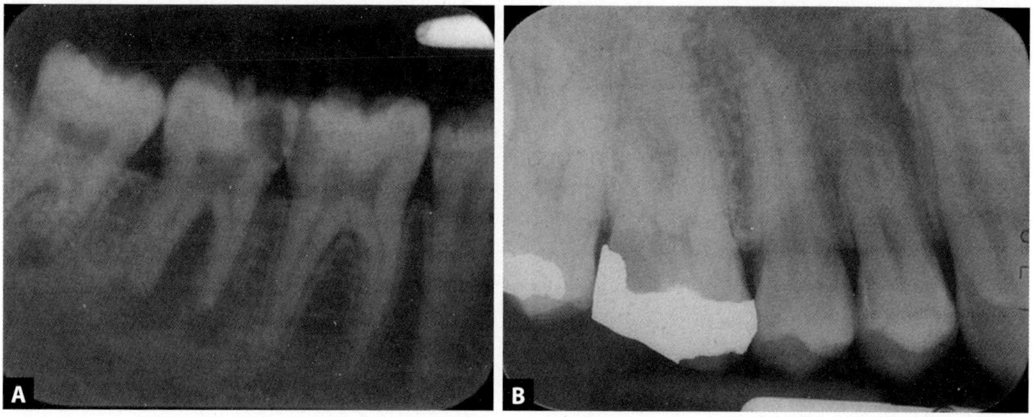

Figs 23.1A and B: (A) Dental caries: Gross caries of the mesial and occlusal surfaces of the LR7 with subsequent periapical infection; (B) Recurrent caries in a heavily restored UR6

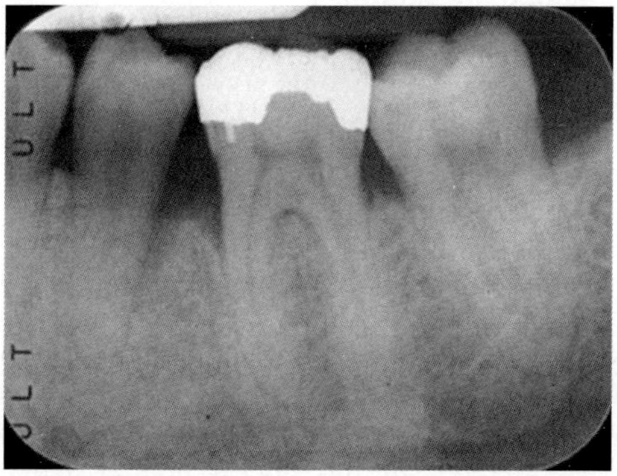

Fig. 23.2: Bone loss in periodontal disease: Horizontal bone loss is noted in relation to the mesial and distal aspect of the LL6

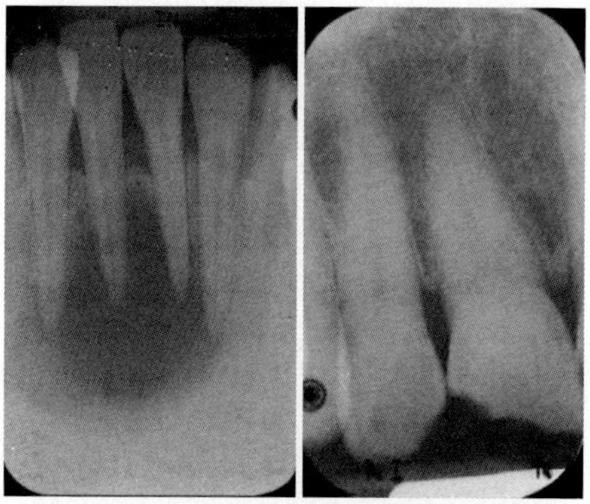

Fig. 23.3: Small radicular cyst surrounding the apices of the clinically nonvital central incisors (left) and traumatic injury to the UR1 and UR2 resulting in tooth substance loss

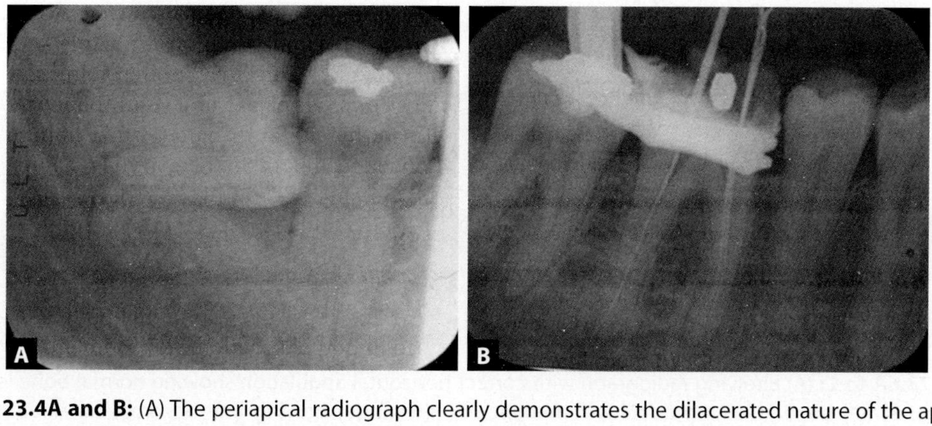

Figs 23.4A and B: (A) The periapical radiograph clearly demonstrates the dilacerated nature of the apices of LR8, close relationship to the ID canal and the coronal bone loss. The intimate relationship to the LR7 is also seen; (B) Endodontic use of periapical radiography of LR6

dose reduction techniques are implemented. These include high-speed films (F-speed), 70 kV machines, rectangular collimation, accurate timer and regular maintenance. It is sometimes necessary to use two films for each side when third molars are fully erupted.

As with periapical radiographs, bitewing radiographs are only able to provide a two dimensional image of the crowns of the teeth and the level of alveolar bone. It is difficult to assess the presence and extent of recurrent caries in the presence of large restorations and to assess bony defects in a buccal-lingual dimension.

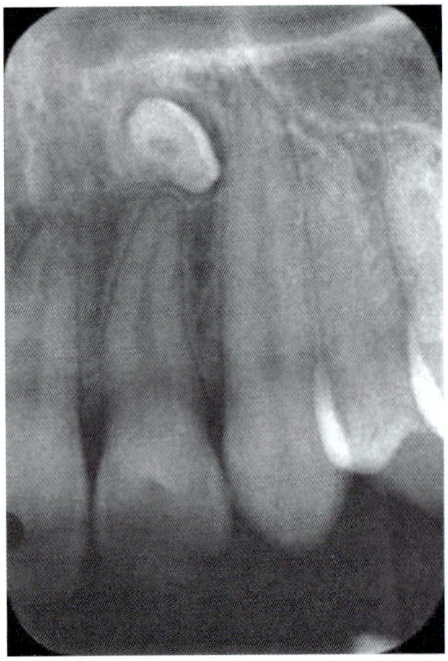

Fig. 23.5: A supernumerary tooth is seen apical to the UL2. There is a clear demonstration of the intact lamina dura at the apex of the UL2

Occlusal Radiography

There are multiple variations of this technique, predominantly based on the site (region of interest) and the angulation of the beam.

In the maxilla the two main types of occlusal radiography are:

1. Upper standard occlusal (USO) aimed at the midline of maxilla.
2. Upper oblique occlusal (UOO) aimed at the posterior region.

In the mandible the three main types of occlusal radiography are:

1. Lower 90 degree occlusal (L90) aimed at the floor of the mouth.
2. Lower 45 degree occlusal (L45) aimed at the lower anterior teeth.
3. Lower oblique occlusal (LOO) aimed at the posterior region.

Applications of occlusal radiography include, but are not limited to:

- Assessment of the periapical region of teeth when it is difficult to obtain a traditional periapical radiograph (USO, L45, UOO, LOO) (**Figs 23.7 to 23.9**)
- Assessment of cystic lesions (**Fig. 23.10**)
- Assessment of the buccal lingual expansion of the bone in the presence of cysts and tumors (L90)
- Assessment of the position and orientation of unerupted teeth using parallax technique (combined with a panoramic radiograph or a periapical radiograph) (US0)

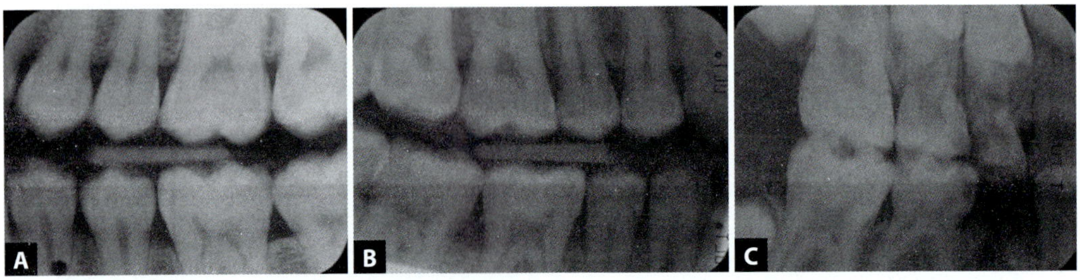

Figs 23.6A to C: (A) Bitewing radiograph with correct horizontal angulation showing normal bone levels; (B) Horizontal bone loss with calculus formation; (C) Bitewings showing interproximal caries affecting URD-URE and LRD-LRE

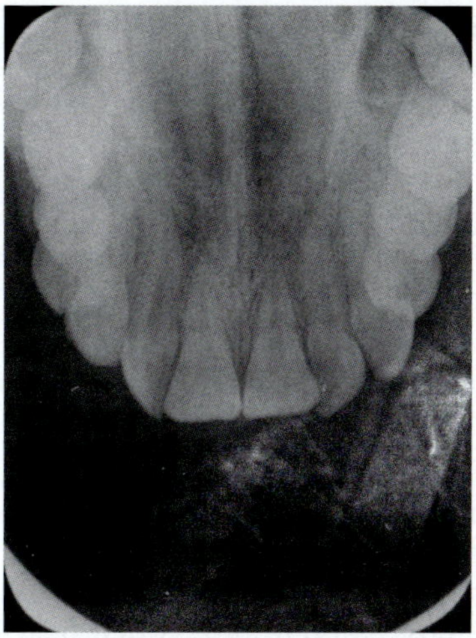

Fig. 23.7: Upper standard occlusal (USO) radiograph demonstrating the apices of the upper anterior incisors

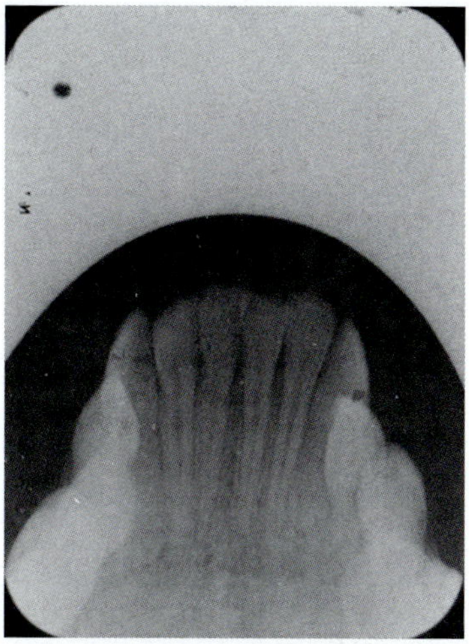

Fig. 23.8: Lower 45 occlusal (L45) radiograph demonstrating the apices of the lower anterior incisors

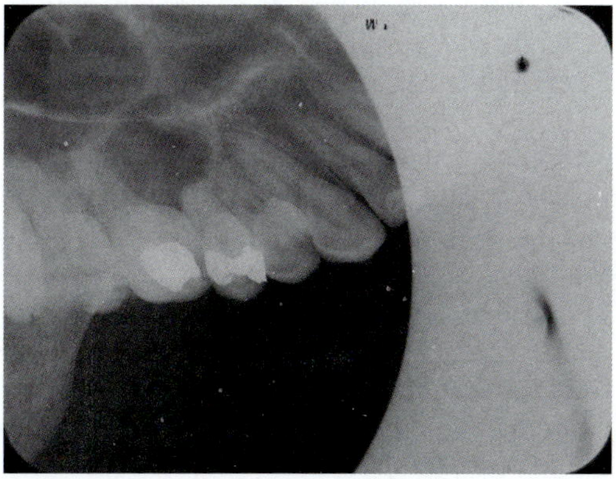

Fig. 23.9: Upper oblique occlusal (UOO) radiograph demonstrating the apices of the upper posterior teeth

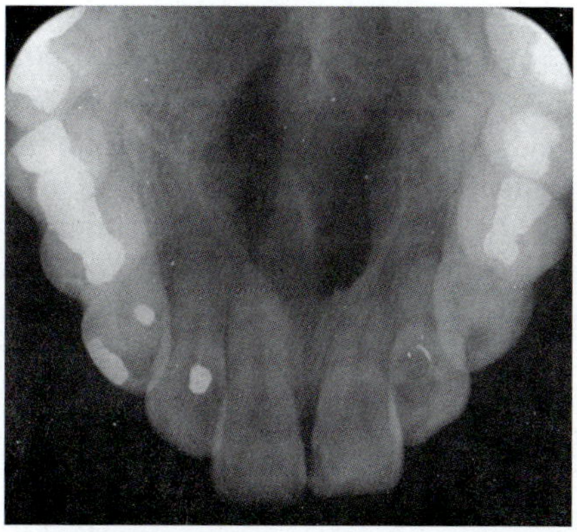

Fig. 23.10: USO radiograph showing a nasopalatine duct cyst in the midline of the anterior maxilla

- Assessment of the orientation and displacement of fractures of the teeth and the alveolar bone in trauma cases (L45, L90)
- Detection of salivary stones within the duct of the submandibular gland (L90) (**Fig. 23.11**).

Panoramic Radiography

Panoramic radiography is a simple, accessible and reasonably accurate imaging modality able to provide an overview of the full dentition and the surrounding supporting structures.

The panoramic image is not strictly conventional. It is based on the principle of narrow beam rotational tomography. The image is acquired by simultaneously rotating the X-ray beam and the sensor/film in opposite directions around the patient. The panoramic machine uses multiple centers of rotation. The image is only able to display accurately structures present within the focal plane (often referred to as the

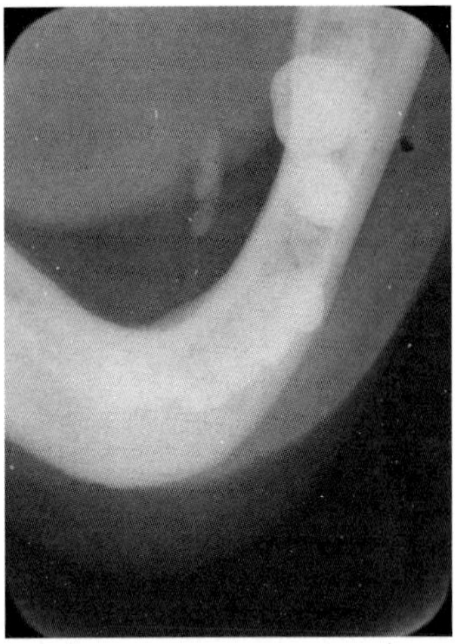

Fig. 23.11: L90 radiograph showing a salivary stone in the duct of the left submandibular gland

focal trough). Most machines are now able to provide a choice of focal plane shapes and sizes to better accommodate patients with different shaped dental arches. Structures present outside this plane are blurred. Correct positioning of the patient will minimize distortion to the final image (**Fig. 23.12A**). Incorrect positioning can lead to misinterpretation of the radiograph (**Figs 23.12B and C**).

Selection criteria for a dental radiography booklet published by the Faculty of General Dental Practice (FGDP) at the Royal College of Surgeons of England (RCS ENG) contains this suggested use for panoramic radiography in dental practice:

- Where a bony lesion is of a size or position that precludes its complete demonstration on intraoral radiographs (**Fig. 23.13A**).
- In the case of a grossly neglected mouth with significant numbers of clinically determined carious lesions and periapical pathology along with established periodontal disease (other than simple gingivitis) and where there is pocketing greater than 6 mm in depth (**Fig. 23.13B**).
- For the assessment of wisdom teeth prior to planned surgical intervention. Routine radiography of unerupted third molars is not recommended (**Fig. 23.13C**).
- As part of an orthodontic assessment where there is a clinical need to know the state of the dentition and presence/absence of teeth (**Fig. 23.13D**).

In a hospital environment the use of panoramic radiography is invaluable when combined with PA mandible (PA Jaws) to assess mandibular fractures (**Fig. 23.14A**). It is also useful in the assessment of postoperative repair of fractures of the mandible to demonstrate the alignment of fragments (**Fig. 23.14B**).

The main advantages of panoramic radiography:

- Simple, accessible with good coverage of the teeth and the supporting structures.
- Relatively low radiation dose (3.85–30 μSv). The dose is even lower when field limitation technique is applied. This allows only the side of interest to be imaged. However, it is important to remember that imaging one side eliminates the ability to compare one side with the other which could pose a diagnostic challenge. It is also possible to limit the exposure to "dentition only", thus excluding part of the ramus and the parotid glands. This reduces the exposure by approximately 50 percent (**Fig. 23.15**).
- Easy to understand by patients.

The main limitations of panoramic radiography are:

- The technique is operator dependent enforcing the importance of adequate training of operators. Film faults can occur during preparation and positioning of patient and also during exposure and processing the film (**Figs 23.16A to D**).
- Preparation errors include dentures, ear rings left *in situ* or the use of a previously exposed cassette.
- Positioning errors have already been described and include rotation, chin-up and down, too-far backwards and too-far forwards.
- Exposure errors include over, and under exposure caused by incorrect kV and mA settings.
- Processing errors can include dirt marks, finger nail marks, and inadequate solution balance (developer and fixer).

The shape of the focal plane (narrow anteriorly and wide posteriorly) does not

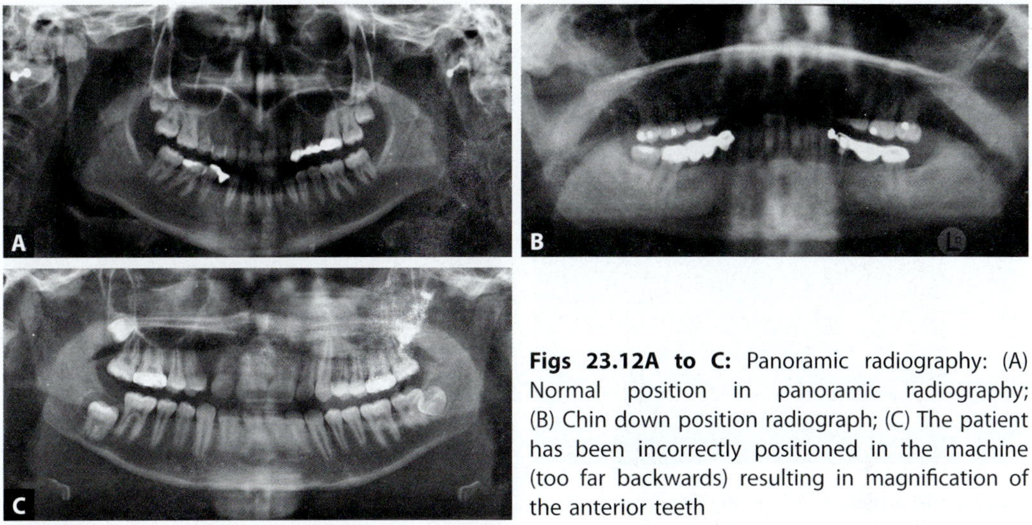

Figs 23.12A to C: Panoramic radiography: (A) Normal position in panoramic radiography; (B) Chin down position radiograph; (C) The patient has been incorrectly positioned in the machine (too far backwards) resulting in magnification of the anterior teeth

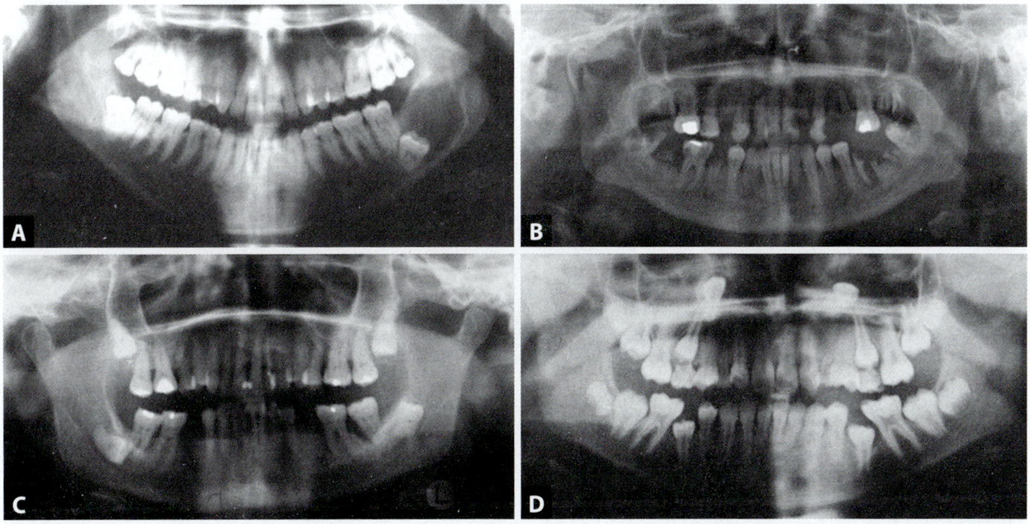

Figs 23.13A to D: (A) A large dentigerous cyst associated with an impacted LL8; (B) Multiple grossly carious teeth and retained roots; (C) Impacted wisdom teeth and their relationship to the adjacent structures; (D) Multiple unerupted teeth during an orthodontic assessment

always fit the shape of the patient's arch leading to significant distortion more often seen in the anterior mandible (**Fig. 23.17**).

The nature of image acquisition leads to multiple ghost shadows on the image. These include the cervical-spine and the contralateral shadow mandible (**Figs 23.18A and B**).

Although the acquisition of the panoramic image is simple, operator training is crucial to overcome simple yet potentially detrimental limitations. Simple deviation from the correct positioning of the patient can have a detrimental effect on the final image.

Skull Radiography

Multiple skull projections have historically been used in the imaging of the maxillofacial

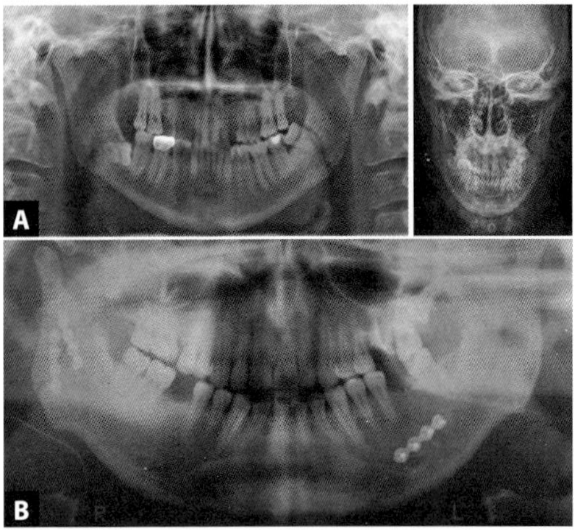

Figs 23.14A and B: (A) Minimally displaced fracture of the left angle of the mandible seen as a well defined radiolucent line; (B) Panoramic radiograph demonstrating the repair to the fractures of the left body and right condylar neck

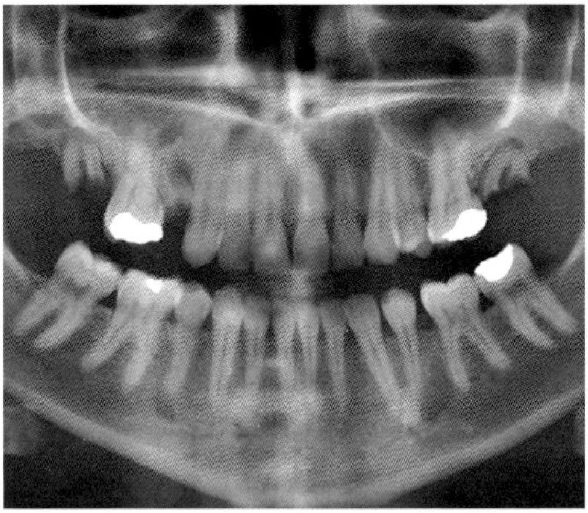

Fig. 23.15: Reduction of radiation dose by excluding parotid glands

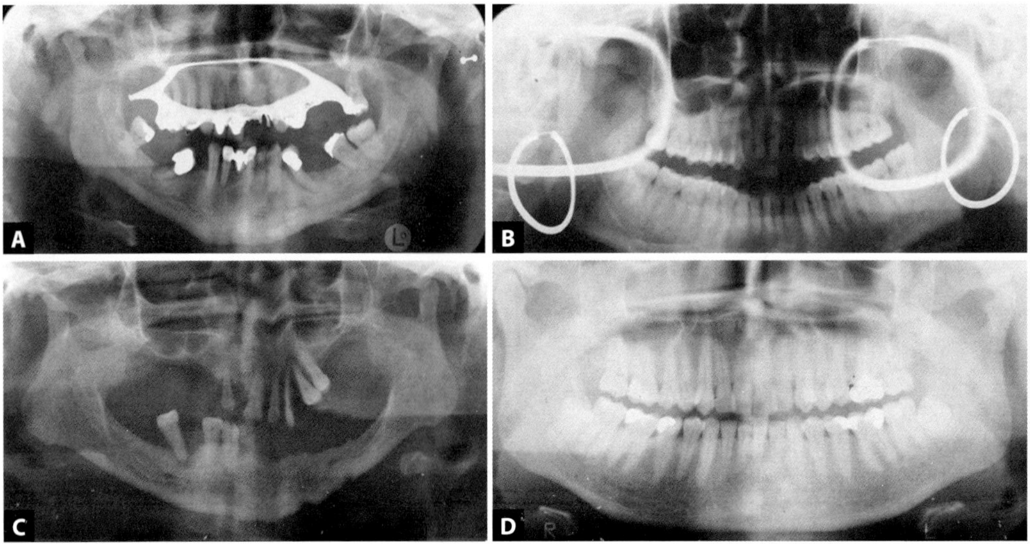

Figs 23.16A to D: (A) Upper denture left *in situ* during the acquisition of the radiograph; (B) Ear-rings left *in situ* causing a strong ghost shadow on the opposite side; (C) Movement artefact in the left mandible; (D) The image is light as result of an exposure error (low mA S) or processing error (weak developer)

region. Due to the two dimensional nature and introduction of new modalities such as cone beam CT, their use appears to be declining. Two projections remain frequently used:

1. Occipital mental (OM) 0° and OM 30°
2. Posteroanterior mandible (PA).

The main use of these radiographs is to help in the assessment of maxillofacial trauma

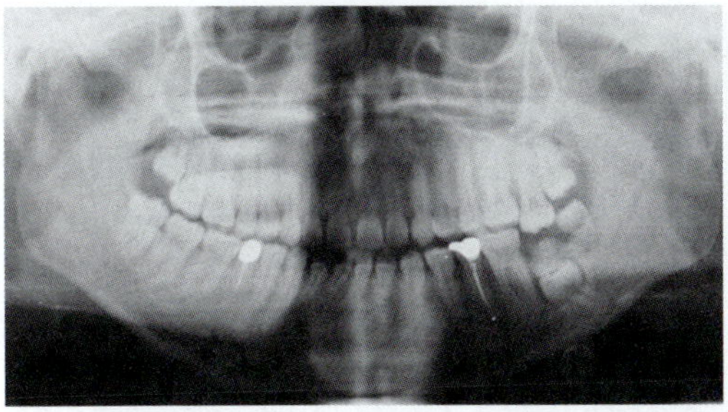

Fig. 23.17: The roots of the lower anterior teeth are out of focus (out of the focal trough) and appear blurred

in the acute setting. OM views are used in the assessment of mid face and zygomatic fractures (**Figs 23.19A to D**). PA mandible is used in the assessment of mandibular fractures combined with panoramic radiography (**Figs 23.20A and B**). These projections are simple and easily accessible with a relatively low radiation dose.

Digital Imaging

The principal of digital imaging relies on substituting the conventional film with a digital sensor. Everything else remains the same as conventional radiography.

There are two main types of digital sensors:

1. Charged coupled device (CCD) or a complimentary metal oxide semi conductor (CMOS). Both CCD and CMOS systems are able to instantly display acquired images on a computer screen.
2. Photo-stimulable phosphor plate (PSP) which requires further digital development in order to display the final image.

The recent years have seen a steady increase in the use of digital imaging in dental practices and hospitals. Although the main driving factor was potentially the lower radiation dose, digital imaging has many other advantages:

- Lower radiation dose which varies between 20 and 90 percent based on the initial equipment used.
- Elimination of processing chemicals and associated hazards and complications.
- Storage of digital imaging lead to saving of physical space.
- Image manipulation including brightness and contrast (**Figs 23.21A to F**).
- Image analysis including bone density and length of root canal (**Fig. 23.22**). Image transfer between practices and hospitals when referring patients or requesting a second opinion. Patient confidentiality and information security should be taken into consideration.

Limitations of Digital Imaging

Image resolution: There is a theoretical reduction in image resolution when switching from conventional films to digital imaging (120 lp/mm for conventional compared to 25 lp/min for digital).

- The naked eye is only able to appreciate 15 lp/mm. The theoretical reduction in the resolution is only appreciated when significant magnification of the image is attempted by

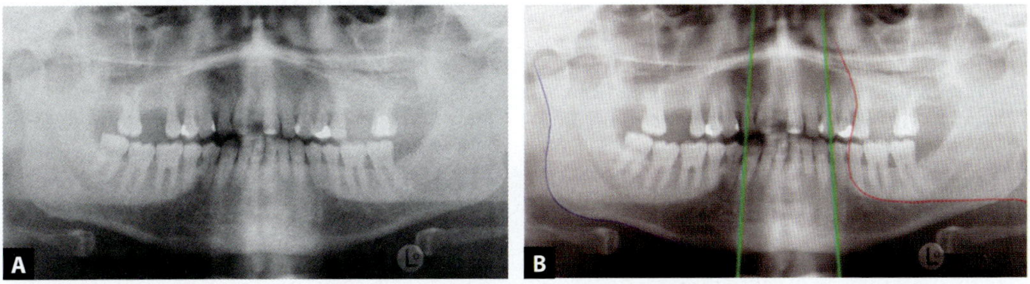

Figs 23.18A and B: The outline of ghost shadow (red line) of the contralateral mandible (blue line) is demonstrated. The outline of the cervical-spine is demonstrated in green lines (*Courtesy*: Dr Ravikiran Pawar)

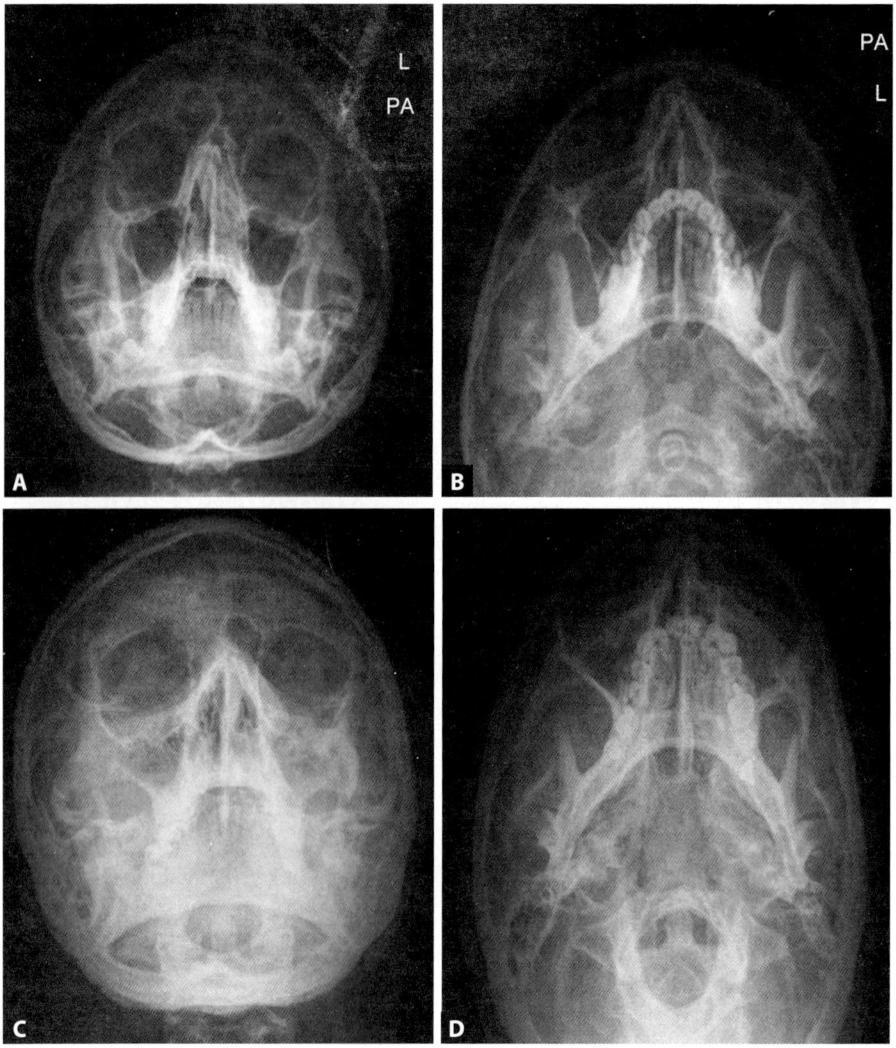

Figs 23.19A to D: Occipital mental view: (A) Normal OM 0° view; (B) Normal OM 30° view; (C and D) OM 0° and OM 30° showing a fracture of the left zygomatic complex

generating a pixelated image (**Figs 23.23A and B**). This does not usually affect the diagnostic quality of digital systems.

- The spatial resolution is comparable between digital and conventional panoramic radiographs.

Sensor size: CCD and CMOS sensors are smaller (**Fig. 23.24**) than conventional films which results in a smaller area covered during radiography. This can result in the need to take two bitewing radiographs per arch to cover all teeth.

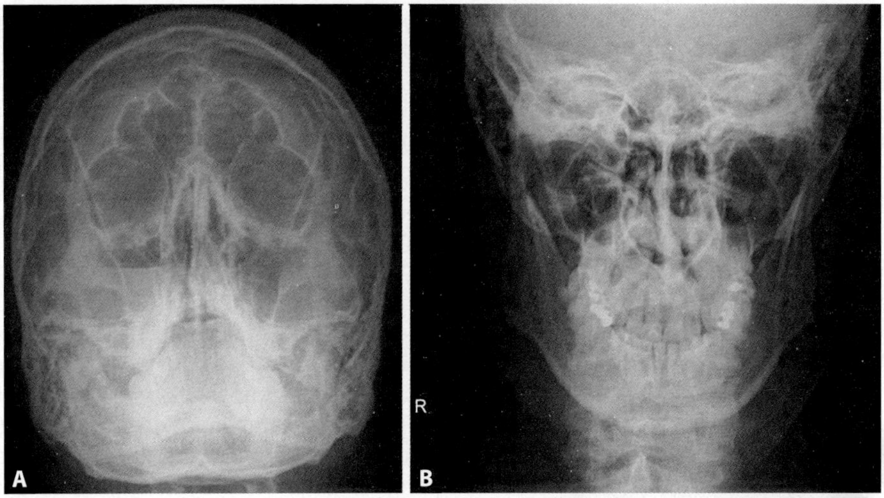

Figs 23.20A and B: (A) OM 0° showing fluid levels in the right maxillary sinus; (B) PA mandible showing a minimally displaced fracture of the right condylar head

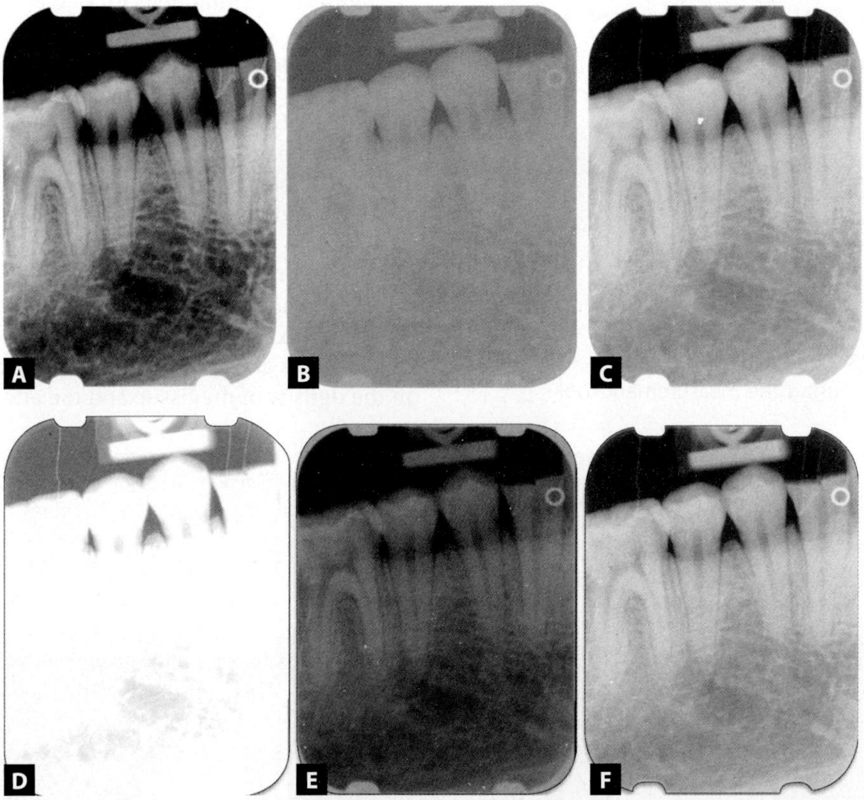

Figs 23.21A to F: The effect of contrast (A to C) and brightness (D to F) on demonstrating different tissues, high (left), low (middle) and good (right) contrast and brightness

The thickness of CCD and CMOS receptors is considerably more when compared to film and phosphor plates making it less tolerable and more difficult to use in patients with challenging anatomical features such as a shallow hard palate or in patients with gag reflex (**Fig. 23.25**). *Cost*: Although there is an initial capital outlay in purchasing a digital system, the long term cost savings are clear when considering the more efficient system of work.

Similar to any other computer system, crashes can occur resulting in loss of data. It is therefore essential to ensure that data is safely and securely backed up to prevent loss of patient information.

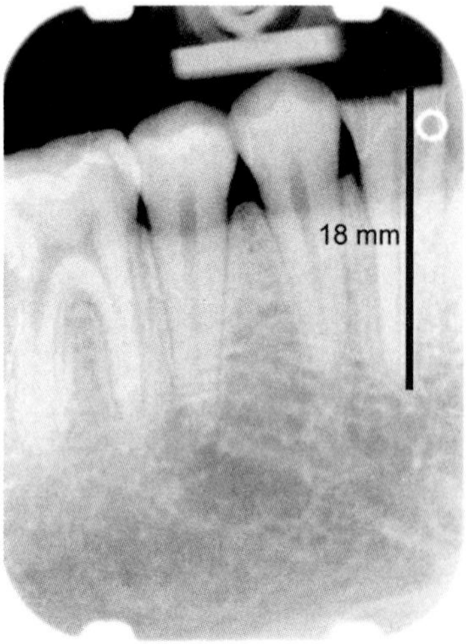

Fig. 23.22: Length of the canal is estimated using the measurement tool

It is important to ensure that selection criteria and a comprehensive quality assurance program are implemented regardless of whether a conventional, or a digital system is used.

COMPUTED TOMOGRAPHY

Computer tomography (CT) utilizes ionizing radiation to produce three-dimensional (3D) images of patients. A rotating narrow fan-shaped X-ray beam is produced by the X-ray source, transmitted through the patient (variably absorbed) and then detected by a ring of sensitive detectors. Spiral CT scanners allow continuous movement of the X-ray source around the patient's table as it mechanically moves within the scanner. Transmitted radiation is detected by a single row of detectors.

Multislice (multidetector) CT scanners utilize spiral technology with multiple (rather than single) rings of detectors. This allows more data to be captured for each beam rotation. More recently dual source CT scanners offered two X-ray beam sources with switching kV to improve efficiency. These do not currently have a widespread role in dental and maxillofacial imaging.

The CT image is made of a matrix of multiple volume elements (voxels) as opposed to picture elements (pixels) usually of isotropic resolution. Each voxel is assigned a Hounsfield unit based on the density of the tissue and the attenuation

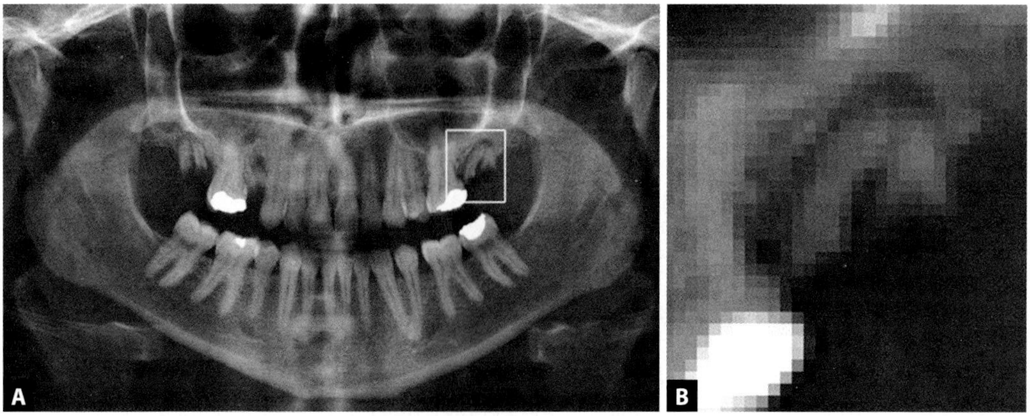

Figs 23.23A and B: Pixelation of the image can occur if significant magnification is attempted

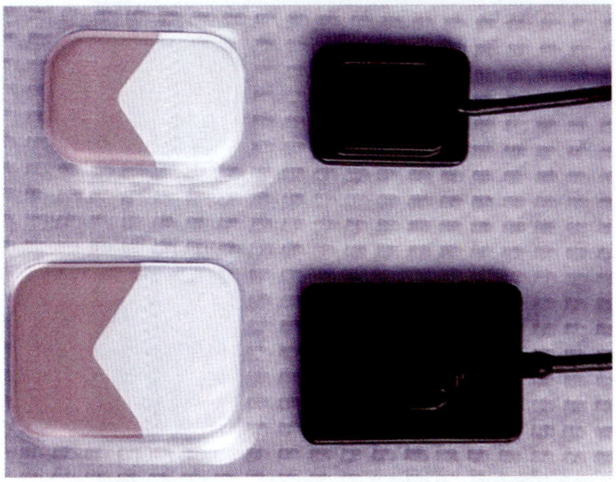

Fig. 23.24: The size difference of digital sensors and conventional films

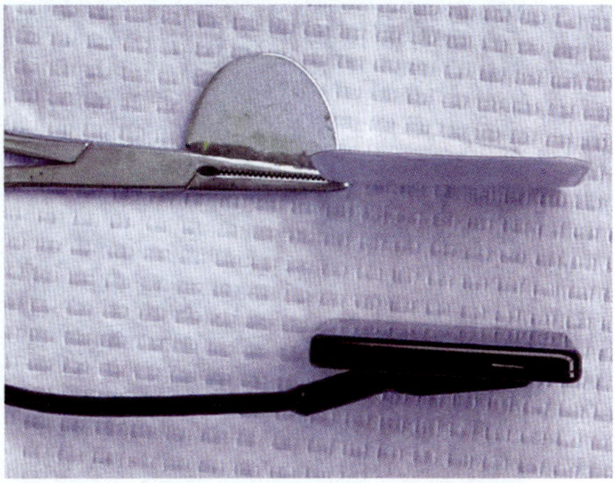

Fig. 23.25: The difference in thickness of digital sensors and conventional film

Table 23.1:
The common tissue and their Hounsfield Unit (HU) values

Tissue	HU value
Air	-1000 HU
Fat	-120 HU
Water	0 HU
Muscle	+40 HU
Contrast	+130 HU
Bone	+1000 HU

of radiation. This unit ranges from -1000 for air to +1000 and more for cortical bone with water at 0 (**Table 23.1**).

Window width (range of Hounsfield Units) and window level (the central value of all Hounsfield Units displayed) adjustments allow selective visualization of bone and soft tissue (**Figs 23.26A and B**) based on the range of Hounsfield units needed for display.

Advantages of CT Scan

- Elimination of superimposition of structures encountered in plain film imaging
- Multiplanar imaging (**Figs 23.27A to C**) allowing objects to be visualized in all three axial, coronal and sagittal planes usually with the benefit of a visual 3D model (**Fig. 23.28**).
- High contrast resolution
- *Speed*: The time taken to scan the full facial skeleton is under 3 seconds. This has a significant benefit in reducing movement artefacts
- *Cost*: CT is relatively cheap to setup and run and more readily available when compared to MRI.
- Patients with ferromagnetic objects can be scanned with CT.

Limitations of CT Scan

- *Radiation dose*: This is significantly higher when compared to plain film radiography. It is estimated at 364–1202 μSv in the Mandible and 100–3324 μSv in the Maxilla.
- Restricted availability within the dental practice.
- Metal streaking artefact from amalgam fillings and other highly dense objects causing significant degradation of the image quality (**Figs 23.29A and B**).

The frequency at which multidetector CT scanning is used in dentistry has decreased due to the introduction of the newer cone beam technology. However, when soft tissue demonstration is needed multidetector CT remains invaluable.

The most common applications of CT:

- Complex polytrauma cases of the head and neck (**Figs 23.30A to C**).
- Assessment of the position of orbital plate reconstruction following trauma when visualization of the intraorbital soft tissue is required.
- Assessment of cortical bone invasion in tumors of the head and neck (**Fig. 23.31A**).

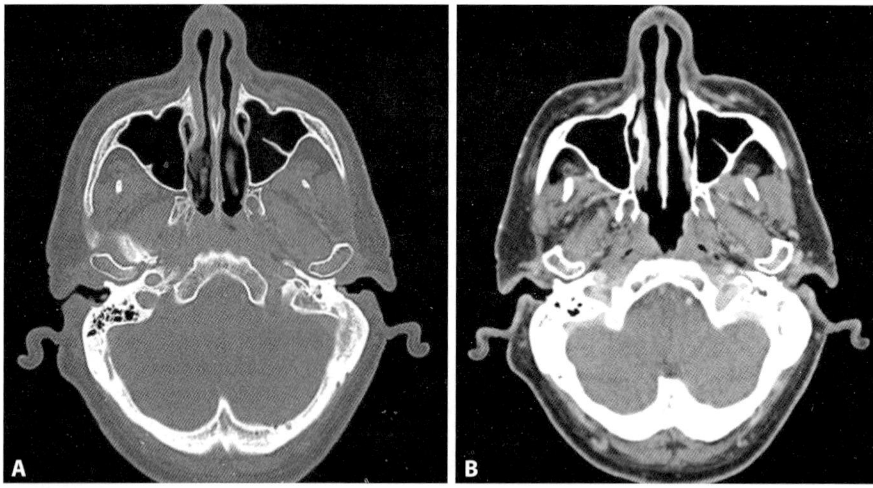

Figs 23.26A and B: CT scan with bone window: (A) Soft tissue window; (B) Setting

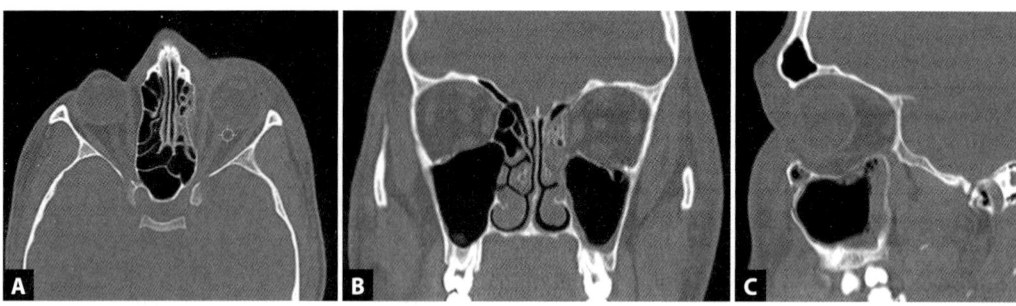

Figs 23.27A to C: Multiplanar display of maxillofacial skeleton in (A) Axial; (B) Coronal; (C) Sagital. These display clear evidence of a medial wall fracture with secondary opacification of ethomoid air cells with minimal disruption of the floor of the orbit seen in both coronal and sagittal planes

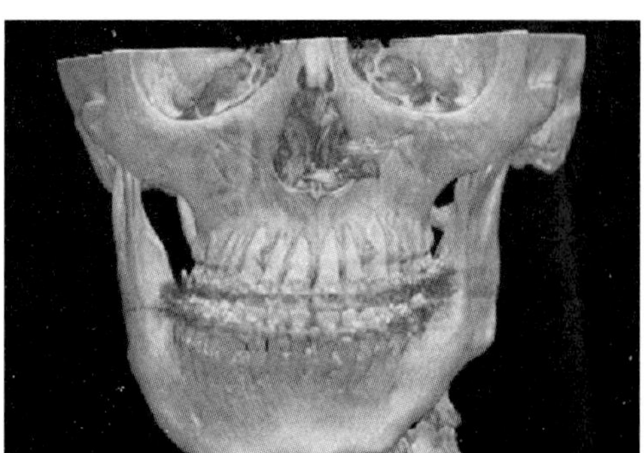

Fig. 23.28: 3D model demonstrating an asymmetry of the right mandible. This represents a strong visual tool demonstrating the severity of the abnormality to both clinicians and patients

- Assessment of osteomyelitis and osteoradionecrosis in the head and neck (**Fig. 23.31B**).

Other applications that utilize multidetector CT scan in the maxillofacial region such as bone assessment prior to dental implant (**Figs 23.32A to E**) placement have now been superseded by cone beam CT.

CONE BEAM COMPUTED TOMOGRAPHY

Cone beam computed tomography (CBCT) has revolutionized the way dental imaging is acquired. The principle of CBCT is based upon utilizing a cone shaped beam aimed at a flat panel detector. Both beam and detector rotate

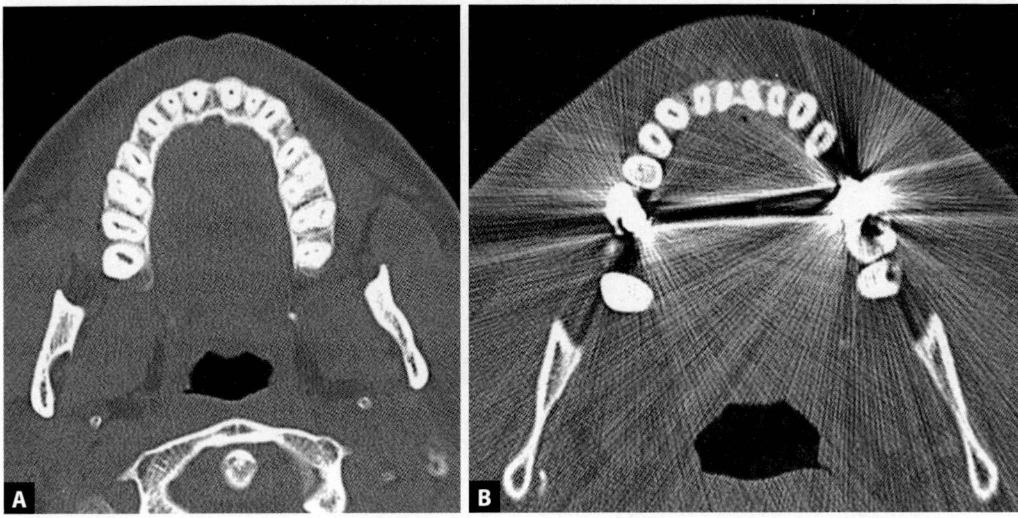

Figs 23.29A and B: (A) Demonstration of clarity in a CT image without metal streaking artefacts; (B) Devastating effect of metal artefacts on the image caused by amalgam fillings

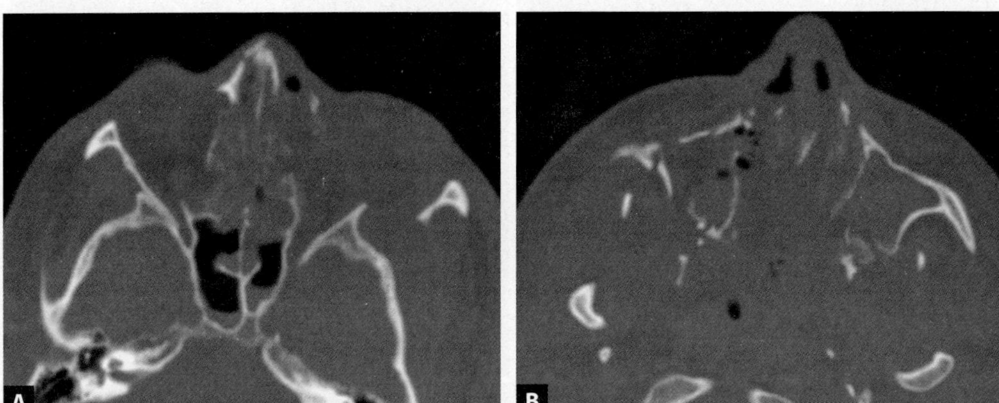

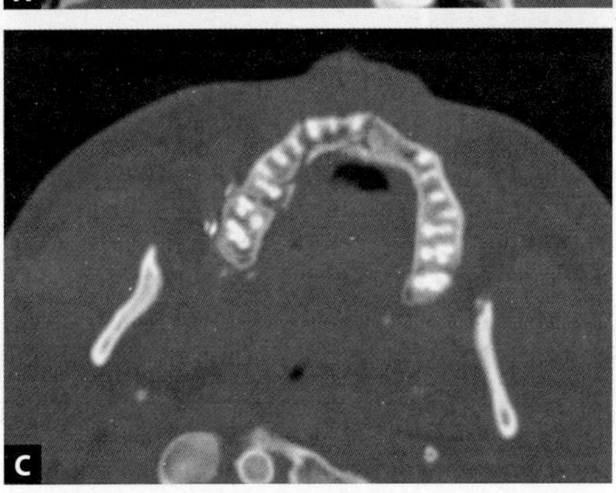

Figs 23.30A to C: (A) Multiple slices through the mid face following trauma demonstrating significantly displaced left zygomatic fracture; (B) Maxillary sinus walls and pterygoid plates; (C) Maxillary alveolar bone

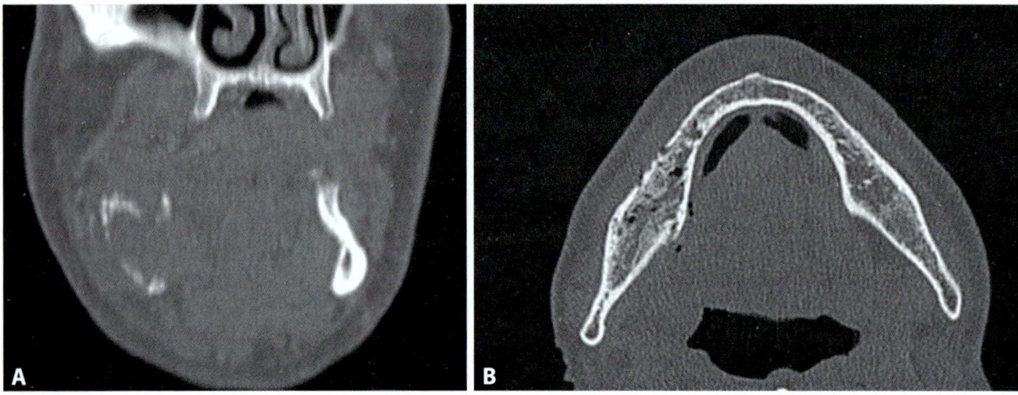

Figs 23.31A and B: (A) Coronal CT image of the mandible demonstrating bone destruction of the cortical plates in osteosarcoma causing of the right mandible; (B) Loss of smooth outline of the right mandible caused by osteoradionecrosis

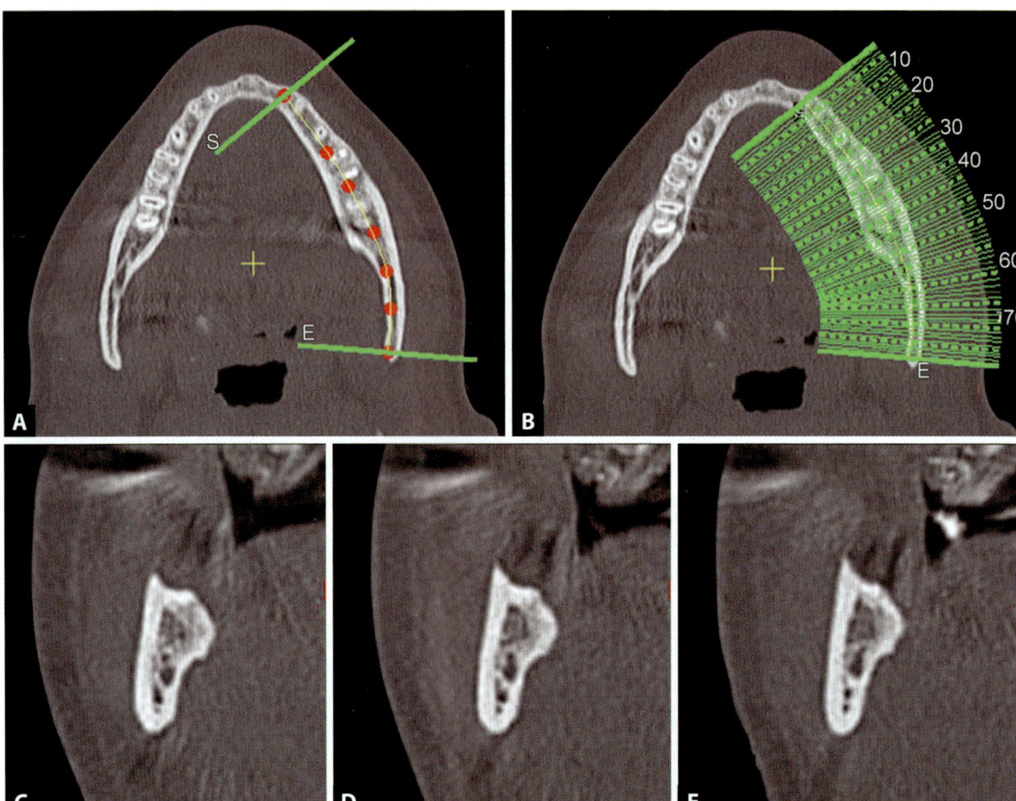

Figs 23.32A to E: Use of CT images in obtaining multiple cross-sectional images

around the patient's head in opposite directions simultaneously. This captures the basic data from the area of interest forming a variable sized cylindrical shaped volume. This limits the exposure to a smaller volume when compared to the traditional fan shaped X-ray beam of the conventional CT.

The acquired data is then reconstructed in multiplanar reformats allowing the visualization of the dental and maxillofacial complex in multiple planes previously unavailable with conventional radiography.

Applications of Cone Beam Computed Tomography

Assessment of impacted and supernumerary teeth: Cone beam computed tomography (CBCT) is able to provide accurate information regarding the number and morphology of the roots, the position and relationship of the ID canal to the roots (**Figs 23.33 to 23.35**).

Complex Cases of Skeletal Abnormalities Requiring Orthodontic and Surgical Management

Endodontics: In selected cases when conventional radiographs provide inadequate information especially in multirooted teeth and in cases complicated by resorption or perforation. CBCT can also be used in planning surgical endodontic procedures.

*Dentoalveolar Trauma (**Figs 23.36A to C**)*

Implant dentistry: CBCT is able to provide information regarding bone width and height in the region of interest and the relationship to the adjacent vital structures, including the ID canal, mental foramen, incisive canal and maxillary sinuses (**Fig. 23.37**).

Facial Trauma

Bony pathology: Large cysts and odontogenic tumors. However, when soft tissue imaging is required conventional CT and/or MRI should be used (**Figs 23.38A to D**).

Advantages of CBCT

- Lower radiation dose. However, optimization of the dose must be considered at all times.
- Accessible technology.
- Small foot print and therefore suitable for dental hospital environment.
- Most machines offer panoramic and cephalometric options.
- There is reduction in metal streaking artefacts compared to the medical CT.

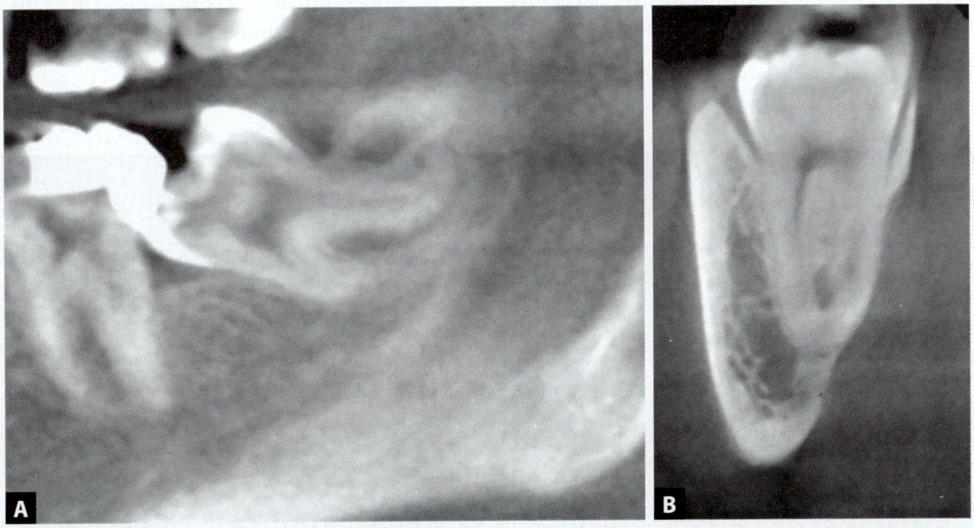

Figs 23.33A and B: (A) CBCT demonstrating dilacerated distal root lower-third molar; (B) Cross-sectional image of a lower-third molar demonstrating the course of the ID canal to be running through the tooth

- Limited volume size reduces unnecessary exposure.
- High isotropic spatial resolution.

Disadvantages of CBCT

- Soft tissue cannot be displayed resulting in limitation in the diagnostic spectrum.
- Lower contrast resolution caused by multiple factors including increased X-ray scatter during acquisition.

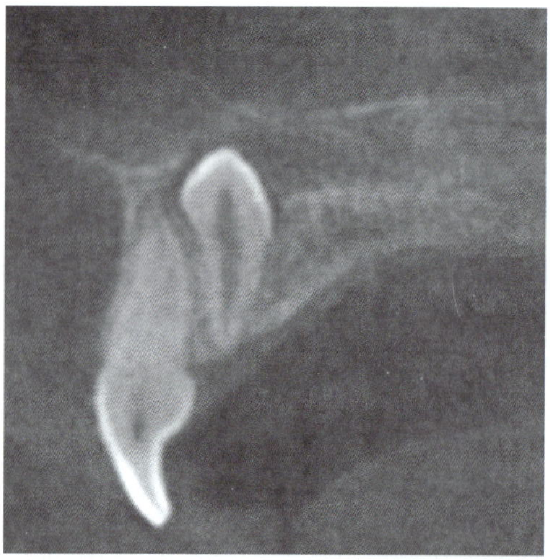

Fig. 23.34: Sagittal slice through the midline of the maxilla demonstrating the inverted supernumerary tooth posterior to the central incisor with no evidence of resorption. The intimate relationship to the floor of the nasal cavity is also demonstrated

MAGNETIC RESONANCE IMAGING

Magnetic resonance imaging (MRI) detects the presence and concentration of hydrogen atoms within the patient's body as they spin randomLy in their own environment. When the patient is placed into a strong magnet, hydrogen protons are aligned parallel to the long access of the magnetic field. At this point no signal can be detected from these protons.

To create a signal, a strong radio frequency (RF) pulse is sent in which the hydrogen protons tilt away from the long access of the magnetic field. These protons continue to spin in the newly created orientation for as long as the radio-frequency signal is on.

When RF is switched off, the protons will now relax, slowly returning to their original alignment, simultaneously emitting a signal.

This principle is now used to detect a signal created from these individual protons in three dimensions thus creating the final image. Changing the strength and angulation of the RF signal change the pattern of tilt of hydrogen protons and alter the resultant final image.

The generated signal intensity variation within the tissues depends on:

- The total number of available hydrogen atoms, as a result water and fat produce a high signal because of their high content of hydrogen protons, as opposed to air, cortical bone and the enamel of teeth that produce

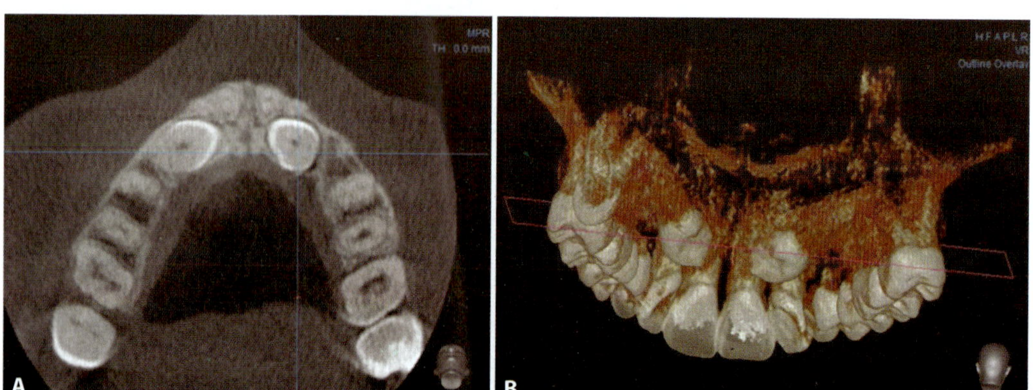

Figs 23.35A and B: Axial slice through the maxilla showing the unerupted canines and their close relationship to the apices of the lateral incisors. 3D model showing the palatal position of the canines

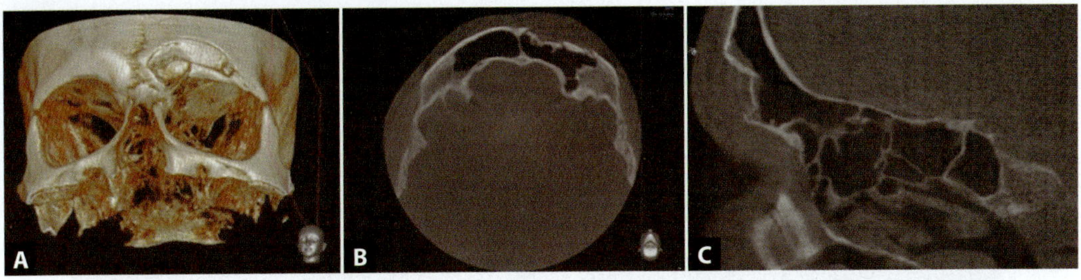

Figs 23.36A to C: Axial, sagittal and 3D model of a displaced fracture of the frontal bone

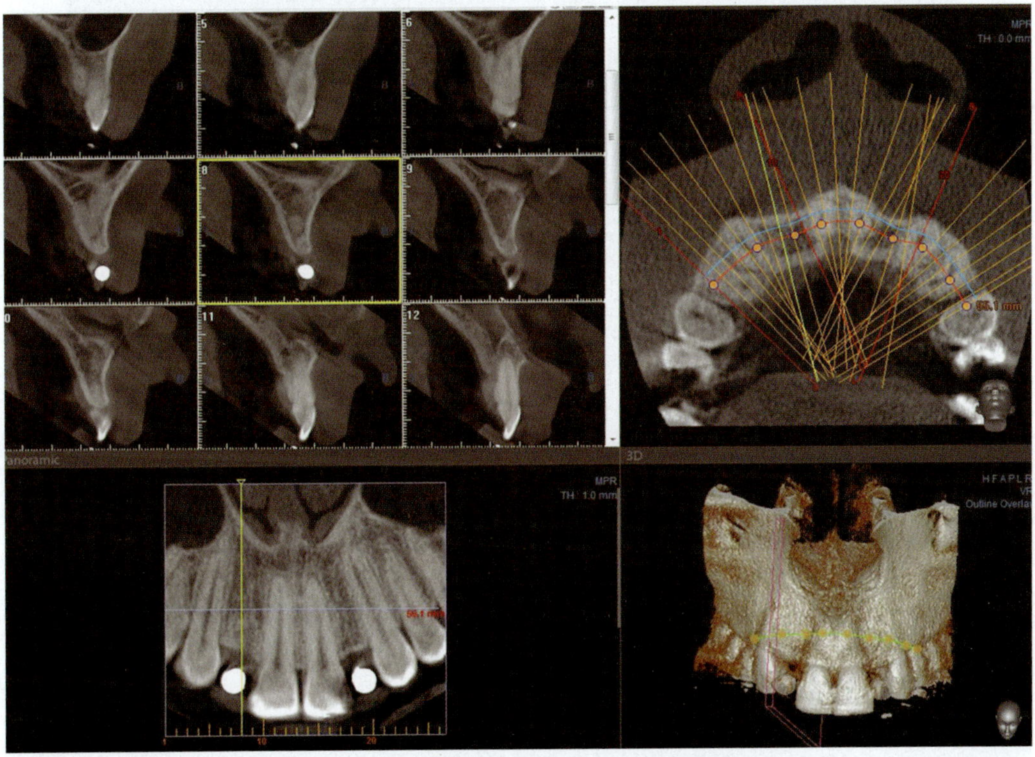

Fig. 23.37: Implant assessment of the missing upper lateral incisors in both cross-sectional and panoramic planes

no signal due to the lack of the hydrogen atoms presence.

- *The strength of the magnet and speed of acquisition*: The majority of available MRI scanners operate a 1.5 Tesla magnet. The more recently introduced 3.0 Tesla magnets offer increase in Signal-to-Noise ratio and speed (**Figs 23.39A and B**).

T1 relaxation time is affected by the strength of the external magnetic field and tissue composition. T1 is approximately 300 to 2000 milliseconds.

T2 relaxation time is affected by the variation within the internal magnetic field. T2 is approximately 150 to 300 milliseconds (**Figs 23.40A and B**).

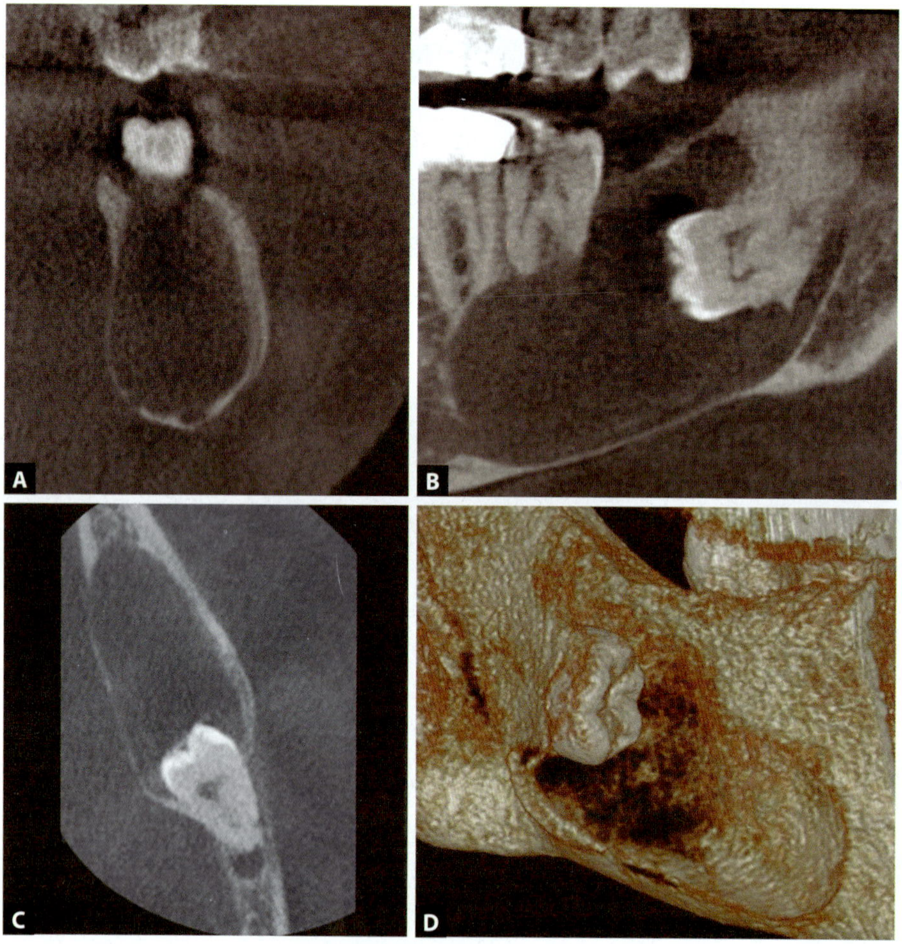

Figs 23.38A to D: Large dentigerous cyst in the mandible associated with unerupted third molar. The ID canal has been displaced inferioly to reach the lower border of the mandible

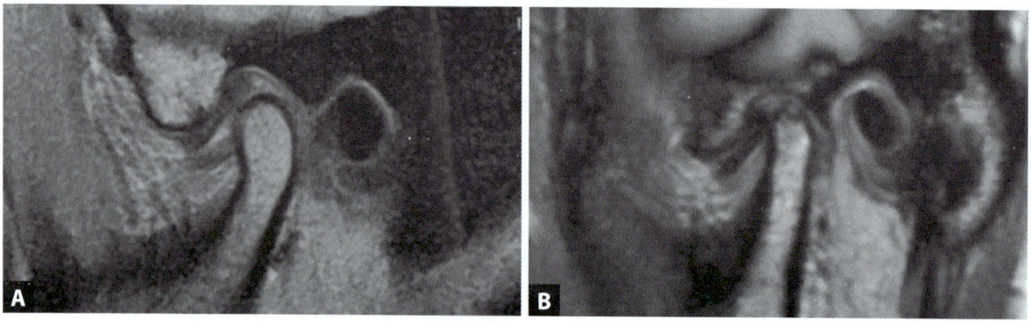

Figs 23.39A and B: Parasagittal MRI images through the condylar head and TMJ using 1.5T: (A) 3T; (B) Scanners

Using the above variations, multiple sequences can be generated when different tissues can appear with a slightly different color.

To improve the quality of the final image, surface coil are often used in the head and neck region to improve the detection of the signal emitted from hydrogen protons.

Clinical Applications of MRI

MRI is widely used in the head and neck. The list below is representative of the common applications but is not exhaustive. The full list is beyond the scope of this chapter.

Examination of soft tissue pathology.

- *Developmental*: Branchial cleft cysts, hemangioma and lymphangioma and venous vascular malformations (**Fig. 23.41A**)
- *Inflammatory*: Osteomyelitis, simple ranula and plunging ranula (**Fig. 23.41B**)
- Benign soft tissue and salivary tumors (**Figs 23.42A to C**)
- *Malignant tumors*: Squamous cell carcinoma (**Figs 23.43A and B**), salivary tumors and nodal staging.
- Functional analysis
- TMJ imaging (**Figs 23.44A to F**)

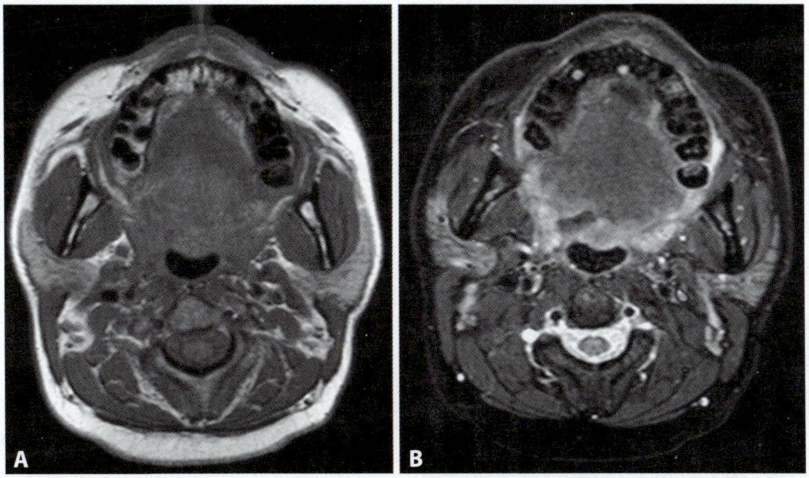

Figs 23.40A and B: Axial slices at the level of mid ramus using (A) T1 sequence; (B) T2 – STIR

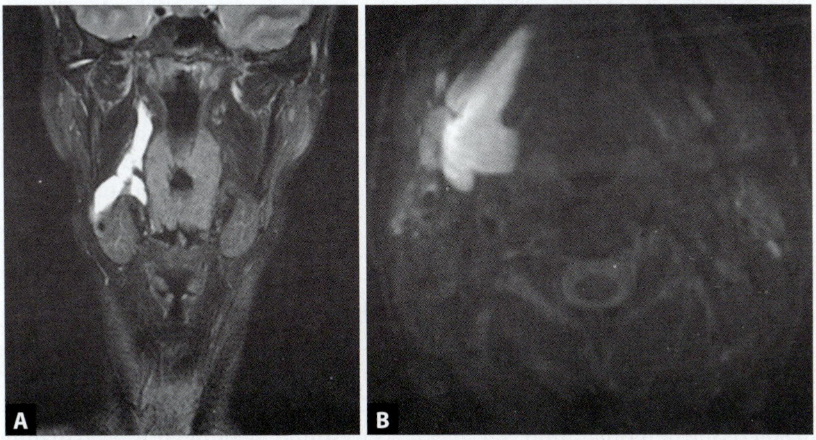

Figs 23.41A and B: (A) Coronal T2 image demonstrating cystic hygroma in the right parapharyngeal and submandibular regions; (B) Axial T2 of the right mandible showing a plunging ranula

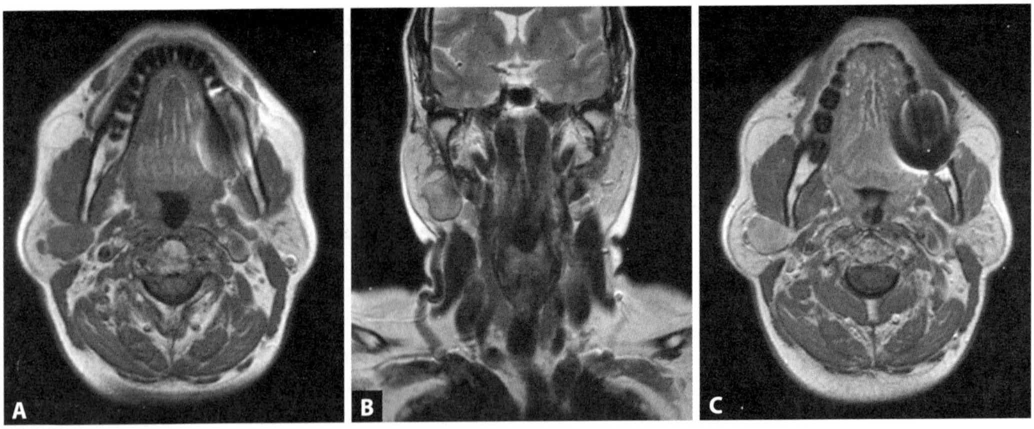

Figs 23.42A to C: Pleomorphic adenoma of the right parotid gland seen on (A) T1 axial; (B) T1 coronal; (C) T1 postcontrast

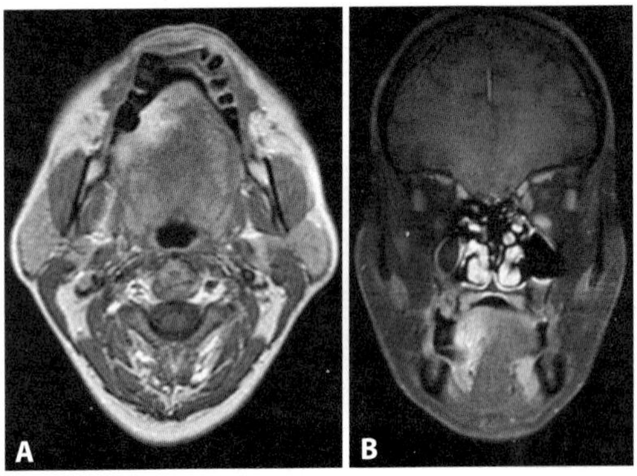

Figs 23.43A and B: High signal intensity showing squamous cell carcinoma of the right tongue seen on (A) Axial; (B) Coronal images

- Masseteric hypertrophy (**Fig. 23.45**)
- Intracranial pathology
- Trigeminal neuralgia (vascular loop) (**Figs 23.46A and B**)
- Exclude intracranial cause of atypical facial pain (**Figs 23.47A and B**).

Advantages of MRI

- There is no ionizing radiation involved, therefore no radiation dose to patients.
- It offers true multiplanar acquisition of data.
- Excellent soft tissue demonstration
- Offers information on bone quality (**Figs 23.48A and B**).

Disadvantages of MRI

- *Speed*: The acquisition of data is slow resulting in increased risk of motion artefacts.
- Limited availability and access when compared to CT.
- Cost is relatively more expensive to set up and train personnel.
- It can be claustrophobic due to the small aperture of magnet. Open MRI can overcome this disadvantage at a cost of reduced signal-to-noise ratio.
- MRI is significantly noisy.

There are strict contra-indications to MRI including the presence of pacemakers and all implanted ferromagnetic objects. It is therefore essential to obtain a comprehensive history and safety questionnaire prior to scanning. Orthodontic brackets and wires are usually made of stainless steel and dental implants are usually made of titanium and therefore do not pose a strict contraindication. They can cause a major metal artefact which can render the images non-diagnostic.

Metal objects cause significant loss of signal (**Fig. 23.49**).

ULTRASOUND

Ultrasound technology is used in different fields of science. The SONAR (Sound Navigation and Ranging) principle has been used for many

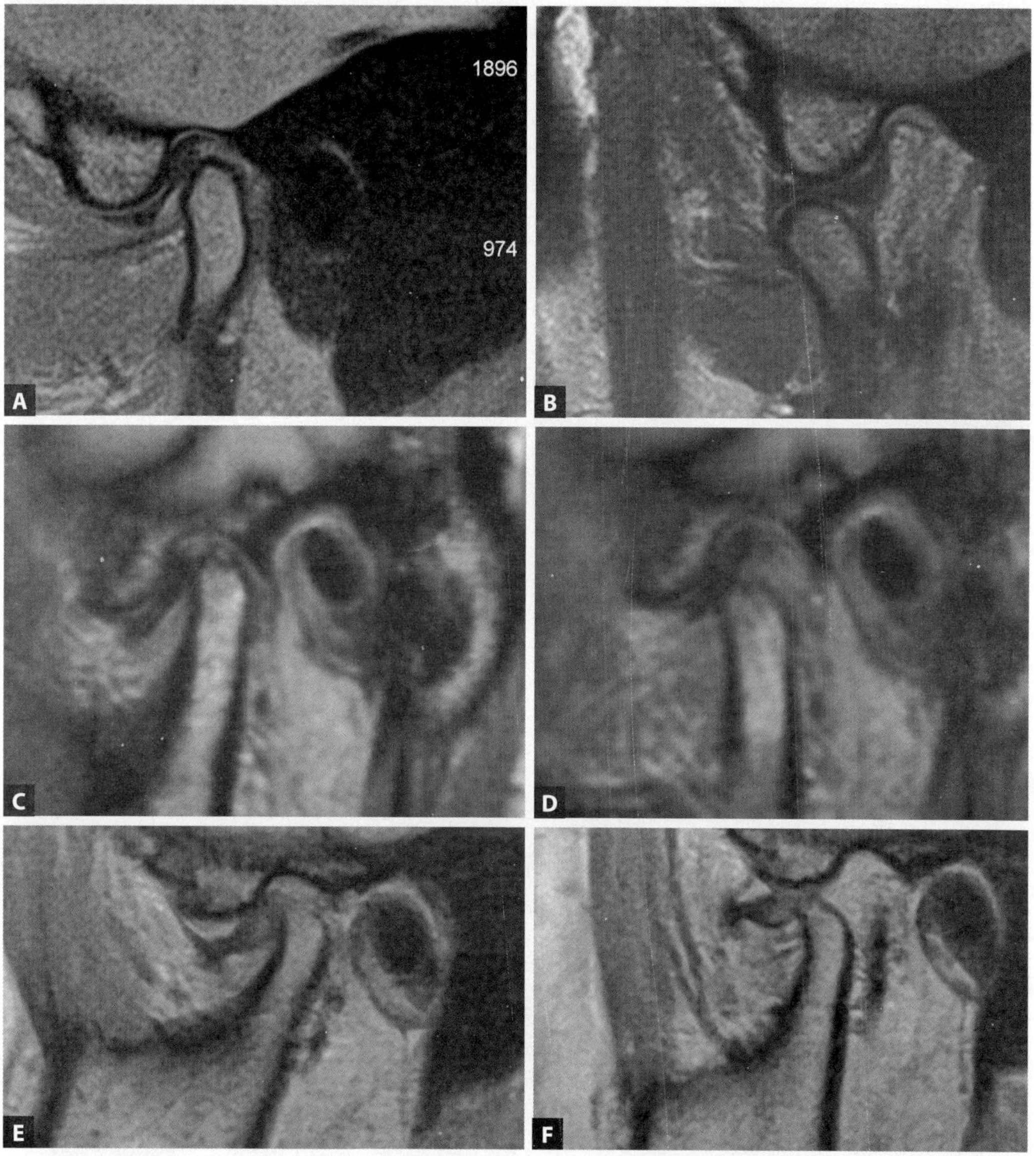

Figs 23.44A to F: Normal TMJ in (A) Closed; (B) Open position, anterior disc displacement with reduction in; (C) Closed; (D) Open anterior disc displacement without reduction; (E) Closed; (F) Open position

years to locate submarines and vessels and to study the sea bed floor.

In medicine, ultrasound utilizes high frequency ultrasonic waves of more than 20 KHz but usually in the range of 5 to 20 MHZ. These waves travel through and interact with tissues of different acoustic characteristics. Higher frequencies are subject to more attenuation and therefore, able to penetrate less tissue. However, they are able to provide better resolution of smaller and more superficial objects. This is an ideal scenario for the imaging of the superficial facial and neck regions.

Ultrasonic waves are unable to travel through vacuum and therefore require a medium. A water base gel is usually adequate.

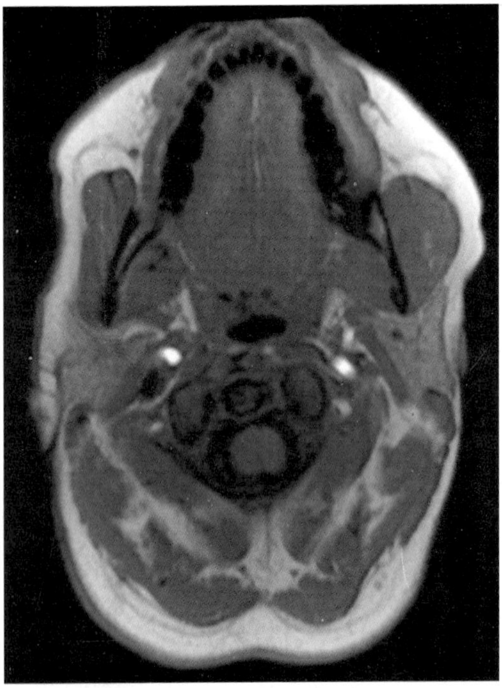

Fig. 23.45: T1 image showing unilateral left sided masseteric hypertrophy

The waves are generated by a transducer made up predominantly among other components, of piezoelectric crystals that are able to convert electrical energy into high frequency ultrasonic waves and vice-versa. The transducer is part of what is generally known as the ultra sound probe. The probe is made in different shapes to adapt to the region of interest. In the head and neck region, extraoral examination is performed using a narrow rectangular shaped high frequency (16 MHZ), whereas intraoral examination can also be carried out using a hockey stick probe of 10 MHZ.

The waves travel through the tissues. Some are absorbed and some are reflected. The reflected waves reach back to the transducer generating an electrical signal which is converted to an image. The processing of these waves by the transducer is fast enough to be able to provide real time imaging. The density of tissues dictates their acoustic characteristics (acoustic impedance) and therefore, their ability to absorb or reflect ultrasonic waves.

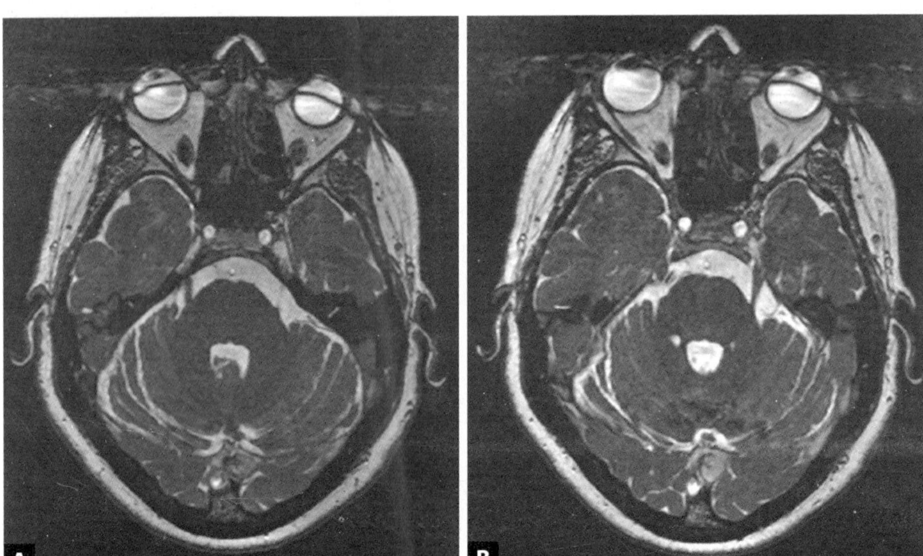

Figs 23.46A and B: (A) Axial slices through the mid brain demonstrating the right trigeminal nerve; (B) Crossed by a vascular loop

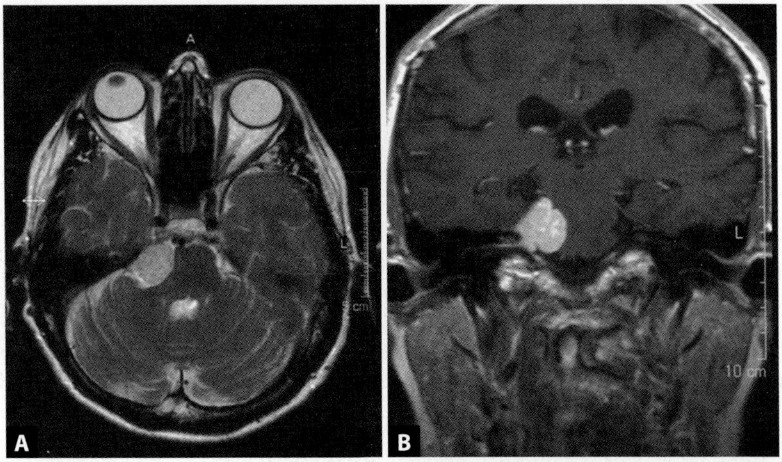

Figs 23.47A and B: Axial and coronal slices demonstrating the presence of an intracranial tumor

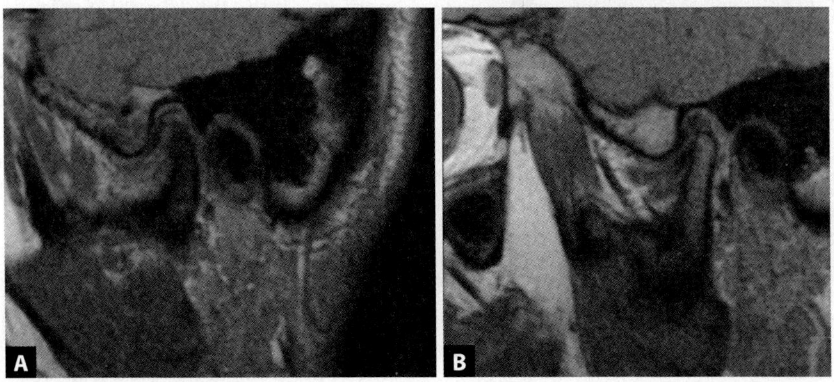

Figs 23.48A and B: (A) Increased sclerosis of condylar head demonstrated as loss of signal intensity of bone marrow; (B) Compared to normal cancellous bone

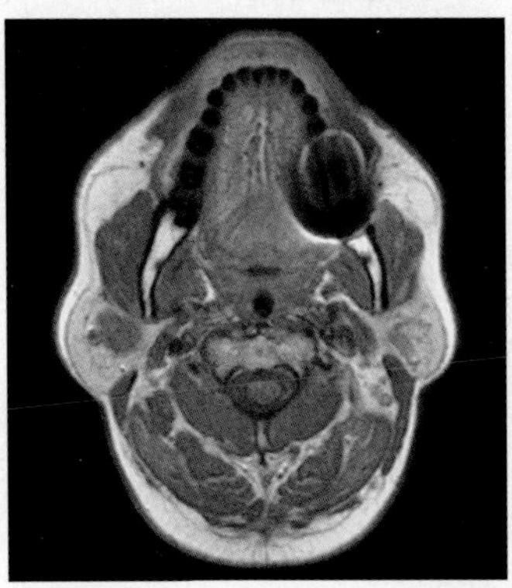

Fig. 23.49: MRI metal artefacts caused by a large metal dental restoration

This is usually described as the echogenecity of a tissue. Highly dense tissues such as bone is highly reflective and therefore described as hyperechoic whereas low density tissues such as cystic cavities are highly absorptive and therefore described as hypoechoic. All hyperechoic objects pose a limitation when performing an ultrasound examination as an acoustic shadow is formed beyond the object and therefore visualization of these tissues becomes limited.

Advantages of ultrasound scan

- Simple, accessible noninvasive technique
- *Portable*: Therefore, nonrestricted to radiology departments

- No ionizing radiation
- Able to examine superficial soft tissue
- Used as guide to carry out fine needle aspiration and core biopsies
- Assess real time vascularity of the tissue using Doppler mode.

Disadvantages of ultrasound scan

- Operator-dependant
- It is considered as an investigation difficult to interpret by clinicians.

Clinical applications

- Obstructive salivary gland disease (**Fig. 23.50**)
- Benign and malignant salivary tumors (**Figs 23.51A and B**)
- Sjögren's syndrome and associated lymphomas (**Fig. 23.52**)
- Sarcoidosis (**Figs 23.53A and B**)
- Superficial swellings in the head and neck regions (**Fig. 23.54**)
- Masseteric hypertrophy
- Nodal characterization and staging (**Figs 23.55A and B**)
- Thyroid gland disease
- Drainage of maxillofacial abscesses
- Vascular malformation (**Figs 23.56A and B**).

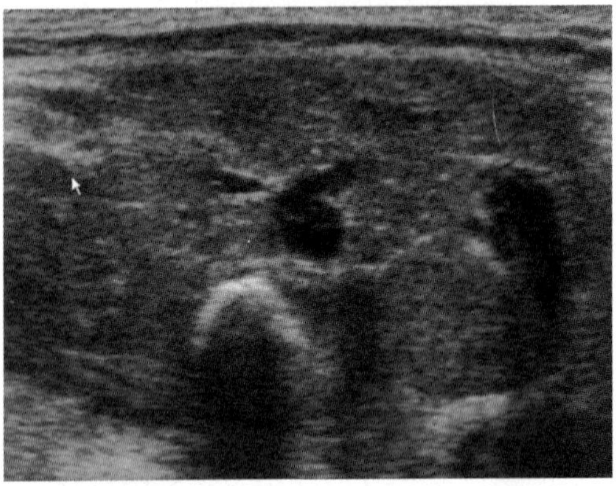

Fig. 23.50: Strong hyperechoic object (arrow) representing a salivary stone with a strong acoustic shadow

SIALOGRAPHY

Sialography is a minimally invasive technique that involves the introduction of contrast medium into the ductal system of major salivary glands (parotid and submandibular glands). This allows the visualization of the ductal architecture of the main duct, the hilum and the intraglandular structure. Water soluble low osmolality contrast media are used with different concentrations of Iodine (140–240 mg I/mL).

The technique is simple and involves the identification of the orifice of the salivary gland. This is situated in the buccal mucosa opposite the upper second molar for the parotid gland and in the floor of the mouth under the tongue

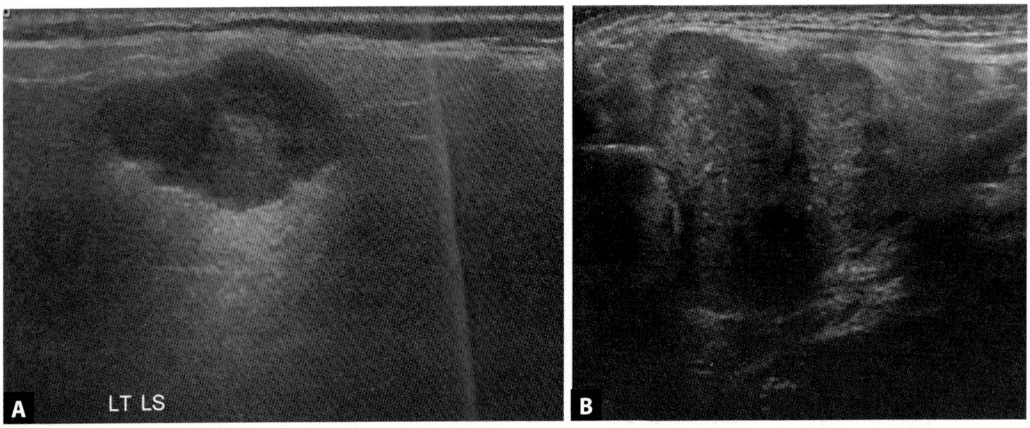

Figs 23.51A and B: (A) Well-defined area in the parotid gland representing a pleomorphic adenoma; (B) Ill-defined area in the submandibular gland representing an adenocystic carcinoma (*Courtesy*: Dr Polly Richards)

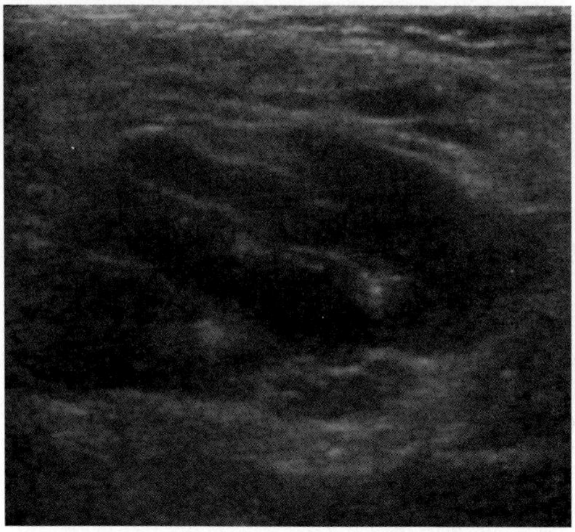

Fig. 23.52: Irregular hypoechoic mass with internal linear striations consistent with a MALT lymphoma

just anterior and to either side of the lingual fraenulum for the submandibular gland. Manual stimulation of the gland will produce saliva from the orifice and therefore help identifying its exact position. A sialogogue can be used.

Once the orifice has been identified a short blunt metal cannula (single-use) filled with approximately 1 to 1.5 mL of contrast medium is inserted. Different sizes are available for parotid and submandibular glands (**Fig. 23.57**). The contrast is slowly injected into the gland under X-ray guidance. Digital subtraction imaging is used to eliminate superimposition of adjacent anatomical structures. This allows a live demonstration of the contrast into the duct which highlights the mobility of the stones and the extent of the presence of mucus plugs.

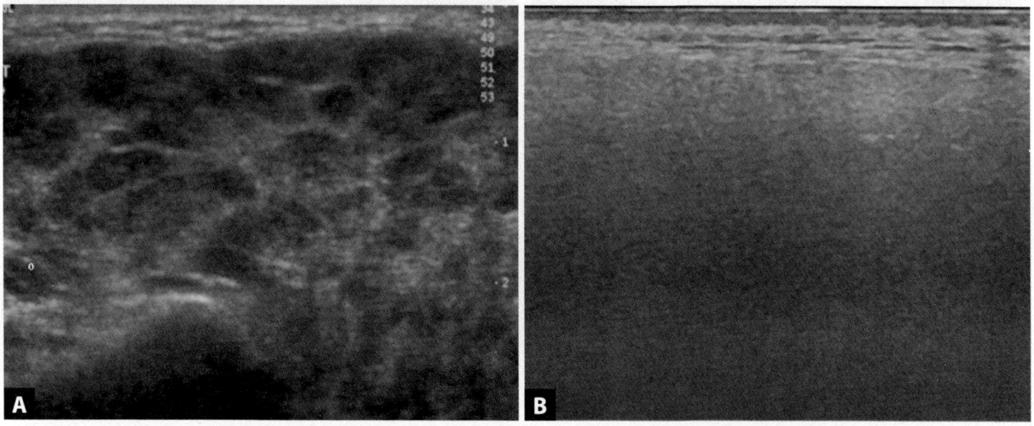

Figs 23.53A and B: (A) Multiple hypoechoic areas within the parotid gland in a patient with sarcoidosis; (B) Normal echogenic appearance of parotid gland

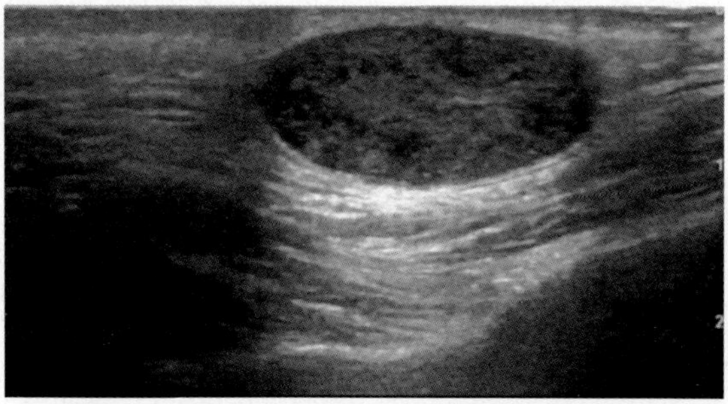

Fig. 23.54: Well-defined area with a strong acoustic enhancement representing a sebaceous cyst (*Courtesy:* Dr Polly Richards)

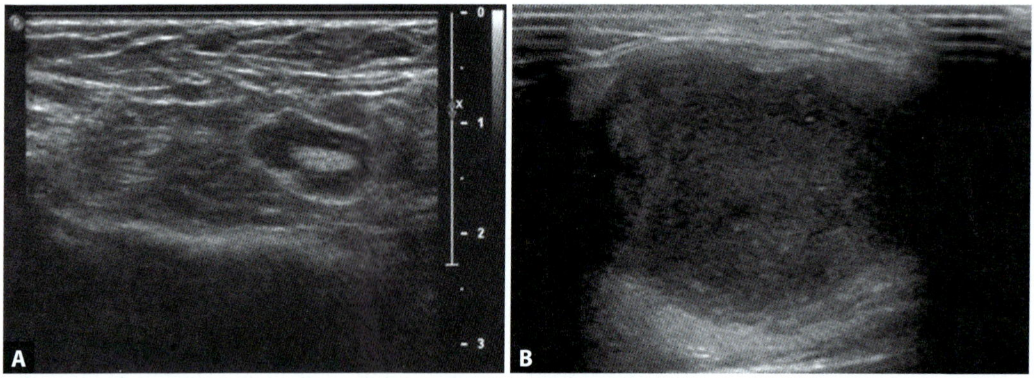

Figs 23.55A and B: Small benign reactive lymph node with well defined outline and a well-defined fatty hilus and malignant lymph node with ill-defined outline and no fatty hilus (*Courtesy*: Dr Polly Richards)

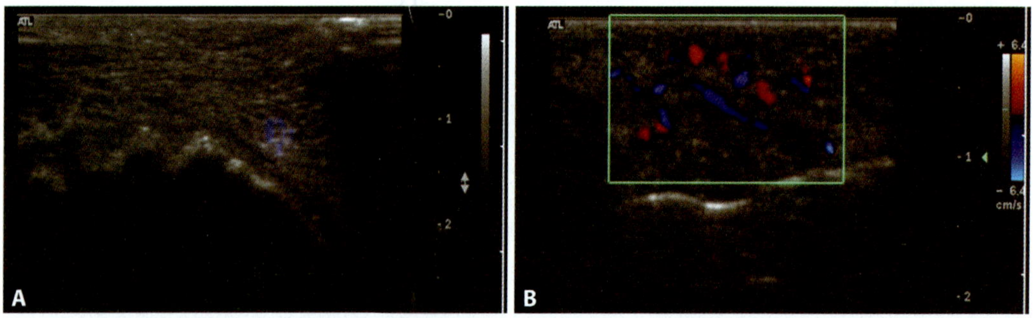

Figs 23.56A and B: Use of color flow capability to demonstrate vascularity in a case of superficial vascular malformation

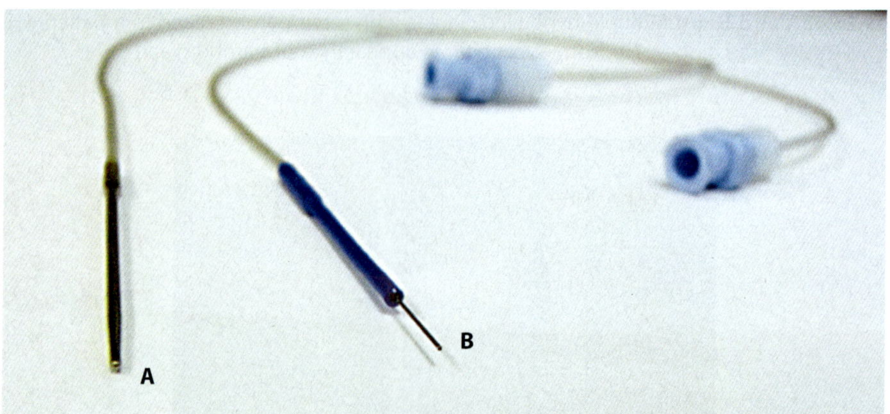

Fig. 23.57: Parotid (A) and submandibular (B) cannula used in sialography

An emptying screen is acquired at the end of the procedure to identify any retention of contrast medium in the duct or the gland.

A normal gland exhibits a uniform main duct of approximately 1 mm diameter (parotid) and 1.5 mm diameter (submandibular) (**Figs 23.58A to D**). The intraglandular structure should be uniformLy represented. There is no evidence of filling defects (stones and mucous plugs) or strictures. Emptying should be rapid and complete following the removal of the cannula. Delayed emptying can be consistent with blockage (stones) or reduced function.

Applications of Sialography

- Obstructive benign salivary gland disease including stones, strictures and mucus plugs (**Figs 23.59A to C**)
- Dry mouth conditions and Sjögren's disease (**Fig. 23.60**) (*see* Chapter 11).

Facilitation of minimally invasive procedures of basket retrieval of stones and balloon dilatation of strictures; this is usually done under local anesthesia and under X-ray guidance (**Figs 23.61A and B**).

Advantages of Sialography

- Visualization of the ductal system and the intraglandular structure.
- Assessment of the size and mobility of stones and therefore whether they are amenable to minimally invasive interventional procedures.
- Washout of mucus plugs.
- Diagnosis of strictures that cannot be clearly seen on ultrasound.

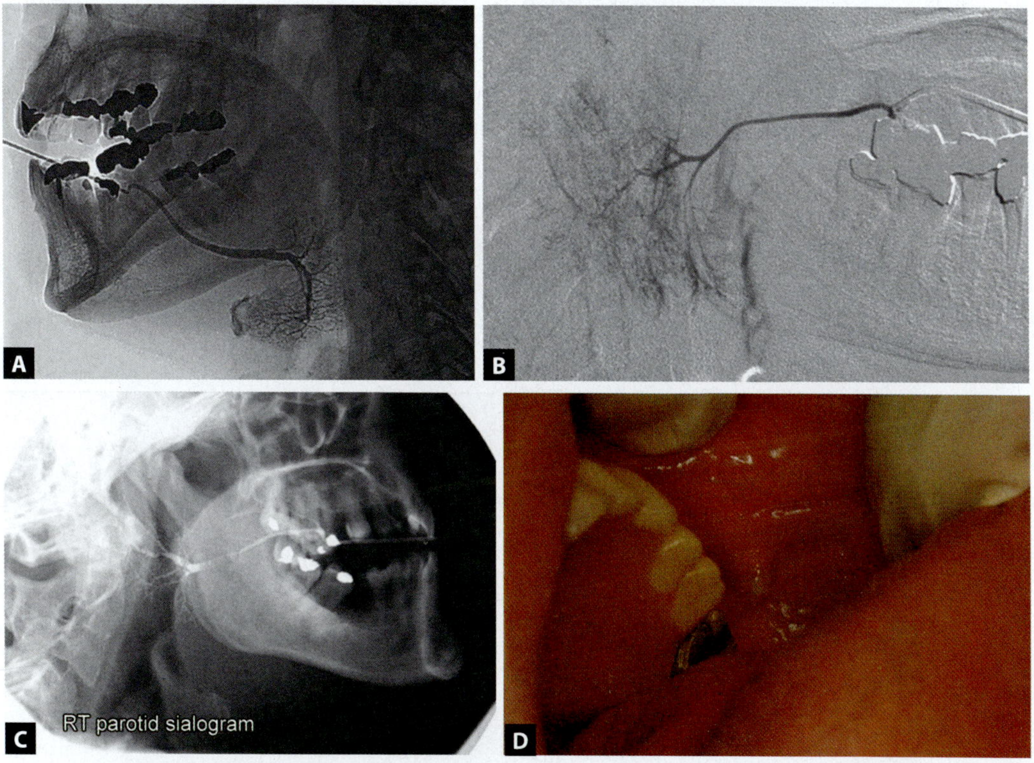

Figs 23.58A to D: (A) Normal sialogram of a submandibular gland using fluoroscopy; (B) Normal sialogram of a parotid gland using digital subtraction imaging; (C) Sialogram demonstrating a filling defect in the middle portion of the main duct representing mucous plugs; (D) Clinical image demonstrating the expulsion of mucus plugs through the orifice of the parotid gland

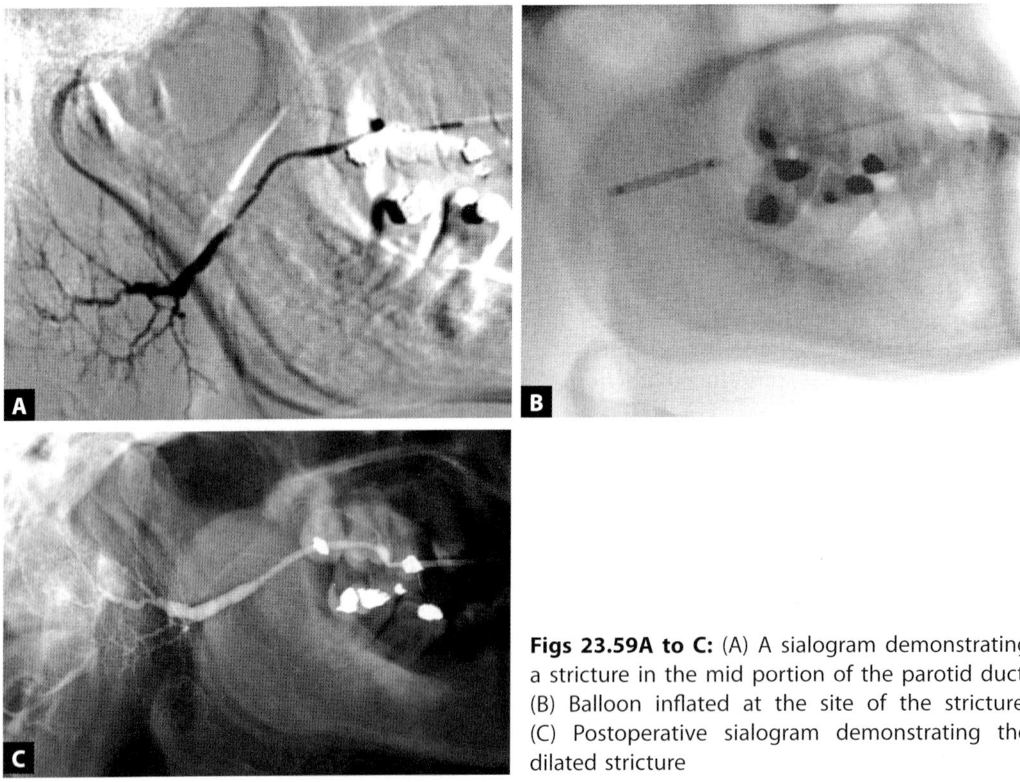

Figs 23.59A to C: (A) A sialogram demonstrating a stricture in the mid portion of the parotid duct; (B) Balloon inflated at the site of the stricture; (C) Postoperative sialogram demonstrating the dilated stricture

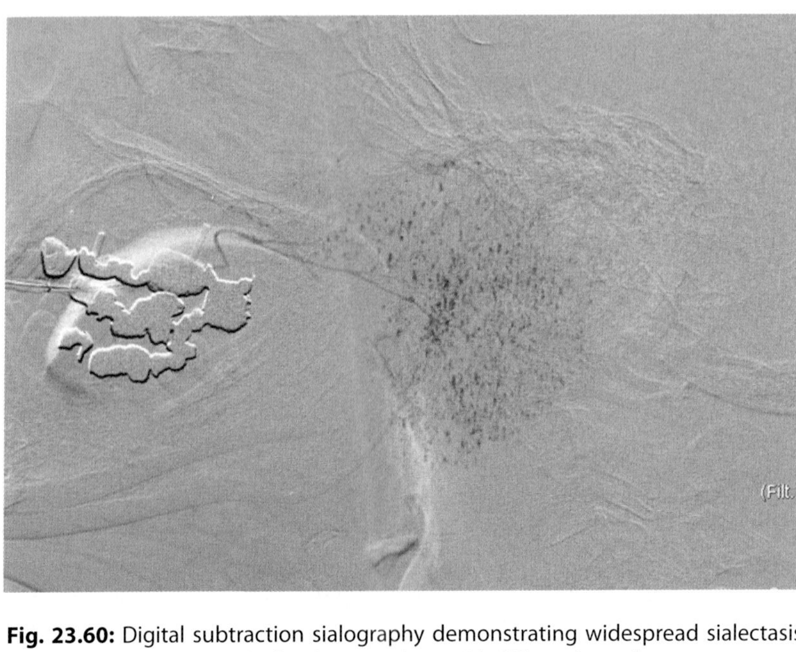

Fig. 23.60: Digital subtraction sialography demonstrating widespread sialectasis of the parotid gland in a patient with Sjögren's syndrome

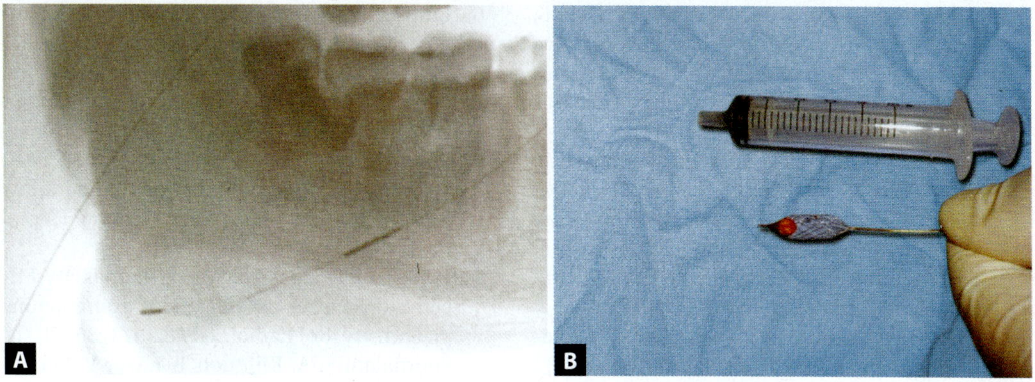

Figs 23.61A and B: (A) Basket *in situ* ready to capture a stone; (B) Stone in the basket

Disadvantages of Sialography

- Not suitable for patients with allergy to iodine. Gadolinium has been suggested as a substitute in these patients
- Not suitable in pregnant patients
- The procedure can be uncomfortable
- Not suitable during the acute phase of sialadenitis.

SIALOENDOSCOPY

Sialoendoscopy is a minimally invasive technique used in the diagnosis and management of benign obstructive salivary gland diseases. It requires the use of semiflexible endoscopes with or without working channels for the introduction of baskets and mini graspers.

Applications of Sialoendoscopy

- Diagnosis of obstructive salivary gland disease including stones and strictures
- Management of obstructive salivary gland disease using baskets, balloons and graspers.

ACKNOWLEDGMENT

I am extremely grateful of the technical help provided by Dr Ravikiran Pawar.

SELF-ASSESSMENT QUESTIONS

1. Discuss the indications for periapical radiographic examination.
2. Discuss the different types of occlusal radiographs and outline their use.
3. Describe the advantages of computerized tomography and outline its limitations.
4. Describe the indications for the use of cone beam computerized tomography (CBCT).
5. Discuss the main advantages and disadvantages of cone beam computerized tomography (CBCT).
6. List the advantages and disadvantages of magnetic resonance imaging (MRI) and add a note on contraindications to its use.
7. Compare and contrast ultrasound and magnetic resonance imaging (MRI) examinations in the diagnosis of superficial maxillofacial lesions.
8. Discuss the use of minimally invasive interventional procedures in the management of obstructive salivary gland disease.
9. List the indications for the use of siaolography and outline the technique.
10. Describe the advantages of digital radiography in comparison to conventional radiography.

SUGGESTED READING

1. Chau AC, Fung K. Comparison of radiation dose for implant imaging using conventional spiral tomography, computed tomography, and cone-beam computed tomography. Oral Surg Oral Med Oral Pathol Oral Radiol Endod 2009;107(4):559-65.

2. Carrafiello G, Dizonno M, Colli V, Strocchi S, Pozzi Taubert S, Leonardi A, et al. Comparative study of jaws with multislice computed tomography and cone-beam computed tomography. Radiol Med 2010;115(4):600-11.
3. Carranza-Pelegrina D, Lomeña-Caballero F, Soler-Peter M, Berini-Aytés L, Gay-Escoda C. The diagnostic possibilities of positron emission tomography (PET): applications in oral and maxillofacial buccal oncology. Med Oral Patol Oral Cir Bucal 2005;10(4):331-42.
4. De Vos W, Casselman J, Swennen GR. Cone-beam computerized tomography (CBCT) imaging of the oral and maxillofacial region: a systematic review of the literature. Int J Oral Maxillofac Surg 2009;38(6):609-25.
5. Ludlow JB, Davies-Ludlow LE, White SC. Patient risk related to common dental radiographic examinations: the impact of 2007 International Commission on Radiological Protection recommendations regarding dose calculation. J Am Dent Assoc 2008;139(9):1237-43.
6. Ludlow JB, Ivanovic M. Comparative dosimetry of dental CBCT devices and 64-slice CT for oral and maxillofacial radiology. Oral Surg Oral Med Oral Pathol Oral Radiol Endod 2008;106(1):106-14.
7. Pendlebury ME, Horner K, Eaton KA. Selection Criteria for Dental Radiography. Second Edition. Faculty of General Dental Practitioners, 2004.
8. Roberts JA, Drage NA, Davies J, Thomas DW. Effective dose from cone beam CT examinations in dentistry. Br J Radiol 2009;82(973):35-40.
9. Suomalainen A, Kiljunen T, Käser Y, Peltola J, Kortesniemi M. Dosimetry and image quality of four dental cone beam computed tomography scanners compared with multislice computed tomography scanners. Dentomaxillofac Radiol 2009;38(6):367-78.
10. Vogl TJ, Harth M, Siebenhandl P. Different imaging techniques in the head and neck: Assets and drawbacks. World J Radiol 2010;2(6):224-9.

Chapter 24

Tobacco Use Prevention and Cessation

Christoph A Ramseier

Chapter Outline

INTRODUCTION

Scientific studies in oral health research in the past have consistently revealed the detrimental effects of smokeless and smoked tobacco on the oral mucosa and the periodontal tissues. For oral care in general, both improving oral hygiene and tobacco use cessation have been identified as necessary measures to gain and maintain long-term periodontal health. This growing evidence has given the dental team a whole new task to tackle when achieving and maintaining oral health with their patients.

The measures carried out to improve the patients' oral hygiene or to support their attempt to quit tobacco use are often referred to as "patient motivation" or "patient education". Improvements of oral hygiene and periodontal stability due to long-term supportive periodontal care have been well studied and presented in the literature. For tobacco use cessation, it has become essential to present suitable approaches to the oral health professionals both adapted for the dental practice and based on the best available evidence in health behavior change.

UNDERSTANDING 'TOBACCO USE DISEASE'

In order to support dental patients to quit tobacco use, it is helpful for the clinician to have a clear understanding of the genesis of 'tobacco use disease' in general. The term 'tobacco use disease' refers to the condition of tobacco users suffering from both psychological tobacco use dependence and physical addiction to nicotine.

Psychological Tobacco Use Dependence

The repeated use of tobacco products can lead to the development of a habit itself. Social contacts to other consumers, altogether with recurring daily repetition, can enhance the development of a consumption habit. Over time, this habit can become part of a person's daily routine. Consequently, if the behavior cannot be carried out for a certain reason, the person experiences symptoms such as restlessness, nervousness or aggression. These reactions are caused by the psychological dependence.

Physical Addiction to Nicotine

Tobacco products contain the drug nicotine which is known to create a pleasant emotional state in tobacco users. In smokers, nicotine from tobacco smoke passes through the lungs or the oral mucosa into the blood circulation, which then transports the molecule to the central nervous system. At this location, nicotine attracts receptors for acetylcholine and prolongs the opening time of the ion channels for the flow of sodium into the target cells. As a result of this additional flow, the concentration of noradrenaline will be raised temporarily in certain areas of the brain, such as the nucleus accumbens and the locus ceruleus, leading to an emotional delight to the consumer. Simultaneously, however, an adaptation will be triggered over time to decrease the sensitivity of the nervous cells to the same stimulus. As a consequence of this adaptation, the tobacco user will increase the nicotine dose (e.g. number of cigarettes per day) in order to experience the same enjoyment from tobacco consumption. Finally, experiences of withdrawal symptoms occur in case the brain cells will not receive the nicotine dose they demand. Once adaptation has proceeded, the tobacco user even requires a minimal dose of nicotine in order to prevent withdrawal symptoms from reoccurring. This process of adaptation by the central nervous system is referred to as the development of the physical nicotine addiction.

Tobacco use disease, again, consists of the psychological dependence and the physical addiction to nicotine. In order to be predictably successful, any approach to support tobacco use cessation should include both behavioral

Box 24.1: Tobacco use disease

Key features of interest

- Tobacco use disease consists of psychological dependence and physical addiction to nicotine.
- Any approach to support tobacco use cessation should include both behavioral support to address the psychological dependence and pharmacotherapy to treat the physical symptoms of withdrawal.

support to address the psychological component of the dependence and pharmacotherapy to treat the physical symptoms of withdrawal.

TOBACCO USE CESSATION

During everyday life, tobacco consumers receive feedback concerning their unhealthy behavior. Numerous articles or programs in the media, "No Smoking" signs at the workplace and in public areas, the strongly expressed wish of friends and family members not to be exposed to the risks of passive smoking: these are only a few of the situations smokers have to contend with on a regular basis. Furthermore, efforts are made to reduce the prevalence of tobacco use by raising taxes on tobacco products and limiting advertizing by the tobacco industry. The support of all health professionals is enlisted for these efforts, which are mounted, among other reasons, in the interest of public health. Although, all these measures taken at the initiative of the public health sector are generally acknowledged, in the final analysis it will always be the consumers who decide whether they are willing to change behavior and terminate their tobacco use addiction. Among those smokers who try to "kick the habit" without support from either professional counseling or self-help groups, the success rate is found to be between 10.2 and 11 percent.

Methods for Tobacco Use Cessation

At present, the evidence-based method for tobacco use cessation consists of professional counseling on behavioral change using the so called "5A Method" ("Ask, Advise, Assess, Assist and Arrange") in combination with pharmacotherapy. It is well known that the success rates achieved by smoking cessation counselling are generally dependent on the amount of time allowed for this counseling. The success rates achieved by counseling lasting for 1 to 3 minutes, 4 to 30 minutes, 31 to 90 minutes and >90 minutes are 1425, 18.8 percent, 26.5 percent and 28.4 percent, respectively. In clinical studies designed to record the success rates achieved by smoking cessation programs, it was observed that the percentage of participants who were still abstinent was relatively high (>50%) around 3 months after quitting. However, this statistic drops dramatically by the end of the first year (<25%) following the quit date as a result of the generally high relapse rate.

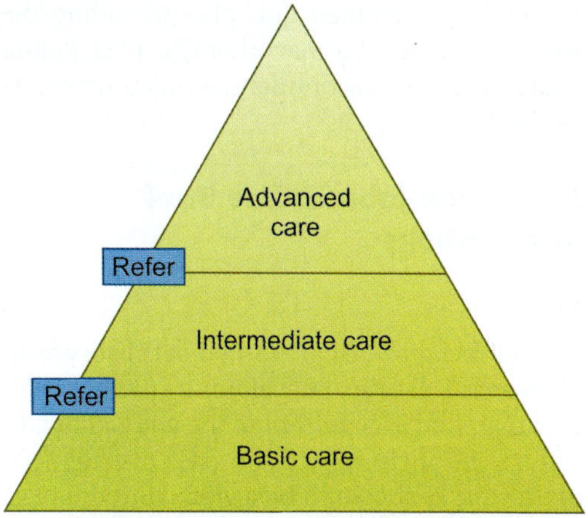

Fig. 24.1: Level of care model (Adapted by Davis et al. 2010)

Given that tobacco use prevention and cessation (TUPAC) in the dental treatment setting occurs in brief interventions over repeated visits, dental practitioners and educators should consider adopting the following level of care model (**Fig. 24.1**).

CATEGORIES OF CARE

The level of care that could be offered would reflect on available facilities, skills of the practitioner and health systems in operation; basic care being affordable at all health service levels.

Basic care: Brief interventions of a few minutes in order to identify tobacco users, assess readiness to quit, request permission to re-address tobacco use at a subsequent visit, and if preferred, refer for further TUPAC counseling.

Intermediate care: Interventions of 5 to 10 or more minutes consisting of (brief) motivational interviewing sessions to build on readiness to quit, enlist resources to support change, and to include cessation medications. If preferred, refer for further TUPAC counseling.

Advanced care: Multiple intensive interventions of 20 or more minutes for complex care patients to develop a detailed quit plan including the use of suitable pharmacotherapy, past failure exploration, and recommendation adjustments as needed.

Basic Care: Tobacco Use Brief Interventions

Ask

It is well recognized that the medical history form plays a critical role in developing an oral health care plan that is cognisant of the general health status. The inclusion of the patients' tobacco use history is shown to be a vital component of the medical history form on a myriad of levels that are integral to the promotion of tobacco use prevention and cessation. For example, if the patient identifies as a never-smoker, it enables the oral health professional to reinforce the benefits of this lifestyle choice.

Particularly in the case of young adults, the opportunity to congratulate their decision to remain tobacco free offers a positive counter to the efforts of peer pressure, advertizing or other adverse influence. Should the patient identify as a former smoker, the opportunity arises again to provide positive reinforcement to the decision to change. The implementation of a tobacco use history form additionally increases the awareness to the patient regarding the detrimental effects of tobacco on oral health. Finally, the tobacco use history form allows a nonthreatening introduction to the ensuing conversation between oral health professional and patient.

Assess

When asked about their readiness to quit smoking, tobacco users often reply that they want to quit smoking "sometime" but that the time is not yet right. There are certain things they need to do first, which are seen as more important than giving up smoking. Even if the patient feels that they are ready to quit smoking, there still may be some uncertainty about the next steps. They may experience a lack confidence or self-efficacy to achieve this goal and feel under prepared to make a quit attempt. Behind this attitude is often the fear of failure, potential change to social habits, or worry about gaining unwanted weight.

Brief Motivational Interviewing

Numerous behavioral studies have demonstrated predictable success in supporting patients to change using Motivational Interviewing (MI). MI is a patient-centred method to enhance the patient's intrinsic motivation to change by exploring and resolving ambivalence. A "short form" of MI known as "Brief Motivational Interviewing" (BMI) appears to be suitable for use during brief interventions for tobacco use prevention and cessation in dental practices. The aim of BMI is to achieve the following objectives within a relative short amount of time:

1. To ask the patient about his or her motivation to change,
2. To ask the patient's self-efficacy to change, and
3. To get the patient's commitment to discuss the change in behavior at the next visit.

As described by Rollnick and co-workers, understanding the current levels of recognized motivation and self-efficacy as indicators of the readiness to change can greatly assist the process of supporting the patient through a quit attempt (**Fig. 24.2**).

For example, asking the patient to use a number scale to rate how motivated he or she is to quit smoking will give a direction for the oral health professional to follow. Using the

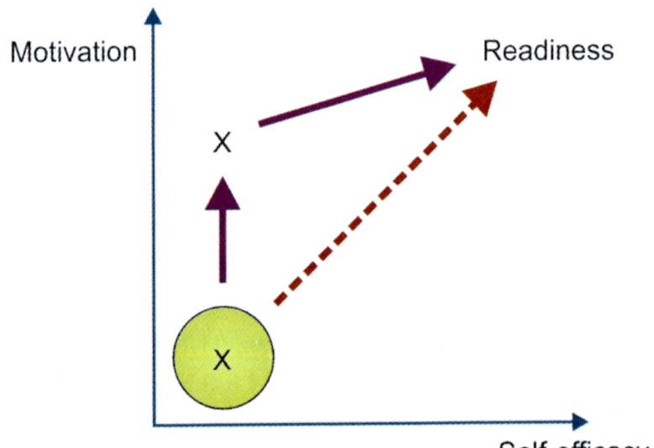

Fig. 24.2: Readiness scale (Adapted by Rollnick et al. 1997)

same number scale to rate how confident they are in achieving this goal will further direct the conversation towards identifying the type of support the patient may need.

Intermediate Care: Behavior Support for Tobacco Use Cessation

Assist

Providing assistance for the patient who wants to quit using tobacco often requires a combination of behavioral modification techniques and pharmacological support. Making arrangements for on-going support either via the dental office or other health agencies provides the patient with a valuable sense of reassurance as they undertake a quit attempt.

When available, refer to TUPAC specialist service, whether in-house (including suitably trained dental personnel) or external (i.e. www.quitline.com). If no TUPAC specialist service is available or patient declines referral consider to offer behavioral support and pharmacotherapy as outlined in the following step-by-step protocol.

Step-by-step Protocol

People who want to kick the smoking habit do not always participate in carefully controlled nicotine withdrawal programs, e.g. in linear fashion and from start to finish. Nevertheless, simple instructions–like those offered in the "Assist" (to help) and "Arrange" (to organize follow-up visits)—can be valuable tools for dental professionals supporting their patients to quit smoking.

Some smokers may even be euphoric about quitting smoking that would therefore tend to quit in a premature, e.g. unprepared manner. Even if this approach works for some smokers, others require varying amounts of support. This support can be given in an individual way manner by adapting the four steps outlined in the following:

Step 1: Ask the Patient to Fill in the Tobacco Use Journal

Every smoker has his or her individual smoking habits. To pinpoint the behavioral changes required in each particular case, it is recommended to fill in a tobacco use journal (**Fig. 24.3**) for several days. The patient will be instructed to fill in every column in the journal.

Instructions for the period up to the patient's next appointment: Fill in each cigarette and the time it is smoked; again, be sure to fill in all four columns of the journal labelled as "Time", "Place or activity", "Companion", "Importance", and "Alternative".

Tobacco use journal — Date:____________

Cig.	Time	Place of activity	Companion	Importance	Alternative
1.					
2.					
3.					
4.					
5.					
6.					
7.					
8.					
9.					
10.					
...					

Fig. 24.3: Tobacco use journal

Step 2: Evaluate the Tobacco Use Journal

Reading through the journal entries at the follow-up appointment may reveal patterns of smoking and assessments of importance which may not have been aware to the patient. This information will serve as the basis for re-assigning new habits for the patient in order to give up smoking (ideally without withdrawal symptoms) and to replace the old habit with new patterns of behavior. During this period, the patient will be advised to reduce tobacco use to a bearable minimum.

The four columns of the journal contain information on four important elements of the cessation protocol:

Time: Patients who smoke regularly throughout the day are primarily advised to alleviate the physical symptoms of withdrawal with sustained-release nicotine patches. On the other hand, patients who only smoke at certain times throughout the day are generally advised to use nicotine gum, sublingual tablets or lozenges. The smoking behavior that has been evaluated can be entered later in the form labelled "Recommendations for Use of Nicotine Replacement Therapy" (see below).

Place or activity and companion: Instructions for the period up to the patient's next appointment—attempt to change situations. Example—spend your work break with different colleagues and at a different location than usual.

Importance: Instructions for the period up to the patient's next appointment: Try to reduce the number of "less important" cigarettes.

Alternative: Instructions for the period up to the patient's next appointment—the patient should try to find his or her own personal alternatives-so-called replacements—which could help them to resist. In this context, they should take care to alternatively distract their mind (mental), their hands (physical) and their mouths (oral). Examples—play a game that requires mental concentration or manual dexterity. Do not select alternatives that simulate smoking. Example: chewing on a stick of liquorice.

Step 3: Behavioral Changes and Nicotine Dependence

The process of successfully replacing smoking habits with other activities can be difficult and time-consuming. Each patient should identify replacements (see above) that contain a personal reward. It might be wise to schedule and arrange additional consultation time as this point so that enough emphasis can be devoted to this important step.

Note the Replacements Identified

Determine the degree of nicotine dependence: This can be assessed easily by asking the following questions (**Table 24.1**).

▪ Table 24.1
Nicotine dependence test adapted from Fagerström, et al. 1978

Have you already attempted to give up smoking?	*How many cigarettes do you smoke per day?*	*How long after waking up in the morning do you smoke your first cigarette?*	*Degree of dependence*
Yes	> 30	< 5 minutes	Very high dependence
Yes	20–30	5–30 minutes	High dependence
Yes	10–20	30–60 minutes	Medium dependence
No	< 10	> 60 minutes	Low dependence

On the basis of the answers to these questions, the patients can be divided into four groups: extremely dependent, very dependent, moderately dependent and slightly dependent. The answer showing the greatest dependency indicates the overall dependency.

Set the quit date.

Step 4: Quit Date

On the quit date, ideally, the patient will be released from the dental practice as a former smoker. It may be worthwhile to give each individual patient a written recommendation for the use of nicotine replacement therapy for the following three months.

Confirm or redefine the replacements that have been identified.

Give the patient a written recommendation on nicotine replacement therapy on the basis of both his and her smoking behavior and degree of nicotine dependence.

Arrange

Experience reveals that smokers have to make several attempts to quit smoking before staying a former smoker. Of the patients who initially succeed in kicking the habit, 50 to 60 percent will suffer a relapse within the next year. Even though there are at present no evidence-based methods for preventing relapses, the dental practice team can continue to offer support during their patients' repeated attempts to quit smoking. Alternatively, the patients can be referred at this time to tobacco use cessation specialists, their family doctors, pharmacists or psychotherapists.

Box 24.2: Care models for dental settings

Key features in management

- Following a level of care model, tobacco use prevention and cessation (TUPAC) in the dental treatment setting occurs in brief interventions over repeated visits.
- All patients visiting a dental practice have to be asked about tobacco use on a regular basis.
- With all tobacco users, the readiness to quit has to be assessed.
- Brief Motivational Interviewing (BMI) appears to be suitable for use during brief interventions for tobacco use prevention and cessation in dental practices.
- With all tobacco users willing to quit either referral to tobacco use cessation specialists or in-house support (behavioral support and pharmacotherapy) has to be arranged.
- Evidence-based guidelines indicate counseling and pharmacotherapy when used in combination are more effective in improving quit rates (Box 24.3) than either alone.

Pharmacotherapy for Tobacco Use Cessation

Nicotine Replacement Therapy

The symptoms of nicotine withdrawal can substantially hamper a person's success to quit smoking. The most common symptoms of nicotine withdrawal are reported to be headache, gastrointestinal complaints, sleeping disorders, depression and increased appetite. Withdrawal usually occurs shortly after the person has smoked his or her last cigarette and occasionally lasts for several days or a few weeks. Withdrawal symptoms can be significantly reduced by pharmacotherapy, e.g. with the replacement of nicotine. It can help former smokers to resist their withdrawal symptoms and to carry out the replacements instead as planned. Nicotine replacement therapy (NRT) is shown to increase success rates by roughly 100 percent. Additionally, research on NRT consistently revealed that comparable success rates were achieved with the use of nicotine gum, nicotine sublingual tablets or lozenges, or nicotine patches.

If there are no medical contraindications for the patient, NRT products can be used without restrictions. Nevertheless, some reservations remain for pregnant women and patients with cardiovascular conditions. Literature suggests, however, that the benefits of NRT for smoking cessation may outweight the detrimental effects from the continued use of tobacco.

Significant success rates from the use of NRT will be achieved when the appropriate product is selected adjusted to:

1. The degree of nicotine dependency and
2. The individual smoking behavior (**Table 24.1**).

In general, patients with "high" or "very high" nicotine dependence are advised to take combinations of NRT. Furthermore, NRT should be used for the entire duration of the therapy (3 months), while the nicotine dose will be reduced every month as suggested by the manufacturer.

Bupropion SR

Sustained-release Bupropion (Bupropion SR) is a non-nicotine-containing drug used for tobacco use cessation therapy (Zyban®, Wellbutrin®, GlaxoSmithKline, USA). With Bupropion, the neuronal uptake of catecholamines will be selectively inhibited in the central nervous system. Consequently, catecholamine levels will increase in certain areas of the brain resulting in the reduction of nicotine withdrawal symptoms.

The manufacturer recommends that Bupropion SR is prescribed for the duration of seven weeks. In order to reach therapeutic levels, Bupropion SR will have to be taken for two weeks. Tobacco use should be ceased only after therapeutic levels have been established. During the first week, it is recommended that 150 mg of Bupropion SR is taken per day. After one week, 150 mg will be taken twice daily for the duration of six weeks.

The efficacy of Bupropion SR either alone or in combination with other nicotine replacement therapy options was evaluated with nondepressed cigarette smokers in placebo-controlled double-blind trials. The abstinence rates for the use of Bupropion SR alone was 23.1 percent following 12 months after the quit date, and 35.5 percent following 12 months when Bupropion SR was used in combination with nicotine replacement therapy.

The most common side effects of Bupropion have been described as insomnia, headaches, and dry mouth. Prior to prescription, it has to be noted that the simultaneous use of psychotropic drugs or cortisone should be avoided. Further contraindications exist in patients with a history of bulimia, anorexia nervosa, and in those who experience epilepsy. Pregnant women are to be advised not to take Bupropion SR, since its safety during pregnancy has not been studied in clinical trials.

Box 24.3: Pharmacotherapy for tobacco addiction

Key features of evidence-based management

- Nictotine replacement therapy (NRT) is the most common medication used to assist tobacco cessation.
- NRT is available in several formulations: transdermal patch, nicotine gum, lozenge, nasal spray and inhaler.
- NRT agents can be combined to obtain a better outcome.
- Medications that can be prescribed via a GP practice includes bupropion and varenicline.
- Several second–line therapies are also available for those who relapse following treatment.

Varenicline

Varenicline has been specifically developed for smoking cessation therapy (Chantix®, Champix®, Pfizer Inc. USA). Varenicline connects as a partial agonist with a high affinity to the $\alpha4\beta2$-nicotinic acetylcholine receptors in the central nervous system. Subsequently, the binding of nicotine will be blocked resulting in the elimination of its addictive effect. Additionally, the binding of Varenicline sufficiently reduces the symptoms of craving and withdrawal.

Varenicline prescription is recommended for the duration of three months and may be extended if necessary by a subsequent three months. In order to reach therapeutic blood plasma levels, 1mg of Varenicline will be taken per day for the duration of one week. Only thereafter, tobacco use should be ceased. After one week, 1mg will be taken twice daily for the duration of 11 weeks.

Five clinical studies involving a total of approximately 4300 patients, mostly heavy, long-term smokers have shown significantly greater success rate following one year after quit date with Varenicline (14.4–23%) and placebo (3.9–10.3%). When taking Varenicline for the duration of six months, one-year success rates of 43.6 percent have been reached.

The most common side effects of Varenicline include dizziness, insomnia, indigestion and vomiting. Patients with renal insufficiency and pregnancy are not recommended for treatment with Varenicline.

Advanced Care

Some smokers eventually relapse while receiving treatment or after quitting for a period of time. Their powerful addiction requires intensive treatment. When first-line treatments have failed or are not tolerated, second-line agents are available for use in addiction specialist centers. These include nortriptiline—a tricyclic antidepressant agent and clonidine—an anti-hypertensive. These may have adverse side effects and should be used under appropriate settings. New medications and nicotine vaccines are also being tried as Phase II trials. New agents include monoamine type B (MAO-B) inhibitors—for example, selegiline, cannabinoid receptor 1 (CB1). These agents are currently under investigation in specialist centers.

DETERMINANTS OF BEHAVIOR CHANGE

The readiness to accomplish behavior change is often described by the so-called trans-theoretical model, according to which a person trying to change his or her behavior passes four different stages: pre-contemplation ("lack of awareness"), contemplation ("gaining of awareness"), preparation ("getting ready") and action ("implementation").

A suitable model for behavioral support in tobacco use cessation would help patients to move from one stage to the next. However, when asked about their readiness to quit smoking, tobacco users frequently respond that they want to quit "sometime" but that this time has not come yet: there would be certain things to be accomplish first, such as to take a final exam or to recover from an emotional trauma. In many ambivalent cases, smokers have learned or created these excuses to continuously justify their tobacco consumption. Behind this attitude, however, there may the fear of failure to quit, an unpleasant memory of a failed past attempt, or a concern about gaining weight. During the kind of skillful counseling, excuses of this kind can be identified in a nonoffensive way. Possibly, the counselor will be able to touch on them without triggering resistance on the part of the smoker.

Fear to Relapse

The fear to relapse is a considerable issue in tobacco use cessation counseling. Many smokers have a significant concern to fail quitting and they often lack self-efficacy. Former smokers frequently report that they successfully quit because they "believed in themselves" and "believed they would make it". It was this belief, many say, which was the key to their success. Through appropriate counseling, self-efficacy can be strengthened, and readiness to quit may be increased. Furthermore, nicotine dependency should be put into perspective: the possible failure to quit smoking should not be interpreted as a weakness, but rather as a function of high nicotine dependency.

Fear to Gain Weight

The concern to gain weight after quitting smoking is a second important issue. In a clinical trial performed in the US. with 5,887 smokers aged 35 to 60, an average weight gain of 9.7 kg was recorded over a period of five years which is significantly higher than the 5.3 kg generally estimated amount of gain in nonsmokers during the same period.

Since the body's metabolism in smokers is increased by regular tobacco consumption,

Box 24.4: Quit rates

Key features on reported outcomes

- The quit rates of smokers without any professional help is found to be 10–11 percent
- Success rates achieved by smoking cessation counseling are generally dependent on the amount of counseling time: 1–3 minutes (14.0%), 4–30 minutes (18.8%), 31–90 minutes (26.5%) and >90 minutes (28.4%), respectively
- Pharmacotherapy has shown to significantly increase tobacco use cessation quit rates
- Nicotine replacement therapy (NRT) is shown to increase success rates by roughly 100 percent
- Reported one-year abstinence are: Nicotine Replacement Therapy (NRT): 20–25 percent, Bupropin SR: 23.1 percent, Varenicline (3 months): 23 percent, and Varenicline (6 months): 43.6 percent.

smokers generally burn up more calories. Conversely, nicotine withdrawal is shown to lower metabolism. Following nicotine withdrawal, therefore, the energy will be stored as body weight even if the individual stays on the same diet. It may be appropriate for the counsellor at this point to mention that pharmacotherapy, e.g. the administration of nicotine substitutes, may lessen weight gain effectively.

BARRIERS TO BE OVERCOME BY THE DENTAL TEAM

We know that most tobacco users are aware of their unhealthy habit. A closer look at the questions of what types of health problems caused by tobacco are generally known, however, reveals that the detrimental effects of tobacco use on the oral mucosa and the periodontal tissues are still substantially underestimated. In the interest of public health, therefore, the dental practice team has to perform an important task—namely, mentioning and discussing the consequences of tobacco use on oral health with all their patients—in addition to assessing their oral hygiene. It is not always easy to integrate this kind of patient briefing into the everyday work of a dental practice. As mentioned above, additionally, a number of tobacco users feel as they remain under social pressure to quit tobacco. Moreover, many patients have visited their dentists on numerous occasions in recent years without members from the dental team addressing the topic of tobacco use, mentioning the consequences for oral health, and assessing the patient's willingness to quit. As a consequence, however, of the scientific knowledge attained over the past 5 to 10 years, the dental practice team was yet assigned an active role in promoting smoking prevention and cessation among their patients.

Reported barriers and obstacles to integrating smoking cessation programs into the daily routine of the dental practice may be listed as:

1. Too little time,
2. Financial considerations,
3. Lack of interest on the part of the patients,
4. Respect for the freedom of the individual,
5. Too little experience in "giving good advice"
6. Fear of losing patients.

In the future these barriers ought to be overcome via appropriate training of dental personnel.

Overcoming Barriers in Practice

On the basis of significant evidence on the recovery of both the oral mucosa and the periodontal tissue following tobacco use cessation the task has been emerged in dentistry to deliver brief interventions and provide counseling for patients who ought to quit tobacco use. Even though success rates from dental counseling are limited at a first glance, it has been found that the support from oral health professionals is yet comparable to that from physicians and psychotherapists. There are several barriers, however, constituting a complex of issues for the dental practice, e.g. the lack of possibilities to charge either patients or insurance companies for such counseling, or the lack of training in tobacco use cessation counseling in the curricula of oral health professionals. Considering the relatively small amount of time for brief interventions (5 minutes each) and for tobacco use cessation counseling (up to 4 session of 15 minutes each), however, these efforts appear to be justified in the longer perspective and may serve not only a benefit for one single individual but have a public health impact to achieve better oral health for all.

SELF-ASSESSMENT QUESTIONS

1. Describe the nature of the 'tobacco use disease.'
2. What are the abstinence rates of smokers who try to quit without professional support? How could this be improved?
3. Describe the level of care model for tobacco use prevention and cessation in the dental practice.
4. "When asked about their readiness to quit smoking, tobacco users often reply that

they wish to quit smoking but there are significant barriers to do so at the present time". Comment on their reply and possible responses by a health professional.
5. Describe the application of "Brief Motivational Interviewing" for tobacco use cessation in the dental practice.
6. What are the four steps enlisted in the Step-By-Step protocol for tobacco use cessation in the dental practice?
7. Concerning pharmacotherapy: what are the common side effects of Nicotine Replacement Therapy (NRT) and precautions needed in prescribing Bupropion SR and Varenicline?
8. Explain the reasons for better success rates achieved in tertiary care facilities compared to primary care.

SUGGESTED READING

1. Casella G, Caponnetto P, Polosa R. Therapeutic advances in the treatment of nicotine addiction: present and future. Ther Adv Chronic Dis. 2010;1:95-106.
2. Davis, et al. Education of tobacco use prevention and cessation for dental professionals: a paradigm shift. Int Dent J. 2010;60:60-72.
3. Fagerstrom. Measuring degree of physical dependence to tobacco smoking with reference to individualization of treatment. Addict Behav. 1978;3:235-41.
4. Fiore, et al. Treating Tobacco Use and Dependence: Update. Clinical Practice Guideline. Rockville, MD: US Department of Health and Human Services. Public Health Service; 2008.
5. Miller and Rollnick. Motivational Interviewing. New York: Guilford Press; 2002.
6. Needleman, et al. Improving the effectiveness of tobacco use cessation (TUC). Int Dent J. 2010;60:50-9.
7. Ramseier CA and Suvan JE. Health behavior change in the dental practice. Ames, Iowa: Wiley-Blackwell; 2010.
8. Ramseier, et al. Consensus report: 2nd European workshop on tobacco use prevention and cessation for oral health professionals. Int Dent J. 2010;60:3-6.
9. Rollnick, et al. Helping smokers make decisions: the enhancement of brief intervention for general medical practice. Patient education and counseling. 1997;31:191-203.
9. Warnakulasuriya, et al. Oral health risks of tobacco use and effects of cessation. Int Dent J. 2010;60:7-30.

Index

Page numbers followed by *f* refer to figure and *t* refer to table

G

H

I

N

O

P